Unwanted effects
of cosmetics and drugs
used in dermatology

UNWANTED EFFECTS OF COSMETICS AND DRUGS USED IN DERMATOLOGY

Second edition

Johan P. Nater
Department of Dermatology, Academic Hospital
State University of Groningen
Groningen, The Netherlands

Anton C. de Groot
Departments of Dermatology
Carolus Hospital and Willem-Alexander Hospital
's-Hertogenbosch, The Netherlands

Co-author for the section on cosmetology:

Dhiam H. Liem
Food Inspection Service
Cosmetics Department
Enschede, The Netherlands

1985

ELSEVIER – Amsterdam – New York – Oxford

ISBN 0 444 90358 5

Published by:
Elsevier Science Publishers B.V.
P.O. Box 1126,
1000 BC Amsterdam

Sole distributors for the USA and Canada:
Elsevier Science Publishing Co. Inc.
52 Vanderbilt Avenue
New York, NY 10017

Printed in the Netherlands by Casparie-Amsterdam

Preface

While preparing the manuscript for the first edition of this book on side effects of cosmetics and (local and systemic) drugs used by the dermatologist, we intended it to become a reference work with the following characteristics: comprehensiveness, easy to use, easy location of relevant information, copiously referenced, and up to date.

We did not know whether and how this 'encyclopaedic approach', providing many alphabetically listed tables while keeping the text to a minimum, so fundamentally different from the major textbooks in this and adjacent areas, would be appreciated. Several reviews in some major dermatological and cosmetical periodicals, as well as many letters from readers proved this 'formula' to be well accepted, and encouraged us in our view that the data provided in this way filled a need.

Stimulated and encouraged by this response and realizing that the fastly increasing amount of information in this field makes it difficult for any reference book to remain up to date, we hereby present a second, enlarged edition, two years after the first edition was released. This second edition has been revised according to new experiences, new publications and helpful advice from many users of the book. Apart from updating and completing the existing text, some important subjects have been added. Chapter 13, 'Drugs used on the oral mucosa', has been extended to the discussion of topical and systemic side effects of drugs used on the vulvo-vaginal mucosa and drugs used in ophthalmological practice. This chapter has accordingly been renamed 'Drugs used on the mucosae'.

Many more topical drugs and cosmetics which were found to have caused systemic side effects are discussed in Chapter 16. We found it appropriate (though it seems somewhat paradoxical) to include in this chapter a section on 'Transdermal drug delivery systems', where percutaneous absorption of topically applied drug, is exploited for therapeutic purposes. Examples are nitroglycerin, scopolamine and clonidine.

Chapter 19 has been updated with a comprehensive survey on adverse effects of oral retinoids. Although there can be no doubt that this group of vitamin-A analogs, notably etretinate and isotretinoin, is a very valuable addition to the therapeutic armamentarium of the dermatologist, he should be conscious of the fact that many side effects, some serious, may occur. Also new in this chapter are ketoconazole and acyclovir, drugs which, thus far, appear to have relatively low toxicity profiles.

Throughout the text, many more patch test concentrations and vehicles have been listed, thus facilitating adequate investigation in cases of suspected contact allergic reactions.

Approximately 800 new references have been added. This should enable easy access to further relevant information for any one wanting to know more about a particular drug or side effect.

Last but not least, an extensive alphabetic index of all compounds mentioned in the text has been compiled, including synonyms and trade names.

The authors wish to acknowledge their indebtedness to the many dermatologists, whose observations have been incorporated in this volume. We hope that the users of this book will continue to share their criticisms and suggestions for improvements with us.

J. P. Nater
A. C. de Groot

Table of contents

1. Contact dermatitis

INTRODUCTION

1.1   Dermatitis and eczema are names used to indicate a special inflammatory state of the skin; when caused by external agents, this reaction is termed contact dermatitis or contact eczema.

1.2   Contact dermatitis may be classified as follows:
– Acute toxic contact dermatitis
– Irritant contact dermatitis
– Allergic contact dermatitis
– Phototoxic contact dermatitis
– Photoallergic contact dermatitis

MORPHOLOGICAL ASPECTS OF CONTACT DERMATITIS

1.3   An *acute allergic* contact dermatitis is characterized by polymorphy of the eruption; in the acute phase the skin reddens, clusters of minute papules, non-umbilicated vesicles and swelling occur, as well as weeping and exudation leading to the formation of crustae. The eruption is usually accompanied by itching, which may vary from moderate to quite severe. In cases of strong reactions the process may be noted to spread. In the subacute phase the polymorphy of the eruption diminishes: the skin becomes dry and scaly and fissures may be noted.

When the eruption becomes chronic, areas of the epidermis thicken, with deepening of the normal skin lines (lichenification); erythema and papules are less prominent. Multiple excoriations indicate the process to itch.

1.4   *Irritant* contact dermatitis often starts with dryness, itching and scaliness of the skin; papules and vesicles may develop later. In some cases it is impossible, on clinical examination, to distinguish between acute irritant dermatitis and acute allergic contact dermatitis.

2. Toxic and irritant contact dermatitis

ACUTE TOXIC CONTACT DERMATITIS

2.1 Acute toxic contact dermatitis may be provoked by single or repeated contacts with strongly toxic substances. The association between the injury and the toxic substance is usually quite obvious from the patient's history.

   This type of reaction occurs frequently as a result of, mostly accidental, contacts with acids, alkalis, cleansers, solvents, etc.; only very rarely, however, is it caused by drugs.

IRRITANT CONTACT DERMATITIS

2.2 Irritant contact dermatitis is a term used to describe a localized, superficial, exudative, non-immunological inflammation of the skin, which is due to the direct influence of one or more external factors [15]. Many substances, including drugs, may after repeated contact with the skin cause irritant dermatitis by a direct action. This occurs without previous sensitization; immunological processes are not involved.

   During and after the first contacts no visual alterations may be observed. After repeated contact, the skin gradually becomes erythematous; drying and cracking occurs, and later, an eczematous reaction with papules and vesicles may develop.

   An irritant substance will cause dermatitis if it is permitted to act in sufficient intensity and quantity and for a sufficient length of time. Irritant reactions may develop in all persons, though the individual susceptibility varies greatly. This probably depends on the thickness of the epidermis. Irritant reactions are more easily provoked under occlusion, e.g. under adhesives and polyethylene, or in skin folds.

Differential diagnosis

2.3 The condition of an already eczematized skin (from whatever cause) is quickly worsened by the application of a mild irritant medicament; the resulting exacerbation may be mistaken for an allergic reaction. In such cases irritant and allergic reactions are often difficult to distinguish. The differential diagnosis between irritant and allergic contact dermatitis must be made by means of patch testing. This is sometimes rather difficult, as patch tests with mild irritants (if insufficiently diluted) may cause false positive patch test reactions, especially when they are performed on patients with an eczematous eruption elsewhere on the skin. In such circumstances even standard test substances in routine concentrations may elicit false positive reactions. The problem of false positive reactions is further discussed in § 3.18.

   Topical drugs that have caused irritant dermatitis are listed in § 2.4.

2.4   Irritant dermatitis due to topical drugs

Drug	Use	Ref.
6-aminonicotinamide	psoriasis therapy	29
ammonium persulfate	hair bleaches	7
benzalkonium chloride	antiseptic	9
benzoyl peroxide	acne therapy	18
cantharidin	wart treatment	6
carmustine (BCNU)	topical cytostatic drug	39
chrysarobin	psoriasis therapy	11
citral	fragrance material	35
clioquinol	antiseptic	12
colchicine	treatment of condylomata acuminata	26
diethyltoluamide	insect repellent	41
dimethyl sulfoxide (DMSO)	solvent	14
dinitrochlorobenzene (DNCB)	treatment of alopecia areata and warts	16
dithranol (cignolin, anthralin)	psoriasis therapy	30, 33
ether	solvent	17
5-fluorouracil	topical cytostatic drug	10, 42
hexachlorophene	antiseptic	2, 28
hydroquinone	skin bleaching agent	24
6-hydroxy-1,3-benzoxathiol-2-one	psoriasis therapy	22
iodine tincture	antiseptic	13
mechlorethamine hydrochloride	treatment of mycosis fungoides	38
mesulfen	scabicide	31
monobenzyl ether of hydroquinone	skin bleaching agent	23
phenol	antipruritic	4, 21
podophyllum resin	treatment of condylomata acuminata	25
propylene glycol	vehicle constituent	27, 34, 36
quaternary ammonium compounds	antiseptics	9
resorcinol	antipruritic, peeling agent	3
retinoic acid	acne therapy	19, 40
salicylic acid	keratolytic drug	11

(continued)

2.4 Irritant dermatitis due to topical drugs

(continuation)

Drug	Use	Ref.
selenium sulfide	dandruff therapy	1
sodium lauryl sulfate	vehicle constituent	8, 32
tar	psoriasis and eczema therapy, in cosmetics	20
urea	keratolytic drug, enhances penetration of chemicals through the skin	5, 37

2.5 REFERENCES

1. Albright, S. D. and Hitch, J. M. (1966): Rapid treatment of tinea versicolor with selenium sulfide. *Arch. Derm., 93,* 460.
2. Baker, H., Ive, F. A. and Lloyd, M. J. (1969): Primary irritant dermatitis of the scrotum due to hexachlorophene. *Arch. Derm., 99,* 693.
3. Becker, S. W. and Obermayer, M. E. (1947): *Modern Dermatology and Syphilology, 2nd Edition.* J. B. Lippincott Co., Philadelphia, London, Montreal.
4. Björnberg, A. (1968): *Skin Reactions to Primary Irritants in Patients with Hand Eczema.* O. Isacsons Tryckeri, Gothenburg.
5. Colin Hindson, M. T. (1971): Urea in the topical treatment of atopic eczema. *Arch. Derm., 104,* 284.
6. Dilaimy, M. (1975): Lymphangitis caused by cantharidin. *Arch. Derm., 111,* 1073.
7. Fisher, A. A. and Dooms-Goossens, A. (1976): Persulfate hair bleach reactions. *Arch. Derm., 112,* 1407.
8. Fisher, A. A. and Pascher, F. (1971): Allergic contact dermatitis due to ingredients of vehicles. *Arch. Derm., 104,* 286.
9. Gall, H. (1979): Toxisches Kontaktekzem auf die quaternäre Ammonium-Verbindung Benzalkoniumchlorid. *Dermatosen Beruf Umw., 27,* 139.
10. Goette, D. K., Odom, R. B. and Owens, R. (1977): Allergic contact dermatitis from topical fluorouracil. *Arch. Derm., 113,* 196.
11. Goodman, L. S. and Gilman, A. (Eds.) (1970): *The Pharmaceutical Basis of Therapeutics, 4th Edition.* The MacMillan Co., London, Toronto.
12. Kero, M., Hannuksela, M. and Sothman, A. (1979): Primary irritant dermatitis from topical clioquinol. *Contact Dermatitis, 5,* 115.
13. Kirchmayr, W. (1957): Zum Problem der sogenannten Jodüberempfindlichkeit. *Wien. klin. Wschr., 69,* 578.
14. Kligman, A. M. (1965): Topical pharmacology and toxicology of dimethylsulfoxide. Part 1 and 2. *J. Amer. med. Ass., 193,* 796 and 923.
15. Malten, K. E. (1981): Thoughts on irritant contact dermatitis. *Contact Dermatitis, 7,* 238.
16. The Merck Index: *An Encyclopedia of Chemicals and Drugs, 9th Edition* (1976): Merck and Co., Inc., Rahway, U.S.A.
17. Michel, P. J. (1952): Les dermites de l'éther. *J. Méd. Lyon, 33,* 741.
18. Pace, W. E. (1965): Benzoyl peroxide-sulfur cream for acne vulgaris. *Canad. med. Ass. J., 93,* 252.
19. Peachy, R. D. G. and Connor, B. L. (1971): Topical retinoic acid in the treatment of acne vulgaris. *Brit. J. Derm., 85,* 462.
20. Rothenborg, H. W. and Hjorth, N. (1968): Allergy to perfumes from toilet soaps and detergents in patients with dermatitis. *Arch. Derm., 97,* 417.
21. Rubin, M. B. and Pirozzi, D. J. (1973): Contact dermatitis from carbolated vaseline. *Cutis, 12,* 52.
22. Schoefinius, H. H. (1972): Kontaktdermatitis mit erhöhter Körpertemperatur unter Behandlung von Psoriasis vulgaris capitilii mit einem Benzoxathiol-Derivat. *Z. Haut- u. Geschl.kr., 47,* 227.
23. Spencer, M. C. (1962): Leukoderma following monobenzylether of hydroquinone bleaching. *Arch. Derm., 86,* 615.
24. Spencer, M. C. (1965): Topical use of hydroquinone for depigmentation. *J. Amer. med. Ass., 194,* 962.
25. Sullivan, M. and King, L. S. (1947): Effects of resin of podophyllum on normal skin, condylomata acuminata and verrucae vulgares. *Arch. Derm. Syph., 56,* 30.

26. Von Krogh, G. and Rudén, A. K. (1980): Topical treatment of penile condylomata acuminata with colchicine at 48-72 hours intervals. *Acta derm.-venereol. (Stockh.)*, *60*, 87.

27. Warshaw, T. G. and Herrmann, F. (1952): Studies of skin reactions to propylene glycol. *J. invest. Derm.*, *19*, 423.

28. Watt, T. L. and Baumann, R. R. (1972): Primary irritant dermatitis caused by pHisohex. *Cutis*, *10*, 363.

29. Zackheim, H. S. (1975): Treatment of psoriasis with 6-amino-nicotinamide. *Arch. Derm.*, *111*, 880.

UPDATE – 2nd Edition

30. Puschmann, M. and Schmersahl, P. (1983): Untersuchungen zur Frage der Nebenwirkungen von Anthralin und seinen beiden Hauptveruntreinigungen an der gesunden Haut. *Z. Hautkr.*, *58*, 410.

31. Meneghini, C. L., Vena, G. A. and Angelini, G. (1982): Contact dermatitis to scabicides. *Contact Dermatitis*, *8*, 285.

32. Bruynzeel, D. P., van Ketel, W. G., Scheper, R. J. and von Blomberg-van der Flier, B. M. E. (1982): Delayed time course of irritation by sodium lauryl sulfate: Observations on threshold reactions. *Contact Dermatitis*, *8*, 236.

33. Kingston, T. and Marks, R. (1983): Irritant reactions to dithranol in normal subjects and psoriatic patients. *Brit. J. Derm.*, *108*, 307.

34. Andersen, K. E. and Storrs, F. J. (1982): Hautreizungen durch Propylenglykol. *Hautarzt*, *33*, 12.

35. Rothenborg, H. W., Menné, T. and Sjølin, K.-E. (1977): Temperature dependent primary irritant dermatitis from lemon perfume. *Contact Dermatitis*, *3*, 37.

36. Trancik, R. J. and Maibach, H. I. (1982): Propylene glycol: irritation or sensitization? *Contact Dermatitis*, *8*, 185.

37. Cramers, M. and Thormann, J. (1981): Skin reactions to an urea-containing cream. *Contact Dermatitis*, *7*, 189.

38. Hamminga, B., Noordijk, E. M. and van Vloten, W. A. (1982): Treatment of mycosis fungoides. *Arch. Derm.*, *118*, 150.

39. Zackheim, H. S., Epstein, E. H. Jr., McNutt, N. et al. (1983): Topical carmustine (BCNU) for mycosis fungoides and related disorders: A 10-year experience. *J. Amer. Acad. Derm.*, *9*, 363.

40. Thomas, J. R. III and Doyle, J. A. (1981): The therapeutic uses of topical vitamin A acid. *J. Amer. Acad. Derm.*, *4*, 505.

41. Reuveni, H. and Yagupsky, P. (1982): Diethyltoluamide-containing insect repellent. *Arch. Derm.*, *118*, 582.

42. Goette, D. K. (1981): Topical chemotherapy with 5-fluorouracil. *J. Amer. Acad. Derm.*, *4*, 633.

3.   Allergic contact dermatitis (general aspects)

IMMUNOLOGICAL ASPECTS

3.1   Two main types of immunological mechanisms are recognized in adverse reactions to topically applied substances: the *immediate* and the *delayed* type of hypersensitivity. In both reactions an important role is played by lymphocytes, of which two main subpopulations may be distinguished:
1. *B-cell lymphocytes;* these are precursors of antibody-producing plasma cells involved in immediate-type reactions, such as allergic contact urticaria.
2. *T-cell lymphocytes;* these cells are important in delayed-type reactions, such as allergic contact dermatitis, the most frequently reported side effect of topical drugs.

3.2   The process of delayed-type hypersensitivity reactions develops in two phases. In the first, or conductive, phase the sensitization process takes place, in the second, or eliciting, phase the hypersensitivity becomes clinically manifest. The minimal interval between these two phases ranges from 5 to 7 days.
         In the conductive phase, a chemical of low molecular weight (the hapten) penetrates the skin and remains there for some time (the minimal contact time). Here, formation of antigen takes place: the hapten forms immunogenic conjugates with various autologous proteins. These conjugates come into contact with immunocompetent antigen-inexperienced T-lymphocytes bearing receptors for the conjugates formed in the skin. The lymphocytes are triggered by this contact. Apparently there are several mechanisms as to how the hapten stimulates the specific lymphocytes [73]:
1. Macrophages take up the hapten in the conjugated or unconjugated form and present it to the lymphocytes.
2. Macrophages are not the only cells with stimulatory capacity. Dendritic cells in the skin known as Langerhans' Cells play an important role in this respect [74].
3. Hapten-coated lymphocytes or erythrocytes stimulate specific lymphocytes (*in vitro*).
4. Specific lymphocytes are stimulated directly by the conjugated hapten or by the hapten bound directly to the receptors.
These mechanisms are not mutually exclusive. The specific lymphocytes stimulated by encountering the antigen migrate to the draining regional lymph nodes. There, in the paracortical or thymus-dependent area, proliferation and differentiation take place. Immunoblasts are formed which further differentiate into small lymphocytes with memory or effector function. *Memory cells* are, upon renewed contact with the antigen, able to proliferate and differentiate further into a new progeny of sensitized lymphocytes; however, they do not produce lymphokines. *Effector T-cells* are able to react upon new contact with the allergen with the release of soluble substances (lymphokines), which induce an inflammatory reaction of the skin; these cells are not capable of further proliferation and differentiation.

6

During the same phase a third generation of specific lymphocytes is generated: suppressor cells. Activated precursors of suppressor cells form active suppressor cells which control the generation of effector cells. Thus active suppressor cells form a mechanism which controls and in an extreme case prevents the development of contact sensitivity. Elimination of precursors of suppressor cells enhances the sensitization.

At the end of the conductive phase memory and effector cells leave the lymph node and circulate in the organism which is now sensitive to the specific hapten. When in the following (eliciting) phase the hypersensitive organism comes into contact with the specific hapten the secondary response occurs, involving both memory and effector cells. The following hypothesis of the mechanism of the eliciting phase has been developed [73]: specific sensitized lymphocytes are attracted to the site of hapten application by the hapten. There they release substances (the nature of which is not known), that are able to stimulate basophils and mast cells. These cells release vasoactive substances which induce the inflammatory skin reaction. At the same time mediators (lymphokines) released by sensitized lymphocytes upon hapten stimulation, attract and activate macrophages which then clear the inflammation.

3.3   Several factors influence the induction of contact allergy:

1. *Genetics:* Experiments in animals indicate that heredity plays a role in all immunological processes, including contact allergy.
2. *The nature of the allergen:* Some chemicals frequently cause contact sensitization, others are virtually non-allergenic.
3. *Age:* Although contact sensitization can be induced in the newborn and in young children, allergic contact dermatitis in individuals under 10 years of age is infrequent. In aged people allergic skin reactivity appears to decrease [4].
4. *The site of contact:* The site of contact with the allergen is of importance in the induction of contact sensitization: contact sensitization for instance readily occurs to ingredients of pharmaceutical preparations used in the treatment of leg ulcers [5].
5. *Concentration of the allergen:* Higher concentrations will more frequently cause contact sensitization. For strong allergens there are no 'safe' concentrations.
6. *The nature of the vehicle:* The vehicle influences the penetration of the allergen into the skin.
7. *Surface-active agents:* Their presence may achieve greater contact with, and penetration of the allergen.
8. *Occlusion:* Occlusion increases penetration and prevents loss of the allergen.
9. *Adjuvants:* In experimental situations sensitization has been potentiated by the use of adjuvants.

For a more extensive discussion of factors influencing the induction of contact sensitivity the reader is referred to the relevant literature on this subject (e.g. Magnusson and Kligman [28]).

THE TECHNIQUE OF PATCH TESTING

3.4   The process of sensitization leads to a specific hypersensitivity of the skin. This can be demonstrated by the application of the causative substance(s) to a normal skin site, which is usually done under occlusion. This procedure, named patch testing, is used for diagnosing allergic contact dermatitis. Although its purpose is primarily the positive identification of a contact allergic reaction and the establish-

7

ment of its cause(s), negative patch test results are nevertheless of similar importance in that allergic contact dermatitis *from the tested substances* can then be ruled out and other possibilities should be considered.

The technique of patch testing has been standardized. The patch tester used for fixation and occlusion of the allergen on the skin consists of a piece of Whatman filter paper affixed to aluminum foil paper, which is coated on one side with polyethylene film. The two main types of patch tester available are:
– the Al test (Imeco, Sweden)
– the Silver Patch (van der Bend, P.O. Box 1518, 9701 BM Groningen, The Netherlands).

The suspected allergen, suitably diluted, is placed on the filter paper disc and the patch tester is applied to the skin with adhesive plaster. Since in cases of contact allergy the entire skin is sensitized, the patch tests can, in principle, be performed anywhere on the body. Generally patch tests are done on the skin of the back. The patch testers are left in place for 48 hours. Some clinics use an exposure time of 24 hours (e.g. the Free University of Amsterdam). Studies comparing patch test results after 24- and 48 hours' exposure have been inconclusive as to the optimal time of exposure [89]. After removal of the patch testers and the occlusive dressing the test sites are marked, and the results are read initially after 15–30 minutes. Sufficient time must elapse for the pressure effects of the dressing to wear off.

Opinions concerning the optimal time for the second (and often conclusive) reading differ. This second reading is performed in St. John's (London) on Day 4. Other clinics (e.g. Groningen, the Netherlands) perform the second reading on the third day, 24 hours after the first reading. It must be appreciated that several allergens (the classic example of which is neomycin) may become positive only after 4 or 5 days, or even considerably later. For further details on the technique of patch testing the reader is referred to the relevant literature [12, 29].

In most centers patch tests are performed with one or more standard patch test series. Testing with these series is in most cases not sufficient and must be supplemented with additional substances, the selection of these depending on the patient's case history.

Finn Chamber test

3.5   Conventional patch testers have some disadvantages which may hamper a reliable reading of the test:
1. Non-porous adhesive tape has to be used for adequate fixation of the testers to the skin. This may cause skin irritation and sweat retention.
2. The polythene covering of aluminum foil may cause erythema and edema around the test filter paper.
3. Strongly positive reactions tend to spread to the adjacent skin.

These disadvantages have led to the development of the so-called (Finn) Chamber test (Epitest Ltd, Oy P.O. Box 943 SF-00101, Helsinki, Finland). The chambers are made of inflexible aluminum. They have a diameter of 8 mm and a depth of 0.5 mm. The round border of the chamber is turned against the skin and causes a tight occlusion of the test materials. A filter paper is only required when solutions are tested. This tight occlusion permits the use of porous (Scanpor) tape.

Advantages of the Finn Chamber are [76]:
1. Better fixation of the testers
2. Smaller reactions without spreading
3. More allergens may be placed on a smaller area of the skin

4. Porous tape can be used with less danger of skin irritation and sweat retention. Disadvantages of the Finn Chamber are:
1. The correctly applied Finn Chamber causes an indented ring around the test area. As this gives the impression that the test area is edematous, false positive readings may be facilitated.
2. As more allergens can be placed on the skin the examiner may be tempted to apply large test series, which bears an increased risk of the development of the so-called 'excited skin syndrome' (formerly called 'angry back syndrome', see § 3.18).

In a comparative study of the Al-test and the Finn Chamber test approximately the same number of positive reactions were found, when the Al-tests were fixated with non-porous leukoplast and the chambers with porous Scanpor. However, when both tests are fixated with Scanpor, more reactions (both irritant and allergic) are seen with the Finn Chamber [75].

3.6   As patch testing in patients with an acute and/or widespread dermatitis may worsen the existing eruption and may furthermore lead to false positive reactions, this procedure should be performed only after the eruption has subsided. The site chosen for patch testing must have been free from dermatitis preferably for at least four weeks, in order to avoid false positive reactions. For other causes of false positive patch test reactions, see § 3.18

CLASSIFICATION OF PATCH TEST REACTIONS

3.7   Patch test reactions are classified and recorded as follows:

+ ?	=	doubtful reaction, possibly caused by a weak irritant effect: the reaction shows only a weak erythema without infiltration
+	=	erythema with infiltration
+ +	=	erythema, infiltration, papules
+ + +	=	the same with formation of vesicles
+ + + +	=	strong positive reaction with marked edema and confluent vesicles/bullae
–	=	negative
IR	=	irritant reaction
NT	=	not tested.

PATCH TESTING WITH TOPICALLY APPLIED MEDICAMENTS

3.8   Allergic contact dermatitis from topically applied drugs or cosmetics can be caused by:
1. The active ingredient
2. The vehicle constituents
3. The additives.

Additives are substances added to the vehicle in order to enhance the quality and tenability. They include preservatives, antioxidants, stabilizers, emulsifiers, solubilizers, coloring agents and perfume ingredients. The nature of a contact dermatitis is seldom determined by the nature of the allergen.

3.9   The first problem for the dermatologist, in cases of suspected contact allergy to topical drugs, is to obtain full information about the composition of the medicament or cosmetic. The identification of a sensitizer in a locally applied preparation can be relatively easy if this sensitizer is already known in the literature and/or is part of routine patch test batteries. However, one should keep in mind that even at universally recommended concentrations several materials can induce false positive reactions, as there is an enormous inter-individual variability in susceptibility to weak irritants [24].

Difficulties occur when a particular substance has never been reported to induce contact allergic reactions. This may happen with materials which have a low sensitizing index or with newly developed drugs, constituents or additives. In such cases the physician has to answer the following questions before adequate patch testing with the drug or cosmetic can be performed:
1. Which concentration of the substance should be used for patch testing (i.e. a non-irritating concentration)?
2. Which vehicle should be used?
3. Are other test methods indicated, e.g. photopatch tests?
4. How should the results of patch tests be interpreted in this particular circumstance?

These problems are discussed in the next Chapters.

THE TEST CONCENTRATION

3.10   Materials for patch testing should be diluted to such a degree that the solution does not provoke reactions in non-sensitized control persons when patch-tested. The ideal is, of course, to select the highest non-irritating concentration. In choosing too high a concentration it is potentially irritating. On the other hand, a too low concentration evokes no response, except in strongly sensitized subjects. The choice of a correct concentration often remains a difficult problem. There is an enormous range of individual susceptibility to irritants. This is due to variables like race, sex, age and skin type. Tests on a few 'normal' control persons may give untrustworthy results. Kligman and Leyden [24] demonstrated that even recommended standard concentrations may cause irritant false positive patch test reactions. In the present situation, patch tests on a sufficiently large group of control persons remain the best method to select an adequate test concentration.

In practice, few materials should be tested in a concentration higher than 10%. Some medicaments are an exception to this rule: higher concentrations are, for instance, used in patch testing with balsam Peru (25%), neomycin (20%), wool alcohols (30%) and lanolin (100%).

THE VEHICLE TO BE USED FOR PATCH TESTING

3.11   The vehicle used should not be sensitizing or irritating. The following vehicles are commonly used: water, ethyl alcohol, amyl alcohol, phenethyl alcohol, ethyl acetate, amyl acetate, acetone, methyl ethyl ketone, diethyl phthalate, olive oil, liquid paraffin, petrolatum. Generally speaking, the most stable and the least volatile solvent or vehicle is the best. Solvents used in daily life (e.g. naphtha) may act as irritants when applied under occlusion.

Attention should be paid to the bioavailability of the substance in the material made up for patch testing, in order to avoid false negative results.

PHOTOPATCH TESTING

3.12   Photopatch tests are indicated when photosensitivity is suspected. This adverse effect should be considered in all patients with a dermatitis occurring on sun-exposed areas.

In photopatch testing a standard patch test with the suspected agent, suitably diluted, is applied to the skin for a period of 48 hours. The area is subsequently exposed to UV radiation (e.g. sunlight) and the reaction is read after 24 to 48 hours. Appropriate non-UV-exposed control tests are necessary to compare the degree of the reaction and the influence of the UV radiation. Phototoxic patch test reactions must be differentiated from photoallergic ones. A phototoxic reaction is a sunburn type of reaction occurring within six hours, and consists of erythema only. A photoallergic reaction has eczematous features (papules, vesicles etc.); combinations occur frequently. Characteristics of phototoxic and photoallergic reactions are listed in § 3.13.

When only the irradiated test site is positive, the diagnosis of photosensitivity is made. When the non-irradiated site is also positive but less positive than the irradiated site, both contact allergy and photosensitivity are present. If both test sites are equally positive there is an allergic contact sensitivity without photosensitization. Numerous techniques and light sources for photopatch testing have been described [e.g. 93, 94].

Drugs having caused phototoxic and/or photoallergic reactions are listed in Chapter 6.

3.13   Some characteristics of phototoxic and photoallergic reactions [27]

Feature	Photoallergy	Phototoxicity
prevalence	low	high
latency between first exposure and response	present	absent
dosage	low	high
action spectrum	wide	narrow, usually short-wave UV radiation
recurrence requires:	– 'light' + photosensitizer, *or:* – 'light' alone, *or:* – photosensitizer alone.	'light' + photosensitizer
lesion morphology	various forms	intensified sunburn
skin flare-up	*a:* at an unirradiated site *b:* at previously affected area	absent
results of photopatch testing	*a:* allergic morphology and histology, response delayed *b:* retested, response more immediate	limited to area of contact, and response more immediate
cross-reactions	may occur to chemically related compounds	–

THE INTERPRETATION OF PATCH TEST RESULTS

Irritant versus allergic patch test reactions

3.14   In order to differentiate between irritant and allergic patch test reactions the following characteristics of both types of reactions may be taken into account:

3.15 Allergic and irritant patch test reactions

Irritant reactions	Allergic reactions
– relatively oligomorphous	– frequently more polymorphous
– reaction not spreading	– round spreading reaction
– sharp delimitation	– vaguely delimited
– commonly no inclination to increase in size and severity after removal: commonly 'decrescendo' course (with exceptions)	– frequently greater and stronger reaction the days after removal: commonly a 'crescendo' course in the days after removal
– smarting	– itching

Irritant reactions usually develop fully earlier than allergic responses. However, it has been shown [80] that some irritant responses are at their maximum after two days, and are consequently very similar to allergic patch test reactions. This makes differentiation more complicated.

Frequently, even after a careful examination, a decisive answer about the character of an observed patch test reaction remains impossible. This is especially the case when low-strength (+ or + +) reactions are obtained. Unfortunately, these are the reactions most frequently observed in the practice of patch testing. In such cases a punch biopsy of the patch test area may be of some help. The following characteristics of the histopathology of allergic and irritant dermatitis may be useful for differentiation between them [25]:

3.15 Distinctive histological criteria between allergic and irritant patch test reactions in man

	Allergic reactions	Irritant reactions
Epidermis:		
spongiosis	+ to + + +	not frequent
exocytosis	+ to + + +	+ + +
vesicles	+ (spongiotic)	+ (not spongiotic)
formation of bullae	facultative (spongiotic)	facultative (not spongiotic)
pustules	–	+ or –
necrosis of epidermal cells	–	+ to + + +
acantholysis of epidermal cells	–	+ or –
Dermis:		
perivascular infiltrate	mononuclear	mononuclear
eosinophilic leukocytes	+ or –	– (rarely +)
dilatation of lymphatic vessels	+ or –	–
dilatation of blood capillaries	+ or –	–
edema	+ or –	not frequent

It must be stressed that even these histological criteria often are insufficient, again especially in low-strength ($+$ or $++$) reactions. Other reported methods for differentiation (e.g. the lymphocyte transformation test) may be useful in individual cases. For routine daily practice they are generally too costly and time-consuming. As yet, the best method to differentiate between allergic and irritant patch test reactions is to test a number of healthy volunteers with the incriminated test substance.

Multiple positive patch test reactions

3.16   When more than one patch test is positive, the following possibilities should be considered:
1. Concomitant sensitization: this means sensitization to two or more substances present in the same product.
2. Simultaneous sensitization: this means sensitization to two or more substances present in different products. A special form of simultaneous sensitization is the so-called 'Ampliative medicament allergy' [82]. It is well-known that patients with chronic venous stasis leg ulcers have a tendency, in the course of time, to develop contact sensitivities to multiple locally applied medicaments [81]. In some leg ulcer patients a propensity may be noted to develop, within a short period of time, contact allergic reactions to a whole series of locally applied immunologically innocuous medicaments. This state has been called ampliative medicament allergy [82]. Probably the dense lymphocytic infiltrate around the ulcers, in combination with the condition of the surrounding skin and the occlusive effect of bandages, provides a good receptor site for the rapid induction of sensitization, even to low-grade allergens in topical medications.
3. Cross-sensitivity: this implies that a secondary allergen, chemically related to the primary allergen, also produces a positive patch test reaction. Cross-sensitivity can only be assumed when the sensitized person has not been in contact with the secondary allergen previously.
4. One allergen is present in different products or substances (e.g. positive reactions to several balsams may be caused by one and the same allergen present in these substances).
5. One or more patch tests are false positive (§ 3.18).

False positive and false negative patch test reactions

3.17   One of the main problems in contact allergy is the occurrence of false positive or false negative reactions to patch tests. These reactions are especially to be expected when materials are tested for which no proper test concentration and vehicle has been established.

False positive reactions are caused by weakly irritant materials. 'Typical' irritant reactions caused by strong irritants are easily recognized. They are characterized by:
– a sharply defined vivid erythema, which quickly (in about 24 hours) fades away
– an erosion
– the formation of a bulla corresponding to the size of the Whatman paper disc.
However, problems occur with mild irritant reactions, which are often characterized by a slightly elevated erythema without a clear infiltration. This kind of reaction is not easily distinguishable from a true but weak allergic reaction.

Causes of false positive reactions to patch tests with drugs

3.18   Several situations may lead to false positive reactions:
1. The drug has (also) an irritant action and the test concentration has been too high. This has been reported, for instance, in patch testing with clioquinol [20].
2. The vehicle (e.g. powder or pieces of powderized pills) causes false positive traumatic reactions.
3. The drug is unevenly dispersed in the vehicle or on the patch tester.
4. The allergen has degraded (e.g. oxidized) into an irritant substance.
5. The vehicle used for testing is an irritant.
6. The diluent is (too) volatile and thus the concentration of the drug on the patch tester becomes higher than intended.
7. The drug is a potent sensitizer, but the patient is not allergic at the moment of patch testing. Sometimes a late reaction (after one or two weeks) to a patch test is noted in such situations, which may indicate that active sensitization by patch testing has taken place. This has for instance been reported in patch testing with phenothiazines.
8. The test is read too quickly after removal of the patch tester. Redness and edema occurring within a few minutes after removal of the adhesive and the patch tester are mistaken for a true positive reaction.
9. The presence of an irritant or allergic dermatitis in an acute phase elsewhere on the skin may increase non-specific reactivity to some (but not all) mild irritants [3].
10. The presence of a severe reaction to adhesive tape makes a reliable reading difficult. The skin in the region of the test has become highly irritated and may elicit reactions to normally correctly diluted but potentially irritating substances.
11. One or more positive patch test reactions may cause false positive reactions to other patch tests. This condition has been termed 'angry back' [38], but as the phenomenon is not restricted to the back, it is preferable to use the name 'excited skin syndrome' (ESS) [83, 84, 88]. Weak positive patch test reactions, concomitant to other weak or strong positive reactions may lose their reactivity in up to 45% when retested [88]. Allergens which are marginal irritants, e.g. formaldehyde, frequently cause weak positive reactions in the ESS, which are lost at retesting. False positive reactivity is often found at the proximity of strong reactions.
12. Patch tests with salts of metals (nickel, copper, arsenic, mercury) may produce a non-specific reaction characterized by small pustules, each with a small erythematous areola. The reaction differs clinically and histopathologically from a true positive patch test reaction.
13. 'Para-allergy': this term has been used to describe reactions which become accentuated as a result of strong allergic test reactions elsewhere. A subject may be strongly sensitized to one agent and weakly to a different one. If both patch tests are applied at the same time, the site exposed to the weaker allergen will react more intensely than when it was applied alone. The concomitant intense allergic dermatitis has exaggerated the reaction. The mechanism is apparently a translocation of the more potent allergen via the blood stream to the site of the weaker one [23].

Causes of false negative reactions to patch tests with drugs

3.19 The following situations may lead to false negative reactions:

1. The amount of the drug tested is too small.
2. The concentration of the allergen in the test substance or in the proprietary preparation is too low. It is sometimes necessary to increase the patch test concentration with a factor of 10 or more to obtain positive allergic patch test reactions. This is for instance the case with neomycin and ethylene diamine.
3. The allergen is degraded or oxidized during storage.
4. The allergic dermatitis has been caused by a photoallergen.
5. The allergen is volatile.
6. The diluent is volatile, rapid evaporization decreases the possibility of penetration of the allergen into the epidermis.
7. The allergen is poorly absorbed. The bioavailability of the allergen in the patch test vehicle (e.g. petrolatum) may be considerably lower than in the original proprietary drug.
8. A 'quenching effect' has occurred: a contact sensitizing substance no longer causes contact sensitization in combination with another substance [42]. This phenomenon has thus far only been observed in the maximization test with the sensitizing aldehydes phenylacetaldehyde, citral and cinnamic aldehyde. This phenomenon probably is of no importance as a cause of false negative reactions.
9. A compound allergy has occurred: a mixture of substances causes an allergic reaction, but the individual ingredients react negatively. Thus the 'allergen' is a combination of more than one ingredient [7].
10. Corticosteroids present in the medication tested decrease the extent as well as the strength of the reaction. It is possible that low-grade patch test reactions are completely masked.
11. The skin of the patient is still in a refractory state immediately after a severe allergic contact dermatitis (presumably all available T-lymphocytes are involved in the clinical reaction).
12. The patient is under corticosteroid treatment. It is generally assumed that doses of 15 mg prednisolone or more may suppress weak positive patch test reactions.
13. The skin has recently been treated with a potent corticosteroid preparation. In view of the fact that a depot of steroid is formed in the skin an interim period of one week is considered necessary in order to obtain trustworthy patch test results. Otherwise, weak positive reactions may be diminished in size and strength, or even completely suppressed. Intermediate-strength topical steroids are said *not* to prevent the detection of contact allergy by patch testing [91, 92].
14. Immunosuppressive drugs inhibit the patch test reaction.
15. There is a slow development of the patch test reaction – the test is read too quickly, e.g. as seen with neomycin testing (positive reactions may sometimes only be noted after several days).
16. The sensitivity to the tested substance is a low-grade one. This may occur in patch tests with cross-reacting substances.
17. The permeability of the skin in the test area is low compared with the site of clinical exposure. Nail polish may cause dermatitis of the face and the neck, whilst the hands are not affected, and the patch tests on the skin of the back remain negative.
18. Technical problems, e.g. insufficient occlusion of the patch tests.

3.20　True positive patch test reactions

The relevance of true positive patch test reactions

3.20　Patch tests are performed primarily to establish the cause of an allergic contact dermatitis. However, a causal relationship between the allergen thus demonstrated and the eruption is not always clear, especially when the patient apparently has not been exposed to the allergen (at least according to his medical history).

The following situations may occur:
1. The patient does not know or does not *remember* having been in contact with the allergen previously.
2. The patient's history is incomplete, e.g. important details concerning his work or his hobbies have been overlooked. Exact and detailed information may provide a satisfactory explanation and subsequently the solution to the cure of the patient's skin problem.
3. The observed patch test reaction is caused by a compound cross-reacting to the allergen that has caused the eruption, but the actual causative allergen has not been tested, and therefore remains unknown. In this case, the patient may rightly deny contact with the allergen demonstrated. In such situations it would be useful to know to which compound(s) the positively reacting substance has been reported to cross-react, as this may possibly indicate the actual causative allergenic substance.

    An alphabetical listing of substances that are known to cross-react is provided in § 3.22, and for every substance the possible primary sensitizer is stated. It must, however, be pointed out that not all reactions listed are true cross-reactions; sometimes the compound mentioned forms part of (or is an ingredient of) the primary sensitizer (see Point 4).
4. The observed patch test reaction is caused by a compound which is an ingredient of the preparation that has caused the contact allergic reaction. When both the patient and the physician are unaware of this, and the sensitizing preparation has not been tested (or the preparation failed to elicit a positive reaction due to the low concentration of the allergen), the significance of the positive patch test reaction may be overlooked.
5. The observed patch test reaction is caused by a complex preparation (e.g. balsam Peru) which contains several allergenic compounds, but the patient has been sensitized by one of its ingredients from *another source*. Again, the patient may (apparently) rightly deny previous contact with the allergen demonstrated by patch testing.

3.21　On the other hand, not every positive patch test reaction may be considered relevant to the existing dermatosis, even when the patient has apparently been exposed to the allergen thus demonstrated.

The following possibilities must be kept in mind:
1. The observed positive reaction is a secondary, complicating and aggravating factor, but not the primary cause of the eruption. This may be seen especially with topical drugs.
2. The reaction is caused by an allergen to which the patient has been exposed in the past, but is not relevant to the present situation.
3. The patient has been in contact with the allergen, but the observed patch test reaction represents a cross-reaction to the actual causative allergen.
4. The patient is allergic to several chemicals, and the allergen demonstrated is unrelated to the eruption.

16

3.22   List of (pseudo) cross-reactions

Compound cross-reacting to the primary sensitizer, or forming part of it	Primary sensitization to:	See §:
abietic acid	colophony	5.16
	dihydroabietyl alcohol	5.39
abietic alcohol	colophony	5.39
alcohols	other alcohols	5.7
amantadine	tromantadine	5.42
ambutyrosin	neomycin	5.25
aminophylline	ethylenediamine hydrochloride	5.22
amodiaquin	clioquinol	5.7
α-amylcinnamic alcohol	α-amylcinnamic aldehyde	5.16
α-amylcinnamic aldehyde	α-amylcinnamic alcohol	5.16
amylocaine	tetracaine	5.20
antazoline sulfate	ethylene diamine hydrochloride	5.22
	tripelennamine	5.30
antidiabetics (para-compounds)	sulfonamide	5.25
aryl salicylates	phenyl salicylate	23.53
atranorin	oak moss	5.16
azo-dyes	p-aminobenzoic acid	25.66
	diacetazotol	5.42
	other azo-dyes	
bacitracin	neomycin (?)	5.25
	polymyxin-B sulfate	5.25
balsam Peru	tiger balm	5.42
	beeswax	5.39
	balsam Tolu	5.16
	benzaldehyde	5.16
	benzyl benzoate	5.41
	benzyl cinnamate	5.16
	benzyl salicylate	5.16
	cinnamic acid	
	cinnamic alcohol	5.16
	cinnamic aldehyde	5.16
	cinnamon oil	5.16
	colophony	5.39
	coniferyl alcohol	5.16
	coumarin	5.16
	eugenol	5.16
	farnesol	5.16
	isoeugenol	5.16
	methyl cinnamate	
	propanidid	5.20
	propolis	5.43
	2-ethoxyethyl-p-methoxycinnamate	25.66
	benzoin tincture	5.39
	storax	5.39
	diethylstilbestrol	5.42

(continued)

17

3.22 (Pseudo) cross-reactions

(continuation)

Compound cross-reacting to the primary sensitizer, or forming part of it	Primary sensitization to:	See §:
balsam Peru/colophony/turpentine oils/wood tars	(some) perfume ingredients	5.12
balsam Tolu	balsam Peru	5.16
	benzyl benzoate	5.41
benzalkonium chloride	cetalkonium chloride (?), cetrimonium bromide	5.7
	benzethonium chloride	5.7
benzestrol	diethylstilbestrol	5.42
benzocaine	parabens	5.7
	butethamine	5.20
	old orthoform	5.20
	glyceryl-p-aminobenzoate	25.66
benzoic acid	balsam Peru	5.16
benzoin	balsam Peru	5.16
	storax	5.39
benzyl alcohol	balsam Peru	5.16
	benzoin tincture	5.39
benzyl benzoate	propolis	5.43
	balsam Peru	5.16
benzyl cinnamate	2-ethoxyethyl-p-methoxycinnamate	25.66
	benzoin tincture,	5.39
	propolis	5.43
benzyl ester of p-hydroxybenzoic acid	diethylstilbestrol	5.42
benzyl penicillin	penethamate hydriodide	5.44
p-benzylphenol	diethylstilbestrol	5.42
bisphenol-A	diethylstilbestrol	5.42
	monobenzyl ether of hydroquinone	5.42
bupivacaine	lidocaine	5.20
cananga oil	benzyl salicylate	5.16
ω-chloracetophenone	chlorphenoxide	5.32
chloramphenicol	azidamfenicol	5.25
4-chloro-m-cresol	p-chloro-m-xylenol	5.7
chlorofluoromethane	freon 11/12	5.22
p-chloro-m-xylenol	4-chloro-m-cresol	5.7
chlorpromazines	chlorprothixene	5.44
chlorquinaldol	clioquinol	5.7
cinnamates	balsam Peru	5.16

(continued)

(continuation)

Compound cross-reacting to the primary sensitizer, or forming part of it	Primary sensitization to:	See §:
cinnamic acid	balsam Peru	5.16
cinnamic alcohol	balsam Peru	5.16
	propolis	5.43
cinnamic aldehyde	cinnamic alcohol, cinnamon oil	5.16
cinnamon oil	propanidid	5.20
cinnamyl alcohol	2-ethoxyethyl-p-methoxycinnamate	25.66
cinamyl cinnamate	propolis	5.43
citronellal	hydroxycitronellal	5.16
clioquinol	dibucaine (?)	5.20
	quinine sulfate (?)	5.44
cocamidopropyl betaine	cocobetaïne	22.7
cocarboxylase	thiamine (vitamin B1)	5.44
colistine	bacitracin	5.25
colophony	balsam Peru	5.16
	dihydroabietyl alcohol	5.16
	wood tars	5.38
cresols	phenol	5.38
cycloheximide	neomycin (?)	5.25
DC yellow 10	DC yellow 11	23.47
dehydroabietic acid	colophony	5.39
demethylchlortetracycline	chlortetracycline	5.25
dextropimaric acid	colophony	5.39
5,7-dibromo-8-hydroxyquinoline (DBO)	clioquinol	5.7
dibucaine	lidocaine	5.20
dichlorophene	hexachlorophene	5.7
dienestrol	diethylstilbestrol	5.42
diethazine hydrochloride	chlorpromazine	5.44
diethylenetetramine	ethylenediamine hydrochloride	5.22
diethylstilbestrol	monobenzylether of hydroquinone (?)	5.42
dihydralazine	hydrazines	5.44
dihydroabietic acid	colophony	5.39
dihydrostreptomycin	streptomycin	5.25
diisopropyl fluorophosphate	epinephrine chloride (?)	5.42

(continued)

3.22 (Pseudo) cross-reactions

(continuation)

Compound cross-reacting to the primary sensitizer, or forming part of it	Primary sensitization to:	See §:
dimercaprol (BAL)	thioglycerol	5.22
N,N'-dimethyl piperazine	piperazine	5.44
p-dinitrobenzene	chloramphenicol (?)	5.25
dinitrochlorbenzene	chloramphenicol (?)	5.25
	pyrrolnitrin (?)	5.32
dioxybenzone	oxybenzone	25.66
diphenylamine	N-phenyl-p-phenylenediamine	22.28
diuretics (para-compounds)	sulfonamide	5.25
econazole	miconazole	5.32
	enilconazole	5.32
epinephrine borate	epinephrine chloride	5.42
essential oils	balsam Peru	5.16
	wood tars	5.38
	propolis	5.43
ethopropazine hydrochloride	chlorpromazine	5.44
ethyl aminobenzoate	parabens	5.6
ethyl chloride	chlorofluoromethane (?)	5.22
ethylenediamine hydrochloride	edetic acid (EDTA)	5.7
	antazoline	5.30
	aminophylline	5.44
	promethazine hydrochloride	5.30
	zinc pyrithione (?)	22.7
	piperazine	5.44
ethylenediamine dihydriodide	ethylenediamine hydrochloride	5.22
eugenol	balsam Peru	5.16
	isoeugenol	5.16
	propanidid	5.20
	benzoin tincture	5.39
evernic acid	oak moss	5.16
formaldehyde	aryl-sulfonamide resin	24.12
	chloroallylhexaminium chloride	5.7
	bronopol [?]	5.7
framycetin	neomycin	5.25
fumarprotocetraric acid	oak moss	5.16
gentamicin	neomycin	5.25
geranium	geranial	5.16
halogenated quinolines	other halogenated quinolines	5.7

(continued)

(continuation)

Compound cross-reacting to the primary sensitizer, or forming part of it	Primary sensitization to:	See §:
halogenated salicylanilides	bithionol	5.7
	trichlorocarbanilide	5.7
hexachlorophene	dichlorophene (?)	5.7
	bithionol	5.7
	halogenated salicylanilides (usually photo-cross-reactions)	
hexamethonium bromide	benzalkonium chloride	5.7
hexestrol	diethylstilbestrol	5.42
hexylresorcinol	resorcinol	5.38
4-homosulfanilamide	parabens	5.7
hydralazine	hydrazines	5.44
hydrochlorthiazide	dibenzthione	5.32
hydroquinone	phenol (?)	5.38
	resorcinol	5.38
hydroxycitronellal	citronellal	5.16
	geranial	5.16
	methoxycitronellal	5.16
	linalool (?)	5.16
hydroxyhydroquinone	resorcinol	5.38
hydroxyzine	zinc pyrithione (?)	22.7
iodine	povidone-iodine	5.7
isobutyl p-aminobenzoate	old orthoform	5.20
isoconazole	enilconazole	5.32
isoeugenol	eugenol	5.16
isoniazid (INH)	hydrazines	5.44
4-isopropylaminodiphenylamine	N-phenyl-p-phenylenediamine	22.28
jasmin oil	benzyl salicylate	5.16
kanamycin	dihydrostreptomycin	5.25
	framycetin (?)	5.25
	gentamicin sulfate	5.25
	neomycin	5.25
	streptomycin	5.25
lanolin	eucerin	5.22
	lanette N	5.22
	lanette wax	5.22
lavender oil	geranial	5.16
levamisole	tetramisole hydrochloride	5.44

(continued)

3.22 (Pseudo) cross-reactions

(continuation)

Compound cross-reacting to the primary sensitizer, or forming part of it	Primary sensitization to:	See §:
levopimaric acid	colophony	5.39
linalool (?)	hydroxycitronellal	23.47
lincomycin	clindamycin	5.25
mafenide	parabens	5.7
maleopimaric acid	colophony	5.39
mepacrine	chloroquine diphosphate	5.44
mepivacaine hydrochloride	lidocaine	5.20
meprylcaine	benzocaine	5.20
mepyramine maleate	ethylenediamine hydrochloride	5.22
mercurials (anorganic, organic, metallic mercury)	other anorganic and organic mercurials, and metallic mercury	5.7
metabutethamine	benzocaine	5.20
metadihydroxybenzenes	resorcinol	5.38
methacycline	oxytetracycline	5.25
methyl abietate	colophony	5.39
methyl cinnamate	2-ethoxyethyl-p-methoxycinnamate	25.66
methyl-2-piperazine	piperazine	5.44
N-methylpiperazine	piperazine	5.44
metoprolol	alprenolol	5.44
miconazole	enilconazole	5.32
monobenzylether of hydroquinone	diethylstilbestrol	5.42
morphine	apomorphine	5.44
moskene	musk ambrette	5.16
neoabietic acid	colophony	5.39
neomycin	streptomycin	5.25
	dihydrostreptomycin	5.25
	framycetin	5.25
	gentamicin	5.25
p-nitrobenzoic acid	chloramphenicol	5.25
nitrofuran derivatives (?)	nitrofurazone (?)	5.25
nitrofurylaminothiadiazoles	2-(5-nitro-2-furyl)-5-amino-1,3,4-thiadiazole	5.38
	ichthyol(?)	5.7

(continued)

(continuation)

Compound cross-reacting to the primary sensitizer, or forming part of it	Primary sensitization to:	See §:
orthoform, new	orthoform, old	5.20
orthoform, old	orthoform, new	5.20
oximetazole chlorhydrate	imidazole chlorhydrate	5.42
oxybenzone	dioxybenzone	25.66
palustric acid	colophony	5.39
parabens	other parabens	5.7
	monobenzylether of hydroquinone	5.42
	para-compounds	
para-compounds	benzocaine	5.20
	procaine	5.20
	promethazine hydrochloride	5.30
	mafenide	5.25
	glyceryl-p-aminobenzoate (?)	25.66
	parabens	5.7
	diacetazotol	5.42
	sulfonamides	5.25
	tetracaine hydrochloride	5.20
	benzidine	5.44
paromomycin	framycetin (?)	5.25
	neomycin	5.25
perfume ingredients (some)	wood tars/colophony/turpentine oil/balsam Peru	
β-phenylethylhydrazine	hydrazines	5.44
phenol	resorcinol	5.38
phenothiazines	chlorpromazine	5.44
	promethazine hydrochloride	5.30
	tripelennamine	5.30
phenylbutazone	oxyphenbutazone	5.42
p-phenylene diamine	parabens	5.7
	diphenylamine (?)	5.22
	p-aminobenzoic acid	25.66
	para-compounds	
phenylhydrazine	hydrazines	5.44
phenylmercuric acetate	parachloromercuriphenol	25.66
α-pinene	benzoin tincture	5.39
piperazine citrate	ethylenediamine hydrochloride	5.22
	zinc pyrithione (?)	22.7
polyethylene glycols	other polyethylene glycols	5.22
polymyxin	polymyxin-B sulfate	5.25
polymyxin-B sulfate	bacitracin	5.25

(continued)

23

3.22   (Pseudo) cross-reactions

(*continuation*)

Compound cross-reacting to the primary sensitizer, or forming part of it	Primary sensitization to:	See §:
potassium iodide (?)	clioquinol	5.7
prilocaine	lidocaine	5.20
pristinamycin	virginiamycin	5.25
procaine	parabens	5.7
	butethamine	5.20
	p-aminobenzoic acid	25.66
promethazine hydrochloride	ethylenediamine hydrochloride	5.22
	triethanolamine (?)	5.22
	chlorpromazine	5.44
	tripelennamine	5.30
propolis	balsam Peru	5.16
pyridine derivatives	nicotinic acid	5.44
pyridoxine hydrochloride	pyridoxine-3,4-dioctanoate	22.65
pyrimidine analogs (brominated, chlorinated)	idoxuridine	5.42
pyrocatechol	resorcinol	5.38
pyrogallol	resorcinol	5.38
quinine	clioquinol	5.7
reindeer lichen	oak moss	5.16
resoquine	clioquinol	5.7
resorcinol	phenol	5.38
resorcinol monoacetate	resorcinol	5.38
ribostamycin	neomycin	5.25
risocaine	old orthoform	5.20
sisomycin	neomycin	5.25
sodium salicylate	methyl salicylate	5.42
sorbic acid	potassium sorbate	5.7
sorbitan mono-oleate	sorbitan sesquiolate (Arlacel 83®)	5.22
sorbitan monostearate	sorbitan sesquiolate (Arlacel 83®)	5.22
spectinomycin	neomycin	5.25
spiramycin	tylosin	5.44
storax	diethylstilbestrol	5.42
	tincture of benzoin	5.39

(*continued*)

(continuation)

Compound cross-reacting to the primary sensitizer, or forming part of it	Primary sensitization to:	See §:
streptomycin	dihydrostreptomycin	5.25
	framycetin (?)	5.25
	neomycin (?)	5.25
sulfapyridine	tripelennamine	5.30
sulfonamides	other sulfonamides	5.25
	p-aminobenzoic acid	25.66
	aryl-sulfonamide resin	24.12
	para-compounds	
sweetening agents (para-compounds)	sulfonamide	5.25
	other para-compounds	
tetracycline	oxytetracycline	5.25
tetrahydroabietic acid	colophony	5.39
tetramethylthiuram disulfide	tetra-ethylthiurammonosulfide	5.44
	tetra-ethylthiuramdisulfide	5.44
thiazinamium	chlorpromazine	5.44
tobramycin	neomycin	5.44
tree moss	oak moss	5.16
triazine-antihypertensive drugs	dibenzthione (?)	5.32
triethanolamine	promethazine hydrochloride (?)	5.30
trifluorthymidine	idoxuridine	5.42
triphenylmethane dyes	other triphenylmethane dyes	5.7
turpentine	colophony	5.39
turpentine oil	lemon oil	5.16
tylosin	spiramycin (?)	5.44
undecylenic acid	zinc undecylenate	5.32
ung. alc. lanae B.P.	xanthocillin (?)	5.25
usnic acid	oak moss	5.16
vanilla	coumarin	5.16
	benzoin tincture	5.39
	balsam Peru	5.16
vanillin	coumarin	5.16
	propolis	5.43
virginiamycin	pristinamycin	5.25
vitamin K3	vitamin K4	5.44
vitamin K4	vitamin K3	5.44

(continued)

(continuation)

Compound cross-reacting to the primary sensitizer, or forming part of it	Primary sensitization to:	See §:
wool alcohols	eucerin	5.22
	lanette N	5.22
	lanette wax	5.22
	other wool alcohols	
ylang-ylang oil	benzyl salicylate	5.16
	geranial	5.16
zinc oxide	zinc sulfate	5.22
zinc undecylenate	undecylenic acid	5.32

RISKS OF PATCH TESTING FOR THE PATIENT

3.23   Patch testing may be considered a fairly innocent method of investigation. Occasionally however the patient is exposed to some serious hazards and inconveniences. Therefore, in every case in which patch testing appears to be indicated, the advantages and disadvantages of this method of investigation should be taken into account. The following problems may present themselves:

A: The patient develops a strong skin reaction to the adhesive. A large part of the skin of the back becomes red and irritated. Apart from the inconvenience to the patient the results of the test are less reliable. Causes of skin reactions to the adhesive are:
- trauma of removal
- irritation
- retention of sweat
- disturbance of bacterial flora
- contact allergic reactions to constituents of the adhesive. The adhesive may contain colophony, rubber chemicals, dammar, lanolin, antiseptics, preservatives, acrylates [18].

Before application, the patient's history on adverse reactions to adhesives should be investigated carefully. In cases of suspected untoward reactions preliminary testing with different brands of adhesive material is imperative.

In most European and US centers patch tests are left in place for a period of 48 hours. When, despite previous testing with different brands of adhesives, irritation is to be expected, an application period of 24 hours should be used. In hot climates a patch test application period of 24 hours generally is to be preferred.

B: Patch tests are performed with a substance which acts as an irritant in the concentration tested. This danger presents itself when materials of unknown composition are tested. Unknown substances presented for patch testing should therefore be investigated carefully and literature data should be collected before the material is applied to the skin. Subsequently, the correct concentration and vehicle for patch testing has to be established. In the first phase of this investigation the substance must be tested in several concentrations, in order to obtain data about the correct non-irritant patch test concentration. These preliminary tests should preferably be performed on the skin of the investigator himself. These tests are not entirely without risk, and the investigator should consider to stop his experiment at once as soon as untoward effects (severe itching or burning, pain) become manifest. In the next phase, patch tests with the substance in this concentration must be performed on a group of at least 20 healthy volunteers. In the correct concentration the allergen will elicit a moderate reaction in the sensitized person, whilst controls will remain negative.

C: Patch testing induces contact allergy to the tested substance. Examples of substances with a strong contact sensitizing capacity are: marfenide (p-amino-methylbenzenesulfonamide), other azo-compounds, and some natural products from trees or plants. Of course, patch testing with well-known contact sensitizers such as 2,4-dinitrochlorobenzene (DNCB) and mechlorethamine carries the same risk.

D: Contact urticarial reactions may be observed occasionally during and due to patch testing [79]. Anaphylactoid reactions greatly endangering the patients have occurred with the application of several allergens. See Chapter 7 on Contact urticaria (especially Refs. 52, 53, and 54), and § 16.2.

E: Strong (+ + +) patch test reactions are often very troublesome to the patient. These reactions may be controlled by application of a corticosteroid preparation. Pigmentation or depigmentation may subsequently develop and constitute a major cosmetic problem.

F: Patch tests with the relevant allergen may induce a recurrence or an exacerbation of the dermatitis.

G: In patients with psoriasis or lichen ruber, a Koebner phenomenon may occur.

H: Very infrequently, keloid formation after patch tests may be noted [54].

I: A case of respiratory symptoms presumably due to a patch test with piperazine has been documented [78]. The patient was strongly allergic to piperazine, and had experienced eczema and respiratory symptoms when being exposed to this chemical.

J: Occasionally lymph node enlargement has been reported in association with a strongly positive patch test reaction [86].

K: An extensive purpuric eruption with papulonodular lesions, lesions en cocarde and bullae with a tendency to necrose was seen in a patient who had a very strong patch test reaction to Frullania [87]. The vasculitis was presumably due to an immune complex reaction.

THE USE OF PATCH TESTS IN DRUG ERUPTIONS

3.24   The value of patch tests with drugs that have caused skin eruptions after systemic administration is sometimes doubted. It is pointed out that positive reactions are only to be expected in cases of Type IV allergic reactions (according to the classification of Gell and Coombs). Still, in the opinion of some authors, there may (at least in some cases) be reasons for performing these tests [1]

1. The patient has developed a systemic eczematous contact-type dermatitis medicamentosa. This possibility is surveyed in Chapter 17.

2. In some cases of fixed drug eruption, patch tests with the incriminated drug are positive, provided they are performed at the site of the fixed eruption [46]. The most well-known cause of this type of reaction is phenolphthalein.

3. In eruptions caused by certain systemic drugs, the value of patch testing has been proven by clinical experience. This is apparently especially the case in maculopapular rashes due to penicillin or its derivatives [50, 58, 59]. Other drug eruptions caused by systemic administration, in which patch testing sometimes yields positive allergic patch test reactions relevant to the diagnosis, are summarized in § 3.25.

3.25   Patch testing in drug eruptions

Drug	Patch test conc. and vehicle	Cross-reactions	Comment	Ref.
amantadine	pure		*photo*patch test positive	72
aminophenazone	10% in DMSO 40%			57
aminophylline	2.5% pet.	ethylenediamine		63
amitriptyline	?			1
amoxicillin	pure	other penicillins		59
ampicillin	pure	other penicillins		59
benzylpenicillin	pure	other penicillins		59
carbamazepine	1% and 5% pet.			17
carbimazole	pure			66
carbromal	?			1
carprofen	5%–10%–20% pet.		*photo*patch test positive	62
cephalosporin	20% pet.		generalized urticarial eruption after ampicillin; patch test with ampicillin negative	64
cephalosporin	pure	penicillins		59
chloramphenicol	50% ?			67
cloxacillin		other penicillins		59
diphenhydramine	2% pet.			61
dipyrone	pure	aminophenazone	contact urticarial patch test reaction	71
ethylenediamine	1% pet.	aminophylline		63
feneticillin	pure	other penicillins		59
hydrochlorothiazide	1% pet.		*photo*patch test positive	68
ketoconazole	pure	econazole	*scratch* tests positive	66
neomycin and other aminoglycosides	?			1
phenacetin	10% in DMSO 40%			57
phenazone	5% pet.		EEM-like eruption	60
phenol	1% aqua			70
phenothiazine	?		*photo*patch test positive	34
practolol	10% and 50% pet.			9
propranolol	pure			51

(continued)

(continuation)

Drug	Patch test conc. and vehicle	Cross-reactions	Comment	Ref.
propyphenazone	pure	aminophenazone, phenylbutazone, dipyrone	contact urticarial patch test reaction	71
quinidine sulfate	1% saline sol.		*photo*patch test positive	65
sulfonamides	?			1

3.26   However, in order to exclude non-specific reactions, a series of control tests on a panel of healthy volunteers remains imperative, as many medicaments applied without dilution and under occlusion in patch test conditions act as mild irritants.

Thus Pevny et al. [43] observed an unexpected series of positive patch test reactions to tricyclic psychopharmaceutical drugs in a patient with a drug eruption caused by a similar drug. The patch tests had been performed with the undiluted drugs. A series of 44 psychopharmaceutical drugs was subsequently tested undiluted in a group of 40 non-allergic control persons. All 40 control persons reacted positively to at least one patch test, 90% reacted positively to two, 65% to five or more, and 40% to ten or more drugs.

It may be concluded that patch tests performed with undiluted drugs or with powderized pills or tablets are unreliable and mistakes are easily made. Control tests in a relatively large group of human volunteers are always indispensable.

PREDICTIVE TESTS TO IDENTIFY ALLERGENS

3.27   The number of chemicals which have proven to be allergenic is steadily increasing and there is an urgent need for a reliable predictive method to determine the allergenic potential of drugs before they are marketed and subsequently used by thousands of persons.

Absolute innocuousness of course does not exist; most pharmaceutical products are neither wholly innocuous nor very dangerous. Topical drugs are more prone to cause contact allergy as they are usually applied to an already pathologically altered skin. The occurrence of untoward side effects will complicate the clinical picture and hamper the recovery.

Reviews of the numerous biological test procedures in humans and animals have been provided by several authors (e.g. by Klecak [95]). Among the human test methods with a predictive value, the so-called maximization provocative patch test method developed by Kligman [22] is well known. This test is intended to classify substances according to their sensitizing capacity under arbitrarily defined experimental conditions. The risk of lasting injury to the test persons involved is still controversial and the test is inadmissible in many countries. The same holds true for the (human) photo-maximization test designed by Kaidbey and Kligman [19] to identify topical photocontact sensitizers.

Animal experiments

3.28   Attention therefore has been centered on animal experiments. When animal models are used as a substitute for dermatotoxicological experiments in humans, structural and biochemical differences between human and animal skin should be taken into account, as they are of importance for the degree of penetration of the chemical into the skin. How much of a potential allergen can pass the skin barrier is of course of paramount theoretical and practical importance. Other factors which influence the amount of the drug penetrating the skin are [31, 33]:

1. The physicochemical properties of the vehicle
2. The physicochemical properties of the active substance
3. The concentration of the active substance at induction and elicitation
4. The duration of the exposure
5. The condition of the skin surface.

Various animal models have been developed in order to try to establish the allergenic potential of new chemicals. Predictive test procedures in guinea pigs include the following methods:

- Draize test and variations
- guinea pig maximization test
- Maguire's modified split adjuvant technique
- Freund's complete adjuvant test
- Bühler test
- open epicutaneous test.

Technical details as well as the merits of each of these test methods have been discussed extensively by Klecak [95]. More recently, a modified guinea-pig technique has been developed for the detection of weak allergens and allergenicity of materials unsuitable for testing by intradermal injection [56]; see also Goodwin et al. [55]. The question as to which technique would appear to be the best and the most reliable, is still in debate. Obviously, as yet a completely satisfactory technique has not been developed. In the present situation the use of several test techniques is necessary in order to obtain a reliable estimation of the allergenicity of the substances tested. Every test procedure presently used has certain drawbacks. Cardinal factors such as the degree and type of daily usage are not simulated closely enough by any of these procedures.

In conclusion, the results of animal predictive testing may serve as guidelines rather than absolute criteria for calculating the margin of safety for the materials tested. In the next phase of such investigations, controlled testing on human subjects would appear to be desirable.

THE PERSISTENCE OF ACQUIRED EPIDERMAL SENSITIVITY

3.29   The course of an acquired epidermal sensitivity is a matter of great practical importance. The results of the investigations on this subject published thus far have been rather contradictory. The relevant literature on the persistence of positive patch test reactions is summarized in § 3.30. The scarceness of available data makes it impossible to restrict this survey to topically applied drugs. Unfortunately, the available reports are difficult to compare due to methodological differences. Some early investigators [14] found that if the offensive agent was removed, the hypersensitivity subsided, or disappeared completely in a large proportion of cases. The results of another investigation [47] led to a more pessimistic view. In ten patients, patch test reactions to clioquinol (vioform) were still unchanged positive after an average interval of 6 years, even though these patients had scrupulously avoided the allergen and related chemicals. The more recent study of Keczkes et al. [77] in which only 14% of patch test reactions were negative after a period of 10–12 years (although admittedly, probably in a biased population) also seems to indicate that allergic contact sensitivity tends to persist for many years, although a proportion of patients show diminution of their sensitivity over the years. The persistence probably does not only depend on renewed contact with the allergen or related substances but also on the nature of the allergen, and possibly the intensity of the acquired hypersensitivity.

3.30   **The persistence of positive patch test reactions**

Allergen	Interval in patch testing (years)	Number of patients	Negative on re-patch testing (%)	Ref.
turpentine	1–3.5	106	3	14
nickel	1.5–11	54	43	39
balsam Peru		18	16	
nickel	4.2 (average)	9	22	6
turpentine		12	66	
balsam Peru		9	44	
nickel	13.5 (average)	11	18	40
turpentine		29	62	
nickel	2–5	40	10	90
bichromate	3–10	20	45	10
p-phenylenediamine	3–10	50	8	
nickel	5.5–7.6	27	4	30
turpentine			6	
chromate	16	?	25	26
parabens			74	
nickel	2	21	38	44
nickel	1.2–5	36	41	37
turpentine			64	
nickel	2–15	105	32	48
balsam Peru			50	
22 allergens	1–3	208	25	35
bichromate	4–7	48	21	49
clioquinol	6	10	0	47
46 allergens	10–12	100	14	77

PATCH TESTING ON THE ORAL MUCOSA

3.31   It is possible to perform patch tests on the oral mucosa: various methods have been described [11, 13, 41, 45]. A positive allergic reaction is characterized by reddening and sometimes also swelling of the area of the mucosa exposed. The patients may also experience a sensation of burning and irritation of the mouth. Vesicles are hardly ever seen, as they rupture easily in the mouth. This is a definite disadvantage of oral patch testing: the differentiation between an irritant and an allergic patch test response is even more difficult than on the skin. Patch testing on the oral mucosa has several other disadvantages in addition: (1) False negative reactions easily occur. This is due to the technical difficulties of patch testing on the oral mucosa: it is not easy to obtain a lasting intimate contact between the allergen and the mucosa, the former being so readily rinsed off by the saliva. (2) The reaction obtained is generally of a duration shorter than that on the skin. (3) The more rapid absorption of the allergen through the mucosal membrane may in some patients cause a generalized eczema-like skin eruption, sometimes combined with heavy itching, headaches, hypersalivation and general malaise [2].

As sensitization of the oral mucosa is nearly always combined with sensitization of the skin, patch testing on the latter may be used in routine allergological examination of patients with a suspected contact allergic reaction of the oral mucosa.

3.32   REFERENCES

1. Agrup, G. (1972): Patch testing in drug allergy. In: *Mechanisms in Drug Allergy*. Editors: C. H. Dash and H. E. H. Jones. Churchill Livingstone, Edinburgh.
2. Bauer, E. (1963): Allergie durch Edelmetallegierungen. *Dtsch. zahnaerztl. Z., 18,* 1023.
3. Björnberg, A. (1968): *Skin Reactions to Primary Irritants in Patients with Hand Eczema.* Thesis, Oscar Isacson, Göteborg, Sweden.
4. Bleumink, E., Nater, J. P., Schraffordt Koops, H. and The, T. H. (1974): A standard method for DNCB sensitization testing in patients with neoplasms. *Cancer, 33,* 911.
5. Brian, R. G. and Nater, J. P. (1973): Ulcus cruris en contacteczeem. *Ned. T. Geneesk., 117,* 561.
6. Bülow, K. (1954): En efterundersögelse of eczempatienter med positive lappepröver. *Ugeskr. Laeg., 18,* 245.
7. Calnan, C. D. (1975): Compound allergy to a cosmetic. *Contact Dermatitis, 1,* 123.
8. Omitted.
9. Felix, R. H. and Comaish, J. S. (1974): The value of patch tests and other skin tests in drug eruptions. *Lancet, 1,* 1017.
10. Fisher, A. A., Pelzig, A. and Kanof, N. B. (1958): The persistence of allergic eczematous sensitivity and the cross-sensitivity pattern to paraphenylenediamine. *J. invest. Derm., 30,* 9.
11. Forlen, H. P. and Stüttgen, G. (1961): Vergleichende Studien über die allergische Reaktion an Haut und Mundschleimhaut. *Dermatologica (Basel), 122,* 417.
12. Fregert, S. (1981): *Manual of contact dermatitis, 2nd Edition,* Munksgaard, Copenhagen, Denmark.
13. Goldman, L. and Goldman, B. (1944): Contact testing of the buccal mucous membrane for stomatitis venenata. *Arch. Derm., 50,* 79.
14. Gomez-Orbaneja, J. and Barrientos, E. (1938): Funktionelle Nachuntersuchungen bei Ekzematikern. *Schweiz. med. Wschr., 24,* 694.
15. Omitted.
16. Omitted.
17. Houwerzijl, J., De Gast, G. C. and Nater, J. P. (1974): Tests for drug allergy. *Lancet, 2,* 655.
18. Jordan, W. P. (1975): Cross-sensitization patterns in acrylate allergies. *Contact Dermatitis, 1,* 13.
19. Kaidbey, K. H. and Kligman, A. M. (1980): Photomaximization test for identifying photoallergic contact sensitizers. *Contact Dermatitis, 6,* 161.
20. Kero, M., Hannuksela, M. and Sothman, A. (1979): Primary irritant dermatitis from topical clioquinol. *Contact Dermatitis, 5,* 115.
21. Omitted.
22. Kligman, A. M. (1966): The identification of contact allergens by human assay. *J. invest. Derm., 47,* 369.
23. Kligman, A. M. and Epstein, W. (1975): Updating the maximization test for identifying contact allergens. *Contact Dermatitis, 1,* 231.
24. Kligman, A. M. and Leyden, J. L. (1979): 'Reactions' to standard patch test materials. *Acta derm.-venereol. (Stockh.), 59,* Suppl. 89, 101.
25. Lachapelle, J. H. (1973): Comparative histopathology of allergic and irritant patch test reactions in man. *Arch. belges Derm., 28,* 83.
26. Lakaye, G. and Lapière, M. (1961): Evolution des eczémas de contact professionel. *Arch. belges Derm., 17,* 130.
27. Magnus, I. A. (1976): *Dermatological Photobiology,* p. 255. Blackwell Scientific Publications, Oxford.
28. Magnusson, B. and Kligman, A. M. (1977): Factors influencing allergic contact sensitization. In: *Advances in Modern Toxicology, Vol. 4: Dermatotoxicology and Pharmacology.* Editors: I. N. Marzulli

and H. I. Maibach. Hemisphere Publishing Corporation, Washington-London; John Wiley and Sons, New York.

29. Malten, K. E., Nater, J. P. and van Ketel, W. G. (1976): *Patch Testing Guidelines*. Dekker en van de Vegt, Nijmegen, the Netherlands.
30. Marcussen, P. (1959): Specificity of patch tests with 5% nickel sulphate. *Acta derm.-venereol. (Stockh.), 39*, 187.
31. Marzulli, F. and Maibach, H. I. (1974): The use of graded concentrations in studying skin sensitizers: experimental contact sensitization in man. *Food Cosm. Toxicol., 12*, 219.
32. Marzulli, F. N. and Maibach, H. I. (Eds.) (1977): In: *Advances in Modern Toxicology, Vol. 4: Dermatotoxicology and Pharmacology*. Hemisphere Publishing Corporation, Washington-London; John Wiley and Sons, New York-London-Sydney-Toronto.
33. Marzulli, F. N. and Maibach, H. I. (1980): Further studies on effects of vehicles and elicitation concentration in experimental contact sensitization testing in humans. *Contact Dermatitis, 6*, 131.
34. Matsuo, I., Ozawa, A., Niizuma, K. and Ohkido, M. (1979): Lichenoid dermatitis due to chlorpromazine phototoxicity. *Dermatologica (Basel), 159*, 46.
35. Meneghini, C. L. and Angelini, G. (1977): Behaviour of contact allergy and new sensitivities on subsequent patch tests. *Contact Dermatitis, 3*, 138.
36. Meneghini, C. L., Rantuccio, F., Riboldi, A. and Hofmann, M. F. (1967): Beobachtungen über das Persistieren der experimentellen ekzematösen Kontaktsensibilisierung auf einige chemische Substanzen beim Menschen. *Berufsdermatosen, 15*, 103.
37. Meneghini, C. L., Rantuccio, F. and Lomuto, M. (1971): Modelli sperimentali della ipersensibilità di tipo ritardato da contatto: Implicazioni cliniche nelle dermatiti eczematose. *Folia allerg., 18*, 317.
38. Mitchell, J. C. (1975): The angry back syndrome: eczema creates eczema. *Contact Dermatitis, 1*, 193.
39. Morgan, J. K. (1953): Observations on the persistence of skin sensitivity with reference to nickel eczema. *Brit. J. Derm., 65*, 84.
40. Nielsen, J. P. and Bang, K. (1954): On the persistence of acquired hypersensitivity, illustrated by re-examination and repetition of standardized patch tests on eczematous patients. *Acta derm.-venereol. (Stockh.), 34*, 110.
41. Nyquist, G. (1952): A study of denture sore mouth. An investigation of traumatic and toxic lesions of the oral mucosa arising from the use of full dentures. *Acta odont. scand., 10, Suppl. 9.*
42. Opdyke, D. (1976): Inhibition of sensitization reactions induced by certain aldehydes. *Food Cosm. Toxicol., 14*, 197.
43. Pevny, I., Mahr, E. and Schröpl, F. (1974): Toxische Hautreaktionen beim Epikutantest mit tricyclischen Psychopharmaka. *Hautarzt, 25*, 430.
44. Rhodes, E. I. and Warner, J. (1966): Contact eczema, follow-up study. *Brit. J. Derm., 79*, 640.
45. Rosenberg, E. W. and Fischer, R. W. (1963): Improved method for intraoral patch testing. *Arch. Derm., 87*, 115.
46. Schulz, K. H. and Schmidt, P. (1967): Fixe Exantheme durch drei verschiedene Arzneimittel mit getrennter Lokalisation. Beitrag zur Frage der Barbituratallergie. *Z. Haut.- u. Geschl.kr., 42*, 561.
47. Soesman-van Waadenoyen Kernekamp, A. and Van Ketel, W. G. (1980): Persistence of patch test reactions to clioquinol (vioform) and cross-sensitization. *Contact Dermatitis, 6*, 455.
48. Te Lintum, J. C. A. and Nater, J. P. (1973): On the persistence of positive patch test reactions to balsam of Peru, turpentine and nickel. *Brit. J. Derm., 89*, 629.
49. Thormann, J., Jespersen, N. B. and Joensen, H. D. (1979): Persistence of contact allergy to chromium. *Contact Dermatitis, 5*, 261.
50. Van Ketel, W. G. (1975): Patch testing in penicillin allergy. *Contact Dermatitis, 1*, 253.
51. Van Ketel, W. G. and Soesman, A. (1977): Een op de ziekte van Lyell gelijkende eruptie door Propranolol. *Ned. T. Geneesk., 121*, 1475.
52. Omitted.
53. Omitted.
54. Calnan, C. D. (1981): Keloid formation after patch tests. *Contact Dermatitis, 7*, 279.
55. Goodwin, B. F. J., Crevel, R. W. R. and Johnson, A. W. (1981): A comparison of three guinea-pig sensitization procedures for the detection of 19 reported human contact sensitizers. *Contact Dermatitis, 7*, 248.
56. Sato, Y., Katsumura, Y., Ichikawa, H. et al. (1981): A modified technique of guinea pig testing to identify delayed hypersensitivity allergens. *Contact Dermatitis, 7*, 225.

UPDATE – 2nd Edition

57. Heise, H. and Mattheus, A. (1982): Dimethylsulfoxid (DMSO) als Vehikel zur perkutanen Auslösung einer Testreaktion bei Arzneimittelexanthemen. *Derm. Mschr., 168,* 402.

58. Van Ketel, W. G. (1979): De betekenis van allergologisch onderzoek bij geneesmiddelenerupties. *Ned. T. Geneesk. 123,* 349.

59. Van Ketel, W. G. and de Haan, P. (1983): Allergologisch onderzoek bij penicilline-overgevoeligheid. *Pharm. Weekbl., 118,* 97.

60. Landwehr, A. J. and van Ketel, W. G. (1982): Delayed-type allergy to phenazone in a patient with erythema multiforme. *Contact Dermatitis, 8,* 283.

61. Lawrence, C. M. and Byrne, J. P. H. (1981): Eczematous eruption from oral diphenhydramine. *Contact Dermatitis, 7,* 276.

62. Merot, Y., Harms, M. and Saurat, J. -H. (1983): Photosensibilisation au carprofène (Imadyl®), un nouvel anti-inflammatoire non-stéroïdien. *Dermatologica, (Basel), 166,* 301.

63. De Shazo, R. D. and Stevenson, H. C. (1981): Generalized dermatitis to aminophylline. *Ann. Allergy, 46,* 152.

64. Valsecchi, R. and Cainelli, T. (1982): Penicillin allergy with positive skin test to cephalosporin alone. *Contact Dermatitis, 8,* 278.

65. Lang, P. G. Jr. (1983): Quinidine-induced photodermatitis confirmed by photopatch testing. *J. Amer. Acad. Derm., 9,* 124.

66. Van Ketel, W. G. (1983): Allergy to carbimazole. *Contact Dermatitis, 9,* 161.

67. Rudzki, E., Grzywa, Z. and Maciejowska, E. (1976): Drug reaction with positive patch test to chloramphenicol. *Contact Dermatitis, 2,* 181.

68. White, I. R. (1983): Photopatch test in a hydrochlorothiazide drug eruption. *Contact Dermatitis, 9,* 237.

69. Van Ketel, W. G. (1983): An allergic eruption probably caused by ketoconazole. *Contact Dermatitis, 9,* 313.

70. Rudzki, E. and Dajek, Z. (1975): Drug eruption with positive patch test to phenol. *Contact Dermatitis, 1,* 322.

71. Maucher, O. M. and Fuchs, A. (1983): Kontakturtikaria im Epikutantest bei Pyrazolonallergie. *Hautarzt, 34,* 383.

72. Van den Berg, W. H. H. W. and van Ketel, W. G. (1983): Fotosensibilisatie door Amantadine (Symmetrel®). *Nieuwsbr. Contactderm., 16,* 221.

73. Polak, L. (1978): Recent trends in immunology of contact sensitivity I and II. *Contact Dermatitis, 4,* 249 and 256.

74. Wolff, K. and Stingl, G. (1983): The Langerhans Cell. *J. invest. Derm., 80,* 175.

75. Peltonen, L. (1981): Comparison of Al-test and Finn Chamber Test. *Contact Dermatitis, 7,* 192.

76. Pirilä, V. (1975): Chamber test versus patch test for epicutaneous testing. *Contact Dermatitis, 1,* 48.

77. Keczkes, K., Basheer, A. M. and Wyatt, E. H. (1982): The persistence of allergic contact sensitivity: a 10-year follow-up in 100 patients. *Brit. J. Derm., 107,* 461.

78. Fregert, S. (1976): Respiratory symptoms with piperazine patch testing. *Contact Dermatitis, 2,* 61.

79. Maucher, O. M. and Fuchs, A. (1983): Kontakturtikaria im Epikutantest bei Pyrazolonallergie. *Hautarzt, 34,* 383.

80. Bruynzeel, D. P., van Ketel, W. G., Scheper, R. J. and von Blomberg-van der Flier, B. M. E. (1982): Delayed time course of irritation by sodium lauryl sulfate: observations on threshold reactions. *Contact Dermatitis, 8,* 236.

81. Angelini, G., Rantuccio, F. and Meneghini, C. L. (1975): Contact dermatitis in patients with leg ulcers. *Contact Dermatitis, 1,* 81.

82. Lawrence, C. M. and Smith, A. G. (1982): Ampliative medicament allergy: concomitant sensitivity to multiple medicaments including yellow soft paraffin, white soft paraffin, gentian violet and Span 20. *Contact Dermatitis, 8,* 240.

83. Bruynzeel, D. P., van Ketel, W. G., von Blomberg-van der Flier, B. M. E. and Scheper, R. J. (1981): The angry back syndrome – a retrospective study. *Contact Dermatitis, 7,* 293.

84. Fisher, A. A. (1982): The 'crazy', 'angry' back has become the 'excited skin syndrome'. *Cutis, 30,* 599.

85. Dahl, M. V. and Jordan, W. P. Jr (1983): Topical steroids an patch tests. (Letter to the Editor). *Arch. Derm., 119,* 3.

86. Wong, G. and Maibach, H. (1982): Axillary lymphadenopathy possibly secondary to a positive patch test on the lower back. *Contact Dermatitis, 8,* 348.

87. Faure, M., Dambuyant, C., Chabeau, G. et al. (1981): Immune complex vasculitis and contact dermatitis to Frullania. *Contact Dermatitis, 7,* 320.

88. Bruynzeel, D. P., van Ketel, W. G., von Blomberg-van der Flier, M. and Scheper, R. J. (1983): Angry back or the excited skin syndrome. A prospective study. *J. Amer. Acad. Derm., 8,* 392.

89. Skog, E. and Forsbeck, M. (1978): Comparison between 24- and 48-hours exposure time. *Contact Dermatitis, 4,* 362.

90. Fisher, A. and Shapiro, A. (1956): Allergic eczematous contact dermatitis due to metallic nickel. *J. Amer. Med. Ass., 161,* 717.

91. Clark, R. A. and Rietschel, R. L. (1982): 0.1% Triamcinolone acetonide ointment and patch test responses. *Arch. Derm., 118,* 163.

92. Dahl, M. V. and Jordan, W. P. Jr. (1983): Topical steroids and patch tests. (Letter.) *Arch. Derm., 119,* 3.

93. Jansén, Ch. T., Wennersten, G., Rystedt, I. et al. (1982): The Scandinavian standard photopatch test procedure. *Contact Dermatitis, 8,* 155.

94. Harber, L. C., Bickers, D. R., Armstrong, R. B. and Kochevar, I. E. (1982): Drug photosensitivity: phototoxic and photoallergic mechanisms. *Semin. Derm., 1,* 183.

95. Klecak, G. (1983): Identification of Contact Allergens: predictive tests in animals. In: *Dermatotoxicology,* 2nd Edition, Editors: N. Marzulli and H. I. Maibach. Ch. 9., pp. 193-236. Hemisphere Publishing Corporation, Washington-London.

4. Unusual manifestations of allergic contact sensitivity

PURPURIC ALLERGIC CONTACT DERMATITIS

4.1   In some cases of allergic dermatitis the development of a definite purpuric component may be noted, even when laboratory studies, including blood count, bleeding time and clot retraction time, are normal. This phenomenon has been reported with contact allergic reactions to paraphenylenediamine (PPD) and the related compound N-iso-propyl-N-phenylenediamine (IPPD) [28]. In these patients patch tests with PPD and IPPD produced a similar purpuric reaction. Contact allergic purpura to wool dust has been reported by Agarwal [38]. In this case nephritis was associated, which disappeared after strict avoidance of exposure to wool dust. Contact purpura to a positive patch test with *Frullania* has been documented; immune complex vasculitis was associated [58]. A purpuric vasculitis-like eruption has also been ascribed to contact allergy to balsam Peru in an antirheumatic ointment [44]. Petechial reactions following patch testing with cobalt are said to occur in 5% of all patients tested [25].

PIGMENTED CONTACT DERMATITIS

4.2   Riehl's melanosis is a non-itching pigmented dermatosis localized on the face and neck, and sometimes on other exposed areas. In Japan a series of patients has been reported presenting with a clinical picture similar to Riehl's melanosis, in some cases with pruritic lesions. These cases of Riehl's melanosis were considered to be 'pigmented cosmetic dermatitis' [30]. This particular type of pigmented dermatitis could be related to contact allergy to coal tar dyes used in cosmetics, particularly to CI 15800 Brilliant Lake Red R (an azo-dye), and other 1-phenylazo-2-naphthol derivatives. Fragrance materials were involved to a lesser degree. The results of patch testing and of photopatch testing indicated that, as in most cases both the non-irradiated and irradiated patch tests were positive, the relevance of UV exposure was less than might have been expected.

4.3   In other Japanese publications [11, 12] the cross-reaction pattern was studied in patients with a pigmented contact dermatitis due to CI 15800 Brilliant Lake Red R. The following reactions were observed:

Positive reaction to:		No positive reaction to:	
CI 12055*	(0.1% pet.)	CI 12120	(1% pet.)
CI 12100	(1% pet.)	CI 12075	(1% pet.)
CI 12175	(1% pet.)	CI 15630	(1% pet.)
CI 11390	(1% pet.)	CI 26100	(1% pet.)
CI 12140	(1% pet.)		

*Sudan I; structurally related contaminant of CI 15800
Test concentrations are given in brackets.

Pigmented contact dermatitis must be differentiated from phototoxic and photoallergic contact dermatitis.

Other causes of pigmented contact dermatitis have included:
– optical whiteners and textiles [9, 19]
– chromium hydroxide used as a pigment in commercial toilet soap [42].

FOLLICULAR CONTACT DERMATITIS

4.4   Sometimes, contact dermatitis may present itself as an itchy papular eruption. In
such cases, the center of the elementary papule is usually pierced by a hair; the
skin between the papules remains normal. This form of follicular allergic contact
dermatitis has been reported in cases of textile contact dermatitis due to formaldehyde. The eruption is presumably caused by the transfollicular absorption of formaldehyde [31]. Follicular contact dermatitis has also been reported in patients
with contact allergy to homomenthyl salicylate [22].

This reaction should be differentiated from non-allergic pustular and papular
reactions which may develop in patch tests with salts of metals (nickel, cobalt and,
especially, copper).

ERYTHEMA MULTIFORME-LIKE ERUPTIONS

4.5   Occasionally a contact allergic reaction to the skin or mucous membranes [24, 40,
43] may manifest itself as an erythema multiforme-like eruption. The eruption
may be bullous and is localized mainly on the face and arms or hands. The oral
mucosa may also be involved. Patch tests with the causative allergens are strongly
positive.

Several allergens have been reported to cause erythema multiforme-like eruptions:
– 9-bromofluorene [20, 37]
– chloramphenicol [44]
– p-chlorbenzenesulfonylglycolic acid nitrile [21]
– clioquinol [44]
– econazole [41]
– ethylenediamine [44]
– formaldehyde [52]
– neomycin [44]
– nickel [48]
– nickel and cobalt [49]
– perfume [51]
– a phenylsulfone-derivative [23]
– primula [7]
– promethazine [44]
– pyrrolnitrin [44, 45, 46]
– scopolamine hydrobromide [6]
– sulfonamide [24, 40, 43, 44]
– terpenes in Sloan's liniment [10]
– toxicodendron radicans (poison ivy) [53]
– tropical woods [8].

CONTACT URTICARIA

4.6   Contact urticaria of immunological or non-immunological nature occurs from numerous sources. Immunological contact urticaria is usually due to an immediate-type hypersensitivity (Type I according to the classification of Gell and Coombs), but several case reports suggest that sometimes the delayed-type variety is also present (and may play a role in the pathogenesis of the contact urticaria?) See Chapter 7 on contact urticaria.

LICHENOID ERUPTIONS

4.7   Allergic contact dermatitis has been reported to change after several weeks into a lichenoid eruption. This has been described in allergic contact sensitivity to substituted paraphenylenediamine derivatives used in the processing of color films [14], and as a manifestation of contact sensitivity to N-isopropyl-N'-phenyl-para-phenylenediamine (IPPD) a rubber antioxidant [50]. Contact allergy to nickel has also been implicated as a cause of lichenoid dermatitis [64]. Both patch tests and oral provocation tests caused lichenoid papules to appear.

CONTACT GRANULOMA

4.8   **Allergic contact granulomas** (see also § 5.43)

Zirconium salts

Axillary granulomas characterized by lesions appearing as firm, shiny papules with a specific histological picture have been described after the use of zirconium salt containing deodorants and antiperspirants. Zirconium oxide or carbonate preparations have also been used in the treatment of Rhus dermatitis. Two types of skin reactions have been identified: one is a non-allergic foreign body inflammation healing spontaneously within a month. This type of reaction has been described in both sensitized and non-sensitized persons. The other reaction has only occurred in individuals sensitized to the zirconium salt. The epithelioid cell granulomas formed in these cases may persist for a year or longer [2].

Beryllium salts

Cutaneous contact with beryllium salts may cause the formation of a cutaneous epithelioid granuloma with positive patch test reactions [29]. Not only localized but also systemic granulomatous reactions have been reported.

Metals in tattoos

Delayed hypersensitivity reactions to mercury, chromium, manganese, cobalt or cadmium salts in tattoos may cause contact granulomata. Various histological patterns have been described (allergic and/or non-allergic) in tattoo reactions:
- a diffuse lymphohistiocytic infiltrate with an admixture of plasma cells and eosinophils [34, 61]
- lichenoid reactions simulating lichen planus [36, 62]
- granulomatous reactions [33, 35]
- pseudolymphomatous reactions in areas containing mercury salts, chrome salts, and cobalt salts [32].

The histology of tattoo reactions has been reviewed by Goldstein [33]; *see also* § 5.43.

4.9   **Non-allergic contact granulomas** have been caused by:

1. Chronic irritation, e.g. by glasses (granuloma fissuratum)
2. Oil, e.g. in cosmetics [1]
3. Talc [16]
4. Sodium stearate [3]
5. Zirconium salts
6. Metals in tattoos [3, 35].

FOCAL CONTACT SENSITIVITY

4.10   According to the basic immunological concept, in allergic contact sensitivity the entire skin is sensitized. Once sensitivity has developed, sensitized T-lymphocytes circulate through the skin, rendering all sites sensitive. In a patient treated for mycosis fungoides the entire skin surface was painted with topical nitrogen mustard (mechlorethamine hydrochloride 1/5000 aqueous). A remarkable focal contact sensitivity developed: the eczematous contact dermatitis was limited precisely to the of clinically identifiable mycosis fungoides, whereas the uninvoled skin, though also painted with nitrogen mustard, showed no response whatsoever [27]. It is hypothesized that a malignant clone of T-cells had become specifically sensitized to nitrogen mustard. Thus sensitization would be restricted to the tumor sites.

TOXIC EPIDERMAL NECROLYSIS (LYELL)

4.11   *Monosulfiram*

Monosulfiram is used in some antiscabietic preparations. A patient developed an extensive skin eruption diagnosed as toxic epidermal necrolysis of Lyell after application of a monosulfiram-containing lotion to her body below the neck as an antiscabietic treatment. According to her history she had developed a rubber dermatitis on her hands while working in a munition factory twenty-eight years earlier [18].

When the eruption had disappeared patch tests were performed. Positive reactions were found to the rubber chemical thiram disulfide and to the chemically related monosulfiram.

Perfume

A young adult female patient, on prolonged corticosteroid therapy for nephrotic syndrome, developed erythema multiforme with progression to toxic epidermal necrolysis and ultimately death following a double exposure to a locally applied unidentified perfume in spray cologne [51].

LYMPHOMATOID CONTACT DERMATITIS

4.12   Two conditions have been described under this name:
1. Orbaneja et al. [56] were the first to use the term 'lymphomatoid contact dermatitis'. They described 4 patients who had infiltrated plaque-like lesions of der-

matitis with some histological similarity to mycosis fungoides or lymphoma. The condition was due to contact allergy from the striker surface of a matchbox, and the special features were ascribed to the *prolonged* contact with the allergen. When contact with the source was avoided, the lesions healed in a relatively short time. A similar case, due to contact sensitivity from ethylenediamine dihydrochloride contained in a trouser pocket was described more recently [57].

2. Ecker and Winkelmann [55] and Buechner and Winkelmann [54] use the term 'lymphomatoid contact dermatitis' to describe patients with a recurrent and progressive erythematous patchy dermatitis with temporary flares of generalized erythema (not unlike actinic reticuloid), in who the histological findings consist of a distinct pattern of lymphocytic dermal reticulosis and chronic epithelial response. Although one or more positive patch test reactions to (unrelated) allergens were found in these patients, a causal relationship with the clinical picture has not been proven, and the eruption does *not* clear after avoidance of the chemicals producing positive patch tests. The authors argue that the similarity of these cases of lymphomatoid contact dermatitis, both clinically and histologically with actinic reticuloid, photosensitive dermatitis and airborne contact dermatitis indicates that these conditions represent a common transitional lymphoproliferative pre-malignant state. Lymphomatoid contact dermatitis is considered to be a potential pre-Sézary state that can be recognized in the course and the histological pattern [55].

ALLERGIC CONTACT DERMATITIS COMPLICATED BY EXTRACUTANEOUS SYMPTOMS

4.13   In extensive, severe, or generalized allergic contact dermatitis, non-specific constitutional symptoms may be observed:
– Headache, fever, anorexia, nausea and malaise have been reported in patients with severe allergic contact dermatitis from lauryl ether sulfate in a dish washing liquid containing an allergenic sultone impurity [13].

In cases of limited dermatitis (e.g. limited to the hands), extracutaneous symptoms are rare:
– *Paresthesia:* paresthesia of the finger tips in the form of a burning sensation, tingling and slight numbness is a phenomenon described in cases of allergic contact dermatitis of the hands due to acrylic monomer. This type of paresthesia accompanying an allergic contact dermatitis and persisting several weeks after the dermatitis had subsided, was reported in orthopedic surgeons sensitized to methylmethacrylate bone cement [4].
– *Gastrointestinal symptoms:* in another case of allergic contact dermatitis of the hands due to hydroxyethylmethacrylate (in a laboratory technician), an association was found with nausea, diarrhea and persistent paresthesia of the finger tips. The gastrointestinal symptoms were reproduced by patch testing! Hydroxyethylmethacrylate was demonstrated to pass through vinyl gloves [15].
– *Respiratory symptoms:* a patient working in a factory where, among other substances, piperazine was processed, developed an eczema of the hands, arms, face and penis as well as respiratory symptoms. A patch test with 1% piperazine in water caused after about 17 hours itching of the piperazine patch test site and respiratory symptoms. The test was strongly positive after 48 hours. The respiratory symptoms disappeared after 5-6 hours [5]. In this case a sufficient amount of piperazine must have been absorbed from the patch test site in order to elicit the respiratory symptoms which, according to the author, probably were allergic (? Type 1 reaction). (Scratch, prick or intracutaneous tests are not mentioned.) Rhinitis has been associated with contact allergy to metals in dentures [65]. Patch tests with nickel and/or cobalt provoked the symptoms in some patients.

– *Fever:* four cases were reported in which treatment of psoriasis localized on the scalp with an ointment containing 3% 6-hydroxy-1,3-benzoxathiol-2-one resulted in a burning and itching erythema with vesiculation and edema, which extended in some cases to the face. In three cases body temperature was raised. Patch testing was impossible owing to the erythematous effect of this benzothiazole derivative on the skin [26].

– *Collapse:* a systemic reaction consisting of cyanosis and collapse after topical application of a mixture of 1% gentian violet (CI 42535) and 1% methyl green (CI 42590) on an ulcus cruris of a previously sensitized individual was described by Michel et al. [17].

– *Immune complex reaction: cutaneous vasculitis and nephritis:* a patient was patch-tested to *Frullania tamarisci* and *Frullania dilatata*. After 2 days a strong positive erythematous reaction was found. On the following day the two reactions were purpuric, and in the next 24–36 hours became bullous and necrotic. At the same time, a purpuric eruption with papulonodular lesions, lesions en cocarde and bullae with a tendency to necrose appeared on the lower limbs, on the pelvis and lower abdomen, and on the arms. Epistaxis accompanied the purpuric eruption. Histoimmunologic and immunologic findings were in favor of an immune complex reaction [58]. In a similar case [59], contact allergy to *Frullania* led to immune complex nephritis. Renal lesions accompanying poison oak dermatitis have been described previously [60]. Allergic contact purpura to wool dust was associated with nephritis in one case [38]; after strict avoidance of exposure to wool dust the nephritis disappeared.

MISCELLANEOUS

4.14   – *Lymphangitis and lymphedema:* two cases have been described in which a recurrent allergic contact dermatitis of the hands led to lymphangitis and the development of a persistent lymphedema [47]. A similar observation was made by Worm et al. [63]. Recurrent bacterial infections may have been a contributory factor.

– *Permanent loss of finger nails:* a patient suffered a severe allergic reaction from sensitization to methylmethacrylate in a mixture of materials designed to make artificial nails. There was marked erythema, edema, and pain of the eponychial and paronychial tissues with persistent paresthesia of the finger tips. Gradual destruction of the nail plates developed, and since no regrowth of the nails resumed in 6 years, the loss of the finger nails was considered to be permanent [39].

4.15   REFERENCES

1. Bergeron, J. R. and Stone, O. J. (1969): Multiple granulomas of the scalp of exogenous origin. *Cutis, 5*, 57.
2. Epstein, W. L., Skahen, J. R. and Krasnobrod, H. (1962): Granulomatous hypersensitivity to zirconium. Localization of allergen in tissue and its role in the formation of epitheloid cells. *J. invest. Derm., 38*, 223.
3. Fisher, A. A. (1973): *Contact Dermatitis.* Lea and Febiger, Philadelphia.
4. Fisher, A. A. (1979): Paresthesia of the fingers accompanying dermatitis due to methylmethacrylate bone cement. *Contact Dermatitis, 5*, 56.
5. Fregert, S. (1976): Respiratory symptoms with piperazine patch testing. *Contact Dermatitis, 2*, 61.
6. Guill, A., Goette, K., Knight, C. G., Peck, C. C. and Lupton, G. P. (1979): Erythema multiforme and urticaria. *Arch. Derm., 115*, 742.
7. Hjorth, N. (1966): Primula dermatitis. *Trans. St. John's Hosp. derm. Soc. (Lond.), 52*, 207.
8. Holst, R., Kirby, J. and Magnusson, B. (1976): Sensitisation to tropical woods giving erythema multiforme-like eruptions. *Contact Dermatitis, 2*, 295.

9.   Josephs, H. and Maibach, H. I. (1967): Contact dermatitis from Spandex brassieres. *J. Amer. med. Ass., 201,* 880.

10. Kirby, D. J. and Darley, C. R. (1978): Erythema multiforme associated with a contact dermatitis to terpenes. *Contact Dermatitis, 4,* 238.

11. Kozuka, T., Tashiro, M., Sano, S., Fujimoto, K., Nakamura, Y., Hashimoto, S. and Nakaminami, G. (1979): Brilliant lake Red R as a cause of pigmented contact dermatitis. *Contact Dermatitis, 5,* 297.

12. Kozuka, T., Tashiro, M., Sano, S., Fujimoto, K., Nakamura, Y., Hashimoto, S. and Nakaminami, G. (1980): Pigmented contact dermatitis from azo-dyes. I. Cross-sensitivity in humans. *Contact Dermatitis, 6,* 330.

13. Magnusson, B. and Gilje, O. (1973): Allergic contact dermatitis from a dishwashing liquid containing lauryl ether sulfate. *Acta derm.-venereol. (Stockh.), 53,* 136.

14. Mandel, E. H. (1960): Lichen planus-like eruptions caused by a color-film developer. *Arch. Derm., 81,* 516.

15. Mathias, C. G. T., Caldwell, T. M. and Maibach, H. I. (1979): Contact dermatitis and gastrointestinal symptoms from hydroxyethylmethacrylate. *Brit. J. Derm., 100,* 447.

16. McCallum, D. I. and Hall, G. F. M. (1970): Umbilical granulomata with particular reference to talc granuloma. *Brit. J. Derm., 83,* 151.

17. Michel, P. J., Buyer, R. and Delorme, G. (1958): Accidents géneraux (cyanose, collapsus cardiovasculaire) par sensibilisation à une solution aqueuse de violet de gentiane et vert de méthyle en applications locales. *Bull. Soc. franç. Derm. Syph., 65,* 183.

18. Monckton Copeman, P. W. (1968): Toxic epidermal necrolysis caused by skin hypersensitivity to monosulfiram. *Brit. med. J., 1,* 623.

19. Osmundsen, B. J. D. (1970): Pigmented contact dermatitis. *Brit. J. Derm., 83,* 296.

20. Powell, E. W. (1968): Skin reactions of 9-bromofluorene. *Brit. J. Derm., 80,* 491.

21. Richter, G. and Scholz, H. (1970): Kontaktekzem und makulöses Exanthem bei p-Chlorbenzosulfonylglykolsäurenitril-Allergie. *Berufsdermatosen, 18,* 70.

22. Rietschel, R. L. and Lewis, Ch. W. (1978): Contact dermatitis to homomenthyl salicylate. *Arch. Derm., 114,* 442.

23. Roed-Petersen, J. (1975): Erythema multiforme as an expression of contact dermatitis. *Contact Dermatitis, 1,* 270.

24. Rubin, A. (1977): Ophthalmic sulfonamide-induced Stevens-Johnson syndrome. *Arch. Derm., 113,* 235.

25. Schmidt, H., Schultz Larsen, F., Ølholm Larsen, P. and Søgaard, H. (1980): Petechial reaction following patch testing with cobalt. *Contact Dermatitis, 6,* 91.

26. Schoefinius, H. H. (1972): Kontaktdermatitis mit erhöhter Körpertemperatur unter Behandlung von Psoriasis vulgaris capillitii mit einem Benzoxathiol-Derivat. *Z. Haut- u. Geschlkr., 47,* 227.

27. Shelley, W. B. (1980): Focal contact sensitivity to nitrogen mustard in lesions of cutaneous T-cell lymphoma (mycosis fungoides). *Acta derm.-venereol. (Stockh.), 61,* 161.

28. Shmunes, E. (1978): Purpuric allergic contact dermatitis to paraphenylenediamine. *Contact Dermatitis, 4,* 225.

29. Sneddon, I. B. (1955): Berylliosis, a case report. *Brit. med. J., 1,* 1448.

30. Sugai, T., Takahashi, Y. and Takagi, T. (1977): Pigmented cosmetic dermatitis and coal tar dyes. *Contact Dermatitis, 3,* 249.

31. Uehara, M. (1978): Follicular contact dermatitis due to formaldehyde. *Dermatologica (Basel), 156,* 48.

UPDATE – 2nd Edition

32. Blumental, G., Okun, M. R. and Ponitch, J. A. (1982): Pseudolymphomatous reaction to tattoos. *J. Amer. Acad. Derm., 6,* 485.

33. Goldstein, A. (1979): Histologic reactions to tattoos, *J. Derm. Surg. Oncol., 5,* 896.

34. Ravits, H. G. (1962): Allergic tattoo granuloma. *Arch. Derm., 86,* 287.

35. Verdich, J. (1981): Granulomatous reaction in a red tattoo. *Acta derm.-venereol. (Stockh.), 61,* 176.

36. Winkelmann, R. and Harris, R. B. (1979): Lichenoid delayed hypersensitivity reactions in tattoos. *J. cutan. Path., 6,* 59.

37. DeFeo, C. P. (1966): Erythema multiforme bullosum caused by 9-bromofluorene. *Arch. Derm., 94,* 545.

38. Agarwal, K. (1982): Contact allergic purpura to wool dust. *Contact Dermatitis, 8,* 281.
39. Fisher, A.A. (1980): Permanent loss of finger nails from sensitization and reaction to acrylic in a preparation designed to make artificial nails. *J. Derm. Surg. Oncol., 6,* 70.
40. Gottschalk, H. R. and Stone, O. J. (1976): Stevens-Johnson syndrome from ophthalmic sulfonamide. *Arch. Derm., 112,* 513.
41. Valsecchi, R., Tornaghi, A., Tribbia, G. and Cainelli, T. (1982): Contact dermatitis from econazole. *Contact Dermatitis, 8,* 422.
42. Mathias, T. C. G. (1982): Pigmented cosmetic dermatitis from contact allergy to a toilet soap containing chromium. *Contact Dermatitis, 8,* 29.
43. Goette, D. K. and Odom, R. B. (1980): Vaginal medications as a cause for varied widespread dermatitides. *Cutis, 26,* 406.
44. Meneghini, C. L. and Angelini, G. (1981): Secondary polymorphic eruptions in allergic contact dermatitis. *Dermatologica (Basel), 163,* 63.
45. Meneghini, C. L. and Angelini, G. (1982): Contact dermatitis from pyrrolnitrin. *Contact Dermatitis, 8,* 55.
46. Valsecchi, R., Foiadelli, L. and Cainelli, T. (1981): Contact dermatitis from pyrrolnitrin. *Contact Dermatitis, 7,* 340.
47. Lynde, C. W. and Mitchell, J. C. (1982): Unusual complication of allergic contact dermatitis of the hands: recurrent lymphangitis and persistent lymphoedema. *Contact Dermatitis, 8,* 279.
48. Calnan, C.D. (1956): Nickel dermatitis. *Brit. J. Derm. 68,* 229.
49. Cook, L. J. (1982): Associated nickel and cobalt contact dermatitis presenting as erythema multiforme. *Contact Dermatitis, 8,* 280.
50. Ancona, A., Monroy, F. and Fernández–Diez, J. (1982): Occupational dermatitis from IPPD in tyres. *Contact Dermatitis, 8,* 91.
51. Thompson, J. A. Jr. and Wansker, B. A. (1981): A case of contact dermatitis, erythema multiforme and toxic epidermal necrolysis. *J. Amer. Acad. Derm., 5,* 666.
52. Nethercott, J. R., Albers, J., Guirguis, S. (1982): Erythema multiforme exudativum linked to the manufacture of printed circuit boards. *Contact Dermatitis, 8,* 314.
53. Mallory, S. B., Miller, O. F. and Tyler, W. B. (1982): *Toxicodendron radicans* dermatitis with black lacquer deposit on the skin. *J. Amer. Acad. Derm., 6,* 363.
54. Buechner, S. A. and Winkelmann, R. K. (1983): Pre-Sézary erythroderma evolving to Sézary syndrome. *Arch. Derm., 119,* 285.
55. Ecker, R. I. and Winkelmann, R. K. (1981): Lymphomatoid contact dermatitis. *Contact Dermatitis, 7,* 84.
56. Orbaneja, J. G., Diez, L., Lozano, J. L. S. and Salazar, L. C. (1976): Lymphomatoid contact dermatitis: a syndrome produced by epicutaneous hypersensitivity with clinical features and a histopathologic picture similar to that of mycosis fungoides. *Contact Dermatitis, 2,* 139.
57. Wall, L. M. (1982): Lymphomatoid contact dermatitis due to ethylenediamine dihydrochloride. *Contact Dermatitis, 8,* 51.
58. Faure, M. Dambuyant, C., Chabeau, G. et al. (1981): Immune complex vasculitis and contact dermatitis to Frullania. *Contact Dermatitis, 7,* 320.
59. Racadot, E. (1978): *Contribution à l'étude des syndromes néphrotiques allergiques. A propos d'un cas d'allergie à Frullania.* Thèse Médecine, Besançon.
60. Devich, K. B., Lee, J. C., Epstein, W. L. et al. (1975): Renal lesions accompanying poison oak dermatitis. *Clin. Nephr., 3,* 106.
61. McGrouther, D. A., Downie, P. A. and Thompson, M. B. (1977): Reactions to red tattoos. *Brit. J. plast. Surg., 30,* 84.
62. Clarke, J. and Black, M. M. (1979): Lichenoid tattoo reactions. *Brit. J. Derm., 100,* 451.
63. Worm, A. -M., Staberg, B. and Thomsen, K. (1983): Persistant oedema in allergic contact dermatitis. *Contact Dermatitis, 9,* 517.
64. Lombardi, P., Campolmi, P. and Sertoli, A. (1983): Lichenoid dermatitis caused by nickel salts? *Contact Dermatitis, 9,* 520.
65. Bork, K. (1978): Fließschnupfen durch Metallteile von Zahnprothesen. *Z. Hautkr. 53,* 814.

5. Allergic contact dermatitis from topical drugs

5.1 This chapter contains alphabetical tabulations of topical drugs and other topically applied substances that have caused contact allergy, as reported in the literature; for each drug one or more relevant references are provided. The drugs have been subdivided into several groups according to their clinical use and functional purposes. The last section in this chapter deals with contact allergy to drugs that are not usually applied topically but have accidentally come into contact with the skin, e.g. in medical and nursing personnel, or in the industry.

Patch test concentration and vehicle (see also Appendix)

5.2 For each drug the vehicle and concentration for patch testing is mentioned; usually this is the generally accepted concentration and vehicle, but sometimes it refers to the way the authors of the report mentioned have patch-tested the particular drug. When there is no consensus about the patch testing dilution, two or more concentrations and vehicles may be stated. Sources may be found in § 27.1– § 27.16.

5.3 **Key to abbreviations**

acet.	=	acetone
alc.	=	alcohol 70%
as is	=	undiluted
BL	=	butyrolactone
c.o.	=	castor oil
comm. ointm. bas.	=	commercial ointment basis
DE	=	detyl extra (isopropyl palmitate)
euc.	=	eucerin
glyc.	=	glycerol
isopropyl alc.	=	isopropyl alcohol
MEK	=	methyl ethyl ketone
m.o.	=	mineral oil
o.o.	=	olive oil
paraff. liq.	=	paraffinum liquidum
pet.	=	petrolatum
prop. glyc.	=	propylene glycol

Estimated frequency of sensitization (EFS)

5.4 Estimated frequency of sensitization (EFS), based both on data from the literature and personal experience, is expressed as follows:
1: contact sensitization is common   3: contact sensitization is uncommon
2: contact sensitization may occur   4: contact sensitization is rare

Cross-reaction

5.5   Cross-reacting chemicals are listed, but only when such compounds have actually cross-reacted and *not* when they might be *expected* to do so on theoretical grounds.

PRESERVATIVES: ANTIMICROBIALS AND ANTIOXIDANTS

5.6   Cosmetic products and other topical preparations must be protected against deterioration caused by microbials (bacteria, yeasts, fungi) or by oxidation of lipid components (air oxygen). The microbial problem is solved by the addition of antimicrobials (preservatives). Usually a combination of two or more (even up to six) compounds is used for preservation.

Concentration levels of the preservatives vary widely. Most compounds (e.g. the paraben esters) are used at levels of 0.1 to 0.5%, but others are active at 0.0025 (25 p.p.m.) levels (e.g. organo-mercurials, methylisothiazolinons). Between these two extremes are the active levels of some important preservatives such as bromonitropropanediol (bronopol: 0.01–0.05%), quaternary ammonium compounds and chlorhexidine.

The antimicrobial level in deodorants is approximately 0.5–%, which is higher than the level necessary for preservation. Antiseptic soaps and lotions contain the highest levels (ca 2%). Cosmetics and other topical pharmaceuticals that do not contain water (salve, lipstick, baby oils and compact powders) do not need preservation.

The problem of oxidation of lipids which leads to rancidity, is solved by the addition of antioxidants. Chelating agents (e.g. EDTA, citric acid) will support antioxidant action by complexing trace heavy metal impurities in the product, which otherwise might catalyze the oxidation reaction.

Contact allergy from preservatives, though well known, must be considered infrequent when related to the widespread presence of these compounds in preparations handled by everyone. As these chemicals have a low sensitizing potential in the concentrations in which they are added to a product, sensitization after contact with *intact* skin, as in cosmetics, is rare; most reports of contact allergy to preservatives are from topical preparations used on eczematous or otherwise damaged skin.

§ 5.7 lists antioxidants, antimicrobials and preservatives that have caused contact allergy. An extensive listing of these compounds is given in § 27.5.

5.7   **Contact allergy to preservatives: antimicrobials and antioxidants**

Drug	Patch test conc. & vehicle (§ 5.2)	EFS (§ 5.4)	Cross-reactions (§ 5.5)	Comment	Ref.
alcohols					181 571
benzyl alcohol	5–10% pet. 10% alc.	4	patients hypersensitive to balsam Peru may cross-react to benzyl alcohol. Other primary alcohols(?)	Preservative in allergen extracts and solutions for injections, also used as solvent, in flavors and perfumes. *Cave:* irritant patch test reactions. For cosmetic allergy, *see* § 23.47	154 575

(continued)

45

5.7 Antimicrobials and antioxidants

(continuation)

Drug	Patch test conc. & vehicle (§ 5.2)	EFS (§ 5.4)	Cross-reactions (§ 5.5)	Comment	Ref.
ethyl alcohol	10% aqua pure	4	other primary alcohols	Has caused systemic eczematous contact-type dermatitis (§ 17.2); systemic side effects (§ 16.30); contact urticaria (§ 7.5) Ethanol in hair spray has caused bronchoconstriction (§ 22.66) For antabuse effects, *see* § 16.31 and § 22.8	444
isopropyl alcohol	10% aqua pure	4		*See also* § 5.22 Has caused contact urticaria (§ 7.5)	283 245
aminacrin	0.1% pet.	4		Aminacrin is an acridine dye	465
ammonium sulfobituminate	1–5% aqua	4	turpentine oil?	Ammonium sulfobituminate consists of sulfur (10%), ammonium sulfate (5–7%), hydrocarbons, nitrogenous bases, acids and derivatives of thiophene 5% ammonium sulfobituminate in mineral oil has comedogenic properties (§ 9.1) *Cave*: irritant patch test reactions with 5% aqua (537) *See also* § 5.38	24 99 537
Ampholyt G®	0.1% sol.	3		Occupational allergy in hospital personnel. The active ingredients are: – 9-lauryl-3,6,9-triazanonanoic acid – 7-lauryl-1,4,7-triazaheptane – 6,9-dilayl-3,6-triazanonanoic acid – 4,7-dilauryl-1,4,7-triaza-heptane The actual allergen is unknown	486
benzoic acid	5–10% pet.	3		Has caused contact urticaria (§ 7.5); also used as antifungal drug (§ 5.32)	564
bithionol	1% pet.	3	cross-reacts to halogenated salicylanilides	Usually photo-allergy (§ 6.5)	329
2-bromo-2-nitro-propane-1,3-diol (bronopol)	0.25–0.5% pet. or aqua	2	formaldehyde (?)	*Cave*: irritant patch test reactions. Usage tests may be necessary. Formaldehyde donor	545 564 583

(continued)

(continuation)

Drug	Patch test conc. & vehicle (§ 5.2)	EFS (§ 5.4)	Cross-reactions (§ 5.5)	Comment	Ref.
butylated hydroxyanisole (BHA)	2 and 5% pet.	4		Antioxidant, primarily used in foods. Has caused systemic eczematous contact-type dermatitis (§ 17.2); contact urticaria (§ 7.5); depigmentation (§ 10.1); vasomotor rhinitis and asthma, with oral challenge reproducing the clinical symptoms and altering the bleeding time	351 156 119 163
butylated hydroxytoluene (BHT)	2 and 5% pet.	4		Antioxidant, primarily used in foods. Has caused systemic eczematous contact-type dermatitis (§ 17.2); contact urticaria (§ 7.5); depigmentation (§ 10.1); vasomotor rhinitis and asthma, with oral challenge reproducing the clinical symptoms and altering the bleeding time	351 163
chloracetamide	0.2% pet. 0.1–1% aqua	2		For cosmetic reactions, *see* § 23.47, § 25.9 and § 25.69	404 258 125
chloramine	0.2% aqua	3		Has caused contact urticaria (§ 7.5) For industrial use, *see* [574]	573 574
chlorbutanol	5% pet.	4			209
chlorhexidine gluconate	1% aqua	3		Has caused photosensitivity (§ 6.5); side effects in mouth washes (§ 13.12); *see also* § 13.14 and § 25.53	456 279 477 478
dibrompropamidine	1% pet.	4			488
1,3-diiodo-2-hydroxy-propane	0.05% alc.	4		Has caused contact urticaria (§ 7.5)	282 228
dodicin	1% aqua	4			409
domiphen bromide	0.1% aqua	4			72
ethacridine	1–2% pet.	2		Ethacridine is an acridine dye Has caused brown dis-coloration of the nails (§ 10.1)	359
ethylenediamine tetra-acetate (EDTA)	1% pet.	4	*not* to ethylenediamine hydrochloride [512, 513]		341 266
fenticlor	1–10% pet.	4		Has caused photosensitivity (§ 5.5) For cosmetic allergy, *see* § 22.65 and § 25.53	129

(continued)

5.7 Antimicrobials and antioxidants

(continuation)

Drug	Patch test conc. & vehicle (§ 5.2)	EFS (§ 5.4)	Cross-reactions (§ 5.5)	Comment	Ref.
formaldehyde	2% aqua	1		*Cave:* irritant patch test reactions. Has caused contact urticaria (§ 7.5) and discoloration of the nails (§ 10.1); photosensitivity (§ 6.5) For cosmetic reactions *see* § 22.7, § 24.12, § 24.13 and § 25.53. Has caused follicular contact dermitis (§ 4.4); EEM-like dermatitis (§ 4.5)	384 115
gallate esters	1% alc. 0.1 and 2% pet.	3		Antioxidants, also in foods (margarine) *Cave:* toxic patch test reactions. For cosmetic allergy, *see* § 23.53 *under* propyl gallate	441 351 62 360
glutaraldehyde	1% aqua (not stable)	2		Has caused discoloration of the skin (§ 10.1); for cosmetic allergy, *see* § 25.53	288 248 285 590
hexahydro-1,3,5-tris(2-hydroxyethyl)triazine	1-2% aqua [562] 5–10% aqua [563]	4			254 562 563
hexamidine	0.15% aqua	3			347
imidazolidinyl urea (Germall 115®)	1% pet.	3		For cosmetic allergy, *see* § 23.47	152 564 584 586
iodine, tincture of	0.5% aqua open test	2		Has caused fatal dermatitis (§ 16.45); irritt dermatitis (§ 2.4); goiter and hypo-thyroidism (§ 16.45) Patch tests may show non-specific papulo-pustular reactions	293
iodoform	5% pet.	3		Use abandoned	242
mercurial compounds			cross-reactions frequently occur between the metal, the organic and the inorganic mercurials [182]	For cosmetic allergy, *see* § 25.25	182
ammoniated mercury	1% pet.	2	other mercurials	Inorganic mercurial compound, formerly used in the treatment of psoriasis and in skin lightening creams Has caused pigmentation and depigmentation (§10.1); systemic toxicity (§ 16.53)	138 564

(continued)

(continuation)

Drug	Patch test conc. & vehicle (§ 5.2)	EFS (§ 5.4)	Cross-reactions (§ 5.5)	Comment	Ref.
merbromin	0.1% aqua	4	other mercurials and the sodium salt of dibromo-hydroxymercuric resorcin-aphthalene	Organic mercurial compound Has caused systemic side effects (§ 16.53)	85 182
mercuric chloride	0.05–0.1% aqua	2	other mercurials	Inorganic mercurial compound *Cave:* irritant patch test reactions	19
mercurous chloride	as is	3	other mercurials	Inorganic mercurial compound, formerly used for the treatment of syphilis and as a diuretic Has caused systemic side effects (§ 16.53)	183
parachloromercuri-phenol	0.067% pet.	4	phenylmercuric acetate		295
phenylmercuric acetate	0.01% aqua/pet. 0.05% pet.	4	other mercurials	Organic mercurial compound Phenylmercuric salts have caused contact urticaria (§ 7.5)	315
phenylmercuric borate	0.01% aqua 0.1% euc.	4	other mercurials	Organic mercurial compound Phenylmercuric salts have caused contact urticaria (§ 7.5)	315
phenylmercuric nitrate	0.01% aqua 0.05% pet. (ICDRG)	4	other mercurials	Organic mercurial compound Phenylmercuric salts have caused contact urticaria (§ 7.5)	315 183
thiomersal	0.1% pet.	2	other mercurials	Organic mercurial compound Also used as preservative in contact lens fluid [540] *Cave:* irritant patch test reactions Some patients are sensitized by the mercury, but the majority by some other component Has caused systemic side effects (§ 16.53); systemic eczematous contact-type dermatitis (§ 17.2); life-threatening laryngeal edema (§ 12.1) *See also* § 13.40	212 383 234 343 166 527 540
N-methylol chloro-acetamide	0.1% aqua	4			4
neutral red chloride	0.1–3% aqua	4		May be carcinogenic (§ 12.1)	312 95
nitrofural	0.1–2% pet.	2	nitrofurantoin	*See also* § 13.18 *under* furazolidine	56 236
nordihydroguaiaretic acid (NDGA)	2–5% pet.	4		Antioxidant in topical preparations, formerly also used in foods	351

(continued)

5.7 Antimicrobials and antioxidants

(continuation)

Drug	Patch test conc. & vehicle (§ 5.2)	EFS (§ 5.4)	Cross-reactions (§ 5.5)	Comment	Ref.
parabens					
esters of p-hydroxy-benzoic acid	15% pet.	3	between the various esters, benzocaine, procaine, p-phenylenediamine and 4-homosulfanilamide	Parabens are also added to certain foods Have caused systemic eczematous contact-type dermatitis (§ 17.2); contact urticaria (§ 7.5) For cosmetic allergy, *see* § 23.47 and § 25.53 *See also* § 13.40	325 381 297 280
– methyl ester	5% pet.				
– propyl ester	5% pet.				
– butyl ester	5% pet.				
– ethyl ester	5% pet.				
– benzyl ester	3–10% pet.				
phenolic compounds					
bismuth tribromophenol	as is	3			175 644
bromochlorophene	2% pet.	4			564
4-chloro-m-cresol	1–5% pet.	3	p-chloro-m-xylenol	For cosmetic allergy, *see* § 25.9	229 70 327 125
p-chloro-m-xylenol	0.5–2% pet.	3	4-chloro-m-cresol	*Cave:* irritant patch test reactions with p-chloro-m-xylenol 1% pet.	69 408
dichlorophene	0.5–1% pet.	3	hexachlorophene?	For cosmetic allergy, *see* § 23.47 *Cave:* irritant patch test reactions to dichlorophene 1% pet.	135 382 564
hexachlorophene	1% pet.	4	dichlorophene may cross-react in cases of primary sensitization to dichlorophene, bithionol, and halogenated salicylanilides (usually photo-cross-reactions)	Has caused irritant dermatitis (§ 2.4); photosensitivity (§ 6.5); systemic side effects (§ 16.36)	139 22 69 603
o-phenylphenol	1% pet.	3		Has caused photosensitivity (§ 6.5) For cosmetic allergy, *see* § 23.47 and § 25.9	530
potassium sorbate	5% pet.	2	sorbic acid	For cosmetic allergy, *see* § 23.47	587
povidone-iodine	10% sol.	3	iodine	PVP-I solution has 10% bound iodine and 1% available iodine. For systemic side effects, *see* § 16.73	520 544
proflavine dihydrochloride	0.1–1% pet.	3		Proflavine is an acridine dye Has caused pigmented allergic contact dermatitis	305
propylene oxide	0.–1% alc.	4			245

(continued)

(continuation)

Drug	Patch test conc. & vehicle (§ 5.2)	EFS (§ 5.4)	Cross-reactions (§ 5.5)	Comment	Ref.
propyl gallate	2% pet.	4		*See also* gallate esters	109 555 564

quaternary ammonium compounds (may be tested 0.1% and 0.01% aqua) [180]

Drug	Patch test conc. & vehicle (§ 5.2)	EFS (§ 5.4)	Cross-reactions (§ 5.5)	Comment	Ref.
benzalkonium chloride	0.05–0.1% aqua	3	other quaternary ammonium compounds, e.g. hexamethonium bromide [534]	Used in ophthalmic solutions (§ 13.40) *Cave:* irritant patch test reactions Has caused irritant dermatitis (§ 2.4) Benzalkonium chloride is a mixture of alkyl-dimethyl-benzyl-ammonium chlorides	3 162 533 534
benzethonium chloride	0.1% aqua	4	benzalkonium chloride	For cosmetic allergy, *see* § 25.53	146
cetalkonium chloride	0.1% aqua	4	benzalkonium chloride (?)	For cosmetic allergy, *see* § 25.53	395
cetrimonium bromide	0.1% aqua	3	benzalkonium chloride [533]	Has caused skin necrosis (§ 8.1); matting of the hair (§ 12.1)	14 206 393
cetyl pyridinium chloride	0.05% aqua	2			694
chloroallylhexa-minium chloride	1% pet. 2% aqua	3	formaldehyde	Chloroallylhexaminium chloride is a formaldehyde releaser For cosmetic allergy, *see* § 23.47	110 584 585
dequalinium chloride	0.01% aqua	4		Has caused skin necrosis (§ 8.1)	368 460 175

quinoline derivatives (halogenated hydroxyquinoles may be tested 5% pet.) [180]   Have caused systemic eczematous contact-type dermatitis (§ 17.2)

Drug	Patch test conc. & vehicle (§ 5.2)	EFS (§ 5.4)	Cross-reactions (§ 5.5)	Comment	Ref.
chlorquinaldol	5% pet.	2	other halogenated quinoline derivatives		57 189 642
clioquinol	5% pet.	2	other halogenated quinoline derivatives, potassium iodide, quinine, chloroquine, amodiaquine	Irritant in a concentration of 3% or more (§ 2.4) Has caused contact urticaria (§ 7.5); a purpuric eruption (§ 12.1); generalized erythema and bronchospasm in a quinine-sensitive patient; discoloration of the nails (§ 10.1); EEM-like eruption (§ 4.5)	257 472
dibromo-8-hydroxy-quinoline (DBO)	5% pet.	2	other halogenated quinoline derivatives	Probably represented a cross-reaction to clioquinol in the reported case	436

(continued)

5.7 Antimicrobials and antioxidants

(continuation)

Drug	Patch test conc. & vehicle (§ 5.2)	EFS (§ 5.4)	Cross-reactions (§ 5.5)	Comment	Ref.
diiodohydroxyquin	5% pet.	2	other halogenated quinoline derivatives		10
sodium benzoate	5% pet.	3		Has caused contact urticaria (§ 7.5)	564
sorbic acid	5% aqua 2% pet.	2		Has caused contact urticaria (§ 7.5); systemic eczematous contact-type dermatitis (§ 17.2)	59 107 539
sulfur	1–5% pet.	4		Has caused contact urticaria (§ 7.5); comedogenic (§ 9.2)	375
tetrachlor salicylanilide	1% alc.	4		Has caused photosensitivity (§ 5.5)	187
tocopherols	10% pet.	3		Patch testing with tocopherols may sensitize *See* for patch testing also § 27.5.1	351 2
DL-α-tocopherol	10% pet.	3		Has caused contact urticaria (§ 7.5) For cosmetic allergy, *see* § 25.53 For patch test sensitization, *see* [607]	351 2
triclocarban	1–2% pet.	3	halogenated salicylanilides	Has caused methemoglobinemia (§ 16.94); photosensitivity (§ 6.5); skin necrosis (§ 8.1) Contact allergy to triclocarban has caused pigmentation of the face (§ 10.1) For cosmetic allergy, *see* § 25.53	287
triclosan (Irgasan DP 300®)	1–2% pet.	3			350 452 564
triphenylmethane dyes (gentian violet, crystal violet, methyl violet, rosaniline, malachite green, brilliant green, chrysoidine and eosin)	2% aqua	3	other triphenylmethane dyes	Gentian violet has caused cyanosis; and shock (§ 16.96) Crystal violet and gentian violet have caused skin necrosis (§ 8.1) Several have caused photosensitivity (§ 6.5) May be carcinogenic and mutagenic (§ 12.1)	44 498
usnic acid	1% pet.	4			564
zinc pyrithione	1% aqua 1–5% pet.	4		Also used as antiseborrheic agent in shampoos (§ 22.7 and § 22.8)	564

CONTACT ALLERGY TO FRAGRANCE MATERIALS

5.8   Not only is fragrance the most important ingredient of perfumes and colognes, it is also a significant part of many other cosmetic products such as creams, lotions, powders, soaps, etc.

A perfume is a creative composition of fragrance materials. On opening a bottle, the most volatile components of the 'top note' will be smelled. After 5–20 minutes the 'heart' or the 'body' of the perfume is perceptible. With a good perfume this heart will last for 2–4 hours. What is left is the 'dry out', which will gradually disappear. There are distinct perfume materials that have a favorable influence on the perfume profile, tempering the top note, refinement and extension of the heart and strengthening the dry out. Such materials are called 'fixatives' and include balsam Peru, balsam tolu, storax, benzoin, coumarin and musk.

The perfumer has approx. 200 fragrance materials of natural origin (e.g. essential oils) and approx. 3000 fragrance compounds, which are either isolates or derivatives of natural materials or synthetics. The most important fragrance materials are listed in § 27.7.

Perfumes contain approx. 12–20% of the so-called 'perfume compound'. It is expensive and actually too concentrated. The more diluted products (perfume lotion, perfume de toilette, eau de toilette, colognes) are therefore much more popular. There are no legally defined concentrations of the perfume compounds for these different products, but in general, colognes will contain 2–5%, perfume lotion and perfume de toilette 5–8% of the perfume compound. Most fragrance products are alcoholic solutions (70–96% ethanol), but perfume creams (sachets) and aerosols are also popular.

5.9   Typical **perfume formulas** are:

Perfume:		*Example:*
4-30%	water	*water*
70–96%	alcohol	*ethanol*
12–20%	perfume compound	*perfume*

Perfume aerosol:		*Example:*
c. 30%	propellant	*chlorfluorocarbon 114*
c. 65%	alcohol	*ethanol*
c. 5%	water	*water*
2–10%	perfume compound	*perfume*

Perfume sachet:		*Example:*
c. 70%	water	*water*
c. 20%	lipid	*glyceryl stearate, cetearyl alcohol*
c. 2%	surfactant: emulsifier	*PEG-25 propylene glycol stearate*
2–10%	perfume compound	*perfume*
c. 0.2%	preservative	*quaternium-15, methylparaben*

5.10   **Incidence of side effects: fragrance materials** (see § 20.17)

	% of total	
US manufacturers' file:	1.6	(35/8399)
US hospitals' file:	4.4	(31/698)
FDA pilot study:	3.6	(21/589)*

(continued)

5.10   Fragrance materials

(continuation)	% of total	
Spanish study:	19.5	(38/210)
Dutch file:	4.5	(9/202)
British consumers' report:	5.0	(31/626)**
Strassburg study:	4.2	(4/96)

* 0 severe	** one of the 'Top 6'
2 moderate	
19 mild	

5.11   **Risk index: fragrance materials** (see § 20.18)

Risk grading according to:
US manufacturers' file: *low risk* (at 1 experience per 1,265,000 estimated units distributed).
FDA pilot study: *medium risk* (at 1 experience per 1,700 person-brand used cosmetics).

IDENTIFICATION OF SENSITIZER

5.12   It is very difficult to establish the specific sensitizer in a perfume. Certain perfumes are both sensitizers and photosensitizers; others are solely photosensitizers. Therefore, patch tests with perfumes must be done, not only with the usual patch testing method but also with photopatch tests. Photosensitization is associated with a number of essential perfume oils, especially bergamot, lavender, cedar wood, neroli and petitgrain. Benzyl alcohol, a perfume solvent, and gum benzoin as well as various balsams and other fixatives may be the actual sensitizers in perfumes [153].

A perfume ingredient which is a sensitizer may become hypoallergenic during the aging process of the perfume. In such cases patch tests with the aged perfume ingredient remain negative, whereas the tests with a freshly prepared solution will give a positive result. This explains for instance the fact that a patient with an allergic sensitivity to cinnamic aldehyde may tolerate an aged perfume containing cinnamic aldehyde, without acquiring a dermatitis [160].

Also, an allergenic perfume ingredient may become non-allergenic, owing to its neutralization by another ingredient of the perfume mixture, or to chemical interchanges between two or more components [35].

The phenomenon that a contact sensitizing substance no longer causes contact sensitization in combination with another compound has been coined as 'quenching effect' [328]. This has been observed in the human maximization test with the contact sensitizing aldehydes phenylacetaldehyde, citral aldehyde and cinnamic aldehyde.

Although nowadays perfumes are considered to be the principal sensitizers in cosmetics [594], fragrance materials as possible sensitizing constituents of cosmetic products have been overlooked for many years. This may largely be explained by the concentrations of fragrances in cosmetics: these are usually too low to elicit a positive patch test result when the cosmetic is tested 'as is', thus leading to false negative results.

It has been shown that contact allergy to certain well-known sensitizers such as balsam Peru, rosin (colophony) and wood tar is frequently associated with a perfume allergy. Therefore, contact allergy to these and/or other so-called 'markers' or 'indicators' of perfume allergy should alert the physician to the possibility of contact allergy to fragrance materials. These indicators are listed in § 5.13. [158].

More recently, a fragrance mixture has been introduced in the ICDRG standard series, which has facilitated testing for fragrance sensitivity. The fragrance mixture is a combination of the most common fragrance allergens detected over the last several years. This mixture will in the future be modified as new fragrance allergens are defined. The fragrances in the mixture are shown in § 5.14.

The fragrance mixture detects possibly 70–80% of fragrance sensitivity, leaving 20–30% undetected [595]. In routine testing positive reactions to the fragrance mix have been noted in 6% [598], 8.2% [597] and 18.7% [596] of patients with contact dermatitis. Most positive reactions are to cinnamic aldehyde, cinnamic alcohol and isoeugenol. One problem with the perfume mixture is that some false positive irritant reactions occur, especially with the Excited Skin Syndrome. Therefore, the patch test concentrations of the 8 individual fragrances in the mix have, in July 1984, been decreased from 2% to 1% each. Although at present this mixture is the most sensitive 'indicator' of perfume allergy, it has not rendered the other indicators obsolete [597].

5.13	**Plant 'indicators' of perfume allergy**	
	balsam Peru	25% pet.
	colophony	10% pet.
	wood tar − pine 3%	
	− beech 3%	
	− juniper 3%	12% pet
	− birch 3%	
	turpentine	10% o.o.
	turpentine peroxides	0.3% pet.
	sesquiterpene lactones	1% pet.
	(costus absolute)	
		1% pet.
	lichen substances	
	(atronin, oak moss)	

5.14	**Fragrance mixture (ICDRG)**	Before July 1984	After July 1984
	cinnamic aldehyde	2% pet.	1% pet.
	cinnamic alcohol	2% pet.	1% pet.
	isoeugenol	2% pet.	1% pet.
	oak moss	2% pet.	1% pet.
	eugenol	2% pet.	1% pet.
	geraniol	2% pet.	1% pet.
	hydroxycitronellal	2% pet.	1% pet.
	α-amylcinnamic aldehyde	2% pet.	1% pet.

5.15   A number of fragrance materials have been reported to cause contact allergy: these are listed in § 5.16. Many other ingredients will probably in future prove to be sensitizers and/or photosensitizers. Individual substances may be tested according to the recommendations of Fisher [153]. The relevant recommended patch test concentrations and vehicles are listed in § 5.17. (See also § 27.7 on fragrance materials.) Contact allergy to various fragrance materials is probably of great importance in the production of the state of persistent light reaction as seen in the photosensitivity dermatitis with actinic reticuloid; some of these allergens are also capable of involving photosensitivity mechanisms [592, 593].

5.16   Contact allergy to fragrance materials

Substance	Patch test conc. & vehicle (§ 5.2)	EFS (§ 5.4)	Cross-reactions (§ 5.5)	Comment	Ref.
amyl cinnamate	32% pet.	4			290
α-amylcinnamic alcohol	2% pet.	2	α-amylcinnamic aldehyde	Commercial forms of α-amylcinnamic alcohol not infrequently contain α-amylcinnamic aldehyde	272 567
α-amylcinnamic aldehyde	2% pet.	3	α-amylcinnamic alcohol		567
anisylidene acetone	2% pet. (fresh)	4			
atranorin	1% pet. 0.1% acet.	2	fumarprotocetraric acid	Present in oak moss perfumes *See also* § 23.47 and § 25.53	116
balsam Peru	25% pet.	1	benzoin, colophony, benzoic acid, benzyl alcohol, cinnamic acid, essential oils, orange peels, eugenol, cinnamon, propolis, cinnamic alcohol, cinnamates, benzyl benzoate, vanilla	Has caused contact urticaria (§ 7.5); photosensitivity (§ 6.5) Perfume allergy indicator Has caused purpuric contact dermatitis (§ 4.1)	226 130 605
balsam Tolu	1–10% alc.	1	balsam Peru	Ingredients are listed by Mitchell [308]	226
benzaldehyde	5–10% pet. 10% alc.	1	balsam Peru	Has caused contact urticaria (§ 7.5)	226
benzyl alcohol	10% alc. 5–10% pet.	4	See § 5.7	Also used as preservative (§ 5.7) Contact allergy to benzyl alcohol has caused pigmentation of the face (§ 10.1) For cosmetic allergy, *see* § 23.47	386 320
benzyl cinnamate	5–8% pet. 10% alc.	1	balsam Peru		226
benzylidene acetone	0.5% pet.	4			51 290
benzyl salicylate	2% pet.	3	ylang-ylang oil, cananga oil, jasmin oil, balsam Peru	Benzyl salicylate is a preservative Contact allergy to this compound has caused pigmentation of the face (§ 10.1) Also used as sunscreen (§ 25.66)	319 357
cananga oil	2% pet.	3		Contact allergy to cananga oil has caused pigmentation of the face (§ 10.1)	320
cinnamic alcohol	2% pet.	1	balsam Peru, cinnamic aldehyde	Contact allergy to cinnamic alcohol has caused pigmentation of the face (§ 10.1) Consumer patch-test sensitization has been investigated [553] *See also* § 23.47 *under* cinnamic alcohol *and under* perfumes in facial tissue	271 319

(continued)

(continuation)

Drug	Patch test conc. & vehicle (§ 5.2)	EFS (§ 5.4)	Cross-reactions (§ 5.5)	Comment	Ref.
cinnamic aldehyde	2% pet.	1	balsam Peru	Has caused depigmentation (§ 10.1); contact urticaria (§ 7.5) Contact allergy from occupational exposure: *see* [483] Has caused contact allergy in a facial tissue (§ 23.47 *under perfume*); photoallergy (§ 6.5) *See also* § 13.3 and § 13.40	385 326 605
cinnamon oil	2% pet.	4	balsam Peru, cinnamic aldehyde	Has caused systemic contact-type dermatitis (§ 17.2) For cosmetic allergy, *see* § 13.3	77
cinnamyl benzoate	10% pet.	4			290
cinnamyl cinnamate	8% pet.	4			290
citral	2% pet. (fresh)	2		Citral is a mixture of geranial and neral At higher temperatures citral may be a strong irritant (§ 2.4)	226
citronellal	2-4% pet.	2	hydroxycitronellal		272
citronella oil				*See* lemon grass oil	255
colophony	20% pet.	1	*See* § 4.40	Perfume allergy indicator	291
coniferyl alcohol	2% pet.	2	balsam Peru		226
costus absolute	1% pet.	3	plants containing sesquiterpene lactones	Principal allergens are sesquiterpene lactones, derived from *Saussurea lappa*, a Compositae plant (§ 26.3) Perfume allergy indicator	306 310
coumarin	5–10% pet. 10% o.o.	2	vanilla, vanillin, balsam Peru	Has caused photosensitivity (§ 6.5)	434
diethyl sebacate	20% alc.	3			376
dihydroabietyl alcohol	1% pet.	3	colophony, abietic acid	*See also* § 23.47	124
dihydrocoumarin	5% pet.	2			290
eugenol	2% pet.	1	balsam Peru, isoeugenol	Has caused contact urticaria (§ 7.5) *See also* § 13.9	226
essential oils	2% pet.	3		For individual oils, *see* § 27.7 *and* § 27.2 ref. [23]	
evernic acid	0.1% acet.	2		Present in oak moss perfumes *See also* § 25.53	116
farnesol	4% pet.	2	balsam Peru		226
fumarprotocetraric acid	0.1% acet.	2	atranorin	Present in oak moss perfumes *See also* § 23.47 *and* § 25.53	116

(continued)

5.16   Fragrance materials

(continuation)

Drug	Patch test conc. & vehicle (§ 5.2)	EFS (§ 5.4)	Cross-reactions (§ 5.5)	Comment	Ref.
geranial	1–5% pet.	2	geranium, lavender oil, ylang-ylang oil, hydroxycitronellal	Contact allergy to geranial has caused (§ 10.1)	272 319
geraniol	2% pet.	2		Has caused patch-test sensitization *See also* § 25.53	557
geranium oil	2% pet.	4			319
cis-3-hexenyl salicylate	3% pet.	4	*not* to hexyl, methyl, phenyl, and benzyl salicylate		475
hydroxycitronellal	2% pet.	1	citronellal linalool [?, 521]	Contact allergy to hydroxycitronellal has caused pigmentation of the face (§ 10.1) and facial psoriasis [521] Consumer patch-test sensitization has been investigated [554] *See also* § 23.47	272 82
ionone	2% pet. 0.5% o.o.	3			386
isoeugenol	2% pet.	1	eugenol, balsam Peru	*See also* § 23.47	226
jasmin oil	2% pet.	3			319
jasmin, synthetic	10% pet.	2		Contact allergy to jasmin has caused pigmentation of the face (§ 10.1)	272
laurel oil	2% pet.	4		*See* § 26.3 *under* Laurus nobilis	170
lavender oil	1–2% pet.	3		Has caused photosensitivity (§ 6.5) Contact allergy to lavender oil has caused pigmentation of the face (§ 10.1)	320
lemon oil	1–2% pet.	4	turpentine oil		255
lemon grass oil	1–2% pet.	3		Citral is the main constituent	298
lilial	1% pet.	4		*See also* § 25.53	557
linalool	30% pet.	3	hydroxycitronellal (?)	Caused facial psoriasis in the reported case *See also* § 23.47	493
o-methoxycinnamic aldehyde	4% pet.	4			290
methoxycitronellal	1% pet.	3	hydroxycitronellal	Contact allergy to methoxycitronellal has caused pigmentation of the face (§ 10.1)	320
methyl anisate	4% pet.	4			289

(continued)

(continuation)

Drug	Patch test conc. & vehicle (§ 5.2)	EFS (§ 5.4)	Cross-reactions (§ 5.5)	Comment	Ref.
6-methyl coumarin	1% alc.	4		Has caused photosensitivity (§ 6.5)	251
methylheptine carbonate	0.5% pet.	3		*See also* § 23.47 and § 23.53	232 290
γ-methylionone	10% pet.	4		The relevance of this reaction was not established; the patient had contact urticaria from rouge of which γ-methylionone was a fragrance ingredient	572
musk ambrette	1–3% alc./pet.	3	moskene	Has caused photosensitivity and persistent light reaction (§ 6.5)	340 264
oak moss	2% pet.	2	atranorin, evernic acid, fumarproto-cetraric acid, d-usnic acid, tree moss, reindeer lichen	Has caused photoallergy (§ 6.5) *See also* § 23.47	487 609
orange oil	1–2% pet.	3			301
patchouli oil	1–2% pet.	4			319
phenylacetaldehyde (hyacinthin)	2% pet. (fresh) 0.5% alc.	1		Patch testing may sensitize	178
rose oil Bulgaria	2% pet. 1% alc.	4			319
sandalwood oil	1–2% pet.	3		Has caused photosensitivity (§ 6.5) Contact allergy to sandalwood oil has caused pigmentation of the face (§ 10.1)	407
ylang-ylang oil	2-5% pet.	3		Contact allergy to ylang-ylang oil has caused pigmentation of the face (§ 10.1)	320

Many other cosmetic (fragrance) materials will probably in future prove to be sensitizers and/or photosensitizers. Individual substances may be tested as follows (adapted from Fisher [153]):

5.17   Recommended patch test concentrations and vehicles for the screening of possible new sensitizers

Cosmetic ingredient	Patch test conc. & vehicle (§ 5.2)	Cosmetic ingredient	Patch test conc. & vehicle (§ 5.2)
p-anisaldehyde	1% pet.	cedartone V	as is
balm oil	1% pet.	trans-cinnamaldehyde	2% pet.
bay rum	as is	citracetal parento	10% DE
carnation oil	10% aqua	citron oil	1% pet.

(continued)

(continuation)

Cosmetic ingredient	Patch test conc. & vehicle (§ 5.2)	Cosmetic ingredient	Patch test conc. & vehicle (§ 5.2)
coniferyl benzoate	1% pet (2% pet.: [180])	mirbane oil (nitrobenzene)	25% c.o. (10% o.o.: [180])
deltyl extra	5% pet.	myristyl alcohol	5% pet.
essential oils	1% alc. or 2% pet.	orange peel oil	1% alc. (2% pet.: [180])
estradiol	5% pet.		
gylan	as is	perfumes	as is (open and closed)
Hamamelis virg.	5% aqua	petitgrain oil	10% o.o.
4-hydroxy azobenzene carboxylic acid	2% pet.	rose 62 ter	as is
		sandela 10	as is
irisone alpha	as is	sassafras oil	1% pet.
isoamyl salicylate	5% pet.	spice oil	5% pet. *(see also § 5.40)*
isopropyl quinolone	as is		
lauryl gallate	5% pet. (0.1% pet.: [180])	storax essence GD	5% pet.
		terpineol extra	25% in BL
lauryl sulfate (ammonium)	5% pet.	tetra-hydromuguol	as is
linalool oil	10% pet.	vanilla (alcoholic extract)	10% acet. (as is: [180])
linalyl acetate	1% pet.	verbena oil	1% pet.
mahogonate Dragoco	as is		
menthanyl acetate	as is	versalide prime	10% pet.
		vetivert rectified	as is
mint oil	1% pet.		

LOCAL ANESTHETICS

5.18   Local anesthetics are widely used in topical preparations for their antipruritic and anesthetic properties, e.g. in the treatment of pruritus ani, hemorrhoids and, occasionally, pruritus vulvae. The efficacy however, rather doubtful. Accidental contact with local anesthetics for injection may occur in medical and dental personnel. The allergenic potency of these drugs largely depends on their chemical structure.

   The main groups of local anesthetics are the benzoic acid derivatives (esters of p-aminobenzoic acid, m-aminobenzoic acid and benzoic acid), the amide derivatives and the quinoline derivatives (see § 5.19). The esters of p-aminobenzoic acid frequently cause contact sensitization, whereas the aminoacyl amides, such as lidocaine, are less allergenic. Cross-sensitization is common, especially between the various benzoic acid derivatives; cross-reactivity with other para-compounds occasionally occurs.

   Anesthetics for topical use that have caused contact allergy are listed in § 5.20.

5.19   Main classes of local anesthetics

A.   BENZOIC ACID DERIVATIVES

p-Aminobenzoic acid esters:
butacaine (butelline)
butethamine (monocaine)
butyl aminobenzoate (butamben, butesin)
ethyl aminobenzoate (benzocaine, anesthesin)
isobutyl p-aminobenzoate (cycloform)
naepaine (amylsine)
orthocaine (orthoform old & new)
procaine (novocaine)
propoxycaine (ravocaine)
risocaine (propaesin)
tetracaine (amethocaine, pantocaine)

Benzoic acid esters:
amylocaine (stovaine)
benoxinate hydrochloride (dorsacaine)
benzamine, β-eucaine
cyclomethycaine (surfacaine, topocaine)
meprylcaine hydrochloride (oracaine)

metabutoxycaine (primacaine)
piperocaine (metycaine, neothesin)

m-Aminobenzoic acid esters:
metabutethamine (unacaine)
proparacaine (alcaine)

B.   ANILIDES OR AMIDE DERIVATIVES
bupivacaine (marcaine)
lidocaine, lignocaine (xylocaine)
mepivacaine (carbocaine)
prilocaine (citanest)

C.   QUINOLINE DERIVATIVES
dibucaine (cinchocaine, percaine, nupercaine)
dimethisoquin (quotane)

D.   OTHER LOCAL ANESTHETICS
pramocaine (pramoxine)
propanidid (intravenous compound)
propipocaine (falicaine)

5.20   Contact allergy to topical anesthetics

Drug	Patch test conc. & vehicle (§ 5.2)	EFS (§ 5.4)	Cross-reactions (§ 5.5)	Comment	Ref.
amylocaine hydrochloride	1% pet.	4			464
benzamine lactate	1% pet.	3			76
benzocaine	5% pet.	1	para-compounds, metabutethamine, meprylcaine [516]	Has caused photosensitivity (§ 6.5); contact urticaria (§ 7.5); chlorpropamide has caused systemic eczematous contact-type dermatitis in a benzocaine-hypersensitive patient (§ 17.2) Has caused systemic side effects (§ 16.5)	89 177
butacaine	1% pet./aqua	3	procaine, benzocaine		270
butethamine	1% aqua	3	procaine, benzocaine		145
butyl aminobenzoate	5% pet.	3			440
dibucaine hydrochloride	1% pet./aqua 5% pet. [180]	2	clioquinol (?)		186 301 464 640
diperocaine	1% pet.	4			83
hydroxypolyethoxy-dodecane	5% pet.	3			80 216

(continued)

5.20 Topical anesthetics

(continuation)

Drug	Patch test conc. & vehicle (§ 5.2)	EFS (§ 5.4)	Cross-reactions (§ 5.5)	Comment	Ref.
lidocaine	2% aqua/ pet.	3	bupivacaine prilocaine mepivacaine dibucaine	Has caused systemic side effects (§ 16.46)	186 524 525 640 641
mepivacaine	1% aqua	4			186
orthoform, new	1% aqua/ pet.	2	orthoform, old		270
orthoform, old	1% aqua/ pet.	2	orthoform, new, benzocaine, isobutyl p-aminobenzoate, risocaine		270
pramocaine	1% aqua	4			442 640
prilocaine	2% aqua	3			186
procaine	1–2% aqua 1–5% pet.	2	para-compounds	Has caused systemic eczematous contact-type dermatitis (§ 17.2)	397 165
propanidid (intravenous anesthetic)	5% pet./ aqua	4	eugenol, balsam Peru, cinnamon oil	Propanidid is an eugenol derivative	27 405 191
proparacaine hydrochloride	2% aqua	4		Used in ophthalmology (§ 13.40)	26
propipocaine	1% pet.	2			377 39
quotane ointment (dimethisoquin hydrochloride)	as is	4			117
tetracaine	1% pet.	2	para-compounds, amylocaine		111 464 252

VEHICLE CONSTITUENTS

5.21   Side effects to constituents of vehicles may manifest themselves in several ways:
1. Itching and redness in the treated area. This reaction may be caused by:
   – a weak toxic effect in the substance (e.g. propylene glycol or sodium lauryl sulfate)
   – a low concentration of an allergenic substance in the vehicle.
2. A severe eczematous reaction. This may be caused by:
   – a potent allergenic substance
   – a combination of several allergenic substances
   – a combination of irritant and allergenic effects.
The testing of vehicles as such is often fruitless because the concentrations of the various ingredients may be so low that epicutaneous tests on healthy skin remain negative. In addition, steroids in ointments may have a negative influence on test

reactions. Classic ointment bases with petrolatum and mineral oils are usually harmless; cream bases contain at least preservatives and emulsifiers, but usually also antioxidants, lanolin or wool alcohols and perfumes as possible allergens (see the various relevant chapters). Synthetic vehicles containing polyethylene glycols, propylene glycol and/or fatty alcohols may also be sensitizers.

Those vehicle constituents that have caused contact allergy are listed in § 5.22.

5.22   Contact allergy to vehicle constituents

Vehicle constituent	Patch test conc. & vehicle (§ 5.2)	EFS (§ 5.4)	Cross-reactions (§ 5.5)	Comment	Ref.
carbowaxes	as is	4	other polyethylene glycols of the same molecular weight	Carbowaxes are solid polyethylene glycols	157
castor oil	pure	4		The offending chemical probably was ricinoleic acid (30% pet. and pure) For cosmetic allergy, *see* § 23.53 *and* § 23.47	558 643
cetyl alcohol	30% pet.	3	other higher fatty alcohols	Cetyl alcohol is an aliphatic alcohol Has caused contact urticaria (§ 7.5) Comedogenic (*see* § 9.2 *under* hexadecyl alcohol)	193 207 50
chlorofluoromethane	pure	4	chemically related chlorofluoromethanes ethyl chloride (?)	For cosmetic allergy, *see* § 25.53 *and* § 22.66 *under* aerosol propellants	437
dibutyl phthalate	5–10% pet.	3		For cosmetic allergy, *see* § 25.53	74
diethyl sebacate	20% alc.	3			376
dimethyl sulfoxide	90% aqua	4		Histamine liberator Has caused contact urticaria (§ 7.5); irritant dermatitis (§ 2.4) systemic side effects (§ 16.24); thickening, hardening and desquamation of the skin (§ 12.1).	303
diphenylamine	1% pet.	4	paraphenylene-diamine (?)	79	
ethylenediamine hydrochloride	1% pet.	2	piperazine citrate, diethylene tetramine, promethazine hydrochloride, antazoline sulfate, mepyramine maleate, aminophylline (consists of 2/3 theophylline and 1/3 ethylenediamine), ethylenediamine dihydroiodide	Has caused systemic eczematous contact-type dermatitis (§ 17.2); contact urticaria (§ 7.5) Inhalation has caused asthma in a sensitized individual (§ 22.66) Has caused EEM-like eruption (§ 4.5)	141 67 458 414 150 155 611
ethyl sebacate	20% alc.	4			43

(continued)

5.22 Vehicle constituents

(continuation)

Drug	Patch test conc. & vehicle (§ 5.2)	EFS (§ 5.4)	Cross-reactions (§ 5.5)	Comment	Ref.
eucerin	as is	3	lanolin, wool alcohols	Eucerin is petrolatum with 6% wool alcohols	23
glycerol	1% aqua pure	4		Has caused systemic eczematous contact-type dermatitis (§ 17.2)	208
glyceryl oleate	30% pet.	4		Glyceryl oleate is an aliphatic alcohol	230
glyceryl stearate	30% pet.	3		Glyceryl stearate is an aliphatic alcohol For cosmetic allergy, *see* § 25.53	209
hexantriol	5% aqua	4		Probably represents a cross-reaction after primary sensitization to stearyl alcohol and/or propylene glycol Has caused contact urticaria (§ 7.5)	333
isopropyl alcohol	10% aqua pure	4		*See also* § 5.7 Has caused contact urticaria (§ 7.5)	283
isopropyl myristate	5% pet.	4		Isopropyl myristate is a synthetic fatty alcohol Has comedogenic properties (§ 9.1) For cosmetic allergy, *see* § 25.53	161
isopropyl palmitate	2% pet.	4			575
jojoba oil	20% o.o./m.o.	3		Lubricant, used in cosmetics	522
lanette N	20% pet.	2	lanolin, wool alcohols	Lanette N is a mixture of cetyl and stearyl alcohol (9 parts) and sodium cetyl stearyl acid ester (1 part)	31 210
lanette O	20% pet.	2	wool alcohols	Lanette O is a mixture of cetyl and stearyl alcohol	31 492
lanette wax	30% paraff. liq.	3	lanolin, wool alcohols	Lanette wax consists of cetyl and stearyl alcohol with 10% sulfated esters of fatty alcohols	210
lanolin	as is	3	other wool alcohols	Lanolin consists of a mixture of sterols (wool alcohols), fatty alcohols and fatty acids; for a discussion of its composition, *see* [374, 541 542] Has comedogenic properties (§ 9.1) Lanolin is considered by some to be an extremely weak sensitizer in the healthy population [543] For cosmetic allergy, *see* § 23.47, § 23.53 *and* § 25.25	316 374 92
lauric acid dialkanolamide	1% pet.	4			209

(continued)

(continuation)

Drug	Patch test conc. & vehicle (§ 5.2)	EFS (§ 5.4)	Cross-reactions (§ 5.5)	Comment	Ref.
lauryl dimethyl amine oxide	3.7% aqua	4		Foaming agent *Cave:* irritant patch test reactions	317 538
myristic acid dialkanolamide	1% pet.	4			209
octyl dodecanol	30% pet. 13.5% aqua	4		For cosmetic allergy, *see* § 25.9	514
p-octylphenyl ethylene oxide	0.1% aqua	4			93
oleyl alcohol	pure and 30% pet.	3	stearyl alcohol	For cosmetic allergy, *see* § 23.53	84 151
olive oil	pure (freshly prepared)	4		The major constituents are: glycerides of oleic acid (85.5%), of palmitic acid (9.4%), of linoleic acid (4%), of stearic acid (2%), and of arachidic acid (0.9%) The exact allergen is unknown Has comedogenic properties (§ 9.2) Oleic acid has irritant properties and has been suspected as a sensitizer	201 536
petrolatum (yellow, white)	pure	4		The sensitizing capacity of yellow and white petrolatum has been investigated [490], and some allergens have been identified [491]. For allergenicity prediction and pharmacopoieal requirements, *see* [599] Red veterinary petrolatum has comedogenic properties Has caused chronic dermatitis and hyperpigmentation (§ 10.1); lipogranuloma and myospherulosis (§ 12.1) For cosmetic allergy, *see* § 22.65	203 286 123
polyethylene glycol	10% aqua	4	cross-reactions between PEG 200, 300 and 400	Has caused contact urticaria (§ 7.5) May be carcinogenic (§ 12.1) Has comedogenic properties (§ 9.2)	157
polyoxyethylene oxypropylene stearate	20% pet.	3			210
polyoxyethylene sorbitan monooleate	5% pet.	4			210
polyoxyethylene sorbitan monopalmitate	5% pet.	4			210
polyoxyethylene sorbitol lanolin derivative	20% pet.	3			210

(continued)

5.22 Vehicle constituents

(continuation)

Drug	Patch test conc. & vehicle (§ 5.2)	EFS (§ 5.4)	Cross-reactions (§ 5.5)	Comment	Ref.
propylene glycol	1 and 10% aqua	3		It is difficult to differentiate between toxic and allergic patch test reactions In doubt, patch tests should be repeated, and usage tests or oral provocation may be necessary for accurate diagnosis [551] Irritant when used under occlusion (§ 2.4) Has caused psoriasis-like reactions (§ 12.1); systemic eczematous contact-type dermatitis (§ 17.2) Has caused contact urticaria (§ 7.5) For cosmetic allergy, *see* § 25.53	211 159 12 551 556
sesame oil	as is	3		Consists of triglycerides of oleic acid (48%), of linoleic acid (40%), and 10% of palmitic acid, stearic acid and arachoic acid; 2% is unsaponifiable and contains sesamol, sesamolin and sesamin Has comedogenic properties (§ 9.2)	424 321
sodium dioctyl sulfosuccinate	10% pet.	3		Anionic surfactant	529
sodium lauryl sulfate	0.1% aqua	4		Well-known irritant, rare sensitizer Has comedogenic properties (§ 9.2) Certain batches of SLS solutions are preserved with formaldehyde [561]	337 561
soft paraffin				*See under* petrolatum	
sorbitan monolaurate	5% aqua	4			144 498
sorbitan monooleate	5% aqua	3			210 499
sorbitan monostearate	5% aqua	3			210
sorbitan sesquiolate	20% pet. 5% aqua	3	sorbitan monostearate and sorbitan monooleate		210
stearyl alcohol	30% pet.	4	oleyl alcohol other higher fatty alcohols	Stearyl alcohol is an aliphatic alcohol Has caused contact urticaria (§ 7.5)	333 47 207 151
thioglycerol	10% aqua	2	dimercaprol (BAL)	*See also* Chapter 22	190

(continued)

(continuation)

Drug	Patch test conc. & vehicle (§ 5.2)	EFS (§ 5.4)	Cross-reactions (§ 5.5)	Comment	Ref.
triethanolamine	2% pet./ aqua	2	promethazine (?)	For cosmetic allergy, *see* § 23.47 *and* § 25.9	420 410 13 552
triethanolamine stearate	5% pet.	3		For cosmetic allergy, *see* § 25.66	210
zinc oxide	pure	4	zinc sulfate	May cause black dermographism in the presence of jewelry (§ 12.1)	423

ANTIBIOTICS AND CHEMOTHERAPEUTICS

5.23 Topical antibiotic-containing preparations have a variety of uses:
– treatment of primary bacterial skin infections
– eradication of pathogens from carrier sites
– lessening infection of granulating surfaces such as leg ulcers and burns

Hazards of topical antibiotic administration

5.24 The main hazards in the use of topical antibiotics are:
– contact sensitivity (either immediate- or delayed-type)
– ecological shifts in the cutaneous microflora
– development of resistant strains of micro-organisms
– systemic effects (see Chapter 16)
– generalized reactions after oral or parenteral administration of antibiotics in previously sensitized individuals (see Chapter 17).

In this chapter only delayed-type hypersensitivity will be discussed. Some antibiotics are out of (topical) use because of their high contact-allergic sensitizing potential, such as penicillin and sulfonamides.

It must be stressed that the development of hypersensitivity to an antibiotic may greatly endanger the patient. Topical antibiotic preparations should therefore be used only on strict indications. Relatively 'safe' antibiotics for topical use are erythromycin, tetracycline, sodium fusidate and polymyxin. The reader is also referred to Chapters 16 and 17, on systemic side effects and systemic eczematous contact-type dermatitis medicamentosa, respectively. Those topical antibiotics that have caused contact-allergic reactions are listed in § 5.25.

5.25 **Contact allergy to antibiotics**

Drug	Patch test conc. & vehicle (§ 5.2)	EFS (§ 5.4)	Cross-reactions (§ 5.5)	Comment	Ref.
ampicillin	5% aqua	?		Occupational exposure in medical personnel Has caused contact urticaria (§ 7.5)	388
azidamfenicol	2% pet.	3	chloramphenicol	Chemically closely related to chloramphenicol	457

(continued)

5.25 Antibiotics

Drug	Patch test conc. & vehicle (§ 5.2)	EFS (§ 5.4)	Cross-reactions (§ 5.5)	Comment	Ref.
bacitracin	20–30% pet.	4	polymyxin B, colistine	Rare primary sensitizer; many reactions are cross-reactions to neomycin Has caused contact urticaria (§ 7.5) *See also* § 13.40	435 45
chloramphenicol	1% alc. 5–10% pet.	2	dinitrochlorbenzene, p-nitrobenzoic acid, p-dinitrobenzene (?)	Has caused aplastic anemia (§ 16.14); contact urticaria (§ 7.5); EEM-like eruption (§ 4.5) In one report chloramphenicol caused a drug eruption, patch tests were positive *See also* § 13.40	262 390 140 364
chlorfenicone	1% pet.	4		Chloramphenicol derivative, used in pessaries	108
chlortetracycline ointment	as is 3% pet.	4	chlortetracycline, demethylchlortetra-cycline		73
clindamycin	1% aqua	4	lincomycin	Has caused systemic side effects (*see* § 16.13)	104 489 511
dihydrostreptomycin	5% aqua 20% pet.	2	streptomycin, neomycin, kanamycin	Accidental contact	398
erythromycin	10% pet.	4		Also immediate-type allergy reported [439]	439 501
framycetin	20% pet.	1	neomycin, kanamycin (?), streptomycin (?), paromomycin (?)	Framycetin consists of neomycin B (99%), neomycin C (1%) and neamine (0.2%) Positive patch tests are usually cross-reactions to neomycin	336 90
gentamicin	5–20% pet.	1	neomycin, kanamycin	Most reports are of cross-sensitivity to neomycin rather than of direct sensitization Has caused systemic side effects (*see* § 16.34)	284 32
4′-homo-sulfanilamide	5% pet.	2	related esters of p-aminobenzoic acid	Has caused systemic side effects (*see* § 16.41)	447 25 23
lincomycin	5–30% pet.	4		Has cross-reacted to clinda-mycin	435

(continued)

(continuation)

Drug	Patch test conc. & vehicle (§ 5.2)	EFS (§ 5.4)	Cross-reactions (§ 5.5)	Comment	Ref.
neomycin	20% pet.	1	gentamicin, kanamycin, tobramycin, framycetin, streptomycin (?), paromomycin, ambutyrosin, sisomycin, cyclohexamide (?) [46], bacitracin, ribostamycin, spectinomycin [516]	Has caused systemic side effects (§ 16.62); contact urticaria (§ 7.5); systemic eczematous contact-type dermatitis (§ 17.2); EEM-like eruption (§ 4.5) Patch tests may become positive after 7 days only Co-reacts with bacitracin Sometimes contact allergy can only be detected with intradermal and usage tests It has been suggested that short-term use (less than 1 week) on non-eczematous skin induces few allergic reactions [570] *See also* § 13.40	334b 379 380 167 45 371 136
nitrofural	0.1–2% pet.	2	related nitrofuran derivatives	*See also* § 13.18 *under* furazolidine	49 56 236
oxytetracycline	3–5% pet.	4	tetracycline, methacycline	Tetracycline has caused yellow staining of the skin (§ 10.1) and contact urticaria (§ 7.5)	313 52
penicillin	10,000 IU/g pet. 100,000 IU/ml aqua	1		Anaphylaxis has occurred (§ 7.5) Has caused systemic eczematous ontact-type dermatitis (§ 17.2) Topical use largely abandoned	58 197 318 638
polymyxin B	3% pet.	4	polymyxin A, bacitracin	*See also* § 13.40	435 313
pristinamycin	5% pet.	4	virginiamycin	Has caused systemic eczematous contact-type dermatitis (§ 17.2); contact urticaria (see § 7.5) Factor IIa of pristinamycin and factor M of virginiamycin are identical	21
sodium fusidate	2% pet.	3			118 503
streptomycin	5% aqua 1% pet.	2	dihydrostreptomycin, kanamycin, neomycin	Has caused contact urticaria (§ 7.5); systemic eczematous contact-type dermatitis (§ 17.2); accidental contact in medical personnel	463 638

(continued)

(continuation)

Drug	Patch test conc. & vehicle (§ 5.2)	EFS (§ 5.4)	Cross-reactions (§ 5.5)	Comment	Ref.
sulfonamide	5% pet. 5% aqua	1	chemically related diuretics, oral antidiabetics and sweetening agents, other sulfonamides and para-compounds	Has caused photosensitivity (§ 6.5); Stevens-Johnson syndrome (§ 12.1); systemic eczematous contact-type dermatitis (§ 17.2) Tolbutamide, chlorpropamide and carbutamide (sulfonyl-urea-type antidiabetic drugs) have caused systemic eczematous contact-type dermatitis in sulfonamide-hypersensive patients (§ 17.2) *See also* § 13.18 *and* § 13.40	260 200
tyrothricin	0.5/5/30% pet.	2			199
variotin P	10–50% pet.	4			204
virginiamycin	2–5% pet.	3	pristinamycin	*See also under* pristinamycin Has caused systemic eczematous contact-type dermatitis (§ 17.2) For industrial contact, see [417]	269 48
xanthocillin	1% pet.	2	ung. alc. lanae. BP (?)		223

ANTIHISTAMINES

5.26   Primarily introduced as anti-allergic agents, antihistamines have also been found useful as tranquillizers, anticonvulsants, decongestants, local anesthetics and hypnotics. Most topical antihistamine preparations are used for their antipruritic properties.

The nucleus of the typical antihistamine structure is a substituted ethylamine ($-CH_2CH_2N=$), which may comprise part of a straight chain or a ring structure, and is present in the histamine molecule as well. The main groups of compounds are (a) ethylenediamines (b) alkylamines, (c) ethanolamines, (d) piperazines and (e) phenothiazines (§ 5.29)

5.27   The antihistamines can readily sensitize the skin following topical application or occupational exposure, especially the ethylenediamine derivatives and the phenothiazines. Cross-sensitization occurs frequently, especially between chemically related antihistamines, or with other related drugs. Phototoxic and photoallergic reactions may be seen occasionally, especially in the phenothiazine group. In addition, the antihistamines or chemically related drugs may cause systemic eczematous contact-type dermatitis medicamentosa in previously sensitized individuals, when administered orally or parenterally (see Chapter 17).

5.28   Antihistamines for topical use include antazoline, bamipine, chlorcyclizine, diphenhydramine, doxylamine succinate, methapyrilene, phenindamine, pheniramine, promethazine, pyrilamine, thonzylamine and tripelennamine. Although the Committee on Drugs of the American Academy of Pediatrics [469] recommended 'to discontinue the use of topical antihistamine preparations because their toxicity exceeds their limited benefit' and the American Medical Association came to the same conclusion [128], topical antihistamine preparations are still widely used and are in many countries available 'over the counter', without prescription.

Antihistamines for topical use that have caused contact allergy are listed in § 5.30.

5.29   **Main classes of anthihistamines** (only some of these are used topically, see § 5.28)

Ethylenediamines	doxylamine
antazoline, phenazoline	trimethobenzamide*
buclizine	
chloropyramine	**Piperazines**
clemizole	chlorcyclizine
methaphenilene	cinnarizine
methapyrilene	cyclizine*
pyrilamine, mepyramine	hydroxyzine
thenyldiamine	meclizine, meclozine
thonzylamine	
tripelennamine	**Phenothiazines**
	chlorpromazine*
Alkylamines	N-hydroxyethyl promethazine
bamipine	chloride
brompheniramine maleate	isothipendyl hydrochloride
chlorpheniramine maleate	oxomemazine
dexbrompheniramine maleate	promethazine hydrochloride
dexchlorpheniramine maleate	thiazinamium methylsulfate
dimethindene maleate	trimeprazine tartrate,
mebhydroline	methylpromazine
pheniramine	
	Miscellaneous
Ethanolamines	cyproheptadine
clemastine hydrogen fumarate	deptropine citrate
dimenhydrinate*	diphenylpyraline
diphenhydramine	phenindamine tartrate

*Antiemetics.

5.30   **Contact allergy to topical antihistamines**

Drug	Patch test conc. & vehicle (§ 5.2)	EFS (§ 5.4)	Cross-reactions (§ 5.5)	Comment	Ref.
antazoline	0.5% aqua 1% pet.	2	ethylenediamine and its derivatives	May produce systemic eczematous contact-type dermatitis in sensitized individuals [148] Aminophylline has caused systemic eczematous contact-type dermatitis in a patient sensitive to antazoline eyedrops (§ 17.2) *See also* § 13.40	394 148
brompheniramine	pure (?)	4		The reaction represented a cross-reaction to other pyridine derivatives	579
chlorcyclizine	1% pet.	4			15
chlorphenoxamine	1.5% pet./aqua	3			438

(continued)

71

5.30 Topical antihistamines

(continuation)

Drug	Patch test conc. & vehicle (§ 5.2)	EFS (§ 5.4)	Cross-reactions (§ 5.5)	Comment	Ref.
chlorpheniramine maleate	5% pet.	4		Little used in topical preparations	301
chlorpromazine	1–2.5% pet.	2	phenothiazines	Accidental contact in medical personnel Has caused photosensitivity (see § 6.5) Has caused systemic eczematous contact-type dermatitis (§ 6.5)	399
diphenhydramine	10% aqua 5% pet.	2	antazoline, dimenhydrinate [148]	Has caused systemic eczematous contact-type dermatitis (§ 17.2) Has caused photosensitivity (§ 6.5)	112 481 301
doxylamine succinate	?	?		No case reports	148
isothipendyl	1% pet.	4	*not* to phenothiazine derivatives	Structurally similar to phenothiazine	600
methapyrilene	2% pet.	3			281
phenindamine tartrate	5% pet.	2			134
phenothiazine antihistamines		2	other phenothiazine derivatives		588
promethazine hydrochloride	2% pet.	1	phenothiazines, triethanolamine (?), ethylenediamine and its derivatives, para-compounds	May produce systemic eczematous contact-type dermatitis in sensitized individuals [148] Has caused photosensitivity (§ 6.5); contact urticaria (§ 7.5); systemic side effects (§ 16.78)	399 148
pyrilamine maleate	2% pet.	3			112
tripelennamine	0.5–2% pet.	2	sulfapyridine, antazoline, promethazine, phenothiazines, ethylenediamine-derived antihistamines [148]	May produce systemic eczematous contact-type dermatitis in sensitized individuals	400 301 148

ANTIMYCOTICS

5.31   Antifungal drugs are becoming more important as the incidence of fungal infections increases. This increase is largely iatrogenic; large-scale employment of broad-spectrum antibiotics, and the increasing use of immunosuppressive therapeutics in patients with malignancies, autoimmune diseases and organ transplants disturb the ecological balance and lead to a rising incidence of fungal diseases. Also, the use of hormonal contraceptives predisposes to candidal infections of the vagina.

Therefore, new antifungal drugs are being developed nearly every year. Recently introduced antimycotics, which may be used both systemically and topically, are the *imidazoles:* miconazole, clotrimazole and econazole. These are being used extensively nowadays for topical treatment, because of their high antifungal activity and lack of side effects; contact allergy to the imidazoles appears to be rare. No allergic reactions to the newer imidazoles sulconazole and tioconazole have yet been reported. Topical antimycotics that have caused contact allergy are listed in § 5.32.

5.32   Contact allergy to antimycotics

Drug	Patch test conc. & vehicle (§ 5.2)	EFS (§ 5.4)	Cross-reactions (§ 5.5)	Comment	Ref.
benzoic acid	5–10% pet.	3		Has caused contact urticaria (§ 7.5) Also used as preservative (§ 5.7)	20
5-bromo-4′-chlorosalicylanilide	2% pet.	2	other halogenated salicylanilides (usually photo-cross reactions)	*Only* photosensitizer (§ 6.5)	66
buclosamide	1% pet.	2	halogenated salicylanilides, sulfonamides, sulfonamide-anti diabetics and diuretics (usually photo-cross-reactions)	*Only* photosensitizer (§ 6.5)	249 68
candicidin	0.05% pet.	4			106
Castellani's solution	as is	3	hexyl resorcinol	Contact allergy to the ingredient resorcinol; has caused systemic side effects (§ 16.81 and § 16.31)	294
1-p-chlorbenzyl-2-methylbenzimidazole	1% pet.	3			233
chlordantoin	0.1–1% pet.	4			218
chlorphenesin	0.5–1% pet.	4			61
clophenoxyde	1% ethyl acetate	4	w-chloracetophenone		168
clotrimazole	1% MEK	4			352
dibenzthione	1% acet. 3% pet.	3	possibly antihypertensive drugs derived from traizines, hydrochlorthiazide	Has caused photosensitivity (§ 6.5)	275 40
3,5-dichloro-4-fluorothiocarbanilide	1% isopropyl alc.	3			426
econazole	2% pet.	4		Has caused EEM-like eruption (§ 4.5)	500
enilconazole	2% pet.	4	econazole, isoconazole, miconazole	Enilconazole is a fungicide for veterinary use All mentioned antimycotics are β-substituted 1-phenylethyl imidazoles	476
etisazole	1% pet.	4		Veterinary fungicide Accidental contact	113 429

(continued)

5.32 Antimycotics

(continuation)

Drug	Patch test conc. & vehicle (§ 5.2)	EFS (§ 5.4)	Cross-reactions (§ 5.5)	Comment	Ref.
haloprogin	1% pet.	4			358
hexetidine	0.1% pet.	4		Used in gargles (§ 13.9) Quaternary ammonium compound	526
isoconazole	2% pet.	4			496 515
mesulfen	5% pet.	3		Has caused irritant dermatitis (§ 2.4)	433 96 502
methyl captan	2% aqua 5% lan-vas	4			401
miconazole nitrate	2% pet.	3	econazole		370 450 497 535
mycanodin	1–2% ?	4		Mycanodin is a combination of 3-(2-oxychlorphenyl)-pycazole and bamipine Has caused photosensitivity (*see* § 6.5)	65
nifuratel	1% acet.	4		Also used for the treatment of thrichomoniasis	479
nifuroxime	?	4		Has caused contact urticaria (§ 7.5) *See also* §13.18	1
nystatin	100,000–-300,000 U/g pet.	4		Has caused systemic eczematous contact-type dermatitis (§ 17.2)	172 101
pecilocin	1% pet.	3			323
phenylmercuric borate	0.1% pet.	2	other mercurials	Mercurial compounds have caused systemic side effect (§ 16.53)	467
pyrrolnitrin	1% pet.	2	possibly dinitrochlorbenzene	The eruption imitates EEM (§ 4.5)	299 353 560
sulconazole nitrate	1% cream basis	4	Contact allergy to sulconazole 1% cream; the actual allergen was not determined		473
tolnaftate	0.01–1% pet.	4			195
undecylenic acid	2–5% pet.	4	zinc undecylenate		194
zinc undecylenate	20% talc	4	undecylenic acid		194

CORTICOSTEROIDS

5.33   Contact dermatitis to topical corticosteroid preparations is an uncommon event. The sensitizing potential of the topical steroids is apparently low. Nevertheless, cases of contact sensitivity are being reported with increasing frequency. Contact allergy to ingredients of topical corticosteroid preparations should be considered in cases of long-standing therapy-resistant dermatitis. In many of the reported cases the dermatitis was localized on the legs.

Patch testing

5.34   In all cases of suspected hypersensitivity reactions to a topical corticosteroid preparation, tests should be carried out with the preparation itself as well as with the corticosteroid and the other ingredients separately. Ingredients in corticosteroid ointment or cream bases which have been identified as sensitizers include:
– benzyl alcohol [634]
– cetyl alcohol [619]
– chlorocresol [327]
– ethylenediamine hydrochloride [635]
– isopropyl palmitate [634]
– lanolin [619]
– parabens [637]
– polyethyleneglycol monostearate
– polysorbate 60 [636]
– propylene glycol [327]
– sorbic acid
– stearyl alcohol [47]

Often there is a concomitant sensitization to the corticosteroid and one or more of the other ingredients of the topical preparation. Several cases have been published in which the patient was allergic to more than one corticosteroid [60, 78, 102, 302, 428, 448, 462, 468, 471, 614, 619, 621, 630]. The possibility of cross-sensitization has not been sufficiently investigated in these studies as the information given on the use of corticosteroid creams is often incomplete. The observed multiple positive reactions might also be caused by concomitant sentizitation. Contamination is another possibility which must be taken into account. A changeover to another corticosteroid preparation in cases of proven allergy should be preceded by patch tests with the intended preparation and its ingredients. The patch test concentrations proposed by different authors differ considerably.

The following patch test concentrations for corticosteroids were proposed by Dooms-Goossens et al. [619]:

5.35   **Corticosteroid patch test battery (the vehicle used is white petrolatum)**

Corticosteroid	Patch test conc.	Pharmaceutical conc.
Betamethasone dipropionate	5%	0.05%
Betamethasone valerate	5%	0.1%
Clobetasol propionate	0.5%	0.05%
Clobetasone butyrate	0.5%	0.05%
Cortisone acetate	25%	0.5–2.5%
Desonide		0.05%

(continued)

5.35   Corticosteroid patch test battery

(continuation)

Corticosteroid	Patch test conc.	Pharmaceutical conc.
Desoximetasone	1%	0.25%
Dexamethasone acetate	1%	0.1%
Dexamethasone sodium phosphate	1%	0.1%
Diflorasone diacetate	1%	0.05%
Diflucortolone valerate	1%	0.1%
Fludrocortisone acetate	5%	0.1–0.25%
Flumetasone pivalate	1%	0.02%
Fluocinolone acetate	1%	0.01–0.02%
Fluocinonide	1%	0.05%
Fluocortolone	1%	0.25–0.5%
Fluocortolone hexanoate	1%	0.25–0.5%
Fluocortolone pivalate	1%	0.25–0.5%
Fluorometholone	1%	0.025–0.1%
Fluprednidene acetate	1%	0.05–0.1%
Formocortal		0.025%
Halcinonide	1%	0.025–0.1%
Hydrocortisone	25%	0.25–2.5%
Hydrocortisone acetate	25%	0.5–2.5%
Hydrocortisone butyrate	1%	0.1%
Methylprednisolone acetate	10%	0.25–1%
Prednisolone	5%	0.5%
Triamcinolone acetonide	1%	0.025–0.1%

It has been pointed out that the low concentration in the commercial preparation may cause false negative reactions, when the corticosteroid formulations used are tested 'as is'. It must be kept in mind that the bioavailability of a corticosteroid in a petrolatum base made up for patch testing is generally considerably lower than in the commercial product.

Reported contact allergy to corticosteroids

5.36   Topical steroids that have caused contact allergy are listed in § 5.37.
Other local and systemic side effects are discussed in Chapters 14 and 16.

5.37   Contact allergy to topical corticosteroids

Corticosteroid	Ref.
betamethasone	5
betamethasone valerate	7, 63, 623, 629, 630
budesonide	428
chlorprednisone acetate	448
clobetasol propionate*	78, 443, 610, 614, 623, 628
clobetasone butyrate	614, 619
cortisone	5, 471
desonide	102, 622
dexamethasone	459

(continued)

(continuation)

Corticosteroid	Ref.
fluocinolone acetonide	471, 630
fluocinonide	102, 622
fluocortolone	302, 611, 625
fluocortolone caproate	302
fluocortolone pivalate	302
fluperolone acetonide	471
halcinonide	102, 622
hydrocortisone**	5, 7, 471, 611, 616, 617, 620, 621, 623, 626, 627, 633
hydrocortisone acetate	5, 462, 613, 615
hydrocortisone 21-diol acetate	615
hydrocortisone alcohol	132, 615, 617
hydrocortisone butyrate	54, 60, 611, 624, 632
hydrocortisone succinate	462, 615, 626
hydrocortisone valerate	622
methylprednisolone	471, 631
methylprednisolone acetate	105, 631
prednisolone	205, 471, 616, 617, 622, 626, 631
prednisone	5, 205, 616
triamcinolone	5, 468, 621
triamcinolone acetonide	5, 30, 102, 416, 459, 468, 622, 624, 634

 * has caused contact urticaria (§ 7.5)
** has caused photosensitivity (§ 6.5)

DRUGS USED IN THE TREATMENT OF PSORIASIS, ACNE, ECZEMA AND PRURITUS

5.38   **Contact allergy to drugs used in psoriasis, acne, eczema and pruritus treatment**

Drug	Patch test conc. & vehicle (§ 5.2)	EFS (§ 5.4)	Cross-reactions (§ 5.5)	Comment	Ref.
6-aminonicotinamide	1% dimethyl sulfoxide open test	4		Rarely used Has caused irritant dermatitis (§ 2.4)	470
ammonium sulfobituminate				*See* § 5.7	
antihistamines, topical				*See* § 4.27–4.32	

(continued)

5.38 Drugs used in psoriasis, acne, eczema, pruritus

(continuation)

Drug	Patch test conc. & vehicle (§ 5.2)	EFS (§ 5.4)	Cross-reactions (§ 5.5)	Comment	Ref.
benzoyl peroxide	0.1–1–5% pet.	2		The main indications for BP are acne and leg ulcers. When used for leg ulcers contact sensitization is very frequent [546, 550], but when used for acne, adverse effects are usually of irritant nature [548] Usage tests may be indicated [549] *Cave:* irritant patch test reactions to the higher concentrations *See also* § 13.9 May have tumor-promoting effects (§ 12.1) Has caused irritant dermatitis (§ 2.4); discoloration (§ 10.1) and contact urticaria (§ 7.5)	274 276 546 547 548 549 550
chrysarobin	0.03% pet.	4		Has caused irritant dermatitis (§ 2.4); discoloration of the skin and finger nails (§ 10.1) No contact allergy reported	149
corticosteroids				*See* § 4.34–4.39	
crotamiton	1% MEK	4		Also used as scabicide	425
dithranol	0.02–0.05% acet.	4		Has caused irritant dermatitis (§ 2.4) and discoloration of the skin and finger nails (§ 10.1); also a fixed drug eruption (§ 16.28) *See also* § 12.1	120 568
menthol	1–2% pet.	4		Has caused contact urticaria (§ 7.5)	86 50
8-methoxypsoralen	1% alc. 0.001% alc./ aqua [180]	4		Used in PUVA therapy for psoriasis (§ 18.1) Has caused photosensitivity (§ 6.5)	367
nitrofurylamino- thiadazoles	1% pet.	4	related compounds		176
phenol	0.5–1% aqua	4	resorcin, cresols, hydroquinone (?)	Has caused systemic side effects (§ 16.68); irritant dermatitis (§ 2.4); contact urticaria (§ 7.5) skin necrosis (§ 8.1)	20 591
polidocanol	3% alc.	4		Also used for ulcus cruris therapy	235 80
resorcinol	2% pet. 5% aqua (?)	3	meta-dihydroxy- benzenes, resorcinol monoacetate, pyrocatechol, phenol, pyrogallol, hydroquinone, hydroxyhydroquinone, hexylresorcinol, orcinol	Has caused irritant dermatitis (§ 2.4); systemic side effects (§ 16.81); darkens fair hair (§ 10.1) *See also* § 22.28 *and* § 22.65	256 294 517 531

(continued)

(continuation)

Drug	Patch test conc. & vehicle (§ 5.2)	EFS (§ 5.4)	Cross-reactions (§ 6.5)	Comment	Ref.
salicylic acid	2% pet. 5% aqua	4		Has caused irritant dermatitis (§ 2.4); systemic side effects (§ 16.83); 'xeroderma pigmentosum' (§ 12.1); atrophic scar (§ 12.1); lymphangitis (§ 12.1); contact urticaria (§ 7.5)	366
sulfur	1–5% pet.	4		Has caused contact urticaria (§ 7.5) Comedogenic (§ 9.2)	461 375
tar, coal	5% pet.	2		Has caused irritant dermatitis (§ 2.4); photosensitivity (§ 6.5); 'pigmented cosmetic dermatitis' (§ 10.1); methemoglobinemia (§ 16.17); multiple keratoacanthomas (§ 12.1) comedogenic (§ 9.1); may be carcinogenic? (§ 12.1)	361 402
tar, wood (pine, beech, juniper, birch)	4 × 3% pet.	1	perfumes, essential oils, balsams, colophony and woods (?)	Perfume allergy indicator Has caused irritant dermatitis (§ 2.4)	357
thioxolone	0.05-0.5% alc.	3		Has also caused contact allergy in a hair product (§ 22.65)	451
tretinoin	0.05% pet. 0.01% alc.	4		Has caused irritant dermatitis (§ 2.4); pigment alterations (§ 10.1); increased susceptibility to sunburn; systemic side effects (?) (§ 16.93)	277 365

PLANT-DERIVED SUBSTANCES IN TOPICAL DRUGS

5.39   Contact allergy to plant-derived substances in topical drugs

Drug	Patch test conc. & vehicle (§ 5.2)	EFS (§ 5.4)	Cross-reactions (§ 5.5)	Comment	Ref.
abietic acid	5% pet.	3		*See also* under balsam Peru	339 453
arnica tincture	20% alc. and pure	2		The main suspected allergens are helenalin and its methacryl acid ester (sesquiterpene lactones) *See § 26.3 under* Arnica montana	363 217
balsam Peru				*See* § 5.16	
balsam Tolu				*See* § 5.16	
beeswax	30% pet. and pure	2	balsam Peru	Contains vanillin and cinnamic acid For cosmetic allergy, *see* § 23.47	332

(continued)

5.39 Plant-derived substances

(continuation)

Drug	Patch test conc. & vehicle (§ 5.2)	EFS (§ 5.4)	Cross-reactions (§ 5.5)	Comment	Ref.
benzoin tincture	2–10% pet. 10% alc.	3	balsam Peru, vanilla, α-pinene, benzyl alcohol, benzyl cinnamate, eugenol and storax	Benzoin tincture is 10% benzoin in alcohol; benzoin contains: benzoic acids, cinnamic acids, vanillin and coniferyl benzoate Has caused non-eczematous exanthema (§ 12.1) For cosmetic reactions, *see* § 22.65, § 23.47, § 25.9 *and* § 26.3 *under* Styrax benzoin	233 147 103
bergamot oil	2–10% pet.	4		Contains 5-methoxypsoralen Has caused photosensitivity (§ 6.5)	213
chamomile oil	25% o.o.	3		The allergen is presumably a sesquiterpene lactone called desacetyl matricarin See also § 26.3 *under* Anthemis nobilis *and* Matricaria chamomilla	36 559
colophony	20% pet.	1	abietic acid, abietic alcohol, balsam Peru, dehydroabietic acid, dihydroabietic acid, dextropimaric acid, levopimaric acid, maleopimaric acid, methylabietate, neoabietic acid, palustric acid, tetrahydroabietic acid	Contains abietic acid, which may be the actual sensitizer For cosmetic allergy, *see* § 22.65 *and* § 23.47	173 566 602
coumarin				*See* § 5.16	
esculin	1% pet.	4		*See also* § 26.3 *under* Aesculus hippocastanum	94
gums (karaya, acacia and tragacanth)	– gum: as is – tragacanth: 0.1% aqua	4			323 506 507
henna (lawsonia)	10 mg henna powder in 100 ml aqua, ether and alcohol	4		Used for hair coloring Has caused immediate-type allergy (§ 7.5) *See also* § 22.28	331
karaya powder	karaya seal ring	4		Used in a drainable polyethylene bag at colostomy sites	88
linseed	as is, raw and cooked	4		Folk medicine, used for hidradenitis axillaris	64
niaouli oil	1% alc.	3	thyme oil	Constituent of biogaze (§ 5.42) The main allergen is limonene	238
storax	2% pet.	2	benzoin, balsam Peru		309

(continued)

(continuation)

Drug	Patch test conc. & vehicle (§ 5.2)	EFS (§ 5.4)	Cross-reactions (§ 5.5)	Comment	Ref.
tar (wood and coal)				*See* § 4.39	
terpineol	5% pet.	3		In e.g. thyme oil and niaouli oil	244
thyme oil	1% alc. 10% pet., 25% c.o.	3	niaouli oil	Constituent of biogaze (§ 5.42) The main allergen is limonene *See also* § 26.3 *under* Thymus vulgaris	238
turpentine, vegetable	– turpentine peroxide 0.3% o.o. – α-pinene 15% o.o. – dipentene 10% MEK/2% pet.	2		*Cave:* irritant patch test reactions Contact allergy to turpentine has become infrequent, as turpentine oil in paints has been replaced by white spirit	335 604

Other plant-derived substances and their test concentrations are provided in § 5.40. See also § 5.8–5.18 on contact allergy to fragrance materials, § 27.7 on fragance materials, and Chapter 26 on plant products in cosmetics.

5.40   **Plant-derived substances and patch testing dilutions** (adapted from Fregert [180])

Substance	Patch test conc. & vehicle (§ 5.2)	Comment
alantolactone	0.1% pet.	Patch testing may sensitize
balsam of pine	20% MEK	
balsam of spruce	20% MEK	
dammar resin	20% alc./pet.	
fruits (orange, citrus peels)	as is	*Cave:* irritant patch test reactions
mirbane oil	10% o.o.	
pentadecyl-catechol	0.1% pet.	Patch testing may sensitize
α-pinene	15% o.o./1% pet.	
plant, leaf, flower, pollen, bulb	as is	*Cave:* irritant patch test reactions
pyrethrum	2% pet.	
spice	as is	
spice oils	5% alc. (*see also* § 5.17)	
storax, oil of	2% pet.	
tobacco	as is	
vanilla	as is	
Venice turpentine (larch turpentine)	20% pet.	
wood, exotic	dry sawdust	*Cave:* irritant patch test reactions
wood, pine and spruce	balsams of pine and spruce	

ANTIPARASITIC DRUGS

5.41   Contact allergy to antiparasitic drugs

Drug	Patch test conc. & vehicle (§ 5.2)	EFS (§ 5.4)	Cross-reactions (§ 5.5)	Comment	Ref.
acetarsol	?	4		Also present in several toothpastes and mouthwashes *See also* § 13.18	346
benzyl benzoate	10% pet.	3	balsam Peru, balsam Tolu	May have caused 'pemphigoid' (§ 12.1) Has caused conjunctivitis [581]	226 502
crotamiton	5% pet.	4		Also used as antipruritic drug	42 425
DDT	5% acet. 1% pet.	4		May produce chloracne and possibly porphyria	37
lindane	1% pet.	4		Has caused systemic side effects (§ 16.47); contact urticaria (§ 7.5)	38
malathion	1% alc. (open test) 0.5% pet. 1% aqua [180]	4		Has caused systemic side effects (§ 16.52)	304
mesulfen	5% pet	3		*See also* § 5.32 Has caused irritant dermatitis (§ 2.4)	502
monosulfiram	1% pet.	4	tetramethylthiuram disulfide, disulfiram	Contact allergy caused epidermal necrolysis in the reported case (§ 4.11)	314

MISCELLANEOUS DRUGS

5.42   Contact allergy to miscellaneous topical drugs

Drug	Use	Patch test conc. & vehicle (§ 5.2)	EFS (§ 5.4)	Cross-reactions (§ 5.5)	Comment	Ref.
biogaze	wound treatment	as is	2		The main allergen is limonene in thyme oil and niaouli oil	238 523
boric acid	in topical remedies	5% glyc. 3% aqua	4		Has caused systemic side effects (§ 16.6)	20
bufexamac	antiinflammatory drug	5% pet.	3			268 300 510 601

(continued)

(continuation)

Drug	Use	Patch test conc. & vehicle (§ 5.2)	EFS (§ 5.4)	Cross-reactions (§ 5.5)	Comment	Ref.
camphor	folk medicine decubitus prevention	10% pet.	4		Has caused systemic side effects (§ 16.9); contact urticaria (§ 7.5)	28
capsicum	antirheumatic drug	0.5% pet.	4			300
carmustine (BCNU)	topical cytostatic drug for mycosis fungoides	1% aqua (?)	2		Has caused irritant dermatitis (§ 2.4); pigmentary changes (§ 10.1); erythema followed by patchy teleangiectasia (§ 12.1), and systemic side effects (§ 16.12)	608
chlorambucil	cytostatic drug	pure	4		Drug was administered systemically No controls used with patch testing	259
collagenase A	treatment of leg ulcers	1.2 mg/g pet.	4			55
dexpanthenol	wound treatment	50% aqua	4		No controls used with patch testing	240
dianabol cream	wound treatment	pure	3			391
diethylstilbestrol	hormone	1% alc.	4	dienestrol, hexestrol, bisphenol-A, benzestrol, p-benzylphenol, monobenzylether of hydroquinone, benzylester of p-hydroxybenzoic acid, storax, balsam Peru	Topical sex hormones have caused systemic side effects (§ 16.87); contact urticaria (§ 7.5: estrogen cream)	185
dihydroxyacetone	tanning agent	1% aqua 10% alc.	4		Has caused brown discoloration of the skin (§ 10.1)	215
diisopropoxyphosphoryl fluoride (DPF)	cholinesterase inhibitor	0.1% o.o.	4	related chemicals		184
diphencyprone (2,3-diphenylcyclopropenone-1)	treatment of alopecia areata	?	1		Diphencyprone 2% in acetone is used for (deliberate) sensitization	482
estradiol benzoate	hormone	0.01% MEK	4	balsam Peru, resorcinol monobenzoate		278
etofenamate	antirheumatic drug	2% pet.	4			430

(continued)

5.42 Miscellaneous topical drugs

(continuation)

Drug	Use	Patch test conc. & vehicle (§ 5.2)	EFS (§ 5.4)	Cross-reactions (§ 5.5)	Comment	Ref.
fluorouracil	cytostatic drug	1% prop. glyc. 1–5% pet.	3		Sometimes patch tests are negative, but scratch tests positive Negative scratch tests have become positive after therapy with fluorouracil Has caused photosensitivity (§ 5.5); irritant dermatiti (§ 2.4); skin necrosis (§ 8.1); pigmentation (§ 10.1); for other side effects, *see* § 12.1 *Cave:* irritant patch test reactions	369 198 137 519 569
gelatin	in adhesives	pure	4			506
heparinoid	treatment of phlebitis	0.5% ?	4			378
idoxuridine	antiviral drug	1% pet.		brominated and chlorinated pyrimidine analogs trifluor-thymidine [91]	May be mutagenic? carcinogenic? and/or teratogenic? (§ 12.1) *See also* § 13.40	11 81 342 419 580
imidazoline chlorhydrate	α-adrenergic sympathomimetic	0.1% pet.	4	oximetazoline chlorhydrate		505
4-isopropyl-catechol	bleaching agent	5% pet.	4		Has caused reticular hyperpigmentation and depigmentation (§ 10.1)	122
mechlorethamine hydrochloride	cytostatic drug	0.02% aqua (open test)	1	mechlorethamine homologs [445]	May be (co)carcinogenic (§ 12.1); has caused contact urticaria and anaphylaxis (§ 7.5); pigmentation (§ 10.1); irritant dermatitis (§ 2.4) *See also* § 12.1	415 18 576 577 578 639
methylsalicylate	counter-irritant	2% o.o. 1–2% pet.	4	sodium salicylate	Taking acetylsalicylic acid tablets in a methyl salicylate-sensitive individual has caused systemic eczematous contact-type dermatitis (§ 17.2)	224

(continued)

(continuation)

Drug	Use	Patch test conc. & vehicle (§ 5.2)	EFS (§ 5.4)	Cross-reactions (§ 5.5)	Comment	Ref.
monobenzylether of hydroquinone	depigmenting agent	1% pet.	2	p-hydroxybenzoic acid ester, bisphenol A, diethylstilbestrol (?)	Has caused pigmentation (§ 10.1); erythema progressing into hyperpigmentation, depigmentation (§ 10.1); ochronosis and colloid milia (§ 12.1; hydroquinone) *See also* § 25.44 *and* § 25.45 For systemic side effects, *see* § 16.60 (monobenzone)	127 41
mustard oil	folk medicine	0.1% pet.	4		Also causes toxic reactions Contains allylisothiocyanate	192
nitroglycerin	coronary vasodilator	0.2 mg/ml aqua 2% comm. ointm. bas.	4		For transdermal delivery system, *see* § 16.100	220 372 589
oxyphenbutazone	anti-inflammatory drug	1% pet.	3	phenylbutazone		263 422
pellidol	wound treatment	2% pet.	2	other azo-dyes, para-compounds		396
phenylbutazone	anti-inflammatory drug	1–5% pet.	3		Has caused systemic eczematous contact-type dermatitis (§ 17.2) *See also* § 7.5	418
potassium iodide	formerly used for diagnosing dermatitis herpetiformis	30% pet.	4			8
propolis	folk medicine	1 and 5% pet. (alc. extracts)	2	Pseudo-cross-reactions to balsam Peru Common constituents are: cinnamyl cinnamate, benzyl benzoate, benzyl cinnamate, cinnamic alcohol and vanillin (Pseudo) cross-reactions to essential oils	Sensitization also occurs during beeswax modelling and in beekeepers *See also* § 23.47	565
solcoseryl	wound treatment	comm. prep.	4			289
tannic acid	adstringent	0.25% aqua	4			273

(continued)

5.42   Miscellaneous topical drugs

(continuation)

Drug	Use	Patch test conc. & vehicle (§ 5.2)	EFS (§ 5.4)	Cross-reactions (§ 5.5)	Comment	Ref.
tattoos					For fuller data, *see* § 5.43	392
thiosinamine	skin massage	0.05% alc.	3		Also used in photography	413
tiger balm	folk medicine	as is	3	balsam Peru		226
triaziquone	cytostatic drug	0.05% euc.	4			219
triethanolamine polypeptide oleate condensate	cerumenolytic drug	1% and 10% prop. glyc. 1% aqua	4			202 53 265
trioxyethylrutin	treatment of venous disorders	2% pet.	4			13
tromantadine	antiviral drug	1% comm. ointm. base	1	amantadine [495]	Contact allergy to the commercial ointment is nearly always caused by the active ingredient tromantadine [474]	142 338

PIGMENTS USED IN TATTOOS

5.43   Contact allergy to tattoos [392]

Color	Pigment	Patch testing	Comment	Ref.
blue	– cobalt blue – indigo	cobalt chloride 2% pet.	Contact allergy to cobalt caused granulomatous skin reactions	356
green	– trivalent chromic oxide – chromic hydrate – hydrated chromium sesquioxide	potassium dichromate 0.5% pet.	No primary sensitization to the pigment. Usually preceded by cement eczema	71
red	– mercuric sulfide (cinnabar)	0.1% pet. (?)	Contact allergy has caused lichenoid and granulomatous reactions; these reactions also occur without mercury sensitivity (§ 4.7)	466 412
yellow	– cadmium sulfide – ochre – curcuma yellow		only phototoxic reactions described from cadmium sulfide (§ 6.5)	
purple	– manganese	manganese oxide pure	contact allergy not proven	322

ACCIDENTAL CONTACTANTS

5.44 Contact allergy to accidental contactants

Drug	Use	Patch test conc. & vehicle (§ 5.2)	Cross-reactions (§ 5.5)	Comment	Ref.
alprenolol	β-adrenergic blocking agent	1.25–10 mg/ml aqua	metoprolol		133
p-aminosalicylic acid	tuberculostatic drug	10% o.o.			421
aminophylline	smooth muscle relaxant	1% aqua	ethylenediamine hydrochloride	Aminophylline consists of theophylline and ethylenediamine Has caused systemic eczematous contact-type dermatitis (§ 17.2) in an ethylenediamine-sensitive subject	17
anileridine	narcotic	anileridine injection undiluted			131
apomorphine	treatment of alcoholism	0.01–0.1 and 1% aqua	morphine	Has also caused rhinitis and respiratory symptoms in the reported cases	114
benzidine	organic intermediate	3% pet. 1% MEK [180]	other p-amino compounds		16 521
1,4-bis-chloromethyl-benzene		?		Possibly related to bis-(4-chlorophenyl)-methyl-chloride	241
bis-(4-chlorophenyl)-methylchloride	DDT substitute	1% chloroform		For other chlorinated methyl derivatives, *see* [241]	34
bromocholine bromide	antihypertensive drug	?			373
butyl acetate	in penicillin preparation	5% o.o.			349
carbocromen	coronary vasodilator	0.8% aqua			239
p-chlorobenzene-sulfonylglycolic acid nitrile	synthesis of benzodiazepines	0.001% acet.		Controls may react to 0.01% and 0.1%	449
chloroquine diphosphate	antimalarial drug	5% aqua	mepacrine		221
chlorpromazine	sedative	1–2.5–10% aqua	diethazine hydrochloride, promethazine hydrochloride, thiazinamium, ethopropazine hydrochloride		345 387
chlorprothixene	tranquillizer	1% aqua	chlorpromazine derivatives	Has caused photosensitivity (§ 6.5)	267

(continued)

5.44 Accidental contactants

(continuation)

Drug	Use	Patch test conc. & vehicle (§ 5.2)	Cross-reactions (§ 5.5)	Comment	Ref.
codeine	analgesic	1% ethanol		Also occupational rhinitis, sinusitis, bronchitis and conjunctivitis	480
cycloheximide	fungicide	1% pet.	possibly cross-reacting to primary sensitization to neomycin		46
dibenzyline	α-adrenergic receptor blocking agent	1% aqua			307
diethylaminoethyl-chloride hydriodide	cleaning of syringes	0.1% aqua			253
dimercaprol	chelating agent	1% o.o.			100
emetine hydrochloride	antiparasitic drug	3% alc.			389
ethoxyquin	antioxidant in animal feed	0.5% alc. 1% o.o./ pet.			485
etisazole	antifungal drug	2% pet.		Used in veterinary medicine	429
hydrazines	various	0.015–1% aqua	isoniazid, hydralazine, dihydralazine, phenylhydrazine, hydralazine sulfate, β-phenylethyl-hydrazine	May cause toxic reactions	188 432 411 579
hydroquinone	antioxidant	1% pet.		For cosmetic reactions, *see* § 25.44 *and* § 25.45	246
isoamylether of phenylaminoacetate	antispasmodic	5% aqua			164
meclofenoxate	improves cerebral uptake of oxygen and glucose	2.5% ?			171
2-[4(5)-methyl-5(4)-imidazolyl-methyl-thio]-C13	H2-antagonist	0.1% and 1% aqueous and ethanol solution			87
morphine	analgesic	1% aqua		Histamine releaser, urticariogenic	126
nicotinic acid	vitamin	1% aqua	possibly other pyridine derivatives	In the reported case, the reaction to nicotinic acid was a cross-reaction to other pyridine derivatives	579
penethamate hydriodide	antibiotic	25% o.o.	benzyl penicillin		227 231

(continued)

(continuation)

Drug	Use	Patch test conc. & vehicle (§ 5.2)	Cross-reactions (§ 5.5)	Comment	Ref.
phenolphthalein	in laxatives	0.5% alc.			403
phenoxybenzamine	α-adrenergic receptor blocking agent	1% aqua	related haloalkylamines		311 9
piperazine	anthelmintic	1–5% aqua	ethylenediamine hydrochloride, N-methyl-piperazine, N,N′-dimethyl-piperazine, methyl-2-piperazine	Patch testing may have caused respiratory symptoms Has caused systemic eczematous contact-type dermatitis in ethylenediamine-sensitive subjects (§ 17.2)	75 179 362 169 504
propranolol	β-adrenergic receptor blocking agent	1% aqua			307
quinidine sulfate	antiarrhythmic	1% aqua			454 143 455
quinine sulfate	antipyretic antimalarial drug, in liquids (tonic)	1% aqua. 1% pet.	clioquinol (?)	Has caused photosensitivity (§ 5.5); systemic eczematous contact-type dermatitis (§ 17.2)	2,4 174
spiramycin	antibiotic in veterinary medicine	10% aqua 5% pet.	tylosin (?)		231 446
tetraethylthiuram disulfide	therapy for alcoholism	1% pet.	thiram and related compounds		250
tetramisole hydrochloride	veterinary anthelmintic	1% (?)	levamisole (1%?)		509
tribromoethanol	anaesthetic	1% aqua			29
tylosin	antibiotic	1–5% aqua 1–5% pet.	spiramycin		231 446 484 494
vincamine tartrate	used for cerebral circulatory disturbance	1% aqua			427
vitamin B1	vitamin	10% pet. 50% aqua	co-carboxylase	Has caused systemic eczematous contact-type dermatitis (§ 17.2)	225
vitamin K1	antidote to anticoagulants	commercial solution for injection			222
vitamin K3 sodium bisulfite	vitamin	0.1% aqua/pet.	vitamin K4	Has caused dark brown staining in factory workers (*see* § 10.1 and [508])	355 508
vitamin K4	vitamin	0.1% o.o.	vitamin K3		247

5.45 REFERENCES

1. Aaronson, C. M. (1969): Generalised urticaria from sensitivity to nifuroxime. *J. Amer. med. Ass.*, *210*, 557.
2. Aeling, J. L., Panagotacos, P. J. and Andreozzi, R. J. (1973): Allergic contact dermatitis to vitamin E in aerosol deodorant. *Arch. Derm.*, *108*, 579.
3. Afzelius, H. and Thulin, H. (1979): Allergic reactions to benzalkonium chloride. *Contact Dermatitis*, *5*, 60.
4. Ågren, S., Dahlquist, J., Fregert, S. and Person, K. (1980): Allergic contact dermatitis from the preservative N-methylol-chloracetamide. *Contact Dermatitis*, *6*, 302.
5. Alani, M. D. and Alani, S. D. (1972): Allergic contact dermatitis to corticosteroids. *Ann. Allergy*, *36*, 203.
6. Alani, S. D. and Alani, M. D. (1976): Allergic contact dermatitis and conjunctivitis from epinephrine. *Contact Dermatitis*, *2*, 147.
7. Alani, S. D. and Alani, M. D. (1976): Allergic contact dermatitis and conjunctivitis to corticosteroids. *Contact Dermatitis*, *2*, 301.
8. Alcon, D. N. (1947): Sensitivity to iodides and bromides in dermatoses other than dermatitis herpetiformis. *J. Invest. Derm.*, *8*, 287.
9. Alexander, S. and Spector, R. G. (1975): Phenoxybenzamine. *Contact Dermatitis*, *1*, 59.
10. Allenby, C. F. (1965): Skin sensitisation to remiderm and cross-sensitisation to hydroxyquinoline compounds. *Brit. med. J.*, *ii*, 208.
11. Amon, R. B., Lis, A. W. and Hanifin, J. M. (1975): Allergic contact dermatitis caused by idoxuridine: pattern of cross-reactivity with other pyrimidine analogues. *Arch. Derm.*, *111*, 1581.
12. Angelini, G. and Meneghini, C. L. (1981): Contact allergy from propylene glycol. *Contact Dermatitis*, *7*, 197.
13. Angelini, G., Rantuccio, F. and Meneghini, C. L. (1975): Contact dermatitis in patients with leg ulcers. *Contact Dermatitis*, *1*, 81.
14. August, P. J. (1975): Cutaneous necrosis due to cetrimide application. *Brit. med. J.*, *i*, 70.
15. Ayres III, S. and Ayres Jr., S. (1954): Contact dermatitis from chlorcyclizine hydrochloride. *Arch. Derm. Syph.*, *69*, 502.
16. Baer, R. L. (1945): Benzidine as cause of occupational dermatitis in a physician. *J. Amer. med. Ass.*, *129*, 442.
17. Baer, R. L., Cohen, H. J. and Neideroff, A. H. (1959): Allergic eczematous sensitivity to aminophyllin. *Arch. Derm.*, *81*, 647.
18. Baer, R. L., Michaelides, P. and Prestia, A. E. (1972): Failure to induce immune tolerance to nitrogen mustard. *J. invest. Derm.*, *58*, 1.
19. Baer, R. L., Ramsey, D. L. and Biondi, E. (1973): The most common contact allergens. *Arch. Derm.*, *108*, 74.
20. Baer, R. L., Serri, F. and Weissenbach-Vidal, Chr. (1955): Studies on allergic sensitization to certain topical therapeutic agents. *Arch. Derm. Syph.*, *71*, 19.
21. Baes, H. (1974): Allergic contact dermatitis to virginiamycin. *Dermatologica (Basel)*, *149*, 231.
22. Baker, H., Ive, F. A. and Lloyd, M. J. (1969): Primary irritant dermatitis of the scrotum due to hexachlorophene. *Arch. Derm.*, *99*, 693.
23. Bandmann, H. J. (1967): Kontaktekzem und Ekzematogene. *Münch. med. Wschr.*, *109*, 1572.
24. Bandmann, H. J. (1971): Ichthyol dermatitis. *Contact Dermatitis Newsl.*, *10*, 224.
25. Bandmann, H. J. and Breit, R. (1973): The mafenide story. *Brit. J. Derm.*, *89*, 219.
26. Bandmann, H. J., Breit, R. and Mutzeck, E. (1974): Allergic contact dermatitis from Proxymetacaine. *Contact Dermatitis Newsl.*, *15*, 451.
27. Bandmann, H. J. and Doenicke, A. (1971): Allergisches Kontaktekzem durch Propanidid bei einem Anesthesisten. *Berufsdermatosen*, *19*, 160.
28. Bandmann, H. J. and Dohn, W. (1967): *Die Epikutantestung*, p. 170. Bergmann, Munich.
29. Bandmann, H. J. and Dohn, W. (1967): *Die Epikutantestung*, p. 288. Bergmann, Munich.
30. Bandmann, H. J., Huber-Riffeser, G. and Woyton, A. (1966): Kontaktallergie gegen Triamcinolonacetonid. *Hautarzt*, *17*, 183.
31. Bandmann, H. J. and Keilig, W. (1980): Lanette O – another test substance for lower leg series. *Contact Dermatitis*, *6*, 227.
32. Bandmann, H. J. and Mutzeck, E. (1973): Contact allergy to gentamycin sulfate. *Contact Dermatitis Newsl.*, *13*, 371.
33. Bandmann, M. (1967): *Zur monovalenten Kontaktallergie gegen Eucerinum anhydricum*. Thesis, Munich.

34. Bang-Pedersen, N., Thormann, J. and Senning, A. (1980): Occupational contact allergy to bis-4(4-chlorophenyl)-methylchloride. *Contact Dermatitis, 6,* 56.
35. Bedoukian, P. Z. (1952): Aspects of aging in perfumes. *Amer. Perfumer Essent. Oil Rev., 22,* 263.
36. Beetz, D., Cramer, H. J. and Mehlhorn, H. Ch. (1971): Zur Häufigkeit der epidermalen Allergie gegenüber Kamille in Kamillenhaltigen Arzneimitteln und Kosmetika. *Derm. Mschr., 157,* 505.
37. Behrbohm, P. (1962): Über allergische Krankheit durch DDT und HCH. *Allergie u. Asthma, 8,* 237.
38. Behrbohm, P. and Brandt, B. (1960): Allergisches Kontaktekzem durch technische und gereinigte Hexachlorcyclohexanpräparate bei der Anwendung im Pflanzenschutz und in der Schädlingsbekämpfung. *Berufsdermatosen, 8,* 95.
39. Behrbohm, P. and Lenzner, M. (1975): Sensitivity to falicain (propoxypiperocainhydrochloride). *Contact Dermatitis, 1,* 187.
40. Behrbohm, P. and Zschunke, E. (1965): Allergisches Ekzem durch das Antimykotikum 'Afungin' (Dibenzthion). *Derm. Wschr., 151,* 1447.
41. Bentley-Phillips, B. and Bayler, M. A. H. (1975): Cutaneous reactions to topical application of hydroquinone. *S. Afr. med. J., 49,* 1391.
42. Bereston, E. S. (1952): Contact dermatitis due to N-ethyl-o-croton-o-toluidine ointment (Eurax®). *Arch. Derm. Syph., 65,* 100.
43. Berlin, A. R. and Miller, F. (1976): Allergic contact dermatitis from ethyl sebacate in Haloprogin cream. *Arch. Derm., 112,* 1563.
44. Bielicky, T. and Novák, M. (1969): Contact group sensitisation to triphenylmethane dyes. *Arch. Dermatol., 100,* 540.
45. Binnick, A. N. and Clendenning, W. E. (1978): Bacitracin contact dermatitis. *Contact Dermatitis, 4,* 181.
46. Black, H. (1971): Allergy to cycloheximide (Actidione). *Contact Dermatitis Newsl., 10,* 243.
47. Black, H. (1975): Contact dermatitis from stearyl alcohol in Metosyn (fluocinonide) cream. *Contact Dermatitis, 1,* 125.
48. Bleumink, E. and Nater, J. P. (1972): Allergic contact dermatitis to virginiamycin. *Dermatologica (Basel), 144,* 253.
49. Bleumink, E., Te Lintum, J. C. A. and Nater, J. P. (1974): Kontaktallergie durch Nitrofurazon (furacin) and Nifurprazin (Carofur). *Hautarzt, 25,* 403.
50. Blondeel, A., Oleffe, J. and Achten, G. (1978): Contact allergy in 330 dermatological patients. *Contact Dermatitis, 4,* 270.
51. Bloom, D. (1940): Eczema venenatum (perfume). *Arch. Derm., 42,* 968.
52. Bojs, G. and Möller, H. (1974): Eczematous contact allergy to oxytetracycline with cross-sensitivity to other tetracyclines. *Berufsdermatosen, 22,* 202.
53. Boxley, J. D. and Dawber, R. P. R. (1967): Contact dermatitis to one ingredient of Xerumenex eardrops. *Contact Dermatitis, 2,* 233.
54. Brandao, F. M. and Camarasa, F. M. (1979): Contact allergy to hydrocortisone 17-butyrate. *Contact Dermatitis, 5,* 354.
55. Braun, W. P. H. (1975): Contact allergy to collagenase mixture (IRUXOL). *Contact Dermatitis, 1,* 241.
56. Braun, W. and Schütz, R. (1968): Kontaktallergie gegen Nitrofurazon (Furacin). *Dtsch. med. Wschr., 93,* 1524.
57. Breit, R. and Bandmann, H. J. (1973): The wide world of antimycotics. *Brit. J. Derm., 89,* 657.
58. Brown, E. A. (1948): Reactions to penicillin. A review of the literature 1943-1948. *Ann. Allergy, 6,* 723.
59. Brown, R. (1979): Another case of sorbic acid sensitivity. *Contact Dermatitis, 5, 268.*
60. Brown, R. (1980): Allergy to hydrocortisone-17-butyrate. *Contact Dermatitis, 6, 504.*
61. Brown, R. (1981): Chlorphenesin sensitivity. *Contact Dermatitis, 7,* 162.
62. Brun, R. (1970): Eczéma de contact á un antioxidant de la margarine (gallate) et changement de metier. *Dermatologica (Basel), 140,* 390.
63. Bunney, M. H. (1972): Contact dermatitis due to betamethasone-17-valerate (Betnovate). *Contact Dermatitis Newsl., 12,* 318.
64. Burckhardt, W. and Hellerström, S. (1932): Sensibilisierung gegen Leinsamen. *Acta Derm.-venereol. (Stockh.), 13,* 712.
65. Burckhardt, W., Mahler, F. and Schwarz-Speck, M. (1968): Photoallergische Ekzeme durch Mycanodin. *Dermatologica (Basel), 137,* 208.
66. Burry, J. N. (1967): Photoallergies to fenticlor and multifungin. *Arch. Derm., 95,* 287.
67. Burry, J. N. (1978): Ethylenediamine sensitivity with a systemic reaction to piperazine citrate. *Contact Dermatitis, 4,* 380.

68. Burry, J. N. and Hunter G. A. (1970): Photocontact dermatitis from Jadit. *Brit. J. Derm., 82,* 224.
69. Burry, J. N., Kirk, J., Reid, J. G. and Turner, T. (1973): Environmental dermatitis: patch tests in 1000 cases of allergic contact dermatitis. *Med. J. Aust., 2,* 681.
70. Burry, J. N. Kirk, J. Reid, J. G. and Turner, T. (1975): Chlorocresol sensitivity. *Contact Dermatitis, 1,* 41.
71. Cairns, R. J. and Calnan, C. D. (1962): Green tattoo reactions associated with cement dermatitis. *Brit. J. Derm., 74,* 288.
72. Calnan, C. D. (1962): Contact dermatitis from drugs. *Proc. Roy. Soc. Med., 55,* 39.
73. Calnan, C. D. (1967): Chlortetracycline sensitivity. *Contact Dermatitis Newsl., 1,* 16.
74. Calnan, C. D. (1975): Dibutyl phthalate. *Contact Dermatitis, 1,* 388.
75. Calnan, C. D. (1975): Occupational piperazine dermatitis. *Contact Dermatitis, 1,* 126.
76. Calnan, C. D. (1975): Sensitivity to benzamine lactate. *Contact Dermatitis, 1,* 56.
77. Calnan, C. D. (1976): Cinnamon dermatitis from an ointment. *Contact Dermatitis, 2,* 167.
78. Calnan, C. D. (1976): Use and abuse of topical steroids. *Dermatologica (Basel), 152* (Suppl. 1), 247.
79. Calnan, C. D. (1978): Diphenylamine. *Contact Dermatitis, 4,* 301.
80. Calnan, C. D. (1978): Oxypolyethoxydodecane in an ointment. *Contact Dermatitis, 4,* 168.
81. Calnan, C. D. (1979): Allergy to idoxuridine ointment. *Contact Dermatitis, 5,* 194.
82. Calnan, C. D. (1979): Unusual hydroxycitronellal perfume dermatitis. *Contact Dermatitis, 5,* 123.
83. Calnan, C. D. (1980): Allergy to the local anaesthetic diperodon. *Contact Dermatitis, 6,* 367.
84. Calnan, C. D. and Sarkany, L. (1960): Sensitivity to oleyl alcohol. *Trans. St. John's Hosp. derm. Soc. (Lond.) 44,* 47.
85. Camarasa, G. (1976): Contact dermatitis from mercurochrome. *Contact Dermatitis, 2,* 120.
86. Camarasa, G. and Alomar, A. (1978): Mentholdermatitis from cigarettes. *Contact Dermatitis, 4,* 169.
87. Camarasa, G. and Alomar, A. (1980): Contact dermatitis to an H2-antagonist. *Contact Dermatitis, 6, 152.*
88. Camarasa, J. M. G. and Alomar, A. (1980): Contact dermatitis from Karaya seal ring. *Contact Dermatitis, 6,* 139.
89. Caro, J. (1978): Contact allergy/photoallergy to glyceryl PABA and benzocaine. *Contact Dermatitis, 4,* 381.
90. Carruthers, J. A. and Cronin, E. (1976): Incidence of neomycin and framycetin sensitivity. *Contact Dermatitis, 2,* 269.
91. Omitted.
92. Clark, E. W. (1975): Estimation of the general incidenec of specific lanolin allergy. *J. Soc. cosmet. Chem., 26,* 323.
93. Comaish, J. S. (1970): Reaction to Triton X 45. *Contact Dermatitis Newsl., 7,* 167.
94. Comaish, J. S. and Kersey, P. J. (1980): Contact dermatitis to extract of horse chestnut (esculin). *Contact Dermatitis, 6, 150.*
95. Conant M. and Maibach, H. I. (1974): Allergic contact dermatitis due to neutral red. *Arch. Derm., 109,* 735.
96. Connor, B. L. (1973): Mesulphen in tineafax ointment. *Contact Dermatitis Newsl., 14,* 417.
97. Bunney, M. H. (1972): Contact dermatitis due to betamethasone-17-valerate (Betnovate). *Contact Dermatitis Newsl., 12,* 318.
98. Dupont, C. (1972): Sensitivity to Fentichlor. *Contact Dermatitis Newsl., 12,* 327.
99. Cooke, M. A. and Hocken Robertson, D. E. (1972): Ichthammol dermatitis. *Contact Dermatitis Newsl., 11, 299.*
100. Cornbleet, T. (1947): Skin sensitization to B. A. L. *J. invest. Derm., 9,* 281.
101. Coskey, R. J. (1971): Contact Dermatitis due to nystatin. *Arch. Derm., 103,* 228.
102. Coskey, R. J. (1978): Contact dermatitis due to multiple corticosteroid creams. *Arch. Derm., 114,* 115.
103. Coskey, R. J. (1978): Contact dermatitis owing to tincture of benzoin. *Arch. Derm., 114,* 128.
104. Coskey, R. J. (1978): Contact dermatitis due to clindamycin. *Arch. Derm., 114, 446.*
105. Coskey, R. J. and Bryan, H. G. (1967): Contact dermatitis due to methylprednisolone. *J. Amer. med. Ass., 199,* 136.
106. Council on Drugs (1966): A new agent for the treatment of candidal vaginitis: Candicidin (Candeptin). *J. Amer. med. Ass., 196,* 1144.
107. Coyle, H. E. Miller, E. and Chapman, R. S. (1981): Sorbic acid sensitivity from unguentum Merck® *Contact Dermatitis, 7,* 56.
108. Cronin, E. (1969) Genetris pessaries. *Contact Dermatitis Newsl., 6,* 134.
109. Cronin, E. (1980): Lipstick dermatitis due to propylgallate. *Contact Dermatitis, 6,* 213.

110. Cronin, E. (1980): Cosmetics. In: *Contact Dermatitis*, p. 149. Churchill Livingstone, Edinburgh.
111. Cronin, E. (1980): Medicaments. In: *Contact Dermatitis*, p. 198. Churchill Livingstone, Edinburgh.
112. Cronin, E. (1980): *Contact Dermatitis*, p. 236. Churchill Livingstone, Edinburgh.
113. Dahlquist, I. (1977): Contact dermatitis to a veterinary fungicide. *Contact Dermatitis, 3*, 277.
114. Dahlquist, I. (1977): Allergic reactions to apomorphine. *Contact Dermatitis, 3*, 349.
115. Dahlquist, I. and Fregert, S. (1978): Formaldehyde releasers. *Contact Dermatitis, 4*, 173.
116. Dahlquist, I. and Fregert S. (1980): Contact allergy to atranorin in Lichens and perfumes *Contact Dermatitis, 6*, 111.
117. Daly, J. F. (1952): Contact dermatitis due to 'Quotane'. *Arch. Derm. Syph., 66*, 393.
118. Dave, V. K. and Main, R. A. (1973): Contact sensitivity to sodium fusidate. *Contact Dermatitis Newsl., 14*, 398.
119. Degreef, H. and Verhoeve, L. (1975): Contact dermatitis to miconazole nitrate. *Contact Dermatitis, 1*, 269.
120. De Groot, A. C. and Nater, J. P. (1981): Contact allergy to dithranol. *Contact Dermatitis, 7*, 5.
121. Omitted.
122. Dong Gil Byun, Young Hoe Kim, Yang Ja Park and Soon Bok Lee (1975): Treatment of hyperpigmented disease with 4-isopropyl catechol (Korean). *Kor. J. Derm., 13*, 5.
123. Dooms-Goossens, A. and Degreef, H. (1980): Sensitization to yellow petrolatum used as a vehicle for patch testing. *Contact Dermatitis, 6*, 146.
124. Dooms-Goossens, A., Degreef, H. and Luytens, E. (1979): Dihydroabietyl alcohol (Abitol), a sensitizer in mascara. *Contact Dermatitis, 5*, 350.
125. Dooms-Goossens, A., Degreef, H., Van Hee, J., Kerkhofs L. and Chrispeels, M. T. (1981): Chlorocresol and chloracetamide, allergens in medications, glues and cosmetics. *Contact Dermatitis, 7, 51*.
126. Dore, S. E. and Prosser Thomas, E. W. (1944): Contact dermatitis in a morphine factory. *Brit. J. Derm., 56*, 177.
127. Dorsey, C. S. (1960): Dermatitic and pigmentary reactions to monobenzylether of hydroquinone. *Arch. Derm., 81*, 245.
128. Drug Evaluations (1971): *Antihistamines*, pp. 367-368. American Medical Association, Chicago, Ill.
129. Dupont, C. (1972): Sensitivity to Fentichlor. *Contact Dermatitis Newsl., 12*, 327.
130. Ebner, H. (1974): Perubalsam und Parfums. Untersuchungen über allergologische Beziehungen zwischen diesen Substanzen. *Hautarzt, 25*, 123.
131. Ecker, R. J. (1980): Contact dermatitis to anileridine. *Contact Dermatitis, 6*, 495.
132. Edwards, M. and Rudner, E. J. (1970): Dermatitis venenata due to hydrocortisone alcohol. *Cutis, 6*, 757.
133. Ekenval, L. and Forsbeck, M. (1978): Contact eczema produced by a β-adrenergic blocking agent (alprenolol). *Contact Dermatitis, 4*, 190.
134. Ellis, F. A. and Bundick, W. R. (1949): Reactions to the local use of thephorin. *J. invest. Derm., 13*, 25.
135. Epstein, E. (1966): Dichlorophene allergy. *Ann. Allergy, 24*, 437.
136. Epstein, E. (1980): Contact dermatitis to neomycin with false negative patch tests: Allergy established by intradermal and usage tests. *Contact Dermatitis, 6*, 219.
137. Epstein, E. (1980): Contact dermatitis to 5-fluorouracil with false negative patch tests. *Contact Dermatitis, 6*, 220.
138. Epstein, E. Rees, W. J. and Maibach, H. I. (1968): Recent experience with routine patch testing screening. *Arch. Derm., 98*, 18.
139. Epstein, J. H., Wuepper, K. D. and Maibach, H. I. (1968): Photocontact dermatitis to halogenated salicylanilides and related compounds. *Arch. Derm., 97*, 236.
140. Eriksen, K. (1978): Cross allergy between paranitro-compounds with special reference to DNCB and chloramphenicol. *Contact Dermatitis, 4*, 29.
141. Eriksen, K. E. (1975): Allergy to ethylenediamine. *Arch. Derm., 111*, 791.
142. Fanta, D. and Miescher, P. (1976): Contact dermatitis from tromantadine hydrochloride. *Contact Dermatitis, 2*, 282.
143. Fernström, A. T. B. (1965): Occupational quinidine contact dermatitis, a concept apparently not yet described. *Acta derm.-venereol. (Stockh.), 45*, 129.
144. Finn, O. A. and Forsyth, A. (1975): Contact dermatitis due to sorbitan monolaurate. *Contact Dermatitis, 1*, 318.
145. Fisher, A. A. (1965): Paraphenylene diamine, one of the 'BIG FIVE' in allergic contact dermatitis. *Cutis, 1*, 171.
146. Fisher, A. A. (1973): Allergic reactions to feminine hygiene sprays. *Arch. Derm., 108*, 801.
147. Fisher, A. A. (1973): *Contact Dermatitis*, 2nd Edition, p. 59. Lea and Febiger, Philadelphia.

5.45 Contact allergy to topical drugs

148. Fisher, A. A. (1973): *Contact Dermatitis, 2nd Edition*, pp. 295-297. Lea and Febiger, Philadelphia.
149. Fisher, A. A. (1973): *Contact Dermatitis*, 2nd Edition, p. 371. Lea and Febiger, Philadelphia.
150. Fisher, A. A. (1973): The broad implications of allergic sensitization to ethylenediamine hydrochloride. *Contact Dermatitis Newsl., 14, 418.*
151. Fisher, A. A. (1974): Contact dermatitis from stearyl alcohol and propylene glycol. *Arch. Derm., 110,* 636.
152. Fisher, A. A. (1975): Allergic contact dermatitis from Germall 115, a new cosmetic preservative. *Contact Dermatitis, 1,* 126.
153. Fisher, A. A. (1975): Patch testing with perfume ingredients. *Contact Dermatitis, 1,* 166.
154. Fisher, A. A. (1975): Allergic paraben and benzyl alcohol hypersensitivity relationship of the 'delayed' and 'immediate' varieties. *Contact Dermatitis, 1,* 281.
155. Fisher, A. A. (1975): Allergic contact dermatitis in animal feed handlers. *Cutis, 16,* 201.
156. Fisher, A. A. (1975): Contact dermatitis due to food additives. *Cutis, 16,* 961.
157. Fisher, A. A. (1978): Immediate and delayed allergic contact reactions to polyethylene glycol. *Contact Dermatitis, 4,* 135.
158. Fisher, A. A. (1980): Perfume dermatitis, part I. *Cutis, 26,* 458.
159. Fisher, A. A. and Brancaccio, R. R. (1979): Allergic contact sensitivity to propylene glycol in a lubricant jelly. *Arch. Derm., 115,* 1451.
160. Fisher, A. A. and Dooms-Goossens, A. (1976): The effect of perfume 'aging' on the allergenicity of individual perfume ingredients. *Contact Dermatitis, 2,* 155.
161. Fisher, A. A., Pascher, F. and Kanof, F. N. B. (1971): Allergic contact dermatitis due to ingredients of vehicles. *Arch. Derm., 104,* 286.
162. Fisher, A. A. and Stillman, M. A. (1972): Allergic contact sensitivity to benzalkoniumchloride (BAK). Cutaneous, ophthalmic and general medical implications. *Arch. Derm., 106,* 169.
163. Fisherman, E. W. and Cohen, G. (1973): Chemical intolerance to butylated hydroxyanisole (BHA) and butylated hydroxytoluene (BHT) and vascular response as an indicator and monitor of drug intolerance. *Ann. Allergy, 31,* 126.
164. Folesky, H. J. and Zschunke, E. (1962): Allergisches Ekzem durch Phenylaminoessigsäure Isoamylester (Aklonin). *Berufsdermatosen, 10,* 337.
165. Förström, L., Hannuksela, M., Idänpään-Heikkilä, J. and Salo, O. P. (1977): Hypersensitivity reactions to Gerovital. *Dermatologica (Basel) 154,* 367.
166. Förström, L., Hannuksela, M., Kousa, M. and Lehmuskallio, E. (1980); Merthiolate hypersensitivity and vaccination. *Contact Dermatitis, 6,* 341.
167. Forström, L. and Pirilä, V. (1978): Cross-sensitivity within the neomycin group of antibiotics. *Contact Dermatitis, 4,* 312.
168. Foussereau, J. and Benezra, Cl. (1970): *Les Eczémas Allergiques Professionnels*, p. 61. Masson et Cie., Paris.
169. Foussereau, J. and Benezra, Cl. (1970): *Les Eczémas Allergiques Professionnels*, p. 63. Masson et Cie., Paris.
170. Foussereau, J., Benezra, C. and Ourisson, G. (1967): Contact dermatitis from Laurel. *Trans. St. John's Hosp. med. Soc. (Lond.), 53,* 141.
171. Foussereau, J. and Lantz, J. P. (1972): Allergy to meclofenoxate. *Contact Dermatitis Newsl., 12,* 321.
172. Foussereau, J., Limam-Mestiri, S. and Khochnevis, A. (1971): Allergy to nystatin. *Contact Dermatitis Newsl., 10,* 221.
173. Foussereau, J., Schlewer, G., Chabeau, G. and Reimeringer, A. (1980): Étude allergologique d'intolérances à la colophane. *Dermatosen, 28,* 14.
174. Frain Bell, W., Johnson, B. E., Gardiner, J. M. and Zaynoun, S. (1975): A study of persistent light reaction in quindoxin and quinine photosensitivity. *Brit. J. Derm., 93,* suppl. 11, 21.
175. Fräki, J. E., Peltonen, L. and Hopsu-Havu, V. K. (1979): Allergy to various components of topical preparations in stasis dermatitis and leg ulcers. *Contact Dermatitis, 5,* 97.
176. Fregert, S. (1968): Cross-sensitization among nitrofurylaminothiadazoles. *Acta derm.-venereol. (Stockh.), 48,* 106.
177. Fregert, S. et al (1969): Epidemiology of contact dermatitis. *Trans. St. John's Hosp. Derm. Soc. (Lond.), 55,* 17.
178. Fregert, S. (1970): Sensitization to phenylacetaldehyde. *Dermatologica (Basel), 141,* 11.
179. Fregert, S. (1976): Respiratory symptoms with piperazine patch testing. *Contact Dermatitis, 2,* 61.
180. Fregert, S. (1981): *Manual of Contact Dermatitis*, 2nd Edition. Munksgaard, Copenhagen.
181. Fregert, S., Groth, O., Gruvberger, B., Magnusson, B., Mobacken, H. and Rorsman, H. (1971): Hypersensitivity to secondary alcohols. *Acta derm.-venereol. (Stockh.), 51,* 271.

182. Fregert, S. and Hjorth, N. (1969): Increasing incidence of mercury sensitivity. The possible role of organic mercury compounds. *Contact Dermatitis Newsl., 5*, 88.

183. Fregert, S. and Hjorth, N. (1979): In: *Textbook of Dermatology*, 3rd Edition, p. 476. Editors: A. Rook, D. S. Wilkinson and F. J. G. Ebling. Blackwell Scientific Publications, Oxford.

184. Fregert, S. and Möller, H. (1962): Hypersensitivity to the cholinesterase inhibitor di-iso-propoxy-phosphorylfluoride. *J. invest. Derm., 38*, 371.

185. Fregert, S. and Rorsman, H. (1962): Hypersensitivity to diethylstilbestrol with cross-sensitization to benzestrol. *Acta derm.-venereol. (Stockh.), 42*, 290.

186. Fregert, S., Tegner, E. and Thelin, I. (1979): Contact allergy to lidocaine. *Contact Dermatitis, 5*, 185.

187. Frenk, E. (1962): Akute Putzmittelekzeme der Hände durch Tetrachlorsalicylanilid. *Dermatologica, (Basel), 124*, 433.

188. Frost, J. and Hjorth, N. (1959): Contact dermatitis from hydrazine hydrochloride in soldering flux. *Acta derm.-venereol. (Stockh.), 39*, 82.

189. Garcia-Perez, A. and Moran. M. (1975): Dermatitis from quinolines. *Contact Dermatitis, 1*, 260.

190. Gasser, E. (1953): Coiffeur-Ekzem, verursacht durch Thioglycerin enthaltende Kaltdauerwellen-wasser. Inaugural Diss. Zürich.

191. Gastelain, P.Y and Piriou, A. (1980): Contact dermatitis due to propanidid in an anesthesist. *Contact Dermatitis, 6*, 360.

192. Gaul, L. E. (1964): Contact dermatitis from synthetic Oil of Mustard (allylisothiocyanate). *Arch. Derm., 90*, 158.

193. Gaul, L. E. (1969): Dermatitis from cetyl and stearyl alcohols. *Arch. Derm., 99*, 593.

194. Gelfarb, M. and Leiden, M. (1960): Allergic eczematous contact dermatitis. *Arch. Derm., 82*, 642.

195. Gellin, G. A., Maibach, H. I. and Wachs, G. N. (1972): Contact allergy to tolnaftate. *Arch. Derm., 106*, 715.

196. Omitted.

197. Girard, J. P. (1978): Recurrent angioneurotic oedema and contact dermatitis due to penicillin. *Contact Dermatitis, 4*, 309.

198. Goette, D. K., Odom, R. B. and Owens R. (1977): Allergic contact dermatitis from topical fluorour-acil. *Arch. Derm., 113*, 196.

199. Goldman, L., Feldman, M. D. and Altemeier, W. A. (1948): Contact dermatitis from topical tyrothricin and associated with polyvalent hypersensitivity to various antibiotics. *J. invest. Derm., 11*, 243.

200. Gottschalk, H. R. and Stone, O. J. (1976): Stevens-Johnson syndrome from ophthalmic sulfon-amide. *Arch. Derm., 112*, 513.

201. Greenberg, L. A. and Lester, D. (1954): *Handbook of Cosmetic Materials*. Interscience, New York.

202. Grice, K. and Johnstone, C. J. (1972): Contact dermatitis from cerumenex. *Brit. med. J., i*, 508.

203. Grimalt, F. and Romaguera, C. (1978): Sensitivity to petrolatum. *Contact Dermatitis, 4*, 377.

204. Groen, J., Bleumink, E. and Nater, J. P. (1973): Variotin sensitivity. *Contact Dermatitis Newsl., 15*, 456.

205. Gutzwiller, P. (1974): Zum Problem der Kortikosteroid-Allergie. *Dermatologica (Basel), 148*, 253.

206. Haidar, Z. (1978): An adverse reaction to a topical antiseptic (cetrimide). *Brit. J. oral Surg., 16*, 86.

207. Hannuksela, M. (1979): Frequent contact allergy to higher fatty alcohols. *IV International Sympo-sion on Contact Dermatitis*. San Francisco, March 29-31, 1979.

208. Hannuksela, M. and Forström, L. (1976): Contact hypersensitivity to glycerol. *Contact Dermatitis, 2*, 291.

209. Hannuksela, M., Kousa, M. and Pirilä, V. (1976): Allergy ingredients of vehicles. *Contact Dermatitis, 2*, 105.

210. Hannuksela, M., Kousa, M. and Pirilä, V. (1976): Contact sensitivity to emulsifiers. *Contact Dermatitis, 2*, 201.

211. Hannuksela, M., Pirilä, V. and Salo, O. P. (1975): Skin reactions to propylene glycol. *Contact Dermatitis, 1*, 112.

212. Hansson, H. and Möller, H. (1970): Patch test reactions to merthiolate in healthy young subjects. *Brit. J. Derm., 83*, 349.

213. Harber, C. L., Harris, H., Leder, M. and Baer, R. L. (1964): Berloque dermatitis. *Arch Derm., 90*, 572.

214. Hardie, R. A., Savin, J. A., White, D. A. and Pumford, S. (1978): Quinine dermatitis: investigation in a factory outbreak. *Contact Dermatitis, 4*, 121.

215. Harman, R. R. M. (1961): Severe contact reaction to dihydroxyacetone. *Trans. St. John's Hosp. derm. Soc. (Lond.)*, *47*, 157.

216. Hartung, J. and Rudolph, P. O. (1970): Epidermale Allergie gegen Hydroxypolyaethoxydodekan. *Z. Haut. u. Geschl.kr. 45*, 547.

217. Hausen, B. M. (1978): Identification of allergens in Arnica Montana. *Contact Dermatitis, 4*, 308.

218. Helander, I., Hollmén, A. and Hopsu-Havu, V. K. (1979): Allergic contact dermatitis to chlordantoin. *Contact Dermatitis, 5*, 54.

219. Helm, F. and Klein, E. (1965): Effects of allergic contact dermatitis on basal cell epitheliomas. *Arch. Derm., 91*, 142.

220. Hendricks, A. A. and Dec, G. W. (1979): Contact dermatitis due to nitroglycerin ointment. *Arch. Derm., 115*, 853.

221. Herrmann, W. P. and Schulz, K. H. (1965): Allergisches Kontaktekzem durch Resochin. *Dermatologica (Basel), 130*, 216.

222. Heydenreich, G. (1977): A further case of adverse skin reaction from vitamin K1. *Brit. J. Derm., 97*, 697.

223. Heyer, A. (1961): Sensitisation to xanthocillin in salve. *Acta derm.-venereol. (Stockh.), 41*, 201.

224. Hindson, C. (1977): Contact eczema from methyl salicylate reproduced by oral aspirin (acetylsalicylic acid). *Contact dermatitis, 3*, 348.

225. Hjorth, N. (1958): Contact dermatitis from vitamin B (thiamine). *J. invest. Derm., 30*, 261.

226. Hjorth, N. (1961): Eczematous allergy to balsams, allied perfumes and flavouring agents. *Acta derm.-venereol. (Stockh.), 41*, suppl. 46.

227. Hjorth, N. (1967): Occupational dermatitis among veterinary surgeons caused by penethamate. *Berufsdermatosen, 15*, 163.

228. Hjorth, N. (1972): Contact dermatitis from 1,3-diiodo-2-hydroxypropane. *Contact dermatitis Newsl., 12*, 322.

229. Hjorth, N. and Trolle-Lassen, C. (1962): Skin reactions to preservatives in creams with special regards to paraben esters and sorbic acid. *Amer. Perf., 77*, 146.

230. Hjorth, N. and Trolle-Lassen, C. (1963): Skin reactions to ointment bases. *Trans. St. John's Hosp. derm. Soc. (Lond.), 49*, 127.

231. Hjorth, N. and Weissmann, K. (1973): Occupational dermatitis among veterinary surgeons caused by spiramycin, tylosin and penethamate. *Acta derm.-venereol. (Stockh.), 53*, 229.

232. Hoffman, M. J. and Peters, J. (1935): Dermatitis due to facial cream, caused by methyl heptine carbonate. *J. Amer. med. Ass., 104*, 1072.

233. Hoffman, Th. E. and Adams R. M. (1978): Contact dermatitis to grease paint make up. *Contact Dermatitis, 4*, 379.

234. Holst, R. and Möller, H. (1975): Merthiolate testing in twins. *Contact Dermatitis, 1*, 370.

235. Huber-Riffeser, G. (1978): Allergic contact dermatitis to polidocanol (Thesit). *Contact Dermatitis, 4*, 245.

236. Hull, P. R. and de Beer, H. A. (1977): Topical nitrofurazone, a potent sensitizer of the skin and mucosae. *S. Afr. med. J., 52*, 189.

237. Hunziker, N. (1961): Réaction eczémateuses aux dérivés de l'oxyquinaléine. *Dermatologica (Basel), 122*, 26.

238. Huriez, C. and Martin, P. (1974): Conséquences pratiques des recherches d'isolement et d'identification chimiques des allergènes végétaux. In: *Actualités allergologiques*, pp 83-87. Expansion Scientifique, Paris.

239. Huriez, Cl., Martin, P., Bétourné, M. and Martin, H. J. (1974): Sensitivity to carbocromène. *Contact Dermatitis Newsl., 15*, 429.

240. Ippen, H. (1981): Kontaktallergie auf Dexpanthenol. *Dermatosen Beruf Umw., 2*, 45.

241. Ippen, H. and Liebeskind, H. (1978): Kontaktekzem durch 1,4-Bis-chlormethylbenzol. *Dermatosen, 26*, 97.

242. Jadassohn, J. (1896): Verhandlungen der Deutschen Dermatologischen Gesellschaft. Bericht über die Verhandlung des V. Kongresses. *Arch. Derm. Syph. (Berl.), 34*, 103.

243. Jannasch, G. (1962): Beitrag zur Kontaktallergie durch moderne Antibiotika. *Z. Haut-u. Geschl.kr., 33*, 158.

244. Jelen, G., Schlewer, G., Chabeau, G. and Foussereau, J. (1979): Eczemas due to plant allergens in manufactured products. *Acta derm.-venereol. (Stockh.), 59*, suppl. 85, 91.

245. Jensen, O. (1981): Contact allergy to propylene oxide and isopropyl alcohol in a skin disinfectant swab. *Contact Dermatitis, 7*, 148.

246. Jirásek, L. and Kalensky, J. (1975): Kontakni alergický ekzém z krmných směsi v živočisné výrobě. *Čs. Derm., 50*, 217.

247. Jirásek, L. and Schwank, R. (1965): Berufskontaktekzem durch Vitamin K. *Hautarzt, 16,* 351.
248. Jordan, W. P., Dahl, M. V. and Albert, H. L. (1972): Contact dermatitis from glutaraldehyde. *Arch. Derm., 105,* 94.
249. Jung, E. G. and Schwarz, K. (1965): Photoallergy from 'Jadit' with photocrossreactions to derivatives of sulfanilamide. *Int. Arch. Allergy, 27,* 313.
250. Kaalund-Jörgensen, O. (1949): Eczem efter ekstern pävirkning of Antabus. *Ugeskr. Laeg., 31/3,* 373.
251. Kaidbey, K. H. and Kligman, A. M. (1978): Photocontact allergy to 6-methyl coumarin. *Contact Dermatitis, 4,* 277.
252. Kalveram, K., Günnewig, W., Wehling, K. and Forck, G. (1978): Tetracaine allergy: cross-reactions with para compounds? *Contact Dermatitis, 4,* 376.
253. Kärcher, K. H. (1957): Zur pathogenese der lokalen Sensibilisierung durch Penicillinester. (Pulmo 500). *Derm. Wschr., 136,* 1071.
254. Keczkes, K. and Brown, P. M. (1976): Hexahydro-1,3,5,tris(2-hydroxyethyl)triazine, a new bactericidal agent as a cause of allergic contact dermatitis. *Contact Dermatitis, 2,* 92.
255. Keil, H. (1947): Contact dermatitis due to oil of citronella. *J. invest. Derm. 8,* 327.
256. Keil, H. (1962): Group reactions in contact dermatitis due to resorcinol. *Arch. Derm., 86,* 212.
257. Kero, M., Hannuksela, M. and Sothman, A. (1979): Primary irritant dermatitis from topical clioquinol. *Contact Dermatitis, 5,* 115.
258. Klaschka, F. (1975): Contact allergy to chloracetamide. *Contact Dermatitis, 1,* 265.
259. Knisley, R. E., Settipane, G. A. and Albala, M. M. (1971): Unusual reaction to chlorambucil in a patient with chronic lymphatic leukaemia. *Arch. Derm., 104,* 77.
260. Kooy, R. and van Vloten, Th. J. (1952): Epidermal sensitization due to sulphonamide drugs. *Dermatologica (Basel), 104,* 151.
261. Kounis, N. G. (1976): Untoward reaction to corticosteroids: intolerance to hydrocortisone. *Ann. Allergy, 36,* 203.
262. Kozáková, M. (1976): Sub-shock state brought on by epidermic skin test for chloramphenicol. *Čs. Derm., 51,* 82.
263. Krook, G. (1975): Contact sensitivity to oxyphenbutazone (Tanderil) and cross-sensitivity to phenylbutazone (Butazolidin). *Contact Dermatitis, 1,* 262.
264. Kroon, S. (1979): Musk ambrette, a new cosmetic sensitiser and photosensitiser. *Contact Dermatitis, 5,* 337.
265. Kroon, S. (1981): Contact dermatitis from oleyl polypeptide in Xerumenex® eardrops. *Contact Dermatitis, 7,* 271.
266. Kruyswijk, M. R. J. and Polak, B. C. P. (1980): Contactallergie na toepassing van oogdruppels en oogzalven. *Ned. T. Geneesk., 124,* 1449.
267. Kull, E. and Schwarz-Speck, K. (1961): Gruppenspezifische Ekzemreaktion bei Largactilsensibilisierung. *Dermatologica (Basel), 122,* 263.
268. Lachapelle, J. M. (1975): Contact sensitivity to bufexamac. *Contact Dermatitis, 1,* 261.
269. Lachapelle, J. M. and Lamy, F. (1973): On allergic contact dermatitis to virginiamycin. *Dermatologica (Basel), 146,* 320.
270. Lane, C. G. and Luikart II, R. (1951): Dermatitis from local anaesthetics. *J. Amer. med. Ass., 146,* 717.
271. Larsen, W. G. (1975): Contact dermatitis due to a perfume. *Contact Dermatitis, 1,* 142.
272. Larsen, W. G. (1977): Perfume dermatitis. *Arch. Derm., 113,* 625.
273. Lewis, G. M. (1944): Dermatitis venenata due to tannins. *Arch. Derm. Syph., 50,* 138.
274. Leyden, J. J. and Kligman, A. M. (1977): Contact sensitisation to benzoyl peroxide. *Contact Dermatitis, 3,* 273.
275. Lidén, S. and Göransson, K. (1975): Contact allergy to dibenzthion. *Contact Dermatitis, 1,* 258.
276. Lindemayr, H. and Drobil, M. (1981): Contact sensitization to benzoyl peroxide. *Contact Dermatitis, 7,* 137.
277. Lindgren, S., Groth, O. and Molin, L. (1976): Allergic contact response to vitamin A acid. *Contact Dermatitis, 2,* 212.
278. Ljunggren, B. (1981): Contact dermatitis to estradiol benzoate. *Contact Dermatitis, 7,* 141.
279. Ljunggren, B. and Möller, H. (1972): Eczematous contact allergy to chlorhexidine. *Acta derm.-venereol. (Stockh.), 52,* 308.
280. Lorenzetti, O. J. and Wernet, T. C. (1977): Topical parabens: benefit and risks. *Dermatologica (Basel), 154,* 244.
281. Loveman, A. B. and Fliegelman, M. T. (1951): Local cutaneous sensitivity to methapyrilene. *Arch. Derm. Syph., 63,* 250.

5.45   Contact allergy to topical drugs

282. Löwenfeld, W. (1928): Überempfindlichkeit gegen Iodthion mit gleichzeitiger urtikarieller Reaktion. *Derm. Wschr., 78,* 502.
283. Ludwig, E. and Hausen, B. M. (1977): Sensitivity to isopropyl alcohol. *Contact Dermatitis, 3,* 240.
284. Lynfield, Y. L. (1970): Allergic contact sensitization to gentamycin. *N. Y. St. J. Med., 70,* 2235.
285. Maibach, H. (1975): Glutaraldehyde: cross-reaction to formaldehyde. *Contact Dermatitis, 1,* 326.
286. Maibach, H. I. (1978): Chronic dermatitis and hyperpigmentation from petrolatum. *Contact Dermatitis, 4,* 62.
287. Maibach, H. I. et al. (1978): Triclocarban: evaluation of contact dermatitis potential in man. *Contact Dermatitis, 4,* 283.
288. Maibach, H. I. and Prystowsky, S. D. (1977): Glutaraldehyde (Pentanedial) allergic contact dermatitis. *Arch. Derm., 113,* 170.
289. Malten, K. E. (1977): Sensitization to solcoseryl and methyl anisate (fragrance ingredient). *Contact Dermatitis, 3,* 219.
290. Malten, K. E. (1979): Four bakers showing positive patch tests to a number of fragrance materials, which can also be used as flavors. *Acta derm.-venereol. (Stockh), Suppl. 85,* 117.
291. Malten, K. E. Nater, J. P. and van Ketel, W. G. (1976): *Patch testing guidelines.* Dekker en van de Vegt, Nijmegen, Holland.
292. Mansell, P. W. A., Litwin, M. S., Ichinose, H. and Krementz, E. T. (1975): Delayed hypersensitivity to 5-fluorouracil following topical chemotherapy of cutaneous cancers. *Cancer Res., 35,* 1288.
293. Marcussen, P. V. (1962): Variations in the incidence of contact hypersensitivities. *Trans. St. John's Hosp. Derm. Soc. (Lond.), 48,* 40.
294. Marks, J. G. and West, G. W. (1978): Allergic contact dermatitis to radiotherapy dye. *Contact Dermatitis, 4,* 1.
295. Mathias, C. G. I., Maibach, H. I. and Chappler, R. R. (1981): Contact dermatitis to parachloromercuriphenol. *Contact Dermatitis, 7,* 117.
296. Omitted.
297. Maucher, O. M. (1974): Beitrag zur Kreuz- oder Kopplungsallergie auf Parahydroxy-benzoe-säureester. *Berufsdermatosen, 22,* 183.
298. Mendelsohn, H. V. (1946): Lemon grass oil. *Arch. Derm., 53,* 94.
299. Meneghini, C. L. and Angelini, G. (1975): Contact dermatitis from pyrrolnitrin (an antimycotic agent). *Contact Dermatitis, 1,* 288.
300. Meneghini, C. L. and Angelini, G. (1979): Contact allergy to antirheumatic drugs. *Contact Dermatitis, 5,* 197.
301. Meneghini, C. L. Rantuccio, F. and Lomuto, M. (1971): Additives, vehicles and active drugs of topical medicaments as causes of delayed-type dermatitis. *Dermatologica, (Basel), 143,* 137.
302. Menne, T. and Andersen, K. E. (1977): Allergic contact dermatitis from fluocortolone, fluocortolone pivalate and fluocortolone caproate. *Contact Dermatitis, 3,* 337.
303. Merck Index (1976): An encyclopedia of chemicals and drugs. Ninth edition. Merck and Co., Inc. Rahway, N.J., U.S.A.
304. Milby, T. H. and Epstein, W. L. (1964): Allergic contact sensitivity to malathion. *Arch. environm. Hlth, 9,* 434.
305. Mitchell, J. C. (1972): Contact dermatitis from proflavine dihydrochloride. *Arch. Derm., 106,* 924.
306. Mitchell, J. C. (1974): Contact sensitivity to costusroot oil, an ingredient of some perfumes. *Arch. Derm., 109,* 572.
307. Mitchell, J. C. (1974): Allergic contact dermatitis from alpha- and beta-adrenergic receptor blocking agents (Dibenzyline and propranolol). *Contact Dermatitis Newsl., 16,* 488.
308. Mitchell, J. C. (1975): Contact hypersensitivity to some perfume materials. *Contact Dermatitis, 1,* 196.
309. Mitchell, J. C. and Dupuis, G. (1972): Allergic contact dermatitis from storax (styrax). *Contact Dermatitis Newsl., 11,* 274.
310. Mitchell, J. C. and Epstein, W. L. (1974): Contact hypersensitivity to a perfume material, Costus Absolute. *Arch. Derm., 110,* 871.
311. Mitchell, J. C. and Maibach, H. I. (1975): Allergic contact dermatitis from phenoxybenzamine hydrochloride. *Contact Dermatitis, 1,* 363.
312. Mitchell, J. C. and Stewart, W. D. (1973): Allergic contact dermatitis from neutral red applied for herpes simplex. *Arch. Derm., 108,* 689.
313. Möller, H. (1976): Eczematous contact allergy to oxytetracycline and polymyxin B. *Contact Dermatitis, 2,* 289.
314. Monkton Copeman, P. W. (1968): Toxic epidermal necrolysis caused by skin hypersensitivity to monosulfiram. *Brit. med. J., i,* 623.

315. Morris, G. E. (1960): Dermatoses from phenylmercuric salts. *Arch. environm. Hlth, 1*, 53.
316. Mortensen, T. (1979): Allergy to lanolin. *Contact Dermatitis, 5*, 137.
317. Muston, H. L., Boss, J. M. and Summerly, R. (1977): Dermatitis from Ammonyx LO, constituent of surgical scrub. *Contact Dermatitis, 3*, 347.
318. Nagreh, D. S. (1976): Contact dermatitis from proprietary preparations in Malaysia. *Int. J. Derm., 15*, 34.
319. Nakayama, H., Hanaoka, H. and Oshiro, A. (1974): *Allergen Controlled System (ACS)*, p. 42. Kanehara Shappan, Tokyo.
320. Nakayama, H., Harada, R. and Toda, M. (1976): Pigmented cosmetic dermatitis. *Int. J. Derm., 15*, 673.
321. Neering, H., Vitányi, B. E. J., Malten, K. E., Van Ketel, W. G. and Van Dijk, E. (1975): Allergens in sesame oil contact dermatitis. *Acta derm.-venereol. (Stockh.), 55*, 31.
322. Nguyen, L. Q. and Allen, H. B. (1979): Reactions to manganese and cadmium in tattoos. *Cutis, 23*, 71.
323. Nilsson, D. C. (1960): Sources of allergenic gums. *Ann. Allergy, 18*, 518.
324. Nørgaard, O. (1977): Pecilocinum-Allergie. *Hautarzt, 25*, 35.
325. North American Contact Dermatitis Group (1973): Epidemiology of contact dermatitis in North America: 1972. *Arch. Derm., 108*, 573.
326. Ogier, M. and Duverneuil, G. (1977): Dermitis allergiques à l'aldehyde cinnamique. *Arch. Mal. prof. Med. Trav. Secur. soc., 38*, 835.
327. Oleffe, J. A., Blondeel, A. and De Coninck, A. (1979): Allergy to chlorocresol and propylene glycol in a steroid cream. *Contact Dermatitis, 5*, 53.
328. Opdyke, D. (1976): Inhibition of sensitization induced by certain aldehydes. *Food Cosm. Toxic., 14*, 197.
329. O'Quinn, S. E., Kennedy, B. C. and Isbell, K. H. (1967): Contact photodermatitis due to bithionol and related compounds. *J. Amer. med. Ass., 199*, 89.
330. Pankok, E. (1964): Iatrogene Kontaktallergie gegen Antimykotika. *Arch. klin. exp. Derm., 219*, 555.
331. Pasricha, J. S., Gupta, R. and Panjwani, S. (1980): Contact dermatitis to Henna (Lawsonia). *Contact Dermatitis, 6*, 288.
332. Petersen, H. O. (1977): Hypersensitivity to propolis. *Contact Dermatitis, 3*, 278.
333. Pevny, I. and Uhlich, M. (1975): Allergie gegen Bestandteile medizinischer und kosmetischer Externa. *Hautartz, 26*, 252.
334a. Pirilä, V., Kilpiö, O., Olkkonen, A., Pirilä, L. and Siltanen, E. (1969): On the chemical nature of the eczematogens in oil of turpentine. V. *Dermatologica (Basel), 139*, 183.
334b. Pirilä, V. and Kajama, H. (1962): Über Neomycinallergie mit besonderer Berücksichtigung der sich anschlieszenden Gruppenallergie. *Hautartz, 13*, 261.
335. Pirilä, V., Kilpiö, O., Olkkonen, A., Pirilä, L. and Siltanen, E. (1969): On the chemical nature of the eczematogens in oil of turpentine. V. *Dermatologica (Basel), 139*, 183.
336. Pirilä, V. and Rouhunkoski, S. (1959): On sensitisation to neomycin and bacitracin. *Acta derm.-venereol. (Stockh.), 39*, 470.
337. Prater, E., Göring, H. D. and Schubert, H. (1978): Sodium lauryl sulfate in contact allergy. *Contact Dermatitis, 4*, 242.
338. Przybilla, B. and Balda, B. R. (1980): Kontaktallergie gegen Tromantadine. *Münch. med. Wschr., 122*, 1195.
339. Rapaport, M. J. (1980): Sensitization to Abitol. *Contact Dermatitis, 6*, 137.
340. Raugi, G. J., Storrs, F. J. and Larsen, W. G. (1979): Photoallergic contact dermatitis to men's perfumes. *Contact Dermatitis, 5*, 251.
341. Raymond, J. Z. and Gross, P. R. (1969): EDTA preservative dermatitis. *Arch Derm., 100*, 436.
342. Reiffers, J. (1981): Allergy to 5-Jodo-2'-desoxyuridine. *Contact Dermatitis, 7*, 125.
343. Reisman, R. (1969): Delayed hypersensitivity to merthiolate preservative. *J. Allergy, 43*, 245.
344. Rietschel, R. L. (1978): Photocontact dermatitis to hydrocortisone. *Contact Dermatitis, 4*, 334.
345. Rives, H. (1956): *Contribution à l'étude des dermatoses profesionnelles provoquées par la chlorpromazine*. Thesis, Lyon.
346. Robin, J. (1978): Contact dermatitis to acetarsol. *Contact Dermatitis, 4*, 309.
347. Robin, J. (1978): Contact dermatitis to hexamidine. *Contact Dermatitis, 4*, 375.
348. Omitted.
349. Roed-Petersen, J. (1980): Allergic contact dermatitis from butylacetate. *Contact Dermatitis, 6*, 55.
350. Roed-Petersen, J., Auken, G. and Hjorth, N. (1975): Contact sensitivity to Irgasan DP 300. *Contact Dermatitis, 1*, 293.

5.45 Contact allergy to topical drugs

351. Roed-Petersen, J. and Hjorth, N. (1976): Contact dermatitis from anti-oxidants. *Brit. J. Derm., 94,* 233.
352. Roller, J. A. (1978): Contact allergy to clotrimazole. *Brit. med. J., ii,* 737.
353. Romaguera, C. and Grimalt, F. (1980): Five cases of contact dermatitis from pyrrolnitrin. *Contact Dermatitis, 6,* 352.
354. Omitted.
355. Romaguera, C., Grimalt, F. and Conde-Salazar, L. (1980): Occupational dermatitis from vitamin K3 sodium bisulfite. *Contact Dermatitis, 6,* 355.
356. Rorsman, H., Brehmer-Andersson, E., Dahlquist, I., Ehinger, B., Jacobsson, S., Lindt, F. and Rorsman, G. (1969): Tattoo granuloma and uveitis. *Lancet, 2,* 27.
357. Rothenborg, H. W. and Hjorth, N. (1968): Allergy to perfumes from toilet soaps and detergents in patients with dermatitis. *Arch. Derm., 97,* 417.
358. Rudolph, R. I. (1975): Allergic contact dermatitis caused by haloprogin. *Arch. Derm., 111,* 1487.
359. Rudzki, E. and Baranowska, A. (1974): Contact sensitivity in stasis dermatitis. *Dermatologica (Basel), 148,* 353.
360. Rudzki, E. and Baranowska, A. (1975): Reactions to gallic acid esters. *Contact Dermatitis, 1,* 393.
361. Rudzki, E. and Grzywa, Z. (1977): Occupational dermatitis partly elicited by coal tar. *Contact Dermatitis, 3,* 54.
362. Rudzki, E. and Grzywa, Z. (1977): Occupational piperazine dermatitis. *Contact Dermatitis, 3,* 216.
363. Rudzki, E. and Grzywa, Z. (1977): Dermatitis from arnica montana. *Contact Dermatitis, 3,* 281.
364. Rudzki, E., Grzywa, Z. and Maciejowska, E. (1976): Drug reaction with positive patch test to chloramphenicol. *Contact Dermatitis, 3,* 181.
365. Rudzki, E. and Grzywa, Z. (1978): Dermatitis from retinoic acid. *Contact Dermatitis, 4,* 305.
366. Rudzki, E. and Koslowska, A. (1976): Sensitivity to salicylic acid. *Contact Dermatitis, 2,* 178.
367. Saihan, E. M. (1979): Contact allergy to methoxsalen. *Brit. med. J., iii,* 20.
368. Salo, O. P. and Pirilä, V. (1968): Sensitisation to topical Dequaline. *Contact Dermatitis Newsl., 4,* 66.
369. Sams, W. M. (1968): Untoward response with topical fluorouracil. *Arch. Derm., 97,* 14.
370. Samsoën, M. and Jelen, G. (1977): Allergy to daktarin gel. *Contact Dermatitis, 3,* 351.
371. Samsoën, M., Metz, R., Melchior, E. and Foussereau, J. (1980): Cross-sensitivity between aminoside antibiotics. *Contact Dermatitis, 6,* 141.
372. Sausker, W. F. and Frederick, F. D. (1978): Allergic contact dermatitis secondary to topical nitroglycerin. *J. Amer. med. Ass., 239,* 1743.
373. Saynisch, F. (1957): Allergische Dermatosen durch beruflichen Kontakt mit Bromcholinbromid und Nitrosomethylharnstoff. *Berufsdermatosen, 5,* 197.
374. Schlossman, M. L. and McCarthy, J. P. (1979): Lanolin and -derivatives chemistry: relationship to allergic contact dermatitis. *Contact Dermatitis, 5,* 65.
375. Schneider, H. G. (1978): Schwefel-allergie. *Hautarzt, 29,* 340.
376. Schneider, K. W. (1980): Contact dermatitis due to diethyl sebacate. *Contact Dermatitis, 6,* 506.
377. Scholz, A. and von Richter, G. (1977): Zur Allergie gegen Falikain (Propipokainhydrochlorid). *Derm. Mschr., 163,* 966.
378. Schöne, K. (1975): Klinische Erfahrungen mit einem Heparinoid-Extermum in hoher Wirkstoff-Konzentration. *Fortschr. Med., 93,* 1565.
379. Schorr, W. (1971): Quoted by Fisher (1973): In: *Contact Dermatitis,* 2nd Edition, p. 294. Lea and Febiger, Philadelphia.
380. Schorr, W. and Ridgway, H. B. (1977): Tobramycin-Neomycin cross-sensitivity. *Contact Dermatitis, 3,* 133.
381. Schorr, W. F. (1968): Paraben allergy. A cause of intractable dermatitis. *J. Amer. med. Ass., 204,* 859.
382. Schorr, W. F. (1970): Dichlorophene (G-4) allergy. *Arch Derm., 102,* 515.
383. Schorr, W. F. (1971): Cosmetic allergy. *Arch. Derm., 104,* 459.
384. Schorr, W. F. (1971): Formaldehyde in shampoo and toiletries. *Contact Dermatitis Newsl., 9,* 220.
385. Schorr, W. F. (1975): Cinnamic aldehyde allergy. *Contact Dermatitis, 1,* 108.
386. Schultheiss, E. (1957): Überempfindlichkeit gegenüber Ionon und Benzylalkohol. *Derm. Wschr., 135,* 629.
387. Schulz, K. H. and Herrmann, W. P. (1955): Allergische Kontaktdermatitis durch Megaphen. *Hautartz, 6,* 542.
388. Schülz, K. H., Schöpf, E. and Wex, O. (1970): Allergische Berufsekzeme durch Ampicillin. *Berufsdermatosen, 18,* 132
389. Schwank, R. and Jirásek, (1952): Skin sensitization due to emetine. *Čs. Derm., 27,* 50.

390.   Schwank, R. and Jirásek, L. (1963): Kontaktallergie gegen Chloramphenicol mit besonderer Berücksichtigung der Gruppensensibilisierung. *Hautarzt, 14,* 24.
391.   Schwarz, K. and Storck, H. (1966): Ekzematöse Sensibilisierung auf Methandrostenolon in Salbenform. *Dermatologica (Basel), 132,* 73.
392.   Scutt, R. and Gotch, C. (1974): *Skin Deep, The Mystery of Tattooing,* p. 135. Peter Davies, London.
393.   Sharvill, D. (1965): Reaction to chlorhexidine and cetrimide. *Lancet, i,* 771.
394.   Sherman, W. B. and Cooke, R. A. (1950): Dermatitis following the use of pyribenzamine and antistine. *J. Allergy, 21,* 63.
395.   Shmunes, E. and Levy, E. J. (1972): Quaternary ammonium compound dermatitis from a deodorant. *Arch. Derm., 105,* 91.
396.   Sidi, E. and Arouette, J. (1959): Hautallergien durch Azofarbstoffe. *Hautarzt, 10,* 193.
397.   Sidi, E. and Dobkevitch-Morrill, S. (1951): The injection and ingestion test in cross-sensitization to the para-group. *J. invest. Derm., 15,* 165.
398.   Sidi, E., Gervais, A. and Gervais, P. (1962): Les sensibilisations cutanées dans la groupe Streptomycine-neomycine-framycetine. *Acta allerg. (Kbh.), 17,* 529.
399.   Sidi, E., Hincky, M. and Gervais, A. (1955): Allergic sensitization and photosensitization to phenergancream. *J. invest. Derm., 24,* 345.
400.   Sidi, E., Melki, G. and Longueville, R. (1952): Dermatitis aux pomades antihistaminiques. *Acta allerg. (Kbh.), 5,* 292.
401.   Simeray, M. A. (1966): Action d'un fongicide agricole (orthocide) dans 250 cas de pityriasis versicolor. *Bull. Soc. franç Derm. Syph., 73,* 337.
402.   Simon, Cl. R. and Brandt, R. (1953): Eczematous hypersensitivity to coal tar. *Arch. Derm., 68,* 584.
403.   Skinner, L. C. (1949): Contact dermatitis due to phenolphthaleine. *Arch. Derm. Syph., 59,* 338.
404.   Smeenk, G. and Prins, F. J. (1972): Allergic contact eczema due to chloracetamide. *Dermatologica (Basel), 144,* 108.
405.   Sneddon, I. B. and Glew, R. C. (1973): Contact dermatitis due to propanidid in an anesthesist. *Practitioner, 211,* 321.
406.   Omitted.
407.   Starke, J. C. (1967): Photoallergy to Sandalwood Oil. *Arch. Derm., 96,* 62.
408.   Storrs, F. (1975): Para-chloro-meta-xylenol allergic contact dermatitis in seven individuals. *Contact Dermatitis, 1,* 211.
409.   Suhonen, R. (1980): Contact allergy to dodecyl-di-(aminoethyl)glycine (Desimex i). *Contact Dermatitis, 6,* 290.
410.   Suurmond, D. (1966): Patch test reactions to phenergancream, promethazine and triethanolamine. *Dermatologica (Basel), 133,* 503.
411.   Suzuki, Y. and Ohkido, Y. (1979): Contact dermatitis from hydrazine. *Contact Dermatitis, 5,* 113.
412.   Taaffe, A., Knight, A. G. and Marks, R. (1978): Lichenoid tattoo hypersensitivity. *Brit. med. J., 1,* 616.
413.   Tarnick, M. (1976): Hautsensibilisierungen gegen Thiosinamin (Aminosin®, Allylthiokarbamid). *Derm. Mschr., 162,* 905.
414.   Tas, J. and Weissberg, D. (1958): Allergy to aminophylline. *Acta allerg. (Kbh.), 12,* 39.
415.   Taylor, J. R. and Halprin, K. M. (1972): Topical use of mechlorethamine in the treatment of psoriasis. *Arch Derm., 106,* 362.
416.   Tegner, E. (1976): Contact allergy to corticosteroids. *Int. J. Derm., 15,* 520.
417.   Tennstedt, D., Dumont-Fruytier, M. and Lachapelle, J. M. (1978): Occupational allergic contact dermatitis to virginiamycin, an antibiotic used as a food-additive for pigs and poultry. *Contact Dermatitis, 4,* 133.
418.   Thormann, J. and Kaaber, K. (1978): Contact sensitivity to phenylbutazone ointment (Butazolidine). *Contact Dermatitis, 4,* 235.
419.   Thormann, J. and Wildenhoff, K. E. (1980): Contact allergy to idoxuridine. *Contact Dermatitis, 6,* 170.
420.   Thyresson, N., Lodin, A. and Nilzén, A. (1956): Eczema of the hands due to triethanolamine in cosmetic hand lotions for housewives. *Acta derm.-venereol. (Stockh.), 36,* 355.
421.   Tzanck, A., Sidi, E. and Herbault (1950): Un cas d'intolérance à l'acide para-amino-salicylique. *Bull. Soc. franç. Derm. Syph., 57,* 504.
422.   Valsecchi, R., Serra, M., Foiadelli, L. and Cainelli, T. (1981): Contact allergy to oxyphenbutazone. *Contact Dermatitis, 7,* 157.
423.   Van der Meer, B. J. (1957): Een geval van contactallergie voor koper en zink. *Ned. T. Geneesk., 101,* 2166.

5.45   Contact allergy to topical drugs

424. Van Dijk, E., Neering, H. and Vitányi, B. E. J. (1973): Contact hypersensitivity to sesame oil in patients with leg ulcers and eczema. *Acta derm.-venereol. (Stockh.)*, *53*, 135.
425. Van Dijk, T. J. A. and Marien, K. (1972): Allergic contact dermatitis from Eurax®, Eurax®. *Contact Dermatitis Newsl.*, *12*, 344.
426. Van Hecke, E. (1969): Contact allergy to the topical antimycotic Fluoro-4-dichloro-3'-5'-thiocarbanilid. *Dermatologica (Basel)*, *138*, 480.
427. Van Hecke, E. (1981): Contact sensitivity to vincamine tartrate. *Contact Dermatitis*, *7*, 53.
428. Van Hecke, E. and Temmerman, L. (1980): Contact allergy to the corticosteroid budesonide. *Contact Dermatitis*, *6*, 509.
429. VanHee, J., Ceuterick, A., Dooms, M. and Dooms-Goossens, A. (1980): Etisazole: an animal antifungal agent with skin sensitizing properties in man. *Contact Dermatitis*, *6*, 443.
430. VanHee, J., Gevers, D. and Dooms-Goossens, A. (1981): Contact dermatitis from an antirheumatic gel containing etofenamate. *Contact Dermatitis*, *7*, 50.
431. Omitted.
432. Van Ketel, W. G. (1964): Contact dermatitis from a hydrazine-derivative in a stain remover. Cross-sensitization to Apresoline and Isoniazid. *Acta derm.-venereol. (Stockh.)*, *44*, 49.
433. Van Ketel, W. G. (1967): Allergic dermatitis caused by Tineafax ointment. *Dermatologica (Basel)*, *135*, 121.
434. Van Ketel, W. G. (1973): Allergy to cumarin and cumarin-derivatives. *Contact Dermatitis Newsl.*, *13*, 355.
435. Van Ketel, W. G. (1974): Polymixin-B-sulphate and Bacitracin. *Contact Dermatitis Newsl.*, *15*, 445.
436. Van Ketel, W. G. (1975): Cross-sensitization to 5,7-Dibromo-8-hydroxy quinoline (D.B.O.) (a compound of synalar + DBO cream). *Contact Dermatitis*, *1*, 385.
437. Van Ketel, W. G. (1976): Allergic contact dermatitis from propellants in deodorant sprays in combination with allergy to ethylchloride. *Contact Dermatitis*, *2*, 115.
438. Van Ketel, W. G. (1976): Sensitivity to chlorphenoxamine hydrochloride. *Contact Dermatitis*, *2*, 121.
439. Van Ketel, W. G. (1976): Immediate- and delayed-type allergy to erythromycin. *Contact Dermatitis*, *2*, 363.
440. Van Ketel, W. G. (1978): Allergic contact dermatitis from butylaminobenzoate. *Contact Dermatitis*, *4*, 55.
441. Van Ketel, W. G. (1978): Dermatitis from octylgallate in peanut butter. *Contact Dermatitis*, *4*, 60.
442. Van Ketel, W. G. (1981): Allergy to pramoxine (pramocaine). *Contact Dermatitis*, *7*, 49.
443. Van Ketel, W. G. and Swain, A. F. (1981): Allergy to clobetasol-17-propionate (Dermovate®). *Contact Dermatitis*, *7*, 278.
444. Van Ketel, W. G. and Tan-Lim, K. N. (1975): Contact dermatitis from ethanol. *Contact Dermatitis*, *1*, 7.
445. Van Scott, E. J. and Yu, R. F. (1974): Antimitotic, antigenic and structural relationships of nitrogen mustard and its homologues. *J. invest. Derm.*, *62*, 378.
446. Veien, N. K., Hattel, T., Justesen, O. and Nørholm, A. (1980): Occupational contact dermatitis due to spiramycin and/or tylosin among farmers. *Contact Dermatitis*, *6*, 410.
447. Velasco, J. E. and Africk, J. A. (1971): Contact dermatitis to mafenide acetate. *Arch. Derm.*, *103*, 61.
448. Vermeulen, C. W. and Malten, K. E. (1963): Contacteczeem door 6-alpha-chloorprednison en neomycine. *Ned. T. Geneesk.*, *107*, 548.
449. Von Richter, G. and Scholz, A. (1970): Kontaktekzem und makulöses Exanthem bei p-Chlorbenzolsulfonyl-glykolsäurenitril-Allergie. *Berufsdermatosen*, *18*, 70.
450. Wade, T. R., Jones, H. E. and Artis, W. A. (1979): Irritant and allergic reactions to topically applied Micatin cream. *Contact Dermatitis*, *5*, 168.
451. Wahlberg, J. E. (1971): Sensitization to thioxolone used for topical treatment of acne. *Contact Dermatitis Newsl.*, *10*, 222.
452. Wahlberg, J. E. (1976): Routine patch testing with Irgasan DP 300®. *Contact Dermatitis*, *2*, 292.
453. Wahlberg, J. E. (1978): Abietic acid and colophony. *Contact Dermatitis*, *4*, 55.
454. Wahlberg, J. E. and Boman, A. (1981): Contact sensitivity to quinidine sulfate from occupational exposure. *Contact Dermatitis*, *7*, 27.
455. Wahlberg, J. E. and Forsbeck, M. (1974): Contact sensitivity to quinidine sulphate – an antiarrhythmic. *Contact Dermatitis Newsl.*, *14*, 412.
456. Wahlberg, J. E. and Wennersten, G. (1971): Hypersensitivity and photosensitivity to chlorhexidin. *Dermatologica (Basel)*, *143*, 376.
457. Wereide, K. (1975): Sensitivity to azidamphenicol. *Contact Dermatitis*, *1*, 271.

458. White, M. I. (1978): Contact dermatitis from ethylenediamine. *Contact Dermatitis, 4*, 291.
459. Wiegel, O. (1968): Kontaktallergie durch Kortikosteroid-haltige Externa. *Med. Welt, 19*, 828.
460. Wilkinson, D. S. (1970): Durch Dequalinium hervorgerufene Hautnekrosen. *Hautarzt, 21*, 114.
461. Wilkinson, D. S. (1975): Sulphur sensitivity. *Contact Dermatitis, 1*, 58.
462. Wilkinson, H. D., McGarry, E. M. and Solomon, S. (1967): Allergic contact dermatitis due to hydrocortisone. *J. invest. Derm., 43*, 295.
463. Wilson, H. T. H. (1958): Streptomycin dermatitis in nurses. *Brit. med. J., i*, 1378.
464. Wilson, H. T. H. (1966): Dermatitis from anaesthetic ointments. *Practitioner, 197*, 673.
465. Wilson, H. T. H. (1971): Dermatitis from an acridine dye. *Contact Dermatitis Newsl., 9*, 212.
466. Winkelmann, R. K. and Harris, R. B. (1979): Lichenoid delayed hypersensitivity reactions in tattoos. *J. cutan. Path., 6*, 59.
467. Wortmann, F. (1972): Erfahrungen mit dem neuen Antimykotikum Exomycol. *Mykosen, 15*, 295.
468. Wulf, K. (1967): Beitrag zur Triamcinolon-Kontaktallergie. *Z. Haut- u. Geschlkr., 42*, 765.
469. Yaffe, J., Bierman, W., Cann, M. et al. (1973): Antihistamines in topical preparations. *Pediatrics, 51*, 299.
470. Zackheim, H. S. (1975): Treatment of psoriasis with 6-nicotinamide. *Arch Derm., 111*, 880.
471. Zina, G. and Bonu, G. (1967): Contact sensitivity to corticosteroids. *Contact Dermatitis Newsl., 2*, 26.
472. Soesman-Van Waadenoyen Kernekamp, A. and Van Ketel, W. G. (1980): Persistence of patch test reactions to clioquinol (vioform) and cross-sensitization. *Contact Dermatitis, 6*, 455.

UPDATE – 2nd Edition

473. Lassus, A., Forström, S. and Salo, O. (1983): A double-blind comparison of sulconazole nitrate 1% cream with clotrimazole 1% cream in the treatment of dermatophytoses. *Brit. J. Derm., 108*, 195.
474. Schneider, K. W. (1982): Tromantadin-Kontaktallergien. *Therapiewoche, 32*, 5691.
475. Van Ketel, W. G. (1983): Sensitization to cis-3-hexenyl salicylate. *Contact Dermatitis, 9*, 154.
476. Van Hecke, E. and De Vos, L. (1983): Contact sensitivity to enilconazole. *Contact Dermatitis, 9*, 144.
477. Shoji, A. (1983): Contact dermatitis from chlorhexidine. *Contact Dermatitis, 9*, 156.
478. Osmundsen, P. E. (1982): Contact dermatitis to chlorhexidine. *Contact Dermatitis, 8*, 81.
479. Bedello, P. G., Goitre, M., Cane, D. and Fogliano, M. R. (1983): Contact dermatitis from Nifuratel. *Contact Dermatitis, 9*, 166.
480. Romaguera, C. and Grimalt, F. (1983): Occupational dermatitis from codeine. *Contact Dermatitis, 9*, 170.
481. Coskey, R. J. (1983): Contact dermatitis caused by diphenhydramine hydrochloride, *J. Amer. Acad. Derm., 8*, 204.
482. Happle, R., Hausen, B. M. and Wiesner-Menzel, L. (1983): Diphencyprone in the treatment of alopecia areata. *Acta derm.-venereol (Stockh.) 63*, 49.
483. Nethercott, J. R., Pilger, C., O'Blenis, L. and Roy, A. M. (1983): Contact dermatitis due to cinnamic aldehyde induced in a deodorant manufacturing process. *Contact Dermatitis, 9*, 241.
484. Jung, H.-D. (1983): Beruflich bedingte Kontaktekzeme durch Tylosin (Tylan[R]). *Derm. Mschr., 169*, 235.
485. Menezes Brandão, F. (1983): Contact dermatitis to ethoxyquin. *Contact Dermatitis, 9*, 240.
486. Foussereau, J., Samsoen, M. and Hecht, M. Th. (1983): Occupational dermatitis to Ampholyt G in hospital personnel. *Contact Dermatitis, 9*, 233.
487. Fregert, S. and Dahlquist, I. (1983): Patch testing with oak moss extract. *Contact Dermatitis, 9*, 227.
488. Wright, S. (1983): Contact allergy to dibrompropamidine cream. *Contact Dermatitis, 9*, 226.
489. Conde-Salazar, L., Guimaraens, D. and Romero, L. V. (1983): Contact dermatitis from clindamycin. *Contact Dermatitis, 9*, 225.
490. Dooms-Goossens, A. and Degreef, H. (1983): Contact allergy to petrolatums. (I). Sensitizing capacity of different brands of yellow and white petrolatums. *Contact Dermatitis, 9*, 175.
491. Dooms-Goossens, A. and Degreef, H. (1983): Contact allergy to petrolatums. (II). Attempts to identify the nature of the allergens. *Contact Dermatitis, 9*, 247.
492. Keilig, W. (1983): Kontaktallergie auf Cetylstearylalkohol (Lanette O) als therapeutisches Problem bei Stauungsdermatitis und Ulcus cruris. *Dermatosen, 31*, 50.

493. De Groot, A. C. and Liem, D. H. (1983): Facial psoriasis caused by contact allergy to linalool and hydroxycitronellal in an after-shave. *Contact Dermatitis, 9*, 230.
494. Verbov, J. (1983): Tylosin dermatitis. *Contact Dermatitis, 9*, 325.
495. Przybilla, B., Wagner-Größer, G. and Balda, B.-R. (1983): Kontaktallergische Kreuzreaktion von Tromantadin und Amantadin. *Dtsch. med. Wschr., 108*, 172.
496. Jelen, G. (1982): Allergie gegen imidazolhaltige Antimykotika: Kreuzallergie? *Dermatosen, 30*, 53.
497. Van Hecke, E. and Van Brabant, S. (1981): Contact sensitivity to imidazole derivatives. *Contact Dermatitis, 7*, 348.
498. Lawrence, C. M. and Smith, A. G. (1982): Ampliative medicament allergy: concomitant sensitivity to multiple medicaments including yellow soft paraffin, white soft paraffin, gential violet and Span 20. *Contact Dermatitis, 8*, 240.
499. Austad, J. (1982): Allergic contact dermatitis to sorbitan monooleate (Span 80). *Contact Dermatitis, 8*, 426.
500. Valsecchi, R., Tornaghi, A., Tribbia, G. and Cainelli, T. (1982): Contact dermatitis from econazole. *Contact Dermatitis, 8*, 422.
501. Lombardi, P., Campolmo, P., Spallanzani, P. and Sertoli, A. (1982): Delayed hypersensitivity to erythromycin. *Contact Dermatitis, 8*, 416.
502. Meneghini, C. L., Vena, G. A. and Angelini, G. (1982): Contact dermatitis to scabicides. *Contact Dermatitis, 8*, 285.
503. De Groot, A. C. (1982): Contact allergy to sodium fusidate. *Contact Dermatitis, 8*, 429.
504. Menezes Brandão, F. and Foussereau, J. (1982): Contact dermatitis to phenylbutazone-piperazine suppositories (Carudol®) and piperazine-gel (Carudol®). *Contact Dermatitis, 8*, 264.
505. Romaguera, C. and Grimalt, F. (1982): Contact dermatitis from nasal sprays and amyl nitrite. *Contact Dermatitis, 8*, 266.
506. Hardie, R. A., Benton, E. C. and Hunter, J. A. A. (1982): Adverse reactions to paste bandages. *Clin exp. Derm., 7*, 135.
507. Nilsson, D. C. (1960): Sources of allergic gums. *Ann. Allergy, 18*, 518.
508. Camarasa, J. G. and Barnadas, M. (1982): Occupational dermatosis by vitamin K3 sodium bisulphite. *Contact Dermatitis, 8*, 268.
509. Pambor, M. and Hein, K. (1982): Tetramisolhaltiges Anthelminthikum (Nilverm®) als berufliches Ekzematogen in der Viehwirtschaft. *Derm. Mschr., 168*, 314.
510. Reiffers, J. (1982): Contact allergy to bufexamac. *Dermatologica (Basel), 164*, 354.
511. De Groot, A. C. (1982): Contact allergy to clindamycin. *Contact Dermatitis, 8*, 428.
512. Fisher, A. A. (1980): The antihistamines. *J. Amer. Acad. Derm., 3*, 303.
513. Fisher, A. A. (1981): Contact dermatitis: Questions and answers. Part 1. *Cutis, 28*, 610.
514. Tucker, W. F. G. (1983): Contact dermatitis to Eutanol G. *Contact Dermatitis, 9*, 88.
515. Frenzel, U. H. and Gutekunst, A. (1983): Contact dermatitis to isoconazole nitrate. *Contact Dermatitis, 9*, 74.
516. Fisher, A. A. (1982): Topical medicaments which are common sensitizers. *Ann. Allergy, 49*, 97.
517. Fisher, A. A. (1982): Resorcinol – A rare sensitizer. *Cutis, 29*, 331.
518. Trancik, R. J. and Maibach, H. I. (1982): Propylene glycol: irritation or sensitization? *Contact Dermatitis, 8*, 185.
519. Goette, D. K., Odom, R. B., Arrott, J. W. et al. (1982): Treatment of keratoacanthoma with topical application of fluorouracil. *Arch. Derm., 118*, 309.
520. Marks, J. G. Jr. (1982): Allergic contact dermatitis to povidone-iodine. *J. Amer. Acad. Derm., 6*, 473.
521. Grimalt, F. and Romaguera, C. (1981): Cutaneous sensitivity to benzidine. *Dermatosen, 29*, 95.
522. Scott, M. J. and Scott, M. J. Jr. (1982): Jojoba oil (Letter to the Editor). *J. Amer. Acad. Derm., 6*, 545.
523. Le Roy, R., Grosshans, E. and Foussereau, J. (1981): Recherche d'allergie de contact dans 100 cas d'ulcère de jambe. *Dermatosen, 29*, 168.
524. Chin, T. M. and Fellner, M. J. (1980): Allergic hypersensitivity to lidocaine hydrochloride. *Int. J. Derm., 19*, 147.
525. Fisher, A. A. (1982): Reaction to local and topical anesthetics. *Cutis, 29*, 16.
526. Merk, H., Ebert, L. and Goerz, G. (1982): Allergic contact dermatitis due to the fungicide hexetidine. *Contact Dermatitis, 8*, 216.
527. Fisher, A. A. (1981): Allergic reactions to Merthiolate® (thimerosal). *Cutis, 27*, 580.
528. Meneghini, C. L. and Angelini, G. (1982): Contact dermatitis from pyrrolnitrin. *Contact Dermatitis, 8*, 55.

529. Staniforth, P. and Lovell, C. R. (1981): Contact dermatitis related to constituent of an orthopaedic wool. *Brit. med. J., 283*, 1297.
530. Adams, R. M. (1981): Allergic contact dermatitis due to o-phenylphenol. *Contact Dermatitis, 7*, 332.
531. Waddell, M. M. and Finn, O. A. (1981): Sensitivity to resorcin. *Contact Dermatitis, 7*, 216.
532. Valsecchi, R., Foiadelli, L. and Cainelli, T. (1981): Contact dermatitis from pyrrolnitrin. *Contact Dermatitis, 7*, 340.
533. Lovell, C. R. and Staniforth, P. (1981): Contact allergy to benzalkonium chloride in plaster of Paris. *Contact Dermatitis, 7*, 343.
534. Huriez, C., Agache, P., Martin, P. et al. (1965): Fréquences des sensibilisations aux ammoniums quaternaires. *Sem. Hôp. Paris, 41*, 2301.
535. Van Hecke, E. and Van Brabandt, S. (1981): Contact sensitivity to imidazole derivatives. *Contact Dermatitis, 7*, 348.
536. Van Joost, Th., Sillevis Smitt, J. H. and Van Ketel, W. G. (1981): Senzitization to olive oil (olea europeae). *Contact Dermatitis, 7*, 309.
537. Lawrence, C. M. and Smith, A. G. (1981): Ichthammol sensitivity. *Contact Dermatitis, 7*, 335.
538. Roberts, D. L., Summerly, R. and Byrne, J. P. H. (1981): Contact dermatitis due to the constituents of Hibiscrub. *Contact Dermatitis, 7*, 326.
539. Göransson, K. and Lidén, S. (1981): Contact allergy to sorbic acid and Unguentum Merck. *Contact Dermatitis, 7*, 277.
540. Rietschel, R. L. and Wilson, L. A. (1982): Ocular inflammation in patients using soft contact lenses. *Arch. Derm., 118*, 147.
541. Motiuk, K. (1979): Wool wax acids. A review. *J. Amer. Oil Chem. Soc., 56*, 91.
542. Motiuk, K. (1979): Wool wax alcohols. A review. *J. Amer. Oil Chem. Soc., 56*, 651.
543. Kligman, A. M. (1983): Lanolin allergy: crisis or comedy. *Contact Dermatitis, 9*, 99.
544. Kunze, J., Kaiser, H. J. and Petres, J. (1983): Relevanz einer Jodallergie bei handelsüblichen Polyvidon-Jod-Zubereitungen. *Z. Hautkr., 58*, 255.
545. Storrs, F. J. and Bell, D. E. (1983): Allergic contact dermatitis to 2-bromo-2-nitropropane-1,3-diol in a hydrophilic ointment. *J. Amer. Acad. Derm., 8*, 157.
546. Vena, G. A., Angelini, G. and Meneghini, C. L. (1982): Contact dermatitis to benzoyl peroxide. *Contact Dermatitis, 8*, 338.
547. Rietschel, R. L. and Duncan, S. H. (1982): Benzoyl peroxide reactions in an acne study group. *Contact Dermatitis, 8*, 323.
548. Cunliffe, W. J. and Burke, B. (1982): Benzoyl peroxide: Lack of sensitization. *Acta derm.-venereol. (Stockh.), 62*, 458.
549. Nater, J. P. and De Groot, A. C. (1984): Drugs used on the skin and cosmetics. In: *Side effects of drugs, Annual 8, Chapter 15*, pp 151–152. Editor M. N. G. Dukes. Elsevier, Amsterdam.
550. Jensen, O., Petersen, S. H. and Vesterager, L. (1980): Contact sensitization to benzoyl peroxide following topical treatment of chronic leg ulcers. *Contact Dermatitis, 6*, 179.
551. Andersen, K. E. and Storrs, F. J. (1982): Hautreizungen durch Propylenglycol. *Hautarzt, 33*, 12.
552. Scheuer, B. (1983): Kontaktallergie durch Triäthanolamin. *Hautarzt, 34*, 126.
553. Steltenkamp, R. J., Booman, K. A., Dorsky, J. et al. (1980): Cinnamic alcohol: A survey of consumer patch-test sensitization. *Food Cosmet. Toxicol., 18*, 419.
554. Steltenkamp, R. J., Booman, K. A., Dorsky, J. et al. (1980): Hydroxycitronellal: A survey of consumer patch test sensitization. *Food Cosmet. Toxicol., 18*, 407.
555. Lidén, S. (1974): Alphosyl sensitivity. *International Symposium on Contact Dermatitis*. Gentofte, Denmark, 1974.
556. Trancik, R. J. and Maibach, H. I. (1982): Propylene glycol: irritation or sensitization? *Contact Dermatitis, 8*, 185.
557. Larsen, W. G. (1983): Allergic contact dermatitis to the fragrance material lilial. *Contact Dermatitis, 9*, 158.
558. Sai, S. (1983): Lipstick dermatitis caused by castor oil. *Contact Dermatitis, 9*, 75.
559. Van Ketel, W. G. (1982): Allergy to Matricaria chamomilla. *Contact Dermatitis, 8*, 143.
560. Balato, N., Lembo, G., Cusano, F. and Ayala, F. (1983): Contact dermatitis from pyrrolinitrin. *Contact Dermatitis, 9*, 238.
561. Fisher, A. A. (1981): Dermatitis due to the presence of formaldehyde in certain sodium lauryl sulfate (SLS) solutions. *Cutis, 27*, 360.
562. Rycroft, R. (1978): Is Grotan BK a contact sensitizer? *Brit. J. Derm., 99*, 346.
563. Dahl, M. G. C. (1981): Patch test concentrations of Grotan BK (letter). *Brit. J. Derm., 104*, 607.
564. Meynadier, J.-M., Meynadier, J., Colmas, A. et al. (1982): Allergie aux conservateurs. *Ann. Derm. Vénéréol., (Paris) 109*, 1017.

565. Rudzki, E. and Grzywa, Z. (1983): Dermatitis from propolis. *Contact Dermatitis, 9,* 40.
566. Hausen, B. M., Kuhlwein, A. and Schulz, K. H. (1982): Kolophonium-Allergie. Part 1 and 2. *Dermatosen Beruf Umw., 30,* 107 and 145.
567. Guin, J. D. and Haffley, P. (1983): Sensitivity to α-amylcinnamic aldehyde and α-amylcinnamic alcohol. *J. Amer. Acad. Derm., 8,* 76.
568. Lawlor, F. and Hudson, C. (1982): Allergy to dithranol. *Contact Dermatitis, 8,* 137.
569. Goette, D. K. (1981): Topical chemotherapy with 5-fluorouracil. *J. Amer. Acad. Derm., 4,* 633.
570. MacDonald, R. H. and Beck, M. (1983): Neomycin: a review with particular reference to dermatological usage. *Clin. exp. Derm., 8,* 249.
571. Fisher, A. A. (1983): Topically applied alcohol as a cause of contact dermatitis. *Cutis, 31,* 588.
572. De Groot, A. C. and Liem, D. H. (1983): Contact urticaria to rouge. *Contact Dermatitis, 9,* 322.
573. Osmundsen, P. (1978): Contact dermatitis due to sodium hypochlorite. *Contact Dermatitis, 4,* 177.
574. Dooms-Goossens, A., Gevers, D., Mertens, A. and Van der Heyden, D. (1983); Allergic contact urticaria due to chloramine. *Contact Dermatitis, 9,* 319.
575. Lazzarini, S. (1982): Contact allergy to benzyl alcohol and isopropyl palmitate, ingredients of topical corticosteroid. *Contact Dermatitis, 8,* 349.
576. Vega, F. A., Halprin, K. M., Taylor, J. R. et al. (1982): Failure of periodic ultraviolet radiation treatments to prevent sensitization to nitrogen mustard: a case report. *Brit. J. Derm., 106,* 361.
577. Vonderheid, E. C., Van Scott, E. J., Johnson, W. C. et al. (1977): Topical chemotherapy and immunotherapy of mycosis fungoides. *Arch. Derm., 113,* 454.
578. Price, N. M. (1977): Topical mechlorethamine: Cutaneous changes in patients with mycosis fungoides after its administration. *Arch. Derm., 113,* 1387.
579. Pevny, I. and Peter, G. (1983): Allergisches Kontaktekzem auf Pyridin- und Hydrazinderivate. *Dermatosen Beruf Umw., 31,* 78.
580. Lombardi, P., Spallanzani, P., Giorgini, S. and Sertoli, A. (1982): Allergic contact dermatitis from idoxuridine. *Contact Dermatitis, 8,* 350.
581. Gattefosse, R. M. (1950): *Formulaire de Parfumerie et de Cosmétologie.* Girardot & Cie, Paris.
582. Neumann, H. (1983): Allergische und toxische Nebenwirkungen von Ethylendiamin. *Allergologie, 6,* 27.
583. Peters, M. S., Connolly, S. M. and Schroeter, A. L. (1983): Bronopol allergic contact dermatitis. *Contact Dermatitis, 9,* 397.
584. Fisher, A. A. (1980): Cosmetic dermatitis, Part. II. Reactions to some commonly used preservatives. *Cutis, 26,* 136.
585. Jordan, W. P., Sherman, W. T. and King, S. E. (1979): Threshold responses in formaldehyde-sensitive subjects. *J. Amer. Acad. Derm., 1,* 44.
586. Mandy, S. H. (1974): Contact dermatitis to substituted imidazolidinyl urea – a common preservative in cosmetics. *Arch. Derm., 110,* 463.
587. Fisher, A. A. (1980): Cutaneous reactions to sorbic acid and potassium sorbate. *Cutis, 25,* 350, 352, 423.
588. Fisher, A. A. (1982): Contact dermatitis from topical medicaments. *Semin. Derm., 1,* 49.
589. Chandraratna, P. A. N. and O'Dell, R. E. (1979): Allergic reactions to nitroglycerin ointment: Report of five cases. *Curr. ther. Res., 25,* 481.
590. Fisher, A. A. (1981): Reactions to glutaraldehyde with particular reference to radiologists and X-ray technicians. *Cutis, 28,* 113.
591. Rudzki, E. and Dajek, Z. (1975): Drug eruption with positive patch test to phenol. *Contact Dermatitis, 1,* 322.
592. Addo, H. A., Ferguson, J., Johnson, B. E. and Frain-Bell, W. (1982): The relationship between exposure to fragrance materials and persistent light reaction in the photosensitivity dermatitis with actinic reticuloid syndrome. *Brit. J. Derm., 107,* 261.
593. Frain-Bell, W. (1982): Photosensitivity dermatitis and actinic reticuloid. *Semin. Derm., 1,* 161.
594. Eiermann, H. J., Larsen, W., Maibach, H. I. et al. (1982): Prospective study of cosmetic reactions: 1977 – 1980. *J. Amer. Acad. Derm., 6,* 909.
595. Larsen, W. G. and Maibach, H. I. (1982): Fragrance contact allergy. *Semin. Derm., 1,* 85.
596. Lynde, C. W. and Mitchell, J. C. (1982): Patch testing with balsam of Peru and fragrance mix. *Contact Dermatitis, 8,* 274.
597. Veien, N. K., Hattel, T., Justesen, O. and Nørholm, A. (1982): Patch testing with perfume mixture. *Acta Derm-venereol. (Stockh.), 62,* 341.
598. Calnan, C. D., Cronin, E. and Rycroft, R. J. G. (1980): Allergy to perfume ingredients. *Contact Dermatitis, 6,* 500.

599. Dooms-Goossens, A. and Dooms, M. (1983): Contact allergy to petrolatums (III). Allergenicity prediction and pharmacopoeial requirements. *Contact Dermatitis, 9*, 352.

600. Tokashima, A. and Yoshikawa, K. (1983): Contact allergy to isothipendyl. *Contact Dermatitis, 9*, 429.

601. Watanabe, K. and Yoshikawa, K. (1983): Contact dermatitis due to bufexamac. *Contact Dermatitis, 9*, 433.

602. Karlberg, A.-T., Boman, A. and Wahlberg, J. E. (1980): Allergenic potential of abietic acid, colophony and pine resin-HA. *Contact Dermatitis, 6*, 481.

603. Romaguera, C. and Grimalt, F. (1980): Statistical and comparative study of 4600 patients tested in Barcelona (1973-1977). *Contact Dermatitis, 6*, 309.

604. Cronin, E. (1979): Oil of turpentine – a disappearing allergen. *Contact Dermatitis, 5*, 308.

605. Collins, F. W. and Mitchell, J. C. (1975): Aroma chemicals. Reference sources for perfume and flavour ingredients with special reference to cinnamic aldehyde. *Contact Dermatitis, 1*, 43.

606. Sugai, T. and Higashi, J. (1975): Hypersensitivity to hydrogenated lanolin. *Contact Dermatitis, 1*, 146.

607. Roed-Petersen, J. and Hjorth, N. (1975): Patch test sensitization from, d,1-alpha-tocopherol (vitamin E). *Contact Dermatitis, 1*, 391.

608. Zackheim, H. S., Epstein, E. H. Jr., McNutt, N. S. et al. (1983): Topical carmustine (BCNU) for mycosis fungoides and related disorders: A 10-year experience. *J. Amer. Acad. Derm., 9*, 363.

609. Thune, P., Solberg, Y., McFadden, N. et al. (1982): Perfume allergy due to oak moss and other lichens. *Contact Dermatitis 8*, 396.

610. Bachmann-Buffle, B. (1983): Allergy to clobetasol-17-propionate (Dermovate®). *Dermatologica (Basel), 167*, 104.

611. Brown, R. (1982): Simultaneous hypersensitivity to 3 topical corticosteroids. *Contact Dermatitis, 8*, 339.

612. Bruning, P. F., Meyer, W. J. and Migeon, C. J. (1979): Glucocorticoid receptor in cultured human skin fibroblasts. *J. Steroid Bioch., 10*, 587.

613. Burckhard, W. (1959): Kontaktekzem durch Hydrocortison. *Hautarzt, 10*, 42.

614. Kark, E. C. (1980): Sensitivity to fluorinated steroids presenting as a delayed hypersensitivity. *Contact Dermatitis, 6*, 214.

615. Chalmers, R. J. G., Beck, M. H. and Muston, H. L. (1983): Simultaneous hypersensitivity to clobetasone butyrate and clobetasol propionate. *Contact Dermatitis, 9*, 317.

616. Church, R. (1960): Sensitivity to hydrocortisone acetate ointment. *Brit. J. Derm., 72*, 341.

617. Comaish, S. (1969): A case of hypersensitivity to corticosteroids. *Brit. J. Derm., 81*, 919.

618. Coskey, R. J (1965): Contact dermatitis due to topical hydrocortisone and prednisone. *Michigan Med., 64*, 669.

619. Dooms-Goossens, A., Degreef, H., Parijs, M. and Kerkhofs, L. (1979): A retrospective study of patch test results from 163 patients with stasis dermatitis or leg ulcers. *Dermatologica (Basel), 159*, 93.

620. Dooms-Goossens, A., Vanhee, J., Vanderheyden, D. et al. (1983): Allergic contact dermatitis to topical corticosteroids: clobetasol propionate and clobetasone-butyrate. *Contact Dermatitis, 9*, 470.

621. Dorn, H. (1959): Kontaktallergie gegenüber Salben-Konservierungsmitteln und Hydrocortison. *Z. Hautkr., 27*, 305.

622. Esser, B. (1983): Beitrag zur Kortisonallergie. *Z. Hautkr., 58*, 29.

623. Fisher, A. A. (1979): Allergic reactions to intralesional and multiple topical corticosteroids. *Cutis, 23*, 564, 708.

624. Förström, L., Lassus, A., Salde, L. and Niemi, K.-M. (1982): Allergic contact eczema from topical corticosteroids. *Contact Dermatitis, 8*, 128.

625. Van Ketel, W. G. (1974): Allergy to Ultralan preparations. *Contact Dermatitis Newsl. 15*, 427.

626. Kooij, R. (1959): Hypersensitivity to hydrocortisone. *Brit. J. Derm., 71*, 392.

627. Krook, G. (1974): Contact dermatitis due to Ficortril® (hydrocortisone 1% ointment, Pfizer). *Contact Dermatitis Newsl. 15*, 460.

628. Kuhlwein, A., Hausen, B. M. and Hoting, E. (1983): Kontaktallergie durch halogenierte Kortikosteroide. *Z. Hautkr., 58*, 796.

629. Malten, K. E. (1973): Betnelan V® lotion contact sensitivity. *Contact Dermatitis Newsl. 13*, 360.

630. Pasricha, J. S. and Gupta, R. (1983): Contact sensitivity to betamethasone 17-valerate and fluocinolone acetonide. *Contact Dermatitis, 9*, 330.

631. Shigemi, F., Tanaka, M. and Ohtsuka, T. (1978): A case of sensitization to oral corticosteroids. *J. Derm. (Tokyo), 5*, 231.

107

5.45   Contact allergy to topical drugs

632.   Soesman-Van Waadenoijen Kernekamp, A. and Van Ketel, W. G. (1979): Contact allergy to hydro-cortisone-17-butyrate. *Contact Dermatitis, 5,* 268.

633.   Sönnichsen, N. (1962): Beitrag zur Hydrocortison-Überempfindlichkeit. *Hautarzt, 13,* 226.

634.   Lazzarini, S. (1983): Contact allergy to benzyl alcohol and isopropyl palmitate, ingredients of topi-cal corticosteroid. *Contact Dermatitis, 8,* 349.

635.   Fisher, A. A. (1983): Allergic reactions to topical corticosteroids or their vehicles. *Cutis, 32,* 122.

636.   Maibach, H. I. and Conant, M. (1977): Contact urticaria to a corticosteroid cream: polysorbate 60. *Contact Dermatitis, 3,* 350.

637.   Fisher, A. A. (1982): Cortaid cream dermatitis and the 'paraben paradox'. *J. Amer. Acad. Derm., 6,* 116.

638.   Fisher, A. A. (1983): Allergic contact dermatitis to penicillin and streptomycin. *Cutis, 32,* 314.

639.   Thestrup-Pedersen, K., Christiansen, J. V. and Zachariae, H. (1982): Precautions for personnel ap-plying topical nitrogen mustard to patients with mycosis fungoides. *Dermatologica (Basel), 165,* 108.

640.   Van Ketel, W. G. (1983): Contact allergy to different antihaemorrhoidal anaesthetics. *Contact Der-matitis, 9,* 512.

641.   Nurse, D. S. and Rosner, S. A. (1983): Contact dermatitis due to lignocaine. *Contact Dermatitis, 9,* 513.

642.   Myatt, A. E. and Beck, M. H. (1983): Contact sensitivity to chlorquinaldol. *Contact Dermatitis, 9,* 523.

643.   Sai, S. (1983): Lipstick dermatitis caused by ricinoleic acid. *Contact Dermatitis, 9,* 524.

644.   Wereide, K., Thune, P. and Hanstad, I. (1983): Contact allergy to xeroform in leg ulcer patients. *Contact Dermatitis, 9,* 525.

6. Phototoxic and photoallergic contact dermatitis

6.1   Photosensitivity is the broad term used to describe abnormal or adverse cutaneous reactions to light energy. Drug-induced photosensitivity refers to adverse cutaneous responses which follow the combined or successive exposure to certain chemicals (photosensitizers) and to light. A subdivision can be made into phototoxic and photoallergic reactions. Phototoxicity is the common response which will occur in everybody if enough light energy of the proper wave lengths and, in the case of a photosensitized system, enough of the photosensitizer, is present in the skin. Thus, phototoxicity can be likened to a primary irritant response [91]. Phototoxicity of topical and systemic agents has been reviewed [98].

6.2   Photoallergy can be defined as an acquired altered photoreactivity dependent on an antigen-antibody or cell-mediated hypersensitivity state [24]. Photoallergy was reviewed by Epstein [25, 99] and Frain-Bell [29]. For the pathogenesis of drug-induced photosensitivity, see Magnus [50]. The history of cutaneous photobiology has been discussed by Urbach et al. [74]. An entire issue of 'Seminars in Dermatology' has been devoted to photodermatoses (1982, *Vol 1*, number 3). See also [97] for a review of drug photosensitivity.

6.3   The broad spectrum of clinical photosensitivity reactions has been classified as follows [24]:

I.   Adverse responses due to a loss or lack of protection
This category includes:
A.   Disorders in which there is a lack of pigment formation, as seen in oculocutaneous albinism, and disorders in which there is a loss of pigment, as seen in patients with vitiligo.
B.   The propensity of light-complexioned individuals with light hair and blue eyes, to sunburn easily and readily develop actinic degeneration, keratoses and skin cancer later on in life.
C.   Xeroderma pigmentosum, a rare, recessively inherited genetic disorder, in which epidermal and other cells have a defect in their ability to enzymatically repair UV-damaged DNA.

II.   Adverse responses due to the presence of a photosensitizer
The photosensitizers comprise:
A.   Endogenous photosensitizers; which play a role in some of the porphyrias.
B.   Exogenous photosensitizers; which are subdivided into:
1. *Topical photosensitizers*. This part of the photosensitivity spectrum will be discussed later on in this chapter.
2. *Systemic photosensitizers* [28]. Well-known systemic photosensitizers are e.g. certain sulfonamides, sulfonylurea derivatives, chlorothiazides, phenothiazines, certain tetracyclines, griseofulvin, nalidixic acid and furocoumarins (see also the chapter on Photochemotherapy). In addition, oral contraceptives, triacetyl-di-

phenolisatin, chlordiazepoxide and cyclamates have been reported to induce photosensitivity.

III. Adverse responses of unknown etiology

This category includes a large number of dissimilar diseases, in which both phototoxic and photoallergic reactions may occur, such as solar urticaria, polymorphous light eruption, autoimmune diseases (lupus erythematosus, dermatomyositis, pemphigus vulgaris, pemphigus foliaceus and pemphigoid), pellagra and pellagra-like reactions, photosensitive eczema, actinic reticuloid, hydroa vacciniforme and many other dermatoses. The action spectra and mechanisms of the photoreactions in these diseases are generally unknown or poorly understood.

PHOTOSENSITIVITY DUE TO TOPICAL PHOTOSENSITIZERS (PHOTOCONTACT DERMATITIS)

6.4   Photosensitivity due to topical photosensitizers may be phototoxic, photoallergic, or a combination of both. It is not always easy to determine whether a particular photosensitivity reaction is phototoxic or photoallergic in nature; a combination of both types of reactions frequently occurs. Photopatch testing has been standardized [92, 97].

The most serious consequence of photocontact-allergy is the development of persistent photosensitivity in a small group of patients, despite strict avoidance of further exposure to the photosensitizer. For this group of patients the term *'persistent light reactors'* has been coined. While there is a reasonable chance to recognize contact sensitizers by a series of appropriate bioassays in animals or humans, existing methods to detect photocontact allergens often are insufficient. The most promising method at present is probably a modification of the human maximization test developed by Kaidbey and Kligman [46]. Some animal tests for predicting photocontact allergenicity have been described [93, 94] and reviewed [96].

In § 3.13 some characteristics of phototoxic and photoallergic types of reactions are given that may help to differentiate these conditions. A comprehensive list of topical photosensitizers is provided in § 6.5.

6.5   **Topical photosensitizers** (see also Epstein [24] and Herman and Sams [36])

Drug	Use	Type of reaction	Comment	Ref.
p-aminobenzoic acid (derivatives)	sunscreens	photoallergic		52 39 78
balsam Peru	fragrance	phototoxic	Relevance not established	90
benzocaine	local anesthetic	photoallergic		22 17 42
benzydamine	analgesic and antipyretic drug	photoallergic		20
betacarotene	sunscreen	photoallergic	Photocontact allergy not proven	10

(continued)

(continuation)

Drug	Use	Type of reaction	Comment	Ref.
bithionol	antiseptic	photoallergic	Has photo-cross-reacted with halogenated salicylanilides and hexachlorophene Has caused persistent light reactions	40 9 57
blankophores	in soaps, detergents and cosmetics	photoallergic		14
brilliant lake red R (DC-R31)	coal tar dye in cosmetics	photoallergic	Has caused 'pigmented cosmetic dermatitis'	70
5-bromo-4'-chlorsalicyl-anilide	antiseptic	photoallergic	Has photo-cross-reacted with other halogenated salicylanilides Has caused persistent light reactions	8
buclosamide	antifungal drug	phototoxic photoallergic	Has cross-reacted with sulfanilamide antidiabetics and diuretics Has caused 'localized persistent light reactions'.	12 56
cadmium sulfide	yellow tattoo pigment	phototoxic	Has produced papular and nodular lesions in tattoos	6
chlorhexidine	antiseptic	photoallergic	Sometimes combined with delayed-type hypersensitivity	75
chlormercaptodicarbox-imide	antiseborrhoic agent	photoallergic		23
chloro-2-phenylphenol	antiseptic	photoallergic	Related compounds	1
chlorpromazine hydrochloride	sedative	photoallergic phototoxic	Occupational contact in medical and nursing professionals, in industry, and in veterinary medicine	71 13 95
chlorprothixene	tranquillizer	photoallergic	Accidental contact in a nurse who was allergic to chlorpromazine	49
cinnamates	sunscreens	photoallergic		33
cinnamic aldehyde	fragrance	photoallergic	Also delayed-type allergy in the reported case	86
cinoxate	sunscreen	photoallergic		72
coal tar (and derivatives, including acridine, anthracene, benzpyrine, fluoranthene, phenanthrene)	psoriasis and eczema therapy, cosmetics	phototoxic photoallergic	Has caused persistent light reaction; photocontact urticaria [90] May cause post-inflammatory hyperpigmentation Vegetable and bituminous tars are *not* phototoxic	4 19 79 43 100
coumarin (derivatives)			See 6-methyl coumarin	
dibenzthione	antifungal drug	photoallergic	Has photo-cross-reacted with hydrochlorthiazide	5

(continued)

6.5 Topical photosensitizers

(continuation)

Drug	Use	Type of reaction	Comment	Ref.
dibromsalan	antiseptic	photoallergic	Has photo-cross-reacted with other halogenated salicylanilides, hexachlorophene, dichlorophene and carbanilides	54 35 26
dibucaine	local anesthetic	photoallergic		38
digalloyltrioleate	sunscreen	photoallergic	Digalloyltrioleate is a mixture of tannic acid derivatives	66
dimethoxane	preservative (in sunscreen)	photoallergic		86
diphenhydramine	topical antihistamine	photoallergic	Some patients may be both allergic and photoallergic	21 37
dyes, e.g.: methylene blue fluorescein eosin rose bengal acridine orange acriflavin neutral red	various	phototoxic		16 55
erythrocine-AL (FDC-R3)	coal tar dye in cosmetics	photoallergic	Has caused 'pigmented cosmetic dermatitis'	70
essential oils: bergamot oil cedar oil citron oil lavender oil lime oil neroli oil petitgrain oil sandalwood oil	perfumes	phototoxic	Have caused post-inflammatory hyperpigmentation Sandalwood oil has caused persistent light reaction	34 69 81
2-ethoxyethyl-p-methoxycinnamate	sunscreen	photoallergic phototoxic		18 89
fenticlor	antifungal drug	photoallergic phototoxic	Has photo-cross-reacted with bithionol and hexachlorophene Has caused persistent light reactions	8 9 62
fluorouracil	cytostatic drug	phototoxic (?)	Accelerates inflammatory processes	67
formaldehyde	preservative	uncertain	Immediate sunburn-like reaction in the test situation	87
furocoumarins	cosmetics containing plant extracts essential oils, colognes direct contact with many plants (Umbelliferae, Rutaceae)	phototoxic photoallergic (?)	Have caused postinflammatory hyperpigmentation (berloque dermatitis) Plants containing furocoumarins may cause dermatitis bullosa striata pratensis	60

(continued)

(continuation)

Drug	Use	Type of reaction	Comment	Ref.
glyceryl-p-aminobenzoate	sunscreen	photoallergic	In the reported cases often also a positive reaction to benzocaine During the manufacture of glyceryl-p-aminobenzoate benzocaine is produced	17 27
hexachlorophene	antiseptic	photoallergic	Rare primary photosensitizer; more often photo-cross-reacts with other compounds, e.g. halogenated phenols	57 53
hydrocortisone	corticosteroid	photoallergic	Patch tests were positive after 96 hrs in the reported case	65
2-hydroxy-4-methoxy-benzophenone	sunscreen	photoallergic	*See also under* mexenone	88
isoamyl-p-N,N-dimethyl-aminobenzoate	sunscreen	phototoxic		78 44
lithol red-CA (DC-R11)	coal tar dye in cosmetics	photoallergic	Has caused 'pigmented cosmetic dermatitis'	70
p-methoxy-isoamyl-cinnamate	sunscreen	photoallergic		86
8-methoxpsoralen	PUVA therapy	phototoxic photoallergic	*See also* Chapter 18 on Photochemotherapy	31
6-methyl coumarin	fragrance	photoallergic	Has photo-cross-reacted with 7-methyl coumarin, coumarin, 7-methoxycoumarin	45 47
mexenone	sunscreen	photoallergic	Has photo-cross-reacted with 2-hydroxy-4-methoxy-benzophenone	10 63
musk ambrette	perfumes	photoallergic	Has caused persistent light reactions A photo-cross-reaction to musk xylol has been reported [84]	64 48 11 32 82 83 84 85
musk xylol	fragrance	photoallergic	Probably represented a photo-cross-reaction to musk ambrette	84
mycanodin	antifungal drug	photoallergic		7
oak moss	fragrance	photoallergic	Photocontact allergy to the ingredients atranorin and evernic acid	101
permanent orange (DC-017)	coal tar dye in cosmetics	photoallergic	Has caused 'pigmented cosmetic dermatitis'	70
2-phenylbenzimidazole sulfate	sunscreen ingredient	photoallergic		86
p-phenylenediamine	various	photoallergic		76

(continued)

6.5 Topical photosensitizers

(continuation)

Drug	Use	Type of reaction	Comment	Ref.
promethazine hydrochloride	(topical) antihistamine	photoallergic	Oral use in sensitized individuals may provoke photosensitivity Has caused persistent light reactions	56 61 73 68
quinine sulfate	antimalarial drug	photoallergic	Accidental contact Has caused persistent light reactions	41
sulfanilamide	chemotherapeutic	photoallergic	Has (photo)-cross-reacted with other para-compounds Has caused persistent light reactions	3
tetrachlorosalicylanilide	antiseptic	photoallergic phototoxic	Has photo-cross-reacted with other halogenated salicylanilides, hexachlorophene Has caused persistent light reactions	15 77
toluidine red (DC-R35)	coal tar dye in cosmetics	photoallergic	Has caused 'pigmented cosmetic dermatitis'	70
tribromsalan	antiseptic	phototoxic photoallergic	Has photo-cross-reacted with other halogenated salicylanilides, triclocarban, hexachlorophene and fenticlor	58 59 35
triclocarban	antiseptic	phototoxic photoallergic	Has photo-cross-reacted with halogenated salicylanilides. Rare primary photosensitizer	30 51 2
zinc pyrithione	dandruff therapy	photoallergic (?)	May lead to photosensitive eczema and actinic reticuloid syndrome	80

6.6 The following test tray of topical photosensitizers has been proposed [92]:

Trichlorcarbanilide (TCC)	1% pet.
Promethazine	1% pet.
Para-aminobenzoic acid (PABA)	5% alc.
Tribromsalicylanilide (TBS)	1% pet.
Chlorpromazine hydrochloride	0.1% pet.
Musk ambrette	1% alc.
Tetrachlorsalicylanilide (TCS)	0.1% pet.
Diphenhydramine hydrochloride	1% pet.
6-Methylcoumarin	1% alc.
Bithionol	1% pet.
Hexachlorophene	1% pet.
Balsam Peru	25% pet.
Chlorhexidine	0.5% aq.
Wood mix[a]	20% pet.
Irgasan DP 300® (triclosan)	2% pet.
Lichen mix[b]	16% pet.
Fenticlor	1% pet.
Perfume mix[c]	6% pet.
Compositae mix[d]	approx. 3% pet.

[a] Pine, spruce, birch and teak, 5% each.
[b] A mixture of *Parmelia*, *Hypogymnia*, *Pseudoevernia*, *Cladonia*, *Plasmatica*, *Physica*, *Umbilicaria* and *Cetraria* species.
[c] Cinnamic alcohol, cinnamic aldehyde, hydroxy-citronellal, eugenol, isoeugenol and geraniol, 1% each.
[d] A mixture of oleoresins from *Chrysanthemum*, *Anthemis*, *Achillea* and *Artemesia* species.

One should bear in mind that photocontact dermatitis to several of these compounds is exceptional (e.g. hexachlorophene), whilst others are well-known photosensitizers and therefore hardly used anymore; several are prohibited in some countries (e.g. several halogenated salicylanilides).

6.7   REFERENCES

1. Adams, R. M. (1972): Photoallergic contact dermatitis to chloro-2-phenylphenol. *Arch. Derm., 106,* 711.
2. Ägren-Jonsson, S. and Magnusson, B. (1976): Sensitisation to propantheline bromide, trichlorocarbanilide and propylene glycol in an antiperspirant. *Contact Dermatitis, 2,* 79.
3. Aokï, K. and Saito, T. (1974): Studies on the mechanism of photosensitivity caused by sulfa drugs. In: *Sunlight and Man, Normal and Abnormal Photobiologic Responses. Ch. 27,* p. 431. University of Tokyo Press, Tokyo.
4. Barefoot, S. W. (1979): Report of a persistent light eruption due to pitch. *Cutis, 24,* 395.
5. Behrbohm, P. and Zschunke, E. (1965): Allergisches Ekzem durch das Antimykotikum 'Afungin' (Dibenzthion). *Derm. Wschr., 151,* 1447.
6. Björnberg, A. (1963): Reactions to light in yellow tattoos from cadmium sulfide. *Arch. Derm., 88,* 267.
7. Burckhardt, W., Mahler, F. and Schwarz-Speck, M. (1968): Photoallergische Ekzeme durch Mycanodin. *Dermatologica (Basel), 137,* 208.
8. Burry, J. N. (1967): Photoallergies to fentichlor and multifungin. *Arch. Derm., 95,* 287.
9. Burry, J. N. (1968): Cross sensitivity between fentichlor and bithionol. *Arch. Derm., 97,* 497.
10. Burry, J. N., (1980): Photoallergies from benzophenones and beta carotene in sunscreens. *Contact Dermatitis, 6,* 211.
11. Burry, J. N. (1981): Persistent light reaction associated with sensitivity to Musk Ambrette. *Contact Dermatitis, 7,* 46.
12. Burry, J. N., and Hunter, G. A. (1970): Photocontact dermatitis from Jadit. *Brit. J. Derm., 82,* 224.
13. Calnan, C. D. (1958): Studies in contact dermatitis. V. Photosensitivity from chlorpromazine. *Trans. St. John's Hosp. derm. Soc. (Lond.), 41,* 26.
14. Calnan, C. D. (1973): Hazards of optic bleaches. *Trans. St. John's Hosp. derm. Soc. (Lond.), 59,* 275.
15. Calnan, C. D., Harman, R. R. M. and Wells, G. C. (1961): Photodermatitis from soaps. *Brit. med. J., ii,* 1266.
16. Calnan, C. D. and Sarkany, J. (1957): Studies in Contact Dermatitis. II. Lipstick cheilitis. *Trans. St. John's Hosp. derm. Soc. (Lond.), 39,* 28.
17. Caro, I. (1978): Contact allergy/photoallergy to glycerol PABA and benzocaine. *Contact Dermatitis, 4,* 381.
18. Cronin, E. (1980): Photosensitisers. In: *Contact Dermatitis,* p. 454. Churchill Livingstone, Edinburgh.
19. Crow, K. D., Alexander, E., Buck, W. H. L., Johnson, B. E., Magnus, I. A. and Porter, A. D. (1961): Photosensitivity due to pitch. *Brit. J. Derm., 73,* 220.
20. De Corres, L. F. (1980): Photodermatitis from benzydamine. *Contact Dermatitis, 6,* 285.
21. Emmett, E. A. (1974): Diphenhydramine Photoallergy. *Arch. Derm., 110,* 249.
22. Epstein, S. (1965): Photocontact dermatitis from benzocain. *Arch. Derm., 92,* 591.
23. Epstein, S. (1968): Photoallergic contact dermatitis: report of a case due to Dangard. *Cutis, 4,* 856.
24. Epstein, J. H. (1971): In: *Year Book of Dermatology,* pp. 5-43. Editors: F. D. Malkinson and R. W. Pearson. Year Book Medical Publishers, Chicago.
25. Epstein, J. H. (1977): Photoallergy. *Aust. J. Derm., 18,* 51.
26. Epstein, J. H., Wuepper, K. D. and Maibach, H. I. (1968): Photocontact dermatitis to halogenated salicylanilides and related compounds. *Arch. Derm., 97,* 236.
27. Fisher, A. A. (1977): The presence of benzocaine in sunscreens containing glyceryl PABA (Escalol 106). *Arch. Derm., 113,* 1299.
28. Fitzpatrick, T. B. et al. (1974): In: *Sunlight and Man, Normal and Abnormal Photobiologic responses,* pp. 10-11. University of Tokyo Press, Tokyo.
29. Frain-Bell, W. (1979): What is that thing called light? *Clin. exp. Derm., 4,* 1.
30. Freeman, R. G. and Knox, J. M. (1968): The action spectrum of photocontact dermatitis. *Arch. Derm., 97,* 130.

6.7 Topical photosensitizers

31. Fulton, J. E. and Willis, I. (1968): Photoallergy to methoxsalen. *Arch. Derm., 98,* 445.
32. Giovinazzo, V. J., Harber, L. C., Bickers, D. R., Armstrong, R. B. and Silvers, D. N. (1981): Photoallergic contact dermatitis to Musk Ambrette. *Arch. Derm., 117,* 344.
33. Goodmann, T. F. (1970): Photodermatitis from a sunscreening agent (letter). *Arch. Derm., 102,* 563.
34. Harber, C. L., Harris, H., Leder, M. and Baer, R. L. (1964): Berloque dermatitis. *Arch. Derm., 90,* 505.
35. Harber, L. C., Targovnik, S. E. and Baer, R. L. (1967): Contact photosensitivity patterns to halogenated salicylanilides. *Arch. Derm., 96,* 646.
36. Herman, P. S. and Sams, W. M. (1972): *Soap Photodermatitis. Photosensitivity to Halogenated Salicylanilides.* Charles C. Thomas, Springfield, Ill.
37. Horio, T. (1976): Allergic and photoallergic dermatitis from diphenhydramine. *Arch. Derm., 112,* 1124.
38. Horio, T. (1980): Photosensitivity reactions to dibucaine. *Arch. Derm., 115,* 973.
39. Horio, T. and Hituchi, T. (1978): Photocontact dermatitis from p-aminobenzoic acid. *Dermatologica (Basel), 156,* 124.
40. Jillson, O. F. and Baughman, R. D. (1963): Contact photodermatitis from bithionol. *Arch. Derm., 88,* 409.
41. Johnson, B. E., Zaynoun, S., Gardiner, J. M. and Frain-Bell, W. (1975): A study of persistent light reaction in quindoxin and quinine photosensitivity. *Brit. J. Derm., 93,* suppl. 11, 21.
42. Kaidbey, K. H. and Allen, H. (1981): Photocontact allergy to benzocaine. *Arch. Derm., 117,* 77.
43. Kaidbey, K. H. and Kligman, A. M. (1977): Clinical and histological study of coal tar phototoxicity in humans. *Arch. Derm., 113,* 592.
44. Kaidbey, K. H. and Kligman, A. M. (1978): Phototoxicity to a sunscreen ingredient. Padimate A. *Arch. Derm., 114,* 547.
45. Kaidbey, K. H. and Kligman, A. M. (1978): Photocontact allergy to 6-methylcoumarin. *Contact Dermatitis, 4,* 277.
46. Kaidbey, K. H. and Kligman, A. M. (1980): Photomaximization test for identifying photoallergic contact sensitizers. *Contact Dermatitis, 6,* 161.
47. Kaidbey, K. H. and Kligman, A. M. (1981): Photosensitization by coumarin derivatives. *Arch. Derm., 117,* 258.
48. Kroon, S. (1979): Musk Ambrette, a new cosmetic sensitizer and photosensitizer. *Contact Dermatitis, 5,* 337.
49. Kull, E. and Schwarz-Speck, K. (1961): Gruppenspezifische Ekzemreaktionen bei Largactilsensibilisierung. *Dermatologica (Basel), 122,* 263.
50. Magnus, I. A. (1976): *Dermatological Photobiology,* pp. 255 and 211. Blackwell Scientific Publications, Oxford.
51. Maibach, H. et al. (1978): Triclocarban. Evaluation of contact dermatitis potential in man. *Contact Dermatitis, 4,* 283.
52. Marmelzat, J. and Rapaport, M. J. (1980): Photodermatitis with PABA. *Contact Dermatitis, 6,* 230.
53. Masuda, T. et al. (1971): Photocontact dermatitis due to bithionol, TBS, diaphene and hexachlorophene. *Jap. J. Derm., 81,* 238.
54. Molloy, J. F. and Mayer, J. A. (1966): Photodermatitis from dibromosalicylanilide. *Arch. Derm., 93,* 331.
55. Morikawa, F., Fukuda, M., Naganuma, M. and Nakayama, Y. (1976): Phototoxic reactions to xanthine dyes induced by visible light. *J. Derm. (Tokyo), 3,* 59.
56. Nagreh, D. S. (1975): Photodermatitis study of the condition in Kuantan, Malaysia. *Contact Dermatitis, 1,* 27.
57. O'Quinn, S. E., Kennedy, C. B. and Isbell, K. H. (1967): Contact photodermatitis from bithionol and related compounds. *J. Amer. med. Ass., 199,* 125.
58. Osmundsen, P. E. (1968): Contact photodermatitis due to tribromsalicylanilide. *Brit. J. Derm., 80,* 228.
59. Osmundsen, P. E. (1970): Contact photodermatitis due to tribromsalicylanilide (cross reaction pattern). *Dermatologica (Basel), 140,* 65.
60. Pathak, M. A. (1974): Phytophotodermatitis. In: *'Sunlight and Man',* p. 502. University of Tokyo Press, Tokyo.
61. Prisco, D. J., Soto, J. M. and Herrera, E. (1968): Phenergan sensitivity. *Contact Dermatitis Newsl., 4,* 63.
62. Ramsay, C. A. (1979): Skin responses to ultraviolet radiation in contact photodermatitis due to fentichlor. *J. invest. Derm., 48,* 255.

63. Ramsay, D. L., Cohen, H. J. and Baer, R. L. (1972): Allergic reactions to benzophenones. *Arch. Derm, 105,* 906.
64. Raugi, G. J., Storrs, F. J. and Larsen, W. G. (1979): Photoallergic contact dermatitis to men's perfumes. *Contact Dermatitis, 5,* 251.
65. Rietschel, R. L. (1978): Photocontact dermatitis to hydrocortisone. *Contact Dermatitis, 4,* 334.
66. Sams, W. M. (1956): Contact photodermatitis. *Arch. Derm., 73,* 142.
67. Sams, W. M. (1968): Untoward response with topical fluorouracil. *Arch. Derm., 97,* 14.
68. Sidi, E., Hincky, M. and Gervais, A. (1955): Allergic sensitisation and photosensitization to phenergan cream. *J. invest. Derm., 24,* 345.
69. Starke, J. C. (1967): Photoallergy to sandalwood oil. *Arch. Derm., 96,* 62.
70. Sugai, T., Takahashi, Y. and Tagaki, T. (1977): Pigmented cosmetic dermatitis and coal tar dyes. *Contact Dermatitis, 3,* 249.
71. Sulser, H., Schwarz, K. and Schwarz, M. (1963): Über Kreuzreaktionen bei experimenteller photoallergischer Chlorpromazinsensibilisierung. *Dermatologica (Basel), 127,* 108.
72. Thompson, G., Maibach, H. and Epstein, J. (1977): Allergic contact dermatitis from sunscreen preparations complicating photodermatitis. *Arch. Derm., 113,* 1252.
73. Tzanck, A., Sidi, E., Mazalton, and Kohen, (1951): Sur deux cas de dermite au phenergan avec photosensibilisation. *Bull. Soc. franç. Derm. Syph., 58,* 433.
74. Urbach, F., Forbes, D., Davies, R. E. and Berger, D. (1976): Cutaneous photobiology: past, present and future. *J. invest. Derm., 67,* 209.
75. Wahlberg, J. E. and Wennersten, G. (1971): Hypersensitivity and photosensitivity to chlorhexidine. *Dermatologica, (Basel), 143,* 376.
76. Wasserman, G. A. and Haberman, H. F. (1975): Photosensitivity: results of investigation in 250 patients. *Canad. med. Ass. J., 113,* 1055.
77. Wilkinson, D. S. (1962): Further experiences with halogenated salicylanilides. *Brit. J. Derm., 74,* 295.
78. Willis, J. and Kligman, A. M. (1970): Aminobenzoic acid and its esters. *Arch. Derm., 102,* 405.
79. Wiskemann, A. and Hoyer, H. (1971): Zur Phototoxizität von Teerpräparaten. *Hautarzt, 22,* 257.
80. Yates, V. M. and Finn, O. A. (1980): Contact allergic sensitivity to zinc pyrithione followed by the photosensitivity dermatitis and actinic reticuloid syndrome. *Contact Dermatitis, 6,* 349.
81. Zaynoun, S. T., Johnson, B. E. and Frain-Bell, W. (1977): A study of oil of bergamot and its importance as a phototoxic agent. *Contact Dermatitis, 3,* 225.
82. Zugerman, C. (1981): Persistent photosensitivity caused by Musk Ambrette. *Arch. Derm., 117,* 432.

UPDATE – 2nd Edition

83. Menezes Brandão, F., Cirne de Castro, J. and Pecegueiro, M. (1983): Photoallergy to musk ambrette. *Contact Dermatitis, 9,* 332.
84. Galosi, A. and Plewig, G. (1982): Photoallergisches Ekzem durch Ambrette Moschus. *Hautarzt, 33,* 589.
85. Kroon, S. (1983): Standard photopatch testing with Musk Ambrette. *Contact Dermatitis, 9,* 1.
86. Fagerlund, V. -L., Kalimo, K. and Jansén, C. (1983): Photocontact allergy from sunscreens. *Duodecim, 99,* 146.
87. Shelley, W. B. (1982): Immediate sunburn-like reaction in a patient with formaldehyde photosensitivity. *Arch. Derm., 118,* 117.
88. Hölzle, E. and Plewig, G. (1982): Photoallergische Kontaktdermatitis durch benzophenonhaltige Sonnenschutzpräparate. *Hautarzt, 33,* 391.
89. Davies, M. G., Hawk, J. L. M. and Rycroft, R. J. G. (1982): Acute photosensitivity from the sunscreen 2-ethoxyethyl-p-methoxycinnamate. *Contact Dermatitis, 8,* 190.
90. Kroon, S. (1983): Standard photopatch testing with Waxtar®, para-aminobenzoic acid, potassium dichromate and balsam of Peru. *Contact Dermatitis, 9,* 5.
91. Epstein, J. H. (1983): Phototoxicity and photoallergy in man. *J. Amer. Acad. Derm., 8,* 141.
92. Jansén, Ch. T., Wennersten, G., Rystedt, I. et al. (1982): The Scandinavian standard photopatch test procedure. *Contact Dermatitis, 8,* 155.
93. Jordan, W. P. Jr. (1982): The guinea pig as a model for predicting photoallergic contact dermatitis. *Contact Dermatitis, 8,* 109.
94. Maurer, Th., Weirich, E. G. and Hess, R. (1980): Predictive animal testing for photocontact allergenicity. *Brit. J. Derm., 103,* 593.

6.7 Topical photosensitizers

95. Ertle, T. (1982): Beruflich bedingte Kontakt – und Photokontaktallergie bei einem Landwirt durch Chlorpromazin. *Dermatosen Beruf Umw., 30,* 120.
96. Harber, L. C., Armstrong, R. B., Walther, R. R. and Ichikawa, H. (1982): Current status of predictive animal models for drug photoallergy and their correlation with humans. In: *Safety and Efficacy of Topical Drugs and Cosmetics, Chapter 10,* pp. 177-192. Eds: A. M. Kligman and J. J. Leyden. Grune and Stratton, New York.
97. Harber, L. C., Bickers, D. R., Armstrong, R. B. and Kochevar, I. E. (1982): Drug photosensitivity: Phototoxic and photoallergic mechanisms. *Semin. Derm., 1,* 183.
98. Maibach, H. I. and Marzulli, F. N. (1983): Phototoxicity (Photoirritation) of topical and systemic agents. In: *Dermatotoxicology, 2nd Edition, Chapter 17,* pp. 375-389. Eds.: F. N. Marzulli and H. I. Maibach. Hemisphere Publishing Corporation, Washington.
99. Epstein, J. H. (1983): Photocontact allergy in humans. In *Dermatotoxicology, 2nd Edition, Chapter 18,* pp. 391-404. Hemisphere Publishing Corporation, Washington.
100. Diette, K. M., Gange, R. W., Stern, R. S. et al (1983): Coal tar phototoxicity: Kinetics and exposure parameters. *J. invest. Derm., 81,* 347.
101. Fernández de Corres, L., Muñoz, D., Leaniz-Barrutía, I. and Corrales, J. L. (1983): Photocontact dermatitis from oak moss. *Contact Dermatitis, 9,* 528.

7.   The contact urticaria syndrome

7.1   Contact urticaria denotes a wheal-and-flare response after cutaneous exposure to certain agents; usually the reaction is elicited within 30–60 minutes, but delayed-onset urticaria (up to 6 hours) may infrequently occur, possibly through slower percutaneous penetration. The broad spectrum of clinical manifestations described justifies the term 'the contact urticaria syndrome'. The subject has been thoroughly reviewed [52–54, 72]; a monograph on non-immunologic contact urticaria has been published [27].

7.2   On the basis of the action mechanisms involved, contact urticaria may be subdivided into three types [30, 36], which are characterized as follows:

Type A: Non-immunologic contact urticaria
– The response may be evoked in many or nearly all exposed individuals.
– Contact with the incriminated chemical induces release of histamine and other vasoactive substances, without involving immunologic processes.
– Passive transfer is not possible.
– This type of contact urticaria occurs frequently.

Type B: Immunologic contact urticaria
– The response may be evoked in previously sensitized individuals only.
– Immunologic mechanisms are involved in releasing histamine and other vasoactive substances.
– Passive transfer is possible.
– This type of contact urticaria occurs less frequently.

Type C: Uncertain mechanism contact urticaria
– The mechanisms involved are not clarified: neither an immunologic nor a non-specific direct release of mediators has been proven.

7.3   On a clinical basis, the following division has been suggested [52]:

Cutaneous reactions only

Stage 1: Localized urticaria
          dermatitis/dermatosis
          non-specific symptoms (e.g. itching, tingling and burning).
Stage 2: Generalized urticaria.

Extracutaneous reactions

Stage 3: Bronchial asthma
          rhinoconjunctivitis
          otolaryngeal
          gastrointestinal.
Stage 4: Anaphylactoid reactions.

7.4 Contact urticaria

7.4   Contact urticaria may be elicited by contact with various foods, plants, animal products, physical influences, textiles, cosmetics and industrial contactants [36, 52–54]. Sometimes a positive delayed test-response may develop subsequent to the initial wheal-and-flare reaction. For patients exhibiting combined reactions in the test situation the term 'contact dermatitis of immediate and delayed type' has been proposed [52]. For test procedures to evaluate the immediate-type responses the reader is referred to the review articles on the subject [52–54].

Table 7.5 lists chemicals used in dermatology and cosmetology, which have caused contact urticaria. In many reported cases the authors believe the contact urticaria to be of immunologic origin, but substantial evidence for this is often lacking. Therefore, the mechanism of action for a particular drug is only then listed as 'immunological' (type B) if passive transfer has been successful or if specific antibodies have been demonstrated.

7.5   **Contact urticaria caused by topical drugs**

Drug	Use	Mechanism involved	Comment	Ref.
acetylsalicylic acid	analgesic	?	Only listed; no references	36
aminophenazone	antipyretic, analgesic	uncertain	Generalized urticaria upon patch testing Also delayed-type allergy Caused also anaphylactic shock Has cross-reacted to propyphenazone and metamizole [62]	7 20 62
ammonium persulfate	in hair bleaches	uncertain	Scratch tests in an atopic patient have caused a mild asthmatic attack May induce urticarial responses to scratch tests in controls Anaphylaxis has occurred	12 5
ampicillin	antibiotic	uncertain	A patch test evoked the urticarial reaction	38
amyl alcohol	solvent	immunologic	The reported patient also reacted to butyl alcohol, ethyl alcohol and propyl alcohol	41
arsphenamine	formerly used for treating syphilis	uncertain		46
bacitracin	antibiotic	immunologic	Anaphylactic reaction Specific reagins were demonstrated	43
balsam Peru	various	non-immunologic	The % of positive reactions depends upon the test concentration A concentration of 12.5% yields the largest number [13] Also positive reactions to cinnamic aldehyde, cinnamic acid, benzoic acid and benzaldehyde in some cases Sometimes also delayed-type allergy	13 48 64

(continued)

(continuation)

Drug	Use	Mechanism involved	Comment	Ref.
benzaldehyde		non-immuno-logic	*See under* balsam Peru	
benzocaine	local anesthetic	uncertain	Scratch tests positive Also anaphylactic reaction Also delayed-type hypersensitivity	24
benzoic acid		non-immuno-logic	*See also under* balsam Peru Benzoic acid in food has caused perioral contact urticaria	63
			See under denatonium benzoate	
benzoyl peroxide	acne therapy	uncertain		59
butyl alcohol		non-immuno-logic	*See under* amyl alcohol	
butylated hydroxyanisole	antioxidant	uncertain	Also delayed-type hypersensitivity in the reported case	42
butylated hydroxytoluene	antioxidant	uncertain	Also delayed-type hypersensitivity in the reported case	42
camphor	rubefacient	probably non-immuno-logic	The patient described also reacted to balsam Peru and cinnamon oil	48
caraway seed oil	in toothpastes	uncertain	Also caused 'sub-shock'	22
cephalosporins	antibiotics	uncertain	Also sneezing, watery nasal discharge, lacrimation and difficulty of breathing in the reported case	50
cetyl alcohol	vehicle constituent	uncertain	Both urticarial response and delayed type hypersensitivity in the reported case with concomitant reaction to stearyl alcohol	16
chloramine	disinfectant	immunologic	Specific IgE antibodies demonstrated Also dyspnea and rhinitis in the reported case	57
chloramphenicol	antibiotic	uncertain	Has caused a 'sub-shock'	26
chlorpromazine	sedative	?	Only listed; no references	36
cinnamic acid		non-immuno-logic	*See under* balsam Peru	

(continued)

7.5 Contact urticaria caused by topical drugs

(continuation)

Drug	Use	Mechanism involved	Comment	Ref.
cinnamic aldehyde	flavoring agent	non-immuno-logic	Some controls were positive on patch testing Was shown to release histamine from human leukocytes	35
cinnamon oil		non-immuno-logic	*See also under* sorbic acid In patients wih urticaria displaying contact urtication to patch tests with cinnamon oil, oral provocation induced urticaria	64
clioquinol	antimicrobial	uncertain		51
clobetasol-17-propionate	corticosteroid	uncertain		61
denatonium benzoate	denaturant in alcoholic preparations	uncertain	Also asthmatic symptoms in the reported patient The patient also had contact urticarial responses to patch testing with benzoic acid and sodium benzoate	3
diethyl toluamide	insect repellent	immunologic	Passive transfer demonstrated	30 58
1,3-diiodo-2-hydroxypropane	antiseptic	uncertain	Also delayed-type hypersensitivity in the reported case	28
dimethyl sulfoxide	solvent	non-immuno-logic	Concentrations below 20% only cause erythema	33 25
estrogen cream	topical hormone preparation	uncertain		8
ethyl alcohol	antiseptic	immunologic	Passive transfer positive only after scratching The patient reported also reacted to amyl alcohol, butyl alcohol and propyl alcohol In another patient [67] who displayed erythema 20 minutes after cutaneous contact with ethyl alcohol, a generalized eruption developed after drinking alcoholic beverages	41 67
ethylenediamine	stabilizer	uncertain	Contact urticarial response upon patch testing in a patient with urticaria	64
ethyl vanillin	flavoring agent	uncertain	Also an urticarial response to balsam Peru in the reported case	44

(continued)

(continuation)

Drug	Use	Mechanism involved	Comment	Ref.
eugenol	fragrance/flavor	uncertain, probably non-immunologic	Contact urticarial response upon patch testing in patients with urticaria Also delayed-type allergy in some cases Oral provocation caused urticaria	64
formaldehyde	preservative	uncertain	The reaction was provoked by contact with gaseous formaldehyde	65
gentian violet	antiseptic	uncertain	The patient was treated with Milian's solution	14
henna	hair dye	uncertain	Also sneezing, wheezing and throat complaints in the reported case Prick tests were positive	9
hexantriol	vehicle constituent	uncertain		47
p-hydroxybenzoic acid	preservative	uncertain		60
isopropyl alcohol	antiseptic	uncertain		68
lanolin alcohol	vehicle constituent	uncertain		51
lemon perfume constituents	perfume	non-immunologic		70
lindane	antiparasitic drug	?	Industrial contactant, also induces asthma Only listed; no references	36
mechlorethamine hydrochloride	cytostatic drug	uncertain	Has also caused anaphylaxis and dyspnea	10 17 18 75
menthol	antipruritic	uncertain		37
metamizole	analgesic	uncertain	Contact urticarial reaction upon patch testing in patients with anaphylaxis after oral administration Cross-reactions occur between pyrazolone derivatives	62
methyl green	antiseptic	uncertain	The patient was treated with Milian's solution, also containing gentian violet	14
monoamylamine	antifungal drug	uncertain	Also delayed-type hypersensitivity to tolnaftate in the same preparation	49

(continued)

7.5 Contact urticaria caused by topical drugs

(continuation)

Drug	Use	Mechanism involved	Comment	Ref.
neomycin	antibiotic	uncertain	Also delayed-type hypersensitivity to neomycin in the reported case, with cross-reaction to paromomycin and kanamycin Anaphylaxis after open test	32
nicotinyl alcohol	vasodilator	uncertain		32
nitrofuroxime	antifungal drug	uncertain	Also delayed-type hypersensitivity in the reported case	1
parabens	preservatives	immunologic and non-immunologic	Passive transfer demonstrated	21 64
penicillin	antibiotic	uncertain	Anaphylaxis after oral administration	32 60
phenol	antipruritic	non-immuno-logic		4
phenylbutazone	analgesic	uncertain	Cross-reaction to propyphenazone in a patient with anaphylaxis after oral propyphenazone Also delayed-type hypersensitivity to phenylbutazone in the reported case	62
p-phenylenediamine	in hair preparations	uncertain	Also difficulty in breathing Scratch tests were positive	6
phenylmercuric compounds	antiseptics	immunologic	Inhalation produced asthma Passive transfer demonstrated	31
polyethyleneglycol 400	vehicle constituent	uncertain		11
polysorbate 60	vehicle constituent	uncertain	Only urticarial response when patch-tested on the forehead	29
pristinamycin	antibiotic	uncertain	Also delayed-type hypersensitivity in the reported patient	2
promethazine hydrochloride	antihistamine	uncertain		20
propyl alcohol	solvent	immunologic	The patient reported also reacted to amyl alcohol, ethyl alcohol and butyl alcohol	41
propylene glycol	vehicle constituent	uncertain		55

(continued)

(continuation)

Drug	Use	Mechanism involved	Comment	Ref.
propyphenbutazone	analgesic	uncertain	Contact urticarial reaction upon patch-testing in patients with anaphylaxis after oral propyphenbutazone Cross-reactions between pyrazolone derivatives	62
pyrazolone derivatives	analgesics	uncertain	Contact urticarial reactions upon patch-testing in patients with anaphylaxis after oral administration *See under* aminophenazone, propyphenbutazone, metamizole *and* phenylbutazone	62
rouge	cosmetic	uncertain	The patient had a delayed-type reaction to γ-methylionone, a perfume ingredient of the cosmetic The relevance of this finding remained uncertain The contact urticarial reaction was limited to the face	56
salicylic acid	keratolytic drug	uncertain		36
sodium benzoate	preservative	non-immuno-logic	*See also under* denatonium benzoate	3
sorbic acid	preservative	non-immuno-logic and immunologic (?) [40]	Also urticarial response to cinnamon oil [40] Sorbic acid in food has caused perioral contact urticaria [63]	40 15
stearyl alcohol	vehicle constituent	uncertain	Also delayed-type hypersensitivity in the reported case, with concomitant reaction to cetyl alcohol	16
streptomycin	antibiotic	uncertain	*See also under* neomycin Rhinitis and conjunctivitis after open test	32 45
sulfur	antiseborrheic drug	uncertain		60
sulisobenzone	sunscreen	uncertain	Also delayed-type hypersensitivity in the reported patient	39
terpinyl acetate	fragrance	uncertain	Terpinyl acetate was a fragrance ingredient in spray starch	74

(continued)

7.5 Contact urticaria caused by topical drugs

(continuation)

Drug	Use	Mechanism involved	Comment	Ref.
tetracycline	antibiotic	uncertain	Also asthma in the reported case Generalized urticaria upon patch-testing	73
thurfyl nicotinate	rubefacient	non-immuno-logic	Histamine releaser	34
α-tocopherol	antioxidant	uncertain		23
tropicamide	anticholinergic ophthalmic preparation	uncertain		19
wheat bran	in baths	immunologic	The patient was an atopic infant whose eczema improved on a gluten-free diet	71

7.6 Cosmetics that have caused contact urticaria include:

- fixation fluid for perma-nent wave [51]
- permanent wave fluid [51]
- hair spray [69]
- hair bleach

- (*see* § 7.5 *under* ammonium persulfate)
- nail varnish [69]
- perfumes [44, 69, 70]
- deodorant [48]

- rouge (*see* § 7.5)
- shampoo [40]
- toothpaste [40] (*see* § 7.5 *under* sorbic acid)

7.7 REFERENCES

1. Aaronson, C. M. (1969): Generalized urticaria from sensitivity to nifuroxime. *J. Amer. med. Ass., 210,* 557.
2. Baes, H. (1974): Allergic contact dermatitis to virginiamycin. *Dermatologica (Basel), 149,* 231.
3. Björkner, B. (1980): Contact urticaria and asthma from denatonium benzoate (BitrexR). *Contact Dermatitis, 6,* 466.
4. Björnberg, A. (1968): *Skin reactions to primary irritants in patients with hand eczema.* O. Isacson Tryckeri, Gothenburg.
5. Brubaker, M. M. (1972): Urticarial reaction to ammonium persulphate. *Arch. Derm., 106,* 413.
6. Calnan, C. D. (1967): Hair dye reaction. *Contact Dermatitis Newsl., 1,* 16.
7. Camarasa, J. M. G., Alomar, A. and Perez, M. (1978): Contact urticaria and anaphylaxis from amin-ophenazone. *Contact Dermatitis, 4,* 243.
8. Cole, H., Marmelzat, W. and Walker, A. (1948): Severe allergic sensitization to an estrogenic cream. *Ohio St. med. J., 44,* 472.
9. Cronin, E. (1980): Immediate-type hypersensitivity to henna. *Contact Dermatitis, 5,* 198.
10. Daughters, D., Zackheim, H. and Maibach, H. I. (1973): Urticaria and anaphylactoid reactions after topical application of mechlorethamine. *Arch. Derm., 107,* 429.
11. Fisher, A. A. (1978): Immediate and delayed allergic contact reactions to polyethyleneglycol. *Contact Dermatitis, 4,* 135.
12. Fisher, A. A. and Dooms-Goossens, A. (1976): Persulfate hair bleach reactions. Cutaneous and respi-ratory manifestations. *Arch. Derm., 112,* 1407.
13. Forsbeck, M. and Skog, E. (1977): Immediate reactions to patch tests with balsam of Peru. *Contact Dermatitis, 3,* 201.
14. François, A., Henin, P., Carli Basset, C. and Ginies, G. (1970): Anaphylactic shock following appli-cation of Milian's solution. *Bull. Soc. franç. Derm. Syph., 77,* 834.

15. Fryklöf, L. E. (1958): A note on the irritant properties of sorbic acid in ointments and creams. *J. Pharm. Pharmacol., 10,* 719.
16. Gaul, L. E. (1969): Dermatitis from cetyl and stearyl alcohol. *Arch. Derm., 99,* 593.
17. Grunnet, E. (1976): Contact urticaria and anaphylactoid reaction induced by topical application of nitrogen mustard. *Brit. J. Derm., 94,* 101.
18. Guilhou, J. -J., Barnéon, G., Malbos, S., Peyron, J. -L., Michel, B. and Meynadier, J. (1980): Mucinose folliculaire perforante et hypersensibilité immédiate à la méchloréthamine chez un malade atteint de mycosis fongoïde. *Ann. Derm. Venereol. (Paris), 107,* 59.
19. Guill, A., Goette, K., Knight, C. G., Peck, C. C. and Lupton, G. P. (1979): Erythema multiforme and urticaria. *Arch. Derm. 115,* 742.
20. Haustein, U. F. (1976): Anaphylactic shock and contact urticaria after the patch test with professional allergens. *Allergie u. Immunol. (Leipzig), 22,* 349.
21. Henry, J. C., Tschen, E. H. and Becker, L. E. (1979): Contact urticaria to parabens. *Arch. Derm., 115,* 1231.
22. Heygi, E. and Doležalóva, A. (1976): Urticarial reaction after patch tests of toothpaste with a sub-shock condition: Hypersensitivity to Caraway seed. *Čs. Derm., 51,* 19.
23. Kassen, B. and Mitchell, J. C. (1974): Contact urticaria from a vitamin E preparation in two siblings. *Contact Dermatitis Newsl., 16,* 482.
24. Kleinhans, D. and Zwissler, H. (1980): Anaphylaktischer Schock nach Anwendung einer Benzocain-haltigen Salbe. *Z. Hautkr., 55,* 945.
25. Kligman, A. M. (1965): Dimethyl Sulfoxide – Part 2. *J. Amer. med. Ass., 193,* 151.
26. Kozáková, M. (1976): Sub-shock brought on by epidermic skin test for chloramphenicol. *Čs. Derm., 51,* 82.
27. Lahti, A. (1980): Non-immunologic contact urticaria. *Acta derm.-venereol. (Stockh.), 60,* Suppl. 91, 1.
28. Löwenfeld, W. (1928): Überempfindlichkeit gegen Iodthion mit gleichzeitiger urtikarieller Reaktion. *Derm. Wschr., 78,* 502.
29. Maibach, H. I. and Conant, M. (1977): Contact urticaria to a corticosteroid cream: polysorbate 60. *Contact Dermatitis, 3,* 350.
30. Maibach, H. I. and Johnson, H. L. (1975): Contact urticaria syndrome. *Arch. Derm., 111,* 726.
31. Mathews, K. P. and Pan, P. M. (1968): Immediate type hypersensitivity to phenylmercuric compounds. *Amer. J. Med., 44,* 310.
32. Maucher, O. D. (1972): Anaphylaktische Reaktionen beim Epikutantest. *Hautarzt, 23,* 139.
33. Merck Index (1976): Ninth Edition, p. 433. Merck and Co., Inc., Rahway, U.S.A.
34. Murrell, T. W. and Taylor, W. M. (1959): The cutaneous reaction to nicotinic acid (niacin) – furfuryl. *Arch. Derm., 79,* 545.
35. Nater, J. P., De Jong, M. C. J. M., Baar, A. J. M. and Bleumink, E. (1977): Contact urticarial skin responses to cinnamaldehyde. *Contact Dermatitis, 3,* 151.
36. Odom, R. B. and Maibach, H. I. (1976): Contact Urticaria: A different contact dermatitis. *Cutis, 18,* 672.
37. Papa, C. M. and Shelley, W. B. (1974): Menthol hypersensitivity. *J. Amer. med. Ass., 189,* 546.
38. Pietzcker, F. and Kuner, V. (1975): Anaphylaxie nach epikutanem Ampicillin-Test. *Z. Hautkr., 50,* 437.
39. Ramsay, D. L., Cohen, H. J. and Baer, R. L. (1972): Allergic reaction to benzophenone. *Arch. Derm., 105,* 906.
40. Rietschel, R. L. (1978): Contact urticaria from synthetic cassia oil and sorbic acid limited to the face. *Contact Dermatitis, 4,* 347.
41. Rilliet, A., Hunziker, N. and Brun, R. (1980): Alcohol contact urticaria syndrome (immediate-type hypersensitivity). *Dermatologica (Basel), 161,* 361.
42. Roed-Petersen, J. and Hjorth, N. (1976): Contact dermatitis from antioxidants. *Brit. J. Derm., 94,* 233.
43. Roupe, G. and Strannegård, C. (1969): Anaphylactic shock elicited by topical administration of bacitracin. *Arch. Derm., 100,* 450.
44. Rudzki, E. and Grzywa, Z. (1976): Immediate reactions to balsam of Peru, cassia oil and ethyl vanillin. *Contact Dermatitis, 2,* 360.
45. Rudzki, E., Rebandel, P. and Rogozinski, T. (1981): Contact urticaria from rat tail, guinea pig, streptomycin and vinyl pyridine. *Contact Dermatitis, 7,* 186.
46. Sikorski, H. (1951): Salvarsan-Allergie der Haut. *Z. Haut- u. Geschlkr., 11,* 341.
47. Tachibana, S., Horio, T. and Hayakawa, M. (1977): Contact urticaria and dermatitis due to fluocinonide cream. *Acta derm. (Kyoto), 72,* 141.

7.7 Contact urticaria

48. Temesvári, E., Soos, G., Podányi, B., Kovács, I. and Nemeth, I. (1978): Contact urticaria provoked by balsam of Peru. *Contact Dermatitis, 4,* 65.
49. Tharp, C. K. (1973): Contact urticaria (monoamylamine). *Arch. Derm., 108,* 135.
50. Tuft, L. (1975): Contact urticaria from cephalosporins. *Arch. Derm., 111,* 1609.
51. Von Liebe, V., Karge, H. J. and Burg, G. (1979): Kontakturtikaria. *Hautarzt, 30,* 544.

UPDATE – 2nd Edition

52. Von Krogh, G. and Maibach, H. I. (1981): The contact urticaria syndrome – an updated review. *J. Amer. Acad. Derm., 5,* 328.
53. Von Krogh, G. and Maibach, H. I. (1983): The contact urticaria syndrome. In: *Dermatotoxicology, 2nd Edition, Chapter 14,* pp. 301-322. Eds: F. N. Marzulli and H. I. Maibach. Hemisphere Publishing Corporation, Washington.
54. Von Krogh, G. and Maibach, H. I. (1982): The contact urticaria syndrome. In: *Safety and Efficacy of Topical Drugs and Cosmetics, Chapter 16,* pp. 249-268. Eds: A. M. Kligman and J. J. Leyden. Grune and Stratton, New York.
55. Maibach, H. I., cited by Andersen, K. E. and Storrs, F. J. (1982): Hautreizungen durch Propylenglykol. *Hautarzt, 33,* 12.
56. De Groot, A. C. and Liem, D. H. (1983): Contact urticaria to rouge. *Contact Dermatitis, 9,* 322.
57. Dooms-Goossens, A., Gevers, D., Mertens, A. and Van der Heyden, D. (1983): Allergic contact urticaria due to chloramine. *Contact Dermatitis, 9,* 319.
58. Von Mayenburg, J. and Rakoski, J. (1983): Contact urticaria to diethyltoluamide. *Contact Dermatitis, 9,* 171.
59. Tkach, J. R. (1982): Allergic contact urticaria to benzoyl peroxide. *Cutis, 29,* 187.
60. Böttger, E. M., Mücke, Chr. and Tronnier, H. (1981): Kontaktdermatitis auf neuere Antimykotika und Kontakturtikaria. *Akta Derm., 7,* 70.
61. Gottmann-Lückerath, I. (1982): Kontakturtikaria nach Dermoxin®. Society Proceedings. *Dermatosen, 30,* 124.
62. Maucher, O. M. and Fuchs, A. (1983): Kontakturtikaria im Epikutantest bei Pyrazolonallergie. *Hautarzt, 34,* 383.
63. Clemmensen, O. and Hjorth, N. (1982): Perioral contact urticaria from sorbic acid and benzoic acid in a salad dressing. *Contact Dermatitis, 8,* 1.
64. Warin, R. P. and Smith, R. J. (1982): Chronic urticaria. Investigations with patch and challenge tests. *Contact Dermatitis, 8,* 117.
65. Lindskov, R. (1982): Contact urticaria to formaldehyde. *Contact Dermatitis, 8,* 333.
66. Ryan, M. E., Davis, B. M. and Marks, J. G. (1980): Contact urticaria and allergic contact dermatitis to benzocaine gel. *J. Amer. Acad. Derm., 2,* 221.
67. Drevets, C. C. and Seebohm, P. M. (1961): Dermatitis from alcohol. *J. Allergy, 32,* 277.
68. Fisher, A. A. (1968): Contact dermatitis. The noneczematous variety. *Cutis, 4,* 567.
69. Fisher, A. A. (1973): *Contact Dermatitis, 2nd Edition,* p. 284. Lea and Febiger, Philadelphia.
70. Rothenborg, H. W., Menné, T. and Sjølin, K.-E. (1977): Temperature dependent primary irritant dermatitis from lemon perfume. *Contact Dermatitis, 3,* 37.
71. Langeland, T. and Nyrud, M. (1982): Contact urticaria to wheat bran bath: a case report. *Acta derm.-venereol. (Stockh.), 62,* 82.
72. Von Krogh, G. and Maibach, H. I. (1982): The contact urticaria syndrome – 1982. *Semin. Derm., 1,* 59.
73. Schwarting, H. H. (1983): Berufsbedingte Tetracyclin-Allergie. *Dermatosen Beruf. Umw., 31,* 130.
74. McDaniel, W. R. and Marks, J. G. (1979): Contact urticaria due to sensitivity to spray starch. *Arch. Derm., 115,* 628.
75. Thestrup-Pedersen, K., Christiansen, J. V. and Zachariae, H. (1982): Precautions for personnel applying topical nitrogen mustard to patients with mycosis fungoides. *Dermatologica (Basel), 165,* 108.

8. Necrosis of the skin and the mucous membranes due to topical drugs

8.1 The following drugs have caused necrosis after contact with the skin or mucous membranes:

Drug	Use	Ref.
arsenious oxide	self medication	5
cetrimonium bromide	antiseptic	1
chlorhexidine	antiseptic	6
crystal violet	antiseptic	9
dequalinium	antiseptic	11
fluorouracil	topical cytostatic	7
fuchsin–silver nitrate	marking patch test sites	3
gentian violet	antifungal drug	4
phenol	antipruritic agent antiseptic	8
povidone iodine	antiseptic	10
triclocarban	antiseptic	2

8.2 REFERENCES

1. August, P. J. (1975): Cutaneous necrosis due to cetrimide application. *Brit. med. J., 1,* 70.
2. Barrière, H. (1973): La dermite cutanéomuceuse caustique du trichlorocarbanilide. *Sem. Hôp. Paris, 49,* 685.
3. Björnberg, A. (1977): Toxic reactions to a patch test skin marker containing fuchsin-silver nitrate. *Contact Dermatitis, 3,* 101.
4. Björnberg, A. and Mobacken, H. (1972): Necrotic skin reactions caused by 1% gentian violet and brilliant green. *Acta derm.-venereol. (Stockh.), 52,* 55.
5. Fakirbhai, M. (1969): Self-medication of herpes zoster with an arsenic paste. *Brit. J. plast. Surg., 22,* 382.
6. Fløtra, L., Gjermo, P., Rølla, G. and Waerhang, J. (1971): Side effects of chlorhexidine mouthwashes. *Scand. J. dent. Res., 79,* 119.
7. Lee, S., Kim, J. C. and Chun, S. I. (1980): Treatment of verruca plana with 5% 5-fluorouracil ointment. *Dermatologica (Basel), 160,* 383.
8. Merck Index (1976): Ninth Edition. Merck and Co., Rahway, N. J., U.S.A.
9. Meurer, H. and Konz, B. (1977): Hautnekrosen nach Anwendung 2%iger Pyoktaninlösung. *Hautarzt, 28,* 94.
10. Shroff, A. P. and Jones, J. K. (1980): Reactions to povidone iodine preparation. *J. Amer. med. Ass., 243,* 230.
11. Wilkinson, D. S. (1970): Durch Dequalinium hervorgerufene Hautnekrosen. *Hautarzt, 21,* 114.

9. Acne-folliculitis

9.1 Contact with a great variety of substances can produce a follicular eruption, in which the comedo is the initiating lesion. This type of eruption is called *acne venenata*. The better known varieties are [3, 4]:
1. Chloracne, acne venenata caused by chlorinated hydrocarbons. This type of eruption has occurred, among others, in workers manufacturing DDT and weed killers, such as 2,4,5-trichlorophenol. Chlorinated hydrocarbons may also be present in paints, varnish, lacquers and various oils.
2. Acne venenata caused by cutting oils
3. Acne venenata caused by petroleum oil
4. Acne venenata caused by coal tars and pitches
5. Acne venenata caused by topical corticosteroid therapy.

Important for the purpose of this book is another particular form of acne venenata, which has been termed *acne cosmetica* by Kligman and Mills [2]. It is usually a mild eruption, consisting mainly of closed comedones. Blackheads are hard to find, sometimes a number of papulopustules may be seen over the cheeks and the chin. The eruption is seen in adult women and is attributed to the acneigenic properties of cosmetics used by these patients, mainly facial creams. It is stressed that cosmetics are very weak acneigens, and that it is their daily use, year after year, that enables them to induce acne in prone subjects.

Pomade acne is a variety of acne venenata, occurring chiefly on the forehead and the temples, seen mostly in adult black males, due to the application of various greases and oils to the scalp as hair grooming aids.

9.2 Assays on the rabbit ear [9] suggested the following compounds for topical use to be comedogenic [2, 5, 8]:

acetylated lanolin alcohols	methyl oleate
ammonium sulfobituminate	myristil myristate
butyl stearate	octanol
coal tar	oleic acid
cocoa butter	olive oil
coconut oil	peanut oil
corn oil	pine tar
hexadecyl alcohol	polyethylene glycol 300
hexane	polyoxyethylene ether of white lanolin
hexylene glycol	red veterinary petrolatum
hydrophilic ointment	safflower oil
isopropyl isostearate	sesame oil
isopropyl myristate	sodium lauryl sulfate
lanolin	stearic acid
lauryl alcohol	sulfur
linseed oil	sunscreens, proprietary preparations [6]

Frank [7] has pointed out that there is no evidence that the rabbit ear model is prophetic of acnegenicity in human subjects, and advised that the dermatologist should reserve judgment as to its prophetic value in the diagnosis and management of the patient with an acne eruption. However, Mills and Kligman [5] have reported a 'reasonably good' correspondence between the animal model and a human test model described by them. The rabbit ear model was more sensitive than the human, and the authors suggested that substances that are weakly comedogenic in the rabbit are probably safe for human use, with the possible exception of acne-prone persons. Premarketing 'in-use' testing of cosmetic formulations intended for use by the postadolescent consumer with mild acne has been suggested [10].

Contact acne has also been reported due to a metal spectacle frame in a patient sensitive to nickel sulfate [1].

9.3   REFERENCES

1. Grimalt, F. and Romaguera, C. (1978): Nickel allergy and spectacle frame contact acne. *Contact Dermatitis, 4*, 377.
2. Kligman, A. M. and Mills, O. H. (1972): Acne cosmetica. *Arch. Derm., 106*, 843.
3. Plewig, G. and Kligman, A. M. (1975): *Acne, Morphogenesis and Treatment.* Springer Verlag, Berlin, Heidelberg, New York.
4. Weirich, E. G. (1980): Die Kontaktakne: Beispiel einer Zivilisationsdermatose. *Dermatosen Beruf Umw., 26*, 7, 45.

UPDATE – 2nd Edition

5. Mills, O.H. and Kligman, A.M. (1982): A human model for assessing comedogenic substances. *Arch. Derm., 118*, 903.
6. Mills, O.H. and Kligman, A.M. (1982): Comedogenicity of sunscreens. Experimental observations in rabbits. *Arch. Derm., 118*, 417.
7. Frank, S.B. (1982): Is the rabbit ear model, in its present state, prophetic of acnegenicity? *J. Amer. Acad. Derm., 6*, 373.
8. Fulton, J.E. Jr., Bradley, S., Agundez, A. et al. (1976): Non-comedogenic cosmetics. *Cutis, 17*, 344.
9. Kligman, A.M. and Kwong, T. (1979): An improved rabbit ear model for assessing comedogenic substances. *Brit. J. Derm., 100*, 1.
10. Epinette, W.W., Greist, M.C. and Ozols, I.I. (1982): The role of cosmetics in postadolescent acne. *Cutis, 29*, 500.

10. Discoloration of the skin and appendages

10.1 Discoloration of the skin and the appendages due to topical drugs and cosmetics

Drug	Use	Side effects	Ref.
ammoniated mercury	formerly used for the treatment of psoriasis	Grey-brown discoloration of the skin and finger nails Also depigmentation	17 29 3 9
amphotericin B	antibiotic	Yellow discoloration of the nails	48
Arning's tincture	antifungal solution	Brownish discoloration of the nails	51
benzoyl peroxide	acne therapy	Discoloration of the hair and post-inflammatory pigmentation Hypopigmentation	32 11
butylated hydroxyanisole	antioxidant	Depigmentation	25
butylated hydroxytoluene	antioxidant	Depigmentation (?)	30
carmustine	cytostatic drug	Pigmentation/hypopigmentation	8 55
chlorhexidine	antiseptic	Discoloration of the teeth and the tongue	7
chrysarobin	psoriasis therapy	Brown-purplish discoloration of the skin, nails and hair	10
cinnamic aldehyde	fragrance compound	Depigmentation	23
clioquinol	antiseptic	Brown discoloration of the nails	48
cloflucarban	antiseptic	Contact allergy has caused pigmentation of the face	24
coal tar dyes	in tar products and cosmetics	'Pigmented cosmetic dermatitis'	28
corticosteroids	various dermatoses	Hyper- and hypopigmentation	22
dihydroxyacetone	tanning agent	Brown discoloration	21
dinitrochlorobenzene	treatment of alopecia areata	Yellow discoloration of grey hair Brownish discoloration of the nails	12 50
dithranol	psoriasis therapy	Brown-purplish discoloration of the skin, nails and hair	47

(continued)

(continuation)

Drug	Use	Side effects	Ref.
essential oils (lemon, lime, orange, mandarin, juniper)	fragrance materials	Red discoloration of the skin caused by terpenes	54
ethacridine	antiseptic	Brownish discoloration of the nails	51
fluorouracil	topical cytostatic	Hyperpigmentation/hypopigmentation	18 42 43
formaldehyde	various, e.g. preservative	Brown discoloration of the nails	48
glutaraldehyde	antiperspirant/anti-mycotic	Brown discoloration of the skin and the nails	14 49
henna	hair dye	Brown discoloration of the nails and skin	48
hydroquinone	bleaching agent	Ochronosis Depigmentation Brown discoloration of the finger nails	40 46 6 35 36 39
hydroxyquinoline sulfate	antiseptic	Leukoderma	4
iron salts	hemostasis	Brown discoloration (sometimes permanent)	2 41
4-isopropylcatechol	bleaching agent	Reticular hyperpigmentation and depigmentation	5
mechlorethamine hydrochloride	topical cytostatic drug	Pigmentation	33 52
monobenzylether of hydroquinone	depigmenting agent	Depigmentation and pigmentation (locally and at a distance)	1 34
monomethyl ether of hydroquinone	depigmenting agent	Depigmentation locally and at a distance	34 37
Perfume ingredients – benzyl alcohol – benzyl salicylate – cananga oil – cinnamic alcohol – geraniol – hydroxycitronellal – jasmin absolute – lavender oil – methoxycitronellal – red zig – sandalwood oil – ylang-ylang oil	in cosmetics	Contact allergy has caused pigmentation of the face	24
petrolatum	vehicle	Hyperpigmentation	20
phenolic compounds	antipruritics, antiseptics	Depigmentation	15

(continued)

10.1 Discoloration due to topical drugs

(continuation)

Drug	Use	Side effects	Ref.
potassium permanganate	wet dressings	Brown discoloration of the skin, brown or yellow discoloration of the nails	48
resorcinol (and -monoacetate)	peeling agent	Darkens fair hair Orange-brown discoloration of (lacquered) nails	19 48
silver nitrate	in solutions for antisepsis	Grey-brown discoloration of the conjunctiva Black discoloration of the fingernails	16 45
stilbestrol	hormone	Brown discoloration of the nipples and the linea alba (systemic effects, caused by percutaneous absorption, *see* § 16.87)	26
tetracycline	(topical) antibiotic	Yellow staining	38
thiotepa	in eye drops	Periorbital leukoderma	13
tretinoin	acne therapy	Hypopigmentation Hyperpigmentation	11 44
triclocarban	antiseptic	Contact allergy has caused pigmentation of the face	24
vitamin K_1	vitamin	Dark-brown staining in factory workers	31 53

10.2 REFERENCES

1. Bentley-Phillips, B. and Bayler, M. A. H. (1975): Cutaneous reactions to topical application of hydroquinone. *S. Afr. med. J., 49,* 1391.
2. Brehm, G. (1976): Pigmentierung nach lokaler Anwendung von Eisenchloridlösung. *Akt. Derm., 3,* 117.
3. Butterworth, T. and Strean, L. P. (1963): Mercurial pigmentation of nails. *Arch. Derm., 88,* 55.
4. Calnan, C. D. (1973): Leucoderma with Quinoderm. *Contact Dermatitis Newsl., 13,* 378.
5. Dong Gil Byen, Young Hoe Kim, Yang Ja Park and Soon Bok Lee (1975): Treatment of hyperpigmented disease with 4-isopropylcatechol (Korean). *Kor. J. Derm., 13,* 5.
6. Findlay, G. H. and De Beer, H. A. (1980): Chronic hydroquinone poisoning of the skin from skin-lightening cosmetics. *S. Afr. med. J., 57,* 187.
7. Fløtra, L. (1973): Different modes of chlorhexidine application and related local side effects. *J. periodont. Res., 8, Suppl. 12,* 41.
8. Frost, P. and DeVita, V. T. (1966): Pigmentation due to a new antitumour agent. *Arch. Derm., 94,* 265.
9. Goeckerman, W. H. (1922): The peculiar discoloration of the skin. *J. Amer. med. Ass., 70,* 605.
10. Goodman, L. S. and Gilman, A. (1970): *The Pharmacological Basis of Therapeutics,* 4th Ed. The MacMillan Company, London-Toronto.
11. Handojo, I. (1979): The combined use of topical benzoyl peroxide and tretinoin in the treatment of acne vulgaris. *Int. J. Derm., 18,* 489.
12. Happle, R., Cebulla, K. and Echternacht-Happle, K. (1978): Dinitrochlorobenzene therapy for alopecia areata. *Arch. Derm., 114,* 1629.
13. Harben, D. J., Cooper, P. H. and Rodman, O. (1977): Thiotepa-induced leukoderma. *Arch. Derm., 115,* 973.
14. Juhlin, L. and Hansson, H. (1968): Topical glutaraldehyde for plantar hyperhydrosis. *Arch. Derm., 97,* 327.
15. Kahn, G. (1970): Depigmentation caused by phenolic germicides. *Arch. Derm., 102,* 177.
16. Koch, H. R. (1977): In: *Arzneimittelnebenwirkungen am Auge,* p. 60. Editors: O. Hockwin and H. R. Koch. Georg Thieme Verlag, Leipzig.

17. Lamar, L. M. and Bliss, B. O. (1966): Localized pigmentation of the skin due to topical mercury. *Arch. Derm., 93*, 450.
18. Lee, S., Kim, J. C. and Chun, S. I. (1980): Treatment of verruca plana with 5% 5-fluorouracil ointment. *Dermatologica (Basel), 160*, 383.
19. Loveman, A. B. and Fliegelman, M. T. (1955): Discoloration of the nails. *Arch. Derm., 72*, 153.
20. Maibach, H. I. (1978): Chronic dermatitis and hyperpigmentation from petrolatum. *Contact Dermatitis, 4*, 62.
21. Maibach, H. I. and Kligman, A. M. (1960): Dihydroxyacetone: a suntan-simulating agent. *Arch. Derm., 82*, 505.
22. Marchand, J.-P., Arnold, J. and Ndiaye, B. (1976): Dépigmentation de la peau du noir africain provoquée par les corticoïdes. *Bull. Soc. franç. Derm. Syph., 83*, 17.
23. Mathias, C. G. T., Maibach, H. I. and Conant, M. A. (1980): Perioral leukoderma simulating vitiligo from use of a toothpaste containing cinnamic aldehyde. *Arch. Derm., 116*, 1172.
24. Nakayama, H., Harado, R. and Toda, M. (1976): Pigmented cosmetic dermatitis. *Int. J. Derm., 15*, 673.
25. Riley, P. A. (1971): Acquired hypomelanosis. *Brit. J. Derm., 84*, 290.
26. Stoppelman, M. R. H. and Van Valkenburg, R. A. (1955): Pigmentaties en gynecomastie ten gevolge van het gebruik van stilboestrol bevattend haarwater bij kinderen. *Ned. T. Geneesk., 99*, 3925.
27. Omitted.
28. Sugai, T., Takahashi, Y. and Tagaki, T. (1977): Pigmented cosmetic dermatitis and coal tar dyes. *Contact Dermatitis, 3*, 249.
29. Summa, J. D. (1975): Chronische Quecksilbervergiftung durch Gebrauch kosmetischer Salben. *Münch. med. Wschr., 117*, 1121.
30. Vollum, D. I. (1971): Hypomelanosis from an antioxidant in polyethylene film. *Arch. Derm., 104*, 70.
31. Watrous, R. M. (1947): Health hazards of the pharmaceutical industry. *Brit. J. industr. Med., 4*, 111.
32. Yong, C. C. (1979): Benzoyl peroxide gel therapy in acne in Singapore. *Int. J. Derm., 18*, 485.
33. Zachariae, H. (1979): Histiocytosis X in two infants treated with topical nitrogen mustard. *Brit. J. Derm., 100*, 433.

UPDATE – 2nd Edition

34. Grojean, M. -F., Thivolet, J. and Perrot, H. (1982): Leucomélanodermies accidentelles provoquées par les topiques dépigmentants. *Ann. Derm. Vénéréol. (Paris), 109*, 641.
35. Smith, T. L. (1981): Depigmentation from 2% hydroquinone cream. *Shoch Letter, 31*, 48.
36. Fisher, A. A. (1982): Can bleaching creams containing 2% hydroquinone produce leukoderma? (Letter). *J. Amer. Acad. Derm., 7*, 134.
37. Colomb, D. (1982): Dépigmentation en confettis après application de Leucodinine B® sur un chloasma (Letter). *Ann. Derm. Vénéréol., (Paris), 109*, 899.
38. Feucht, C. L. (1981): Response to a letter to the Editor. *J. Amer. Acad. Derm., 5*, 457.
39. Mann, R. J. and Harman, R. R. M. (1983): Nail staining due to hydroquinone skin-lightening creams. *Brit. J. Derm., 108*, 363.
40. Findlay, G. H. (1982): Ochronosis following skin bleaching with hydroquinone. *J. Amer. Acad. Derm., 6*, 1092.
41. Olmstead, P. M. et al. (1980): Monsel's solution: A histologic nuisance. *J. Amer. Acad. Derm., 3*, 492.
42. Goette, D. K. and Odom, R. B. (1977): Allergic contact dermatitis to topical fluorouracil. *Arch. Derm., 113*, 1058.
43. Goette, D. K. (1981): Topical chemotherapy with 5-fluorouracil. *J. Amer. Acad. Derm., 4*, 633.
44. Plewig, G. and Kligman, A. M. (1975): *Acne: Morphogenesis and Treatment.* Springer Verlag, Berlin.
45. Krebs, A. (1983): Veränderungen der Nägel durch Arzneimittel. *Dtsch. Apoth. Ztg., 123*, 557.
46. Cullison, D., Abele, D. C. and O'Quinn, J. L. (1983): Localized exogenous ochronosis. Report of a case and review of the literature. *J. Amer. Acad. Derm., 8*, 882.
47. Ashton, R. E., Andre, P., Lowe, N. J. and Whitefield, M. (1983): Anthralin: Historical and current perspectives. *J. Amer. Acad. Derm., 9*, 173.
48. Daniel, C. R. III, and Osment, L. S. (1982): Nail pigmentation abnormalities. Their importance and proper examination. *Cutis, 30*, 348.

10.2 Discoloration

49. Swinga, D. W. (1970): Treatment of superficial onychomycosis with topically applied glutaraldehyde. *Arch. Derm., 102,* 163.
50. Daniel, C. R. III (1982): Nail pigmentation abnormalities: An addendum. *Cutis, 30,* 364.
51. Runne, U. and Orfanos, C. E. (1981): The human nail. *Akt. Probl. Derm., 9,* 102.
52. Hamminga, B., Noordijk, E. M. and van Vloten, W. A. (1982): Treatment of mycosis fungoides. *Arch. Derm., 118,* 150.
53. Camarasa, J. G. and Barnadas, M. (1982): Occupational dermatosis by vitamin K3 sodium bisulphite. *Contact Dermatitis, 8,* 268.
54. Shapiro, W. B. (1982): The safety, stability, and compatibility of fragrances in skin and hair products. *J. Toxic. -Cut. Ocular Toxic., 1,* 211.
55. Zackheim, H. S., Epstein, E. H. Jr., McNutt, N. S. et al. (1983): Topical carmustine (BCNU) for mycosis fungoides and related disorders. A 10-year experience. *J. Amer. Acad. Derm., 9,* 363.

11. Stinging sensation due to ingredients of cosmetics and topical pharmaceutical preparations

11.1 Many topical preparations may cause transient burning or itching, especially when applied to diseased skin. Some individuals, mostly women, may experience a stinging sensation due to cosmetics, lasting for up to fifteen minutes and then subsiding. The following ingredients of cosmetics and pharmaceuticals were identified as stinging compounds by Frosch and Kligman [2]:

benzene	1%	phosphoric acid	1 %
benzoyl peroxide gel	10%	hydrochloric acid	1.2%
benzoyl peroxide lotion	5%	phenol	1%
coal tar	5%	propylene glycol	
diethyltoluamide	50%	propylene glycol diacetate	
dimethylacetamide	undiluted	resorcinol	5%
dimethylformamide	undiluted	salicylic acid	5%
dimethyl phthalate	50%	sodium carbonate	15%
dimethyl sulfoxide	undiluted	sodium hydroxide	1.3%
ethoxyethyl-methoxy-cinnamate	[1]	trisodium phosphate	5%
2-ethyl-1,3-hexane diol	50%		

Irritation and/or burning may also be caused by benzylidene acetone, hydroxycitronellal, aurantiol, and cinnamates [3].

11.2 REFERENCES

1. Calnan, C. D. (1978): Stinging sensation from ethoxyethyl-methoxycinnamate. *Contact Dermatitis, 4,* 294.
2. Frosch, P. J. and Kligman, A. M. (1977): A method for appraising the stinging capacity of topically applied substances. *J. Soc. cosmet. Chem., 28,* 197.
3. Anonis, D.P. (1973): Perfume and shampoos. *Drug Cosm. Ind., 112,* 32.

12. Miscellaneous side effects

12.1   Miscellaneous side effects of topical drugs

Drug	Use	Side effects	Ref.
acrylic bone cement	fixation of prostheses	Paresthesia of the fingers	11
benzoin	in cosmetics, adhesives and perfumes	Non-eczematous exanthema	36
benzoyl peroxide	in cosmetics and pharmaceuticals	Skin-tumor promoting activity (?)	35
benzyl benzoate	antiscabietic drug	Pemphigoid (?)	41
cantharidin	treatment of warts	Lymphangitis	7
carmustine (BCNU)	topical cytostatic drug	Erythema, followed by patchy teleangiectasia; lichenified dermatitis	56
cetrimonium bromide	antiseptic	Matting of the hair	5
chlorhexidine	antiseptic in mouthwashes	Disturbance of taste sensations, swelling of the parotid glands	29
clove oil	topical dental anodyne	Permanent local anesthesia and anhydrosis	46
coal tar	psoriasis therapy	Multiple keratoacanthomas	43 44
cobalt blue	in tattoos	Granulomatous skin reaction with and without cobalt-sensitivity	26
diethyltoluamide	insect repellent	Bullous eruption healing with scar formation	50
dimethyl sulfoxide	solvent	Thickening, hardening and desquamation of the skin	18
dinitrochlorobenzene	treatment of alopecia areata and common warts	Potentiates sensitization to non-related allergens	6
		Mutagenic (?), carcinogenic (?) (possibly due to mononitrochlorobenzene contamination?)	45
dithranol	psoriasis therapy	Bullous pemphigoid (?)	52
		Tumor promotion	53

(continued)

(continuation)

Drug	Use	Side effects	Ref.
fluorouracil	topical cytostatic drug	Onycholysis	30
		Onychodystrophy	49
		Bullous pemphigoid	54
			2
		'Mental depression'	24
		Telangiectasiae, exacerbation of herpes labialis	4
		Pain, edema and dermatitis of the erythema livedo reticularis-type	20
		Hypertrophic scarring	55
hydroquinone	bleaching agent	Ochronosis and colloid milia (sun exposure was required)	10
8-hydroxyquinoline	antimicrobial	Purpuric eruption	34
idoxuridine	antiviral drug	Mutagenic? teratogenic? carcinogenic?	38
			13
			48
mechlorethamine hydrochloride	topical cytostatic drug	(co)Carcinogenic?	9
			19
			47
		Focal contact sensitivity on mycosis fungoides plaques	31
		Extensive telangiectasia	51
mercurial compounds	in tattoos	Granulomatous and lichenoid reaction, both with and without mercury-sensitivity	40
			37
monosulfiram	antiseptic	Toxic epidermal necrolysis complicating contact allergy	25
neutral red	protodye therapy for herpes simplex	Carcinogenic?	3
petrolatum	vehicle	Lipogranuloma, myospherulosis	8
		Decrease of inflammatory response in damaged skin	57
p-phenylenediamine	various	Purpuric allergic contact dermatitis	33
podophyllum resin	therapy for condylomata acuminata	Infiltrated hyperplasia reaction	23
polyethylene glycol	vehicle constituent	Carcinogenic?	14
propylene glycol	vehicle constituent	Psoriasis-like reactions	22
salicylic acid	keratolytic drug	Lymphangitis, 'Xeroderma pigmentosum'	7
			39
salicylic acid 15% lactic acid 15% collodion	wart therapy	Atrophic and partially depigmented scar	12
scopolamine hydrobromide	anticholinergic drug used in ophthalmology	Erythema multiforme	17

(continued)

12.1   Miscellaneous side effects

(continuation)

Drug	Use	Side effects	Ref.
selenium sulfide	dandruff medication	Reversible hair loss, oiliness of the scalp	16
sulfonamide	chemotherapeutic in ophthalmic solution	Stevens-Johnson syndrome	28
tar	psoriasis and eczema therapy	Carcinogenic? *See* Chapter 18 *and under* coal tar	15 42
thiomersal	antiseptic	Acute laryngeal obstruction caused by contact allergy to thiomersal spray	21
triphenylmethane dyes	antiseptics	Carcinogenic? mutagenic?	27
zinc oxide	in topical remedies	Black dermographism in the presence of jewelry	1
zirconium compounds	in antiperspirants	Allergic granulomatous skin reactions	32

12.2   REFERENCES

1. Andersen, K. E. and Maibach, H. I. (1980): Allergic reactions to drugs used topically. *Clin. Toxicol., 16,* 415.
2. Bart, B. J. and Bean, S. F. (1970): Bullous pemphigoid following the topical use of fluorouracil. *Arch. Derm., 102,* 457.
3. Berger, R. P. and Papa, C. M. (1977): Photodye herpes therapy: Cassandria confirmed? *J. Amer. med. Ass., 238,* 133.
4. Burnett, J. W. (1975): Two unusual complications of topical fluorouracil therapy. *Arch. Derm., 111,* 398.
5. Dawber, R. P. R. and Calnan, C. D. (1976): Bird's nest hair, matting of the scalp hair due to shampooing. *Clin. exp. Derm., 1,* 155.
6. De Groot, A. C., Nater, J. P., Bleumink, E. and De Jong, M. C. J. M. (1981): Does DNCB therapy potentiate epicutaneous sensitization to non-related contact allergens? *Clin. exp. Derm., 6,* 139.
7. Dilaimy, M. (1975): Lymphangitis caused by cantharidin. *Arch. Derm., 111,* 1073.
8. Dunlap, C. L. and Barker, B. F. (1980): Myospherulosis of the jaws. *Oral Surg., 50,* 238.
9. Du Vivier, A., Vonderheid, E. C., Van Scott, E. J. and Urbach, F. (1978): Mycosis fungoides, nitrogen mustard and skin cancer. *Brit. J. Derm., 99,* 61.
10. Findlay, G. H., Morrison, J. G. L. and Simson, I. W. (1975): Exogenous ochronosis and pigmented-colloid milium from hydroquinone bleaching creams. *Brit. J. Derm., 93,* 613.
11. Fisher, A. A. (1979): Paresthesia of the fingers accompanying dermatitis due to methacrylate bone cement. *Contact Dermatitis, 5,* 56.
12. Gaisin, A. (1976): Facial scarring due to topical wart treatment. *Arch. Derm., 112,* 1791.
13. Green, J. and Staal, S. (1976): Questionable dermatologic use of iododeoxyuridine. *New Engl. J. Med., 295,* 111.
14. Greene, M. H., Young, T. I. and Eisenbarth, G. S. (1980): Polyethylene glycol in suppositories: Carcinogenic? (letter). *Ann. intern. Med., 93,* 78.
15. Greither, A., Gisbertz, C. and Ippen, H. (1967): Teerbehandlung und Krebs. *Z. Haut- u. Geschlkr., 42,* 463.
16. Grover, R. W. (1956): Diffuse hair loss associated with selenium (Selsun) sulfide shampoo. *J. Amer. med. Ass., 160,* 1397.
17. Guill, A., Goette, K., Knight, C. G., Peck, C. C. and Lupton, G. P. (1979): Erythema multiforme and urticaria. *Arch. Derm., 115,* 742.
18. Kligman, A. M. (1965): Topical pharmacology and toxicology of dimethyl sulfoxide. I and II. *J. Amer. med. Ass., 193,* 796 and 923.

19. Kravitz, P. H. and McDonald, C. J. (1978): Topical nitrogen mustard induced carcinogenesis. *Acta derm.-venereol. (Stockh.), 58,* 421.
20. Lubowe, J. J. (1977): Fluorouracil for skin blemishes and lines. *J. Amer. med. Ass., 237,* 1312.
21. Maibach, H. I. (1975): Acute laryngeal obstruction presumed secondary to thiomersal (merthiolate) delayed hypersensitivity. *Contact Dermatitis, 1,* 221.
22. Maibach, H. I. (1980): Topical corticoid therapy: a round table discussion. V. The base as a vehicle. *Cutis, 25,* 441.
23. Maxwell, T. B. and Lamb, J. H. (1954): Unusual reaction to application of podophyllum resin. *Arch. Derm. Syph. (Chic.), 70,* 510.
24. Milstein, H. G. (1980): Mental depression secondary to fluorouracil therapy for actinic keratoses. *Arch. Derm., 116,* 1100.
25. Monkton Copeman, P. W. (1968): Toxic epidermal necrolysis caused by skin hypersensitivity to monosulfiram. *Brit. med. J., 1,* 623.
26. Rorsman, H., Brehmer-Andersson, E., Dahlquist, I., Ehinger, B., Jacobsson, S., Linell, F. and Rorsman, G. (1969): Tattoo granuloma and uveitis. *Lancet, 2,* 27.
27. Rosenkranz, H. S. and Carr, H. S. (1971): Possible hazard in use of gentian violet. *Brit. med. J., iii,* 5776.
28. Rubin, A. (1977): Ophthalmic sulfonamide induced Stevens-Johnson syndrome. *Arch. Derm., 113,* 235.
29. Rushton, A. (1977): Safety of Hibitane. II. Human experience. *J. clin. Periodont., 4,* 73.
30. Shelley, W. B. (1972): Onycholysis due to topical 5-fluorouracil. *Acta derm.-venereol. (Stockh.), 52,* 320.
31. Shelley, W. B. (1981): Focal contact sensitivity to nitrogen mustard in lesions of cutaneous T-cell lymphoma (mycosis fungoides). *Acta derm.-venereol. (Stockh.), 61,* 161.
32. Shelley, W. B. and Hurley, H. J. (1958): The allergic origin of zirconium deodorant granulomas in man. *Brit. J. Derm., 70,* 75.
33. Shmunes, E. (1978): Purpuric allergic contact dermatitis to paraphenylenediamine. *Contact Dermatitis, 4,* 225.
34. Sidi, E. and Hincky, M. (1956): *Les manifestations atypiques de l'allergie de contact.* Communication faite à la Société française d'allergie. Séance du 20 Novembre, p. 283.
35. Slaga, T. J., Klein-Szanto, A. J. P., Triplett, L. L. et al. (1981): Skin tumor-promoting activity of benzoyl peroxide, a widely used free radical-generating compound. *Science, 213,* 1023.
36. Spott, D. A. and Shelley, W. B. (1970): Exanthema due to contact allergen (Benzoin) absorbed through skin. *J. Amer. med. Ass., 214,* 1881.
37. Taffee, A., Knight, A. G. and Marks, R. (1978): Lichenoid tattoo hypersensitivity. *Brit. med. J., 1,* 616.
38. Thomson, J. and O'Neill, S. M. (1976): Idoxuridine in dimethyl sulfoxide: is it carcinogenic in man? *J. cutan. Path., 3,* 269.
39. Weber, G. and Riegel, A. (1968): 'Xeroderma Pigmentosum' e medicamento. *Z. Haut- u. Geschlkr., 43,* 829.
40. Winkelmann, R. K. and Harris, R. B. (1979): Lichenoid delayed hypersensitivity reactions in tattoos. *J. cutan. Path., 6,* 59.
41. Wzanicz, A. and Czernielewski, A. (1974): Pemfigoid sprowokowany nowoskabina. *Przegl. derm., 61,* 693.
42. Zackheim, H. S. (1978): Should therapeutic coal-tar preparations be available over the counter? *Arch. Derm., 114,* 125.

UPDATE – 2nd Edition

43. Reid, B. J. and Cheesbrough, M. J. (1978): Multiple keratoacanthoma. *Acta derm.-venereol. (Stockh.), 58,* 169.
44. Vickers, C. F. G. and Ghadially, F. N. (1961): Keratoacanthoma associated with psoriasis. *Brit. J. Derm., 73,* 120.
45. Doubleday, C. W. and Wilkin, J. K. (1982): The role of mononitrochlorobenzene as a contaminant in dinitrochlorobenzene. *J. Amer. Acad. Derm., 6,* 325.
46. Isaacs, G. (1983): Permanent local anaesthesia and anhidrosis after clove oil spillage (letter). *Lancet, 1,* 882.
47. Lee, L. A., Fritz, K. A., Golitz, L. et al. (1982): Second cutaneous malignancies in patients with mycosis fungoides treated with topical nitrogen mustard. *J. Amer. Acad. Derm., 7,* 590.

12.2 Miscellaneous side effects

48. Koppang, H. S. and Aas, E. (1983): Squamous carcinoma induced by topical idoxuridine therapy? (letter). *Brit. J. Derm., 108,* 501.
49. Krebs, A. (1983): Veränderungen der Nägel durch Arzneimittel. *Dtsch. Apoth.-Ztg., 123,* 557.
50. Reuveni, H., Yagupsky, P. (1982): Diethyltoluamide-containing insect repellent. *Arch. Derm., 118,* 582.
51. Hamminga, B., Noordijk, E. M. and van Vloten, W. A. (1982): Treatment of mycosis fungoides. *Arch. Derm., 118,* 150.
52. Koerber, W. A., Price, N. M. and Watson, W. (1978): Coexistent psoriasis and bullous pemphigoid. *Arch. Derm., 114,* 1643.
53. Ashton, R. E., Andre, P., Lowe, N. J. and Whitefield, M. (1983): Anthralin: Historical and current perspectives. *J. Amer. Acad. Derm., 9,* 173.
54. Tanenbaum, M. H. (1961): Onychodystrophy after topically applied 5-FU for warts. *Arch. Derm., 103,* 225.
55. Kaplan, L. A., Walter, J. F. and Macknet, K. D. (1979): Hypertrophic scarring as a complication of fluorouracil therapy. *Arch. Derm., 115,* 1452.
56. Zackheim, H. S., Epstein, E. H. Jr. and McNutt, N. S. (1983): Topical carmustine (BCNU) for mycosis fungoides and related disorders: A 10-year experience. *J. Amer. Acad. Derm., 9,* 363.
57. Penneys, N. S., Eaglstein, W. and Ziboh, V. (1980): Petrolatum: interference with the oxidation of arachidonic acid. *Brit. J. Derm., 103,* 257.

142

13. Drugs used on the mucosae

DRUGS USED ON THE ORAL MUCOSA

General and local effects

13.1   Drugs coming into contact with the oral mucosa may cause (1) general effects, through absorption, and (2) local effects; the latter may consist of:

Irritant reactions
Though the oral mucosa appears to be more resistant to irritants than the skin, chemical injury may occur. This may be produced by contact of undiluted drugs with the mucosa, e.g. aspirin, hydrogen peroxide, silver nitrate. Accidental contact with drugs and subsequent irritation also occurs, especially in children.

Allergic reactions
Many drugs inducing contact allergy when applied to the skin, may also cause contact sensitization when applied to the mucous membranes. Allergic reactions in the oral cavity are relatively rare. This is explained by [1]:
1. Rapid disposal and absorption of the drug
2. Short period of contact with the mucosa
3. Dilution and removal by saliva
4. Lack of recognition of the drug as an allergen.

Other adverse reactions
These are discussed elsewhere in this book.

TOOTHPASTES

13.2   Toothpastes may contain abrasives, flavors, colors, preservatives, antiseptics and fluorides. Contact allergic reactions to the constituents of toothpastes seem to be rare. Symptoms may include stomatitis, cheilitis, and eczema of the hand holding the toothbrush.
    The main sensitizers are the flavoring agents (§ 13.3).

13.3   **Contact allergy to ingredients of toothpastes**

Ingredient	Patch test conc. & vehicle (§ 5.2)	Ref.
anethole	2–5% pet	1
carvone	2–5% pet.	1

(continued)

13.3   Contact allergy to toothpastes

(*continuation*)

Ingredient	Patch test conc. & vehicle (§ 5.2)	Ref.
cinnamic aldehyde	2% pet.	15 21 11
cinnamon oil	2% pet.	17 13
dichlorophene	0.5–1% pet.	8
fluorides	toothpaste as is (?)	25
hexylresorcinol	0.5–2% pet.	28
italian peppermint	2% pet.	1
laurel oil	2% pet.	27
menthol	1–2% pet.	19
oil of anise	10–25% o.o.	14
oleum menthae piperitae	25% o.o.	26 13
propolis	'natural extract'	121
salol (phenyl salicylate)	2% pet.	122
spearmint oil	2% pet., 1% alc.	1
thymol	1% pet.	2

One case of immediate-type hypersensitivity to caraway seed in a toothpaste has been reported [10].

13.4   Incidence of side effects: Toothpastes (see § 20.17)

	% of total	
US manufacturers' file:	1.5	(130/8399)
US hospitals' file:	2.4	(17/698)**
FDA pilot study:	2.4	(14/589)*
Spanish study:	5.1	(10/210)
Dutch file:	2.0	(4/202)
British consumers' report:	no data available	
Strassburg study:	0	(0/96)

*   1 severe   ** including mouth fresheners
     2 moderate
     11 mild

13.5   Risk index: Toothpastes (see § 20.18)

Toothpaste is graded as a *low-risk* cosmetic according to the following reports: US manufacturers' file: at 1 experience per 937,000 estimated units distributed. FDA pilot study: at 1 experience per more than 5,000 person-brand used cosmetics.

144

OTHER ORAL MEDICATION

Fluorides

13.6   The possible side effects of fluorides in toothpaste are still subject to discussion. The occurrence of acne-like eruptions due to fluorides has been reported [23], but was doubted by other investigators [6]. Ulcerous stomatitis caused by fluorides has been reported by Douglas [5]. Another documented side effect is discoloration of the teeth [3]. The National Registry of possible drug-induced ocular side effects has received two separate case reports of pigmentary macular degeneration in children following dental treatments with fluoride gel [82].
     The possibility of contact allergic reactions to fluorides in toothpastes is still in discussion. Seven cases of contact allergy were reported by Shea et al. [25]. Patch tests with fluoride-containing toothpaste were positive (2 +) in one case, but control tests were not mentioned.

Cinnamic aldehyde

13.7   Contact allergy to cinnamic aldehyde in toothpaste has been reported to cause perioral leukoderma [16].

13.8   Many other chemicals and drugs may come into contact with the oral mucosa, e.g. chemicals and drugs used in dentistry. Their side effects are listed in § 13.9.

13.9   **Side effects of other oral contactants**

Contactant	Use	Side effects	Patch test conc./ vehicle	Comment	Ref.
benzoyl peroxide	dentures (catalyst)	stomatitis	pure (!?)	Patch test conc. not correct	34
chlorphenolcamphor	anti-inflammation	stomatitis	?		35
chrome and cobalt	removable partial denture	generalized dermatitis	metal pure		32
cinnamic aldehyde	in mouthwash	swelling of lip and tongue	2% pet. (open test) reading after 15 min.	Contact urticarial reaction	47
clove oil	topical dental anodyne	permanent local anesthesia and anhidrosis after spillage over the infraorbital skin	–	Possible neurotoxic effect of eugenol in clove oil	42
cobalt chloride	dentures	denture sore mouth	1% pet.		43
cobalt chloride	dentures	rhinitis	1% pet.	Rhinitis 3–24 hours after applying dentures	31
copper	dentures	oral lichen planus	metallic copper		39
dimethyl-p-toluidine	dentures	denture sore mouth	30% o.o.		43

(continued)

13.9 Other oral contactants

(continuation)

Contactant	Use	Side effects	Patch test conc./vehicle	Comment	Ref.
epoxy resin	dentures	stomatitis	cured resin		50
eugenol	impression paste surgical packing cement	dermatitis	2% pet.	Contact allergy in patients and dental personnel	12
formaldehyde	dentures	denture sore mouth	2% aqua		43
gold	dentures	stomatitis	auric trichloride 0.1% aqua	Cave: irritant patch test reactions	51
gold	dentures	stomatitis	auric trichloride 0.5% aqua	Cave: irritant patch test reactions	36
gold	dentures	stomatitis	potassium dicyano-aurate 0.001% (w/v) $(3.5 \cdot 10^{-5}\,mol/l)$ ethanol	Cave: irritant patch test reactions	38
hexetidine	fungicide	stomatitis	0.1% pet.		48
hydroquinone	dentures	denture sore mouth	1% pet.		43
mercury amalgam	dental fillings	swelling of the face, pruritic/erythematous/ urticarial rash on trunk and flexures of the limbs	mercuric chloride 0.1% in ? silver amalgam pure		29
mercury amalgam	dental fillings	allergic contact dermatitis on face, neck and thorax	'mercury'		7 52
mercury amalgam	dental fillings	rash in flexures spreading over extremities	mercurochrome 2% aqua mercuric chloride 0.05% aqua thiomersal 0.1% pet. phenylmercuric nitrate 0.05% pet. ammoniated mercury 1% pet.		49
methyldichloro-benzene sulfate	catalyst in impression material (Impregum)	stomatitis dermatitis	0.1% dibenztoluol	Contact allergy in patients and dental personnel	40 53
methylmethacrylate monomer	dentures	stomatitis	25% o.o. 5% acetone	Patch test conc. of 25% may sensitize!	37 46
methyl-p-toluene sulfonate	catalyst in material for temporary crowns and bridges (Scutan®)	stomatitis dermatitis	0.1% dibenztoluol	Contact allergy in patients and dental personnel	40 45 53
nickel sulfate	dentures	denture sore mouth	5% pet.		43
nickel sulfate	dentures	rhinitis	2.5% pet.	Rhinitis 3–24 hours after applying dentures	31

(continued)

(continuation)

Contactant	Use	Side effects	Patch test conc./vehicle	Comment	Ref.
palladium	dental alloys	swelling of cheek, pain in mouth, generalized itching, dizziness	palladium dichloride 2% aqua		44
p-phenylenediamine	dentures	denture sore mouth	1% pet.		43
pigment	dentures	denture sore mouth	pure	Patch test conc. not correct	34
(heat cured) polymethyl methacrylate	dentures	denture sore mouth	fillings of the prostheses acrylic monomer conc.?		33
potassium bichromate	dentures	denture sore mouth	0.5% pet.		43
potassium bichromate	dentures	generalized eczematoid dermatitis, intraoral erythema	0.5% pet.		41

MOUTH FRESHENERS

13.10   A few drops of a mouth freshener to a glass of water makes a mouthwash, which is capable to induce a clean and refreshing feeling to the oral cavity. Mouthwashes can be classified as follows:

1. Cosmetic mouthwashes consisting of water (and usually ethyl alcohol), flavor and color.
2. Antibacterial mouthwashes: these may contain quaternary ammonium compounds, phenolic derivatives or other antibacterial agents.
3. Astringent mouthwashes: these are formulated for the purpose of flocculating and precipitating proteinacious materials, so that these can be removed by flushing. The most widely used astringents are zinc and aluminum compounds such as zinc chloride, zinc acetate and aluminum potassium sulphate.
4. Buffered mouthwashes: these depend on their pH for their action. Alkaline mouthwashes may be useful in reducing stringy saliva or in reducing mucinous deposits by dispersion of the protein.
5. Mouthwash concentrates: these must be diluted before use.
6. Deodorizing mouthwashes: these contain antibacterial agents.
7. Therapeutic mouthwashes: these are formulated for specific purposes, e.g. for relieving infection or preventing dental caries.

13.11   A typical formula of a **mouth freshener** is:

Ingredient:		*Example:*
20%	water	*water*
70%	alcohol	*ethanol*
0.1%	sweetener	*saccharin*
2–10%	active ingredients:	
	– astringents	*myrrha tincture*
		ratanhia tincture

13.12 Mouth fresheners

– essential oils and fragrances	*phenyl salicylate, peppermint oil, thymol, eugenol, clove oil*
– antimicrobials	*benzalkonium chloride, chlorhexidine digluconate*

13.12 Patch tests with toothpastes and mouthwashes may produce false positive reactions when the preparations are tested undiluted. Dilution and control tests are necessary.

Side effects of mouthwashes

13.13 *Systemic side effects:* Accidental ingestion of mouthwash solution in children has been reported to lead to hypoglycaemia, induced by the ethyl alcohol component [30]. *Local side effects* of ingredients of mouthwashes are listed in § 13.14.

13.14 **Local side effects of mouthwashes**

Ingredient	Side effect	Ref.
chlorhexidine	discoloration of the teeth	3
	discoloration of the dorsum of the tongue	20
	disturbance of taste sensations, with burning, soreness, dryness	18
	desquamation and ulceration of the oral mucosa	9
	swelling of the parotid glands (reversible)	22
hexetidine	disturbance of taste sensations	24
peppermint oil (2% pet.) – D-limonene (2% pet.) – L-limonene (2% pet.) – α-pinene (15% c.o.)	allergic contact dermatitis	4

13.15 **Incidence of side effects: Mouth fresheners** (see § 20.17)

	% of total	
US manufacturers' file:	0.1	(9/8399)
US hospitals' file:	no data available	
FDA pilot study:	0.1	(1/589)*
Spanish study:	0	(0/210)
Dutch file:	0	(0/202)
British consumers' report:	no data available	
Strassburg study:	0	(0/96)

* 0 severe
  0 moderate
  1 mild

13.16   **Risk index: Mouth fresheners** (see § 20.18)

Mouth fresheners are graded as *low-risk* cosmetics according to the following reports:
US manufacturers' file: at 1 experience per 5,346,000 estimated units distributed.
FDA pilot study: at 1 experience per more than 5,000 person-brand used cosmetics.

DRUGS USED ON THE VAGINAL MUCOSA

13.17   Vulvovaginal drugs may cause:
1. Local side effects in and around the vagina, perineum and thighs. Drugs used on the vaginal mucosa that have caused contact allergy are listed in § 13.18.
2. Systemic side effects. These include:
   a. Systemic eczematous contact-type dermatitis (Chapter 17)
   b. Urticarial eruptions
   c. Erythematous rashes
   d. Other systemic effects.

Other systemic effects: Hydrocortisone and dexamethasone cream were associated with vulvar inflammation and the 'toxic shock syndrome' [112]. The local steroid may have facilitated overgrowth of pathogenic staphylococci. The cream also caused irritation which may have enhanced absorption of enterotoxins. Transient eosinophilic pneumonia (Loeffler's syndrome) has been attributed to a vaginal cream containing sulfonamides [116, 117].

13.18   **Contact allergy to vulvovaginal medication**

Ingredient	Type of medication	Side effect	Patch test conc./ vehicle	Comment	Ref.
acetarsol	vaginal tablet	dermatitis of the thigh	not mentioned		114
carbason	vaginal tablet	irritation of vulva and vagina; generalized eruption	1% and 5% pet.		115
furazolidone and nifuroxime	vaginal tablet	pruritus and irritation of vulvar and perineal area; generalized eruption	tablet as is	Further testing not performed	113
nifuroxime	vaginal tablet	severe itching around vagina; generalized urticaria with laryngeal edema	not mentioned	Basophil degradation test positive Combination of type I and IV allergy suggested	111
sulfanilamide	cream	urticarial lesions on vulva, perineum and thighs; generalized eruption		Patch tests not performed	113

(continued)

13.18   Contact allergy to vulvovaginal medication

(continuation)

Contactant	Use	Side effects	Patch test conc./ vehicle	Comment	Ref.
sulfanilamide	cream	vulvar eczema and spreading dermatitis	sulfanilamide 5% pet.	Systemic eczematous contact-type dermatitis caused by an oral sulfonylurea derivative (Orinase®, an antidiabetic)	118
sulfanilamide and dienoestrol	cream	itching, perivulvar eruption and photodermatitis	cream as is	Positive *photo*patch test	113

DRUGS USED IN OPHTHALMOLOGICAL PRACTICE

13.19   Systemic and local side effects of topical ophthalmic preparations may strictly speaking not be primarily the concern of the dermatologist. However, in case of local side effects of ophthalmic drugs the advice of a dermatologist is frequently sought. Therefore we have included a text on unwanted effects of ophthalmic preparations; both local and systemic reactions are discussed. A review of systemic effects of topical ophthalmic medication has been documented [100, 110].

Topically applied ophthalmic drugs

13.20   Topically applied ophthalmic drugs:
1. Are intended to exert a local therapeutic effect on the eye, to penetrate the cornea and act on internal ocular structures
2. May cause local side effects
3. May cause general effects. After being placed in the conjunctival sac a significant amount of the ophthalmic drug may be absorbed and give rise to systemic effects [98].

Absorption takes place by several routes:
1. The drug diffuses into the circulation via conjunctival, episcleral and intra-ocular vessels. These vessels drain by facial and ophthalmic veins and the sinus cavernosus into the vena cava superior and the right atrium.
2. The drug is absorbed through the mucous membranes. The ophthalmic sac is connected with the nasal mucosa by the nasolacrimal duct and the puncta of the eye. Absorption across the nasal mucous membranes takes place rapidly, in the case of phenylephrine HCl almost as rapid as by intravenous injection [73, 105]
3. After the drug has traversed the nasolacrimal duct and the nasopharynx, access to the gastrointestinal tract occurs; if the drug survives the acidity of the stomach, the gastrointestinal tract forms an important pathway of absorption.

The amount of absorption is influenced by several factors:
1. The dosage and the concentration of the drug
2. The condition of the conjunctival sac: the lax eyelids of older people makes more retention possible [81]
3. The condition of the eye. If it is dry (which happens under general anesthesia), hyperemic or in a pathologic condition, absorption will be increased [95]
4. Pediatric and geriatric patients are more prone to develop symptoms of systemic effects [86]

150

5. The position of the patient. In the upright position an approximately tenfold loss of drug occurs [101]
6. Simultaneous use of other ophthalmic medications
7. Degradation of the drug in the course of time
8. Alteration of the potency, e.g. by the addition of preservatives [91].

Among the most useful pharmacologic agents in ophthalmic practice are the topically applied autonomic drugs that produce mydriasis, miosis and cycloplegia. These drugs (§ 13.21) are commonly used for examination of the eye, control of glaucoma, and relief of minor symptoms.

13.21   Topical ophthalmic autonomic drugs

I. Adrenergic
   A. Sympathomimetic
      1. Epinephrine (adrenaline)
      2. Phenylephrine
   B. Anticholinergic
      1. Atropine
      2. Scopolamine
      3. Homatropine
      4. Cyclopentolate
      5. Tropicamide
II. Parasympathomimetic, cholinergic
   A. Direct acting
      1. Pilocarpine
      2. Carbachol
   B. Indirect acting
      1. Reversible
         a. Physostigmine
      2. Irreversible
         a. Echothiopate
         b. Demecarium bromide
III. Beta-adrenergic antagonist
   A. Timolol

SYSTEMIC EFFECTS

Sympathomimetic drugs

13.22   Epinephrine (adrenaline)

Epinephrine is used topically in a 1–2% solution. Systemic side effects from ocular instillation are most frequently cardiovascular. Hypertension, tachycardia, arrhythmias, headache, tremor, pallor, perspiration and faintness have been reported [77, 95]. Most serious systemic side effects occur in older patients suffering from hypertension, hyperthyroidism, coronary artery disease, advanced cerebral arteriosclerosis or diabetes mellitus. Patients with primary open-angle glaucoma may be more responsive to ocular and systemic side effects of epinephrine. If they also have a preexisting cardiac disease, they should be monitored for premature ventricular contractions [105].

13.23   Phenylephrine hydrochloride

Phenylephrine hydrochloride differs from epinephrine only in the lack of a hydroxyl group on the benzene ring. Systemic absorption from the nasal mucosa is almost as rapid as by intravenous injection [105]. Systemic side effects of phenylephrine are dose-dependent. Severe hypertension, sometimes accompanied by palpitations, tachycardia, bradycardia, severe occipital headaches and tachypnea have been reported [95, 105]. The systemic effects are more marked if phenylephrine hydrochloride is instilled in an eye affected by conjunctival hyperemia, extensive bleeding or some disruption of corneal epithelium. Patients with cardiac disease, hypertension, advanced cardiovascular or cerebral arteriosclerosis and/or cerebral aneurysm are particularly susceptible to develop an acute increase in systolic and diastolic blood pressure. Phenylephrine has been reported as the cause of hypertension leading to severe and sometimes fatal myocardial infarctions, primarily in older patients with preexisting cardiac disease. It has also been incriminated as the cause of subarachnoid hemorrhage [81, 82], ventricular arrhythmias, and cardiac arrest [103]. More details and literature data are given by Selvin [100].

Anticholinergic drugs

13.24   Atropine

In children receiving eyedrops containing 1% atropine the following systemic side effects have been noted: dryness of skin and mouth, fever, tachycardia, irritability, and flushing of the face [103]. Other reported side effects in children are: abdominal distension, arrhythmias, loss of neuromuscular coordination, ataxia, dysarthria, mental aberrations, delirium and visual hallucinations [89], precipitation of asthma and convulsions [103]. In adults fever and tachycardia have been reported. The confusional psychosis with ataxia, dysarthria and visual hallucinations which can be observed after parenteral administration of belladonna derivatives has also been reported after (repeated) ocular topical administration of atropine [75].

13.25   Scopolamine

Elderly patients may exhibit a severe confusional state after instillation of scopolamine-containing eyedrops. The central nervous system syndrome includes confusion, disorientation, hallucinations and disturbances in the level of consciousness [84] (*see also* § 16.101).

13.26   Homatropine

Homatropine is in its actions and systemic side effects similar to atropine. It is, however, a weaker drug with about 1/50 the toxicity of atropine [93].

13.27   Cyclopentolate

There is a great similarity in the effects and side effects of atropine and cylopentolate. Side effects of cyclopentolate include central nervous system symptoms: slurred speech, ataxia, hallucinations, hyperactivity, seizures and syncope [92]. These side effects are particularly seen in the very young and very old. Nonspecific psychotic behavior (hallucinations, confusion and disturbances of affect and gait) have also been reported in the elderly [92]. In children the symptoms include clouding of the sensorium, hallucinatory phenomenons and disorganization [92]. Symptoms develop about 30–45 minutes after instillation of the drug.

13.28   Tropicamide

Systemic side effects of this parasympatholytic drug include hallucinations and psychotic behavior (in children and in adults), nausea, vomiting, pallor, headache, tachycardia, muscle rigidity, and even vasomotor and cardiorespiratory collapse [103].

Parasympathomimetic drugs

13.29   Pilocarpine

Pilocarpine, used in a 4% eyedrop solution, is rapidly absorbed in the systemic circulation. Reports on systemic reactions are rare. Systemic side effects are characterized by exaggeration of the parasympathomimetic effects. In asthmatic patients a reduction of the vital capacity due to bronchial musculature stimulation occurs; a typical asthmatic attack may even be precipitated. Other effects are increased tone and motility of the intestines resulting in nausea, vomiting and/or diarrhea; enhanced tone and motility of the ureter, urinary bladder, gallbladder and biliary tract. Also diaphoresis, salivation and lacrimation occur as well as muscle tremors. The cardiovascular symptoms are hypotension and bradycardia [80].

13.30   Carbachol

The systemic side effects of carbachol are similar but more severe than those of pilocarpine [77].

13.31   Physostigmine

Physostigmine is readily absorbed from the nasal mucosa and the gastrointestinal tract. The action of physostigmine is similar to that of acetylcholine; side effects include bronchoconstriction, increased tracheal, bronchial and salivary secretion, autonomic stimulation and symptoms of the central nervous system [89]

13.32   Echothiopate

Echothiopate is an anticholinesterase drug which is rapidly absorbed by all routes: the conjunctiva, the gastrointestinal tract, mucous membranes and the skin. Toxicity is generally cumulative and the toxic systemic symptoms generally do not appear for weeks or months after the start of the therapy. The relation between the systemic toxic symptoms and the ocular use of echothiopate is frequently unrecognized. The toxic symptoms include [100]:
1. Gastrointestinal disturbances: diarrhea, nausea, abdominal cramps, weakness. This may simulate an acute abdominal condition

2. Cardiovascular symptoms. They reflect both the ganglionic and postganglionic effects of accumulated acetylcholine. The wide variety of hemodynamic effects include bradycardia, hypotension and a predomination of decreased cardiac output. Cardiac arrest has occurred
3. Respiratory symptoms are rhinorrhea, cough, dyspnea, laryngospasm, bronchoconstriction, bronchorrhea, pulmonary edema, central respiratory depression and failure
4. Central nervous system symptoms include confusion, slurred speech, ataxia, loss of reflexes, Cheyne-Stokes respiration, central respiratory depression and coma
5. Neuromuscular effects are fatigability, generalized to severe weakness, fasciculation, convulsion and paralysis. Further details and data are given by Selvin [100].

13.33   Demecarium bromide

Demecarium bromide is a cholinesterase inhibitor for local ophthalmological use. Absorption and adverse systemic effects are identical to echothiopate.

Beta-adrenergic antagonists

13.34   Timolol

Eyedrops containing timolol, a β-adrenergic antagonist of both β-1 and β-2 receptors, may cause undesirable systemic side effects. Timolol is absorbed from the conjunctiva and reaches the systemic circulation bypassing the liver, where it is normally metabolized. Timolol reaches the pulmonary circulation and may produce a beta-blockade. This may result, especially in patients with preexisting pulmonary problems, in dyspnea, airway obstruction, bronchospasm, respiratory failure and death [82]. Adverse central nervous system effects are depression, anxiety, fatigue, confusion, anorexia, dysarthria and/or hallucinations [82]. Tinnitus, diplopia and aberrations in taste perceptions also occur. For further details, see Selvin [100].

13.35   Topical ocular anesthetic drugs

Topical ocular anesthetic drugs rarely cause systemic adverse reactions. In markedly apprehensive or emotionally agitated persons symptoms like fainting, convulsions or personality changes may occur, probably an idiosyncratic or exaggerated emotional response [82].

13.36   Corticosteroids

Topically applied ocular corticosteroids may, after absorption, infrequently give rise to systemic effects. More details are given by Nutsall [66] and Burch [67].

13.37   Chloramphenicol

Topical ocular chloramphenicol rarely produces systemic symptoms of hematopoietic toxicity [68].

13.38   Sulfacetamide sodium

A case of Stevens-Johnson syndrome from an ophthalmic preparation containing sulfacetamide sodium 10% has been reported [90].

LOCAL SIDE EFFECTS

13.39   Contact allergy

Drugs that have caused contact allergy in topical ophthalmic preparations are listed in § 13.40. *Other local side effects* of drugs used in topical ophthalmic preparations are listed in § 13.41.

13.40   Contact allergy to topical ophthalmic preparations

Drug	Patch test conc./ vehicle	Cross-reactions	Comment	Ref.
antazoline phosphate	0.5% aqua/1 % pet.	aminophylline	Injection of aminophylline caused generalized dermatitis	72
atropine sulfate	1% pet.			79
bacitracin	20–30% pet.			123
benzalkonium chloride	0.05% aqua		Cave: irritant patch test reactions *See also under* cinnamic aldehyde.	54 85 97
betamethasone valerate	5% pet.			74
chloramphenicol	1% alc./ 5–10% pet.			123
chlorhexidine gluconate	1% aqua		In preserving liquids for soft contact lenses	109
cinnamic aldehyde	2% pet.		Contact allergy and irritation from benzalkonium chloride, cinnamic aldehyde, parabens, neomycin and thiomersal has caused drug-induced cicatrization of the conjunctiva (§ 13.41)	197
echothiopate iodide	0.25–1% aqua			96
edetic acid (EDTA)	1% pet./aqua			123
ephedrine	1% alc./pet.			102
epinephrine bitartrate	1% aqua			99

(continued)

13.40   Contact allergy to topical ophthalmic preparations

(continuation)

Drug	Patch test conc./ vehicle	Cross-reactions	Comment	Ref.
epinephrine chloride	0.1–1% aqua	epinephrine borate, diisopropyl fluorophosphate (?)	Has caused melanosis (§ 13.41)	74 88
idoxuridine	1% pet.			108
metoprolol	3% aqua	propranolol, practolol, timolol		94
neomycin	20% pet.	*see* § 5.25	*See under* cinnamic aldehyde	97
parabens	5% pet.		*See under* cinnamic aldehyde	97
phenylephrine	1–5% aqua			96 124
polymyxin B	3% pet.			123
proparacaine hydrochloride	2% aqua			76
sulfonamides	5% pet./aqua			123
thiomersal	0.1% pet.		Also in preserving liquids for soft contact lenses *See also under* cinnamic aldehyde	104 64 107 109 97
trifluorthymidine	1% comm. eyedrops		The allergy in the case presented probably represents a cross-reaction to primary IDU sensitization	78
wool wax alcohols	pure			123

13.41   Other local side effects of topical ophthalmic preparations

Drug	Side effect	Comment	Ref.
benoxinate	keratitis		70
benzalkonium chloride	corneal damage		87
	cicatrization of the conjunctiva due to allergy and irritation		97
cinnamic aldehyde	cicatrization of the conjunctiva due to allergy and irritation		97
corticosteroids	glaucoma		71
cromoglycate disodium	acute chemotic reaction: redness, swelling, and itching of the conjunctiva	Allergy tests inadequately performed	63

(continued)

(continuation)

Drug	Side effect	Comment	Ref.
epinephrine	melanosis of the conjunctiva and staining of the cornea		69
isofluorophate	depigmentation around one eye		60
neomycin	cicatrization of the conjunctiva due to allergy and irritation		97
parabens	cicatrization of the conjunctiva due to allergy and irritation		97
thiomersal	cicatrization of the conjunctiva due to allergy and irritation		97
thiotepa	periorbital leukoderma		58

13.42 REFERENCES

1. Andersen, K. E. (1978): Contact allergy to toothpaste flavors. *Contact Dermatitis, 4,* 195.
2. Beinhauer, L. G. (1940): Cheilitis and dermatitis from toothpaste. *Arch. Derm., 41,* 892.
3. Dolles, O. K., Eriksen, H. M. and Gjermo, P. (1979): Tooth staining during 2 years' use of chlorhexidine- and fluoride-containing dentifrices. *Scand. J. dent. Res., 87,* 268.
4. Dooms-Goossens, A., Degreef, H., Holvoet, C. and Maertens, M. (1977): Turpentine-induced hypersensitivity to peppermint oil. *Contact Dermatitis, 3,* 304.
5. Douglas, T. E. (1957): Fluoride dentifrice and stomatitis. *Northw. Med. (Seattle), 56,* 107.
6. Epstein, E. (1976): Fluoride toothpastes as a cause of acne-like eruptions. *Arch. Derm., 112,* 1033.
7. Feuerman, E. (1975): Dermatitis due to amalgam dental fillings. *Contact Dermatitis, 1,* 191.
8. Fisher, A. A. and Tobin, I. (1953): Sensitivity to compound G-4 ('Dichlorophene') in dentifrices. *J. Amer. med. Ass., 151,* 998.
9. Fløtra, L., Gjermo, P., Rølla, G. and Waerhaug, J. (1971): Side effects of chlorhexidine mouth washes. *Scand. J. dent. Res., 79,* 119.
10. Heygi, E. and Dolezalova, A. (1976): Urticarial reaction after patch tests of toothpaste with a sub-shock condition: Hypersensitivity to carawayseed. *Čs. Derm., 51,* 19.
11. Kirton, V. and Wilkinson, D. S. (1975): Sensitivity to cinnamic aldehyde in a toothpaste. 2. Further studies. *Contact Dermatitis, 1,* 77.
12. Koch, G., Magnusson, B. and Nyquist, G. (1971): Contact allergy to medicaments and materials used in dentistry. *Odont. Revy, 22,* 275.
13. Laubach, J. L., Malkinson, F. D. and Ringrose, E. J. (1953): Cheilitis caused by cinnamon (Cassis) oil in toothpaste. *J. Amer. med. Ass., 152,* 404.
14. Loveman, A. B. (1938): Stomatitis venenata, report of a case of sensitivity of the mucous membranes and the skin to oil of anise. *Arch. Derm. Syph., 37,* 70.
15. Magnusson, B. and Wilkinson, D. S. (1975): Cinnamic aldehyde in toothpaste. 1. Clinical aspects and patch tests. *Contact Dermatitis, 1,* 70.
16. Mathias, C. G. T., Maibach, H. I. and Conant, M. A. (1980): Perioral leukoderma simulating vitiligo from use of a toothpaste containing cinnamic aldehyde. *Arch. Derm., 116,* 1172.
17. Millard, L. (1973): Acute contact sensitivity to a new toothpaste. *J. Dentistry, 1,* 168.
18. O'Neil, T. C. A. (1976): The use of chlorhexidine mouthwash in the control of gingival inflammation. *Brit. dent. J., 141,* 276.
19. Papa, C. M. and Shelley, W. B. (1964): Menthol hypersensitivity. *J. Amer. med. Ass., 159,* 546.
20. Prayitno, S. and Addy, M. (1979): An in vitro study of factors affecting the development of staining associated with the use of chlorhexidine. *J. periodont. Res., 14,* 397.
21. Romaguera, C. and Grimalt, F. (1978): Sensitization to cinnamic aldehyde in toothpaste. *Contact Dermatitis, 4,* 377.
22. Rushton, A. (1977): Safety of hibitane. II. Human experience. *J. clin. Periodont., 4,* 73.
23. Saunders, M. A. (1975): Fluoride toothpastes: a cause of acne-like eruptions. *Arch. Derm., 111,* 793.

24.   Schaupp, H. and Wohnaut, H. (1978): Geschmackstörungen durch Munddesinfizienten. *HNO (Berl.)*, *26*, 335.
25.   Shea, J. J., Gillespie, S. M. and Waldbott, G. L. (1967): Allergy to fluoride. *Ann. Allergy*, *25*, 241.
26.   Smith, I. L. F. (1969): Acute allergic reaction following the use of toothpaste. *Brit. dent. J.*, *125*, 304.
27.   Spier, H. W. and Sixt, I. (1953): Laurel as a hitherto little recognized allergen in contact eczema. *Derm. Wschr.*, *128*, 805.
28.   Templeton, H. J. and Lunsford, C. J. (1932): Cheilitis and stomatitis from ST 37 toothpaste. *Arch. Derm. Syph.*, *41*, 892.
29.   Thomson, J. and Russel, J. A. (1970): Dermatitis due to mercury following amalgam dental restoration. *Brit. J. Derm.*, *82*, 292.
30.   Varma, B. V. (1978): Mouthwash-induced hypoglycemia. *Amer. J. Dis. Child.*, *132*, 930.

UPDATE – 2nd Edition

31.   Bork, K. (1978): Fließschnupfen durch Metallteile von Zahnprothesen. *Z. Hautkr.*, *53*, 814.
32.   Brendlinger, D. L. and Tarsitano, J. J. (1970): Generalized dermatitis due to sensitivity to a chrome cobalt removable partial denture. *J. Amer. Dent. Ass.*, *81*, 392.
33.   Crissey, J. T. (1965): Stomatitis, dermatitis and denture materials. *Arch. Derm.*, *92*, 45.
34.   Danilewicz-Stysiak, Z. (1971): Allergy as a cause of denture sore mouth. *J. prosth. Dent.*, *25*, 16.
35.   Datschev, B. (1971): Allgemeine und Kontakt-Allergie in der Mundhöhle verursacht durch stomatologische Medikamente und Materialen. *Allergie u. Immunol.*, *17*, 239.
36.   Elgart, M. L. and Higdon, R. S. (1971): Allergic contact dermatitis to gold. *Arch. Derm.*, *103*, 649.
37.   Fisher, A. A. (1956): Allergic sensitization of the skin and the oral mucosa to acrylic resin denture materials. *J. prosth. Dent.*, *6*, 593.
38.   Fregert, S., Kollander, M. and Poulsen, J. (1979): Allergic contact stomatitis from gold dentures. *Contact Dermatitis*, *5*, 63.
39.   Frykholm, K. O., Frithiof, L., Fernström, A. I. B. et al. (1969): Allergy to copper derived from dental alloys as a possible cause of oral lesions of lichen planus. *Acta derm.-venereol. (Stockh.)*, *49*, 268.
40.   Van Groeningen, G. and Nater, J. P. (1975): Reactions to dental impression materials. *Contact Dermatitis*, *1*, 373.
41.   Hubler, W. R. Jr. and Hubler, W. R. Sr. (1983): Dermatitis from a chromium dental plate. *Contact Dermatitis*, *9*, 377.
42.   Isaacs, G. (1983): Permanent local anaesthesia and anhidrosis after clove oil spillage. *Lancet*, *1*, 882.
43.   Kaaber, S., Thulin, H. and Nielsen, E. (1979): Skin sensitivity to denture base materials in the burning mouth syndrome. *Contact Dermatitis*, *5*, 90.
44.   Van Ketel, W. G. and Nieboer, C. (1981): Allergy to palladium in dental alloys. *Contact Dermatitis*, *7*, 331.
45.   Kulenkamp, D., Hausen, B. M. and Schulz, K. H. (1977): Berufliche Kontaktallergie durch neuartige, zahnärztlich verwendete Abdruckmaterialien. *Hautarzt*, *28*, 353.
46.   Malten, K. E. (1960): Allergische reacties op kunstharsen. *T. Tandheelk.*, *67*, 827.
47.   Mathias, C. G. T., Chappler, R. R. and Maibach, H. I. (1980): Contact urticaria from cinnamic aldehyde. *Arch. Derm.*, *116*, 74.
48.   Merk, H., Ebert, L. and Goerz, G. (1982): Allergic contact dermatitis due to the fungicide hexetidine. *Contact Dermatitis*, *8*, 216.
49.   Nakayama, H., Niki, F., Shono, M. and Hada, S. (1983): Mercury exanthema. *Contact Dermatitis*, *9*, 411.
50.   Nathanson, D. and Lockhart, P. (1979): Delayed extraoral hypersensitivity to dental composite materials. *Oral Surg.*, *47*, 329.
51.   Schöpf, E., Wex, O. and Schulz, K. K. (1970): Allergische Kontaktstomatitis mit spezifischer Lymphocytenstimulation durch Gold. *Hautarzt*, *21*, 422.
52.   Feuerman, E. J. (1975): Recurrent contact dermatitis caused by mercury in amalgam dental fillings. *Int. J. Derm.*, *14*, 657.
53.   Kulenkamp, D., Hausen, B. M. and Schulz, K. H. (1976): Berufliche Kontaktallergie durch neuartige Abdruckmaterialen in der zahnärztlichen Praxis (Scutan und Impregum). *Zahnärztl. Prax.*, *66*, 968.

54. Afzelius, H. and Thulin, H. (1979): Allergic reactions to benzalkonium chloride. *Contact Dermatitis, 5,* 60.
55. Barber, K. A. (1983): Allergic contact eczema to phenylephrine. *Contact Dermatitis, 9,* 274.
56. Fratto, C. (1978): Provocation of bronchospasm by eye-drops. *Ann. intern. Med., 88,* 362.
57. Fraunfelder, F. T. and Scafidi, A. F. (1978): Possible adverse effects from topical ocular 10 % phenylephrine. *Amer. J. Ophthal., 85,* 447.
58. Harben, D. J., Cooper, P. H. and Rodman, O. (1977): Thiotepa-induced leukoderma. *Arch. Derm., 115,* 973.
59. Henkes, H. E. and Waubke, T. N. (1978): Keratitis from abuse of corneal anaesthetics. *Brit. J. Ophthal., 62,* 62.
60. Koldys, K. W. and Frye, L. (1973): A perplexing pigmentary problem. *Cutis, 12,* 420.
61. Lipmann, M. and Rogoff, R. C. (1974): Clinical evaluation of pyridostigmine biomide in the reversal of pancuronium. *Anesth. Analg. curr. Res., 53,* 20.
62. Morton, W. R., Drance, S. M. and Fairclough, M. (1969): Effect of echothiopate iodide on the lens. *Amer. J. Ophthal., 68,* 1003.
63. Ostler, H. B. (1982): Acute chemotic reaction to cromolyn. *Arch. Ophthal., 100,* 412.
64. Rietschel, R. L. and Wilson, L. A. (1982): Ocular inflammation in patients using soft contact lenses. *Arch. Derm., 118,* 147.
65. Velez, G. J. (1968): Jaundice and Floropryl. Report of a case. *J. Pediat. Ophthal., 5,* 179.
66. Nursall, J. F. (1965): Systemic effects of topical use of ophthalmic corticosteroid preparations. *Amer. J. Ophthal., 59,* 29.
67. Burch, P. G. and Migeon, C. J. (1968): Systemic absorption of topical steroids. *Arch. Ophthal., 79,* 174.
68. Carpenter, G. (1975): Chloramphenicol eye-drops and marrow aplasia. *Lancet, 2,* 326.
69. Schuster, H. (1974): Uber eine seltene Nebenwirkung von Adrenalin-Augentropfen. *Klin. Mbl. Augenheilk., 165,* 517.
70. Henkes, H. E. and Waubke, T. N. (1978): Keratitis from abuse of corneal anaesthetics. *Brit. J. Ophthal., 62,* 62.
71. Eisenlohr, J. E. (1983): Glaucoma following the prolonged use of topical steroid medication to the eyelids. *J. Amer. Acad. Derm., 8,* 878.
72. Berman, B. A. and Ross, R. N. (1983): Ethylenediamine: systemic eczematous contact-type dermatitis. *Cutis, 31,* 594.
73. Adriani, J. and Campbell, D. (1956): Fatalities following topical application of local anesthetics to mucous membranes. *J. Amer. med. Ass., 162,* 1527.
74. Alani, S. D. and Alani, M. D. (1976): Allergic contact dermatitis and conjunctivitis from epinephrine. *Contact Dermatitis, 2,* 147.
75. Baker, J. P. and Farley, J. D. (1958): Toxic psychosis following atropine eyedrops. *Brit. med. J., 2,* 390.
76. Bandmann, H. J., Breit, R. and Mutzeck, E. (1974): Allergic contact dermatitis from Proxymetacaine. *Contact Dermatitis Newsl., 15,* 451.
77. Benjamin, K. W. (1979): Toxicity of ocular medications. *Int. ophthal. Clin., 19,* 199.
78. Cirkel, P. K. S. and van Ketel, W. G. (1981): Allergic contact dermatitis to trifluorthymidine eyedrops. *Contact Dermatitis, 7,* 49.
79. Dobkevitch, S. and Sidi, E. (1948): Eczéma de la face provoqué par un collyre au sulfate d'atropine. *Bull. Soc. franç. Derm. Syph., 55,* 60.
80. Epstein, E. and Kaufman, I. (1965): Systemic pilocarpine toxicity from overdosage. *Amer. J. Ophthal., 59,* 109.
81. Fraunfelder, F. T. (1976): Extraocular fluid dynamics: how best to apply topical ocular medication. *Trans. Amer. ophthal. Soc., 74,* 457.
82. Fraunfelder, F. T. (1979): Interim report: national registry of possible drug-induced ocular side-effects. *Amer. J. Ophthal., 86,* 126.
83. Fregert, S. and Möller, H. (1962): Hypersensitivity to the cholinesterase inhibitor di-iso-propoxyphosphorylfluoride. *J. invest. Derm., 38,* 371.
84. Freund, M. and Merin, S. (1970): Toxic effects of scopolamine eye-drops. *Amer. J. Ophthal., 70,* 637.
85. Fisher, A. A. and Stillman, M. A. (1972): Allergic contact sensitivity to benzalkonium chloride. *Arch. Derm., 106,* 169.
86. Friedman, T. S. and Patton, T. F. (1976): Differences in ocular penetration of pilocarpine in rabbits of different ages. *J. pharm. Sci., 65,* 1095.
87. Gasset, A. R. (1977): Benzalkonium chloride toxicity to the human cornea. *Amer. J. Ophthal., 84,* 169.

88. Gibbs, R. C. (1970): Allergic contact dermatitis to epinephrine. *Arch. Derm., 101,* 92.
89. Goodman, L. S. and Gilman, A. (Eds) (1980): *The Pharmacological Basis of Therapeutics,* 6th ed., MacMillan Publishing Co., New York.
90. Gottschalk, H. R. and Stone, O. J. (1976): Stevens-Johnson syndrome from ophthalmic sulfonamide. *Arch. Derm., 112,* 513.
91. Haddad, N. J., Moyer, N. and Riley, F. (1970): Mydriatic effect of phenylephrine hydrochloride. *Amer. J. Ophthal., 70,* 729.
92. Havener, W. H. (1979): *Ocular Pharmacology,* 4th ed., pp. 40-50. C. V. Mosby Co, St. Louis.
93. Hoefnagel, D. (1961): Toxic effects of atropine and homatropine eye-drops in children. *New Engl. J. Med., 264,* 168.
94. Van Joost, Th., Middelkamp Hup, J. and Ros, F. E. (1980): Dermatitis as a side-effect of long-term topical treatment with certain beta-blocking agents. *Brit. J. Derm., 101,* 171.
95. Lansche, R. K. (1966): Systemic reactions to topical epinephrine and phenylephrine. *Amer. J. Ophthal., 61,* 95.
96. Mathias, C. G. T., Maibach, H. I., Irvine, A. and Adler, W. (1979): Allergic contact dermatitis to echothiopate iodide and phenylephrine. *Arch. Ophthal., 97,* 286.
97. Ostler, H. B., Okumoto, M., Daniels, T. and Conant, M. A. (1983): Drug-induced cicatrisation of the conjunctiva. *Contact Dermatitis, 9,* 155.
98. Patton, T. F. and Francoeur, M. (1978): Ocular bioavailability and systemic loss of topically applied ophthalmic drugs. *Amer. J. Ophthal., 85,* 225.
99. Romaguera, C. and Grimalt, F. (1980): Contact dermatitis from epinephrine. *Contact Dermatitis, 6,* 364.
100. Selvin, B. L. (1983): Systemic effects of topical ophthalmic medications. *Sth. med. J., 76,* 349.
101. Sieg, J. W. and Robinson, J. R. (1974): Corneal absorption of fluoromethalone in rabbits. *Arch. Ophthal., 92,* 240.
102. Spencer, G. A. (1945): Hypersensitivity to ephedrine. *Arch. Derm. Syph., (Chic.), 51,* 48.
103. Stokes, H. R. (1979): Drug reactions reported in a survey of South Carolina. *Amer. Ophthal., 86,* 161.
104. Suzuki, H., (1972): Allergic conjunctivitis and blepharo-conjunctivitis caused by thiomersal used as a preservant. *Jap. J. Ophthal., 26,* 783.
105. Vaughan, R. W. (1973): Ventricular arrhythmias after topical vasoconstrictors. *Anesth. Analg., 52,* 161.
106. Alani, S. D. and Alani, M. D. (1976): Allergic contact dermatitis and conjunctivitis to corticosteroids. *Contact Dermatitis, 2,* 301.
107. Bang Pedersen, N. (1978): Allergic contact conjunctivitis from merthiolate in soft contact lenses. *Contact Dermatitis, 4,* 165.
108. Van Ketel, W. G. (1979): Allergy to idoxuridine eyedrops. *Contact Dermatitis, 5,* 106.
109. Van Ketel, W. G. and Melzer-van Riemsdijk, F. A. (1980): Conjunctivitis due to soft lens solutions. *Contact Dermatitis, 6,* 321.
110. Palmer, E. A. (1982): Drug toxicity in pediatric ophthalmology. *J. Toxic.-Cut. Ocul. Toxic. 1,* 181.
111. Aaronson, Ch. M (1969): Generalized urticaria from sensitivity to nifuroxime. (Letter). *J. Amer. med. Ass., 210,* 557.
112. Dutton, A. H., Hayes, P. C., Shepherd, A. N. and Geirsson, R. (1983): Vulvovaginal steroid cream and toxic shock syndrome. *Lancet, 1,* 938.
113. Goette, D. K. and Odom, R. B. (1980): Vaginal medications as a cause for varied widespread dermatitides. *Cutis, 26,* 406.
114. Robin, J. (1978): Contact dermatitis to acetarsol. *Contact Dermatitis, 4,* 309.
115. Verburgh-van der Zwan, N. and van Ketel, W. G. (1981): Contactallergie voor een arseen bevattend intravaginaal toegepast geneesmiddel. *Ned. T. Geneesk., 125,* 1718.
116. Donlan, Ch. J. Jr. and Scutero, J. V. (1975): Transient eosinophilic pneumonia secondary to use of a vaginal cream. *Chest, 67,* 232.
117. Klinghoffer, J. F. (1954): Loeffler's syndrome following the use of a vaginal cream. *Ann. intern. Med., 40,* 343.
118. Fisher, A. A. (1982): Systemic contact dermatitis from Orinase® and Diabinese® in diabetics with para-amino hypersensitivity. *Cutis, 29,* 551.
119. Mathias, C. G. T., Chappler, R. R. and Maibach, H. I. (1980): Contact urticaria from cinnamic aldehyde. *Arch. Derm., 116,* 74.
120. Merk, H., Ebert, L. and Goerz., G. (1982): Allergic contact dermatitis due to the fungicide hexetidine. *Contact Dermatitis, 8,* 555.

121. Monti, M., Berti, E., Carminati, G. and Cusini, M. (1983): Occupational and cosmetic dermatitis from propolis. *Contact Dermatitis, 9,* 163.

122. Marchand, B., Barbier, P., Ducombs, G., et al. (1982): Allergic contact dermatitis to various salols (phenyl salicylates). *Arch. derm. Res., 272,* 61.

123. Kruijswijk, M. R. J. and Polak, B. C. P. (1980): Contactallergie na toepassing van oogdruppels en oogzalven. *Ned. T. Geneesk., 124,* 1449.

124. Barber, K. A. (1983): Allergic contact eczema to phenylephrine. *Contact Dermatitis, 9,* 274.

14. Local side effects of corticosteroids

14.1   Topical steroids have the following effects on the skin [32, 33, 22], in that they:

1. inhibit proliferation and regeneration of epidermis (inhibition of DNA synthesis);
2. inhibit collagen synthesis;
3. inhibit elastin synthesis;
4. cause atrophy of adipose tissue;
5. cause vasoconstriction;
6. seal and stabilize the cell walls;
7. cause follicular hyperkeratosis;
8. cause focal degeneration of follicular epithelium;
9. stimulate hair growth;
10. inhibit antigen-antibody reactions;
11. inhibit leukocyte migration and proliferation;
12. inhibit antibody production and proliferation of immunocompetent cells;
13. depress or stimulate melanogenesis.

Table 14.2 provides a guide to the clinical potency of commonly used topical steroids [27, 28].

14.2   **Potency of topical corticosteroids***

Corticosteroid	Group 1 (very potent)	Group 2 (potent)	Group 3 (moderately potent)	Group 4 (weak)
beclomethasone dipropionate	0.5%	0.025%	–	–
betamethasone benzoate	–	0.025%	–	–
betamethasone dipropionate	–	0.05%	–	–
betamethasone valerate	–	0.1%	–	–
clobetasole propionate	0.05%	–	–	–
clobetasone butyrate	–	–	0.05%	–
desonide	–	0.05%	–	–
desoximetasone	–	0.25%	–	–
dexamethasone	–	–	–	0.01%
diflorasone diacetate	–	0.05%	–	–

(continued)

(continuation)

Corticosteroid	Group 1 (very potent)	Group 2 (potent)	Group 3 (moderately potent)	Group 4 (weak)
diflucortolone valerate	0.3%	0.1%	–	–
fluclorolone acetonide	–	0.025%	–	–
fludroxycortide (flurandrenolone)	–	0.05%	0.0125 à 0.025%	–
flumethasone pivalate	–	–	0.02%	–
fluocinolone acetonide	0.2%	0.025%	0.01%	–
fluocinonide	–	0.05%	–	–
fluocortin butylester	–	–	0.75%	–
fluocortolone	–	0.5%	0.2%	–
fluoprednidene acetate	–	0.1%	–	–
halcinonide	–	0.1%	–	–
hydrocortisone	–	–	–	0.1–1%
hydrocortisone butyrate	–	0.1%	–	–
methylprednisolone	–	–	–	0.25%
triamcinolone acetonide	–	0.1%	–	–

* This is a rough guide, since no direct comparison has been made between all these preparations.

TOPICAL CORTICOSTEROID PREPARATIONS

14.3 The activity of topical corticosteroid preparations has been investigated by various methods. One of the most important bioassay methods is the vasoconstrictor test. This assay is based on an alleged relationship between the ability of a corticosteroid to induce vasoconstriction and its clinical effectiveness. Differences in concentration of a particular corticosteroid are not always reflected as significant differences in vasoconstrictor potency [45]. Other bioassay methods are: in vitro fibroblast inhibition, antimitotic effect on human epidermis, the effect on damaged skin, the reaction to inflammation induced by various sources (UV light, croton oil, kerosene, allergic contact dermatitis) and the reduction of the size of histamine-induced wheals. A review of bioassays used in the development of topical steroid preparations has been provided by Haleblian [15]. Although the results of these methods may serve as a useful guide to topical anti-inflammatory and antimitotic activity, clinical assessment remains necessary.

Penetration and effectiveness

14.4 Factors influencing the penetration and clinical effectiveness (and also the possible occurrence of side effects) include [27]:
1. *Anatomical site.* Corticosteroids penetrate the skin through hair follicles and

163

by transepidermal routes [31]: absorption is increased in regions with large or numerous hair follicles. The scalp absorbs 3.5 times, the forehead 6 times and the scrotum 36 times the quantity of hydrocortisone as compared to the ventral aspect of the forearm. Absorption is decreased in regions of the skin having thickened stratum corneum [13].

2. *Vehicle formulation.* Improper formulation may diminish or completely abolish the clinical activity of the corticosteroid [5]. The addition of penetrants may facilitate absorption, e.g. salicylic acid: [30]; urea: [9].

3. *Concentration of the corticosteroid.* A 10-fold increase in concentration induces a 4-fold increase in hydrocortisone absorption from the skin of the forearm [21].

4. *Occlusive (polyethylene) dressing.* This may enhance penetration approximately 10 to 100-fold, lessens the differences in potency between the corticosteroids and reduces the influence of the vehicle on the penetration [24, 18]. In skin folds, occlusion from the anatomical situation also increases penetration.

5. *Age.* The thin skin of children and aged people enhances precutaneous absorption.

6. *Chemical structure of the steroid.*

14.5   The question whether the side effects of corticosteroids are related to the incorporation of halogens in the molecule is still in debate. Dermatitis perioralis (a frequently reported side effect of halogenated corticosteroids) has also been reported after the use of non-halogenated steroids [6]. It must furthermore be stressed that less potent steroids may produce many of the same side effects as do more potent ones. Even prolonged application of 1% hydrocortisone, generally considered innocuous, may cause local side effects in vulnerable skin areas, though generally less than found following use of the more potent corticosteroids [14]. The skin of the face seems to be particularly susceptible to the effects of corticosteroids [7].

Side effects

14.6   The following side effects of locally applied corticosteroids have been reported [32, 33, 16].

1. *Effects on the pilosebaceous unit*
– Perioral dermatitis [25, 38]: This condition is characterized by a symmetric eruption of erythematous papules, papulo-pustules and vesicles on the skin and the nasolabial folds, with a clear perilabial zone. When stopping the application of the topical corticosteroid a rebound phenomenon may frequently be noted. Some authors believe that the *halogenated* corticosteroids play an important part in the pathogenesis of perioral dermatitis. The dermatosis has, however, also been reported in patients treated with hydrocortisone and hydrocortisone butyrate [14, 6]. Perioral dermatitis is not always associated with the topical application of corticosteroids. Three cases have been observed after ingestion of the spices marjoram, bay leaf and cinnamon. The eruption cleared on a diet without these spices [12]. Some authors [44] prefer to restrict the term 'perioral dermatitis' to those patients presenting with the well-known perioral rash who have *not* used topical corticosteroids. If dermal steroids have been used, Cohen [44] prefers the term 'rosacea-like dermatitis'.
– Rosacea-like dermatitis: This term has been used as a synonym to perioral dermatitis, but Cohen [44] distinguishes it from (not steroid-induced) perioral dermatitis by the presence of teleangiectasia and a reddish hue. Steroid-induced papulo-pustular lesions, morphologically similar to perioral dermatitis but located on other parts of the face, may also be termed rosacea-like dermatitis.

– Steroid acne: This side effect of topical corticosteroids is not necessarily limited to the area of application. Steroid acne may also be induced by systemic administration of corticosteroids. The eruption is characterized by crops of inflammatory papules in the same stage of development, sometimes followed by crops of comedones; its onset is usually rather sudden [29].
– Exacerbation of pre-existing rosacea: also, prerosacea may become manifest under corticosteroid treatment.
– Hypertrichosis of the face.
– Perianal comedones [42].

2. *Atrophy of underlying tissues*
There is clinical and experimental evidence that the initial atrophy caused by topical steroids is reversible [41], but long-term application may lead to more permanent changes. The presently available in vitro data do not permit the development of a unifying hypothesis for steroid-induced dermal atrophy [40]. Clinical manifestations of steroid-induced atrophy include:
– 'Cigarette paper wrinkling' of the skin
– Teleangiectasias
– Petechiae, ecchymoses
– Striae rubrae distensae, mainly occurring in the inguinal and axillary region (occlusion effect)
– Susceptibility of the skin to minor trauma
– Fragile skin in surgery
– Delayed wound healing
– Exacerbation of existing ulceration

3. *Effects on skin color* [1]
– Hypopigmentation
– Hyperpigmentation

4. *Effects on the immunological system*
– Masking of the pre-existing disease
– Aggravation of pre-existing disease
– Inhibition of immunological mechanisms

Clinical examples of the effects on the immunological system are:

– Aggravation of pre-existing folliculitis
– Development of extensive, but unrecognized dermatophytic infections, so-called tinea incognito [17]
– Perpetuation of masked infections with candida albicans
– Conversion of scabies into the 'Norwegian' type [26]
– Extensive mollusca contagiosa eruption
– 'Galloping' impetigo
– Development of generalised pustular psoriasis
– Spreading of malignant skin lesions [7]
– Suppression of pruritus

5. *Ocular and nasal effects* [39, 3]
– Ocular hypertension
– Open angle glaucoma [46]
– Uveitis
– Posterior subcapsular cataracts
– Nasal septal perforation (steroid aerosol)

6. *Allergic effects* [35] (see also Chapter 4):
– Allergic contact dermatitis (*cave:* allergic reactions to vehicle constituents, pre-servatives, etc.)
– Generalized urticaria

7. *Miscellaneous side effects*
– Tachyphylaxis [8]: This is acute tolerance to the vasoconstriction effect of topi-cally applied corticosteroids.
– Milia [34]: degeneration of collagen probably plays a role in the pathogenesis.
– Granuloma gluteale infantum [2]: this condition is characterized by multiple red or reddish-brown nodules in the napkin area in young infants. Local steroid treatment as well as candidiasis are held responsible.
– Pseudo-cicatrices stellaires spontanées: This condition is characterized by scarring purpura and skin atrophy on the back of the forearms of elderly people after long-term steroid application [4].
– Elastoidosis cutanée nodulaire à cystes et à comédons Favre-Racouchot: This dermatosis is localized mainly in the periorbital and neck region and is presum-ably caused by solar or senile degeneration of the skin; in addition, it has been reported after topical application of corticosteroids [33].
– Erythrosis interfollicularis colli. This entity is localized on the sides of the neck and upper breast and is usually caused by actinic degeneration. Topical applica-tion of corticosteroids may worsen these changes [33].
– Cutis linearis punctata colli or 'stippled skin': Prominent sebaceous glands on atrophic skin are the cause of this condition. It has also been reported as side effect of systemic steroid therapy [11].
– Photosensitivity: Long-term topical corticosteroid treatment leads to an atro-phy of the epidermis which in turn increases its sensitivity to light [33].
– Erythema craquelé: This effect occurred after *cessation* of long-term continuous steroid application to normal skin [43].

TOPICAL CORTICOSTEROID-ANTIBIOTIC PREPARATIONS

14.7   The use of topical corticosteroid-antibiotic preparations in the treatment of der-matoses is still in debate. Critics state that the use of such combinations is not without hazards. The risks are [19]:
– Shifts in the existing ecological situation, with the possible establishment of pathogenic organisms
– Proliferation of resistant organisms
– Development of resistance of such organisms to antibiotics related to the one used
– Sensitization to the antibiotic in the topical preparation.
– Masking of the sensitization to the antibiotic or other ingredients of the prepa-ration
– Development of cross-sensitization to related antibiotics.
In fact, most of these events may also develop after use of a topical antibiotic preparation alone.

14.8   Topical corticosteroid-antibiotic preparations may be used in the treatment of:
– Primary pyodermic skin diseases (e.g. impetigo, folliculitis).
– Chronic skin diseases in which a shift in the ecological situation has resulted in the invasion of pathogens.
In primary pyodermic skin diseases the addition of a corticosteroid to an antibi-otic preparation adds nothing to the efficacy of the therapy. In cases of chronic

skin diseases secondarily infected by pathogens, the use of combined preparations has been advocated [23]. Other authors are not convinced that the benefi of this addition outweighs the possible risks.

14.9   The discussion is complicated by the fact that the diagnosis of secondary infection of a skin disease is not always easily made. This leads to the question whether the isolation of a pathogen may be considered sufficient evidence for the presence of 'infection'. The lesions of eczema, particularly in atopic subjects, are very readily colonized by staphylococci, and even the normal skin of patients with eczema carries a larger bacterial population than that of controls. It has been assumed that the moist conditions in the lesions favor bacterial multiplication and that treatment should be 'directed at the skin lesions rather than at eradication of micro-organisms'. Eczema does indeed favor colonization and multiplication, but the critical question is whether such colonization increases the severity or duration of the lesions so that they can logically be regarded as 'infected' [10]. The traditional clinical criteria for judging infection are considered unreliable for this purpose. The diagnosis is only possible with certainty by performing a quantitative bacteriological analysis [20]. It is, however, seldom possible to obtain quantitative bacteriological reports, but semi-quantitative reports a re often provided.

14.10   The following directions for the management secondarily infected dermatoses have been given [20, 36, 10]:
1. Clinical evidence of secondary infection of eczema as impetiginous crusting or pustulation, or a report that *Staphylococcus aureus* is present in abundance, may justify the use of a steroid-antibiotic combination. The application should be of short duration, e.g. 7-10 days.
2. The choice of the antibiotic depends on the nature and the sensitivity of the micro-organism.
3. Intermittent resumption of the combination therapy may be justified, e.g. in atopic subjects.
4. Prolonged continuous application must always be avoided.
5. It must be kept in mind that the risk of contact sensitization is especially present in the treatment of eczema or ulcus of the lower legs.
6. The corticosteroid in the preparation may mask the development of contact sensitization.

14.11   REFERENCES

1. Allen, B. R. and Hunter, J. A. A. (1975): Abnormal facial pigmentation associated with the prolonged use of topical corticosteroids. *Scot. med. J.*, *20*, 277.
2. Altmeyer, P. (1973): Die Bedeutung fluorierter Glucocorticoide in der Aetio-pathogenese der Granuloma gluteale infantum (Tappeiner und Pfleger). *Hautarzt, 22,* 383.
3. Bevis Cubey, R. (1976): Glaucoma following the application of corticosteroid to the skin of the eyelids. *Brit. J. Derm., 95,* 207.
4. Braun-Falco, O. and Balda, B. R. (1970): Sogenannte pseudo-cicatrices stellaires spontanées. *Hautarzt, 21,* 509.
5. Burdick, K. H., Poulsen, B. and Place, U. A. (1970): Extemporaneous formulation of corticosteroids for topical usage. *J. Amer. med. Ass., 211,* 462.
6. Cotterill, J. A. (1979): Perioral dermatitis. *Brit. J. Derm., 101,* 259.
7. Deakins, M. J. (1976): Current danger and problems in the topical use of steroids. *Med. J. Aust., 1,* 120.
8. Du Vivier, A. and Stoughton, R. B. (1975): Tachyphylaxis to the action of topically applied corticosteroids. *Arch. Derm., 111,* 58.
9. Dykes, P. J. and Marks, R. (1977): The atrophogenicity of 1% hydrocortisone plus 10% urea. *Clin. Trials J., 14,* 139.

14.11   Local side effects of corticosteroids

10. Editorial (1977): Steroid-antibiotic combinations. *Brit. med. J., 1*, 1303.
11. Even-Paz, Z. and Sagher, F. (1963): Cutis punctata linearis colli: stippled skin. *Dermatologica (Basel), 126*, 1.
12. Farkas, J. (1981): Perioral dermatitis from marjoram, bay leaf and cinnamon. *Contact Dermatitis, 7*, 121.
13. Feldmann, R. J. and Maibach, H. I. (1967): Regional variation in percutaneous penetration of 14C cortisol in man. *J. invest. Derm., 48*, 181.
14. Guin, J. D. (1981): Complications of topical hydrocortisone. *J. Amer. Acad. Derm., 4*, 417.
15. Haleblian, J. K. (1976): Bioassays used in the development of topical dosage forms. *J. pharm. Sci., 65*, 1417.
16. Hill, C. J. H. and Rostenberg, A. (1978): Adverse effects from topical steroids. *Cutis, 21*, 624.
17. Ive, F. A. and Marks, R. (1968): Tinea incognito. *Brit. med. J., 3*, 149.
18. Kaidbey, K. H. and Kligman, A. M. (1976): Assay of topical corticosteroids. *Arch. Derm., 112*, 808.
19. Leyden, J. J. and Marples, R. R. (1973): Ecologic principles and antibiotic therapy in chronic dermatoses. *Arch. Derm., 107*, 208.
20. Leyden, J. J. and Kligman, A. M. (1977): The case for steroid-antibiotic combinations. *Brit. J. Derm., 96*, 179.
21. Maibach, H. I. and Stoughton, R. B. (1973): Topical corticosteroids. In: *Steroid Therapy*, pp. 174-190. Editor: D.L. Azarnoff. W. B. Saunders, Philadelphia.
22. Marghescu, S. (1976): Wirkung und Nebenwirkung örtlich angewandter Glucocorticosteroide in der Dermatotherapie. *Ther. d. Gegenw., 115*, 2044.
23. Marples, R. R., Peborn, A. and Kligman, A. M. (1973): Topical steroid-antibiotic combinations. *Arch. Derm., 108*, 237.
24. Mckenzie, A. W. (1962): Percutaneous absorption of steroids. *Arch. Derm., 86*, 2611.
25. Mihan, R. and Ayres Jr., S. (1964): Perioral dermatitis. *Arch. Derm., 89*, 803.
26. Millard, L. G. (1977): Norwegian scabies developing during treatment with fluorinated steroid therapy. *Acta derm.-venereol. (Stockh.), 57*, 86.
27. Miller, J. A. and Munro, D. D. (1980): Topical steroids, clinical pharmacology and therapeutic use. *Drugs, 19*, 119.
28. Nater, J. P. (1981): Dermale toepassing van corticosteroiden. *Geneesmiddelenbulletin, 15*, 29.
29. Plewig, G. and Kligman, A. M. (1973): Induction of acne by topical steroids. *Arch. derm. Forsch., 247*, 29.
30. Polano, M. K. and Ponec, M. (1976): Dependance of corticosteroid penetration in the vehicle. *Arch. Derm., 112*, 675.
31. Schaefer, H., Zesch, A. and Stüttgen, G. (1975): Penetration von Medikamenten in die Haut. *Hautarzt, 26*, 449.
32. Schöpf, E. (1972): Nebenwirkungen externer Corticosteroidtherapie. *Hautarzt, 23*, 295.
33. Schöpf, E. (1975): Side effects from topical corticosteroid therapy. *Ann. clin. Res., 7*, 353.
34. Smith, M. A. (1977): Localized milia formation on pinna due to topical steroid application. *Clin. exp. Derm., 2*, 285.
35. Tegner, E. (1976): Contact allergy to corticosteroids. *Int. J. Derm., 15*, 520.
36. Wachs, G. N. and Maibach, H. I. (1976): Co-operative double-blind trial of an antibiotic/corticoid combination in impetiginized atopic dermatitis. *Brit. J. Derm., 95*, 323.
37. Weber, S. (1976): Perioral dermatitis, an important side-effect of corticosteroids. *Dermatologica (Basel), 152, Suppl. 1*, 161.
38. Wilkinson, D. S., Kirton, V. and Wilkinson, J. D. (1979): Perioral dermatitis: a 12-year review. *Brit. J. Derm., 101*, 245.
39. Younnessian, S. (1970): Glaucome et cataracte après corticothérapie par voie générale et locale. *Advanc. Ophtal., 23*, 74.

UPDATE – 2nd Edition

40. Booth, B. A., Tan, E. M. L., Oikarinen, A. and Uitto, J. (1982): Steroid-induced dermal atrophy. Effects of glucocorticosteroids on collagen metabolism in human skin fibroblast cultures. *Int. J. Derm., 21*, 333.
41. James, M. D., Black, M. M. and Sparkes, C. G. (1977): Measurement of dermal atrophy induced by topical steroids using a radiographic technique. *Brit. J. Derm., 96*, 303.

42. Oliet, E. J. and Estes, S. A. (1982): Perianal comedones associated with chronic topical fluorinated steroid use. (Letter to the Editor). *J. Amer. Acad. Derm., 7*, 405.
43. Björnberg, A. (1982): Erythema craquelé provoked by corticosteroids on normal skin. *Acta Derm.,-venereol. (Stockh.), 62*, 147.
44. Cohen, H. J. (1981): Perioral dermatitis (Letter to the editor). *J. Amer. Acad. Derm., 4*, 739.
45. Gibson, J. R., Kirsch, J., Dartey, C. R. and Burke, C. A. (1983): An attempt to evaluate the relative clinical potencies of various diluted and undiluted proprietary corticosteroid preparations. *Brit. J. Derm., 109, (Suppl. 25)*, 114.
46. Eisenlohr, J. E. (1983): Glaucoma following the prolonged use of topical steroid medication to the eyelids. *J. Amer. Acad. Derm., 8*, 878.

15. Percutaneous absorption of topically applied drugs

15.1　Several drugs for topical use on the skin and mucous membranes are capable of producing systemic side effects. Whether such events happen or not and, if so, to what extent, usually largely depends on the degree of absorption of the chemical through the skin or mucous membranes. In this chapter the factors influencing the absorption of topically applied drugs will be discussed on the basis of data from Malkinson and Gehlman [2] and Rasmussen [3].

15.2　Although the surface of the skin is only slightly permeable, many substances are capable of penetrating the skin to some degree. Absorption is greatly increased if the epidermis is diseased or damaged. The stratum corneum layer of the epidermis acts as the skin's main barrier; a few substances, however, may encounter a second barrier in the dermal-epidermal basement membrane. Though absorption mainly depends on the transepidermal route, follicular orifices and sweat gland ducts may provide alternate or additional pathways for absorption.

FACTORS INFLUENCING ABSORPTION

15.3　Several factors influence the degree of absorption of a particular substance:

1. **Physicochemical properties of the substance**
   Of importance are:
   - Molecular size – usually, with increasing molecular size, absorption decreases.
   - Water- and lipid-solubility of the drug.
   - Solubility of the penetrant within the vehicle: greater solubility in the stratum corneum than in the vehicle promotes penetration.

2. **Use of occlusive dressings**
   An occlusive covering over the skin enhances the penetration of topical drugs by a factor of 10 or more, caused by:
   - Increased water retention in the stratum corneum layer
   - Increased blood flow
   - Increased temperature
   - Increased surface area after prolonged occlusion.

3. **The vehicle in which the substance is incorporated**
   Of importance are:
   - The degree of affinity of the vehicle for the drug – increased affinity reduces percutaneous absorption.
   - The physical properties of vehicles, especially the degree of occlusion they produce – greases, oils and collodion are very occlusive vehicles (see under 'use of occlusive dressings').
   - Structural or chemical damage in the barrier layer, caused by the vehicle used.

170

In this respect, percutaneous absorption is increased by using vehicles such as dimethyl sulfoxide, dimethyl acetamide and dimethyl formamide. Certain solvents such as acetone, ethanol, methanol and ether may also cause damage.

4. Drug concentration
In general, high concentrations enhance penetration.

5. Site of application
Regional differences in permeability of skin largely depend on the thickness of the intact stratum corneum. According to the findings of a study by Feldman and Maibach [1], the highest total absorption of hydrocortisone is that from the scrotum, followed (in decreasing order) by absorption from the forehead, scalp, back, forearms, palms and plantar surfaces.

6. Age
The impression exists that the skin of children, whether normal or inflamed, is more permeable than in adults.

7. Temperature
Increasing temperature of the skin usually enhances penetration (see under 'use of occlusive dressings').

8. Integrity of the barrier
Increase of percutaneous absorption may result from the loss of barrier integrity caused by:
- Removal of the stratum corneum layer (e.g. 'stripping').
- Damage due to alkalis, acids, etc.
- Irritation or endogeneous inflammation of the skin, e.g. in psoriasis, atopic dermatitis, seborrheic dermatitis and exfoliative dermatitis.

15.4   REFERENCES

1. Feldman, R. J. and Maibach, H. I. (1967): Regional variation in percutaneous penetration of 14C-cortisol in man. *J. invest. Derm., 48*, 181.
2. Malkinson, F. D. and Gehlman, L. (1977): Factors affecting percutaneous absorption. In: *Cutaneous Toxicity*, pp. 63-81. Editors: V. A. Drill and P. Lazar. Academic Press Inc., New York.
3. Rasmussen, J. E. (1979): Percutaneous absorption in children. In: *Year Book of Dermatology*. Editor: R. L. Dobson. Year Book Medical Publishers, Chicago.

16. Systemic side effects caused by topically applied drugs and cosmetics

16.1 Some systemic side effects are the result of the *toxic action* of the chemicals applied, whereas others require an acquired *hypersensitivity state* of the organism, as seen e.g. in contact urticaria and anaphylaxis caused by bacitracin and the insect repellent diethyltoluamide.

ANAPHYLACTIC REACTIONS TO TOPICALLY APPLIED DRUGS AND COSMETICS

16.2 Several topical drugs and cosmetic ingredients have caused anaphylactic shock reactions, usually as part of the 'contact urticaria syndrome' (see § 7.1).

Such reactions have been reported from contact with:
– aminophenazone
– ammonium persulfate
– ampicillin
– bacitracin
– benzocaine
– caraway seed oil
– chloramphenicol
– mechlorethamide hydrochloride
– Millan's solution
  (gentian violet and methyl green)
– neomycin

For further information on this subject, the reader is referred to Chapter 7 on contact urticaria.

TOXIC ACTION OF TOPICALLY APPLIED DRUGS AND COSMETICS

16.3 Systemic side effects have been reported on the topical application of a number of chemicals, which will be discussed below.

Arsenic

16.4 Arsenical keratoses and malignancies are well-recognized long-term adverse reactions to oral administration of arsenic, previously employed widely in the treatment of psoriasis. However, Roemeling et al. [127] have reported on the development of consecutive multifocal malignancies of the large bowel, bladder, rectum and skin of a psoriatic patient who had been treated *externally* with Fowler's solution more than 20 years before. According to the authors, this may indicate that arsenic can be absorbed percutaneously in amounts sufficient to lead to later occurrence of internal cancers.

Benzocaine

16.5   Methemoglobinemia has been reported following the topical application of benzocaine on both the skin [254] and the mucous membranes [217, 219, 255, 256]. However, this is an uncommon occurrence [253]. The preponderance of reported cases occurred in infants and it has been suggested that this might be due to a deficiency of DPNH-dependent methemoglobin reductase, resulting in a diminished capacity to physiologically protect against methemoglobin-inducing foreign compounds. Cases of methemoglobinemia in older children [217] and adults [218] have also been reported.

Boric acid

16.6   Boric acid (H_3BO_3) is a colorless, odorless compound available as crystals, granules and as a white powder.

It is usually prepared by the action of sulfuric acid on borax (sodium borate, $Na_2B_4O_7 \cdot 10H_2O$).

Boric acid was first employed as an antiseptic by Lister in 1875 and for many years it enjoyed great popularity in medical practice; although it had an unwarranted reputation as a germicide, it is, however, only mildly bacteriostatic, even in saturated aqueous solution.

In the past, boric acid was erroneously considered a relative non-toxic substance; nevertheless, it has often proved poisonous, both on ingestion and following topical use. Little boric acid penetrates the intact skin, but it is readily absorbed through inflamed or otherwise damaged skin or through mucous membranes.

Valdes-Dapena and Arey [158] collected 172 cases of boric acid intoxication from the literature, including 83 fatal cases (see § 16.7). In this series there were 37 deaths after external use of boric acid, including 23 children with napkin rashes.

16.7   **Summary of 172 cases of boric acid intoxication**

	Fatal (n = 83)	Non-fatal (n = 89)	Total (n = 172)
Patients:			
adults	28	50	78
children	55	39	94
Exposure:			
diaper area	23	7	30
accidental ingestion (in formula or as medicine or infusion)	35	36	71
other routes (deliberate)	25	46	71

16.8   The most common clinical side effects of boric acid, independent of the route of administration, are seen on the skin, in the gastrointestinal tract and in the central nervous system [64, 89, 136, 198].

The *skin rash* consists of an intense erythematous eruption, often covering the entire body, and followed in one to two days by extensive desquamation. The palms and soles are often particularly red. Some authors observed an initial erythema around the mouth, buttocks and perineum. Mucous membranes are often involved, especially in young infants, in whom the mouth, pharynx and conjunctivae are inflamed. The skin lesions may resemble Ritter's disease [178], Leiner's disease or scarlet fever, and may be confused with these affections.

Cyanosis may be present in the most severe cases. Other skin signs of borate intoxication include psoriasiform lesions and bullae [198].

Gastrointestinal symptoms have been described after topical use of boric acid; the incidence via this route of intoxication is unknown. After ingestion, a typical clinical picture starts with persistent vomiting which terminally becomes bloody, and diarrhea (mucous and bloody, with a bluish-green color). Nausea, vomiting, and epigastric pain have been reported.

Central nervous system manifestations, particularly in the younger patients, consist of signs of meningeal irritation, convulsions, delirium and coma; in the infant, a high-pitched cry, exaggerated startled reflex, opisthotonus and apprehensive facial expression have been noted.

Also, acute *tubular necrosis* with oliguria or anuria may occur, followed by hyperthermia, a fall in blood pressure, tachycardia and shock.

Occupational *toxic alopecia* due to absorption of borax from a hand washing powder containing nearly 80% crystalline borax was reported by Tan [146]. Ingestion of boric acid has also caused alopecia [249].

Undoubtedly the use of borates should be abandoned because of their very limited therapeutic value and high toxicity. Few cases of borate intoxications seem to have been published recently, which may reflect the rapid disappearance of these chemicals from medical use, or greater awareness of the possible adverse effects to those still employing the drug.

Camphor

16.9   Camphor is a pleasant-smelling cyclic ketone of the hydroaromatic terpene group. When rubbed on the skin, camphor is a rubefacient but, if not vigorously applied, produces a feeling of coolness. It is an ingredient of a large number of over-the-counter remedies (with a camphor content of 1–20%), taken especially for symptomatic relief of 'chest congestion' and muscle aches, but its effectiveness is rather dubious.

Camphor is readily absorbed from all sites of administration, including topical application to the skin.

The compound is classified as a Class IV chemical, i.e. a very toxic substance. Hundreds of cases of intoxications have been reported, usually after accidental ingestion in children [26, 209]. The symptomatology of camphor poisoning is provided in § 16.10 [26].

16.10   **Symptomatology of camphor poisoning**

1. nausea and vomiting
2. feeling of warmth, headache
3. confusion, vertigo, excitement, restlessness, delirium and hallucinations
4. increased muscular excitability, tremors, and jerky movements
5. tremors, progression to epileptiform convulsions, followed by depression
6. coma, CNS depression, and finally either:
7. death from respiratory failure or from status epilepticus, or:
8. slow convalescence.

16.11   Skoglund et al. [137] documented systemic adverse reactions after *cutaneous* contact with camphor: a 15-month-old child had crawled through spirits-of-camphor, containing 10% camphor. Over the ensuing 48 hours the child became progressively ataxic and had some brief generalized major motor seizures. The seizures persisted for two days despite appropriate therapy. Over a 15-day period he slowly improved; recovery in motor and mental function was complete. The child had no further seizures until one year later, when a camphorated vaporizer preparation containing 4.81% camphor was administered by the mother. Concurrent with this inhalation, a brief major motor seizure occurred. Two other children of 4 and 6 weeks old have been described showing signs of camphor intoxication from topical camphor-containing preparations due to percutaneous absorption. Signs and symptoms included: paleness, cyanosis, shallow breathing, apnea, and muscular dystony [209]. Gossweiler warns that repeated applications of camphor-containing ointments to young babies has led to poisonings with coma, convulsions, and breathing difficulties. These preparations should therefore not be used in newborns and small infants [209].

Carmustine (BCNU)

16.12   Topical carmustine (BCNU) has been used for the treatment of mycosis fungoides, lymphomatoid papulosis and parapsoriasis en plaques [288]. Percutaneous absorption of BCNU has been demonstrated in man [289]. Zackheim et al. [288] treated 91 patients with mycosis fungoides and related disorders with topical BCNU. Mild to moderate reversible bone marrow depression occurred in 3 patients. Their data suggest that hematological toxicity arises primarily from the shorter intensive schedules; the prolonged use of up to 100 mg/week appears to be safe. Although an occasional mild elevation in the blood urea nitrogen or serum glutamic oxaloacetic transaminase (SGOT) was noted in patients treated with courses exceeding 600 mg, no such changes were seen with lower doses. In the study of Zackheim et al. [288] there were no apparent long-term harmful effects on the hematopoietic system or internal organs.

Castellani's solution

16.13   Castellani's solution (or paint) is an old medicine, mainly used for the local treatment of fungal skin infections. It contains boric acid 5.0, fuchsin 5.0, resorcinol 100.0, water 705.0, phenol 40.0 (90%), acetone 50.0 and spirit 100.0.

Lundell and Nordman [95] reported a case in which two applications of Castellani's solution severely poisoned a 6-week old boy. The infant became cyanotic with 41% of methemoglobin. According to the authors, this case history demonstrates that the application of Castellani's solution to napkin eruptions and other areas where it can be rapidly absorbed may cause serious complications.

Another case report states that hours after the application of Castellani's paint to the entire body surface, except the face, of a six-week old infant for severe seborrhoic eczema, the child became drowsy, had shallow breathing and was passing blue urine. Phenol was detected in the urine of 4 out of 16 children treated with Castellani's paint [128].

The reader is also referred to the paragraphs on resorcinol (§ 16.81), boric acid (§ 16.6), and phenol (§ 16.68), in this chapter.

Chloramphenicol

16.14 Oral administration of chloramphenicol may lead to aplastic anemia. This condition is quite rare, occurring about once in every 18,000 to 50,000 subjects thus treated [164]. Although it has been stated that parenteral administration of chloramphenicol does not induce aplastic anemia [174], at least 4 such cases have been described [50].

A case of marrow aplasia with a fatal outcome after *topical* application of chloramphenicol in eye ointment has been described by Abrams et al. [2]. It is remarkable that very small amounts of chloramphenicol could induce such very serious adverse reactions. There have been 3 earlier reports of bone marrow aplasia after the use of chloramphenicol-containing eyedrops.

Clindamycin

16.15 Topical antibiotics are widely used for the treatment of acne vulgaris. A recent survey indicated that topical clindamycin, erythromycin, tetracycline, and lincomycin hydrochloride are considered more or less efficacious and without significant systemic side effects [144]. However, it is estimated that an average of 4–5% clindamycin (hydrochloride) is absorbed systemically, but greater amounts may be absorbed in some individuals [204]. The degree of absorption largely depends on the vehicle, ranging from 0.13% (acetone) to 13.92% (DMSO) in one study [221]. Several cases of topical clindamycin-associated diarrhea have been reported [144, 163, 220].

16.16 Pseudomembranous colitis is a well-recognized side effect of systemic administration of clindamycin [147] as well as of other antibiotics such as ampicillin, erythromycin, tetracyclines and cephalosporins.

A case of pseudomembranous colitis after *topical* administration of clindamycin has been reported by Milstone et al. [103]. Abdominal cramping and diarrhea developed in a 24-year-old woman with facial acne vulgaris five days after she had started local therapy with 1% clindamycin hydrochloride.

A stool specimen contained a significant titer of a toxin produced by *Clostridium difficile*. Findings from sigmoidoscopy and a colonic biopsy specimen were consistent with pseudomembranous colitis. The patient became asymptomatic after 10 days of supportive care and oral vancomycin hydrochloride therapy. The authors conclude that all patients receiving topical clindamycin should be warned to discontinue therapy and consult their physician if intestinal symptoms occur.

Coal tar

16.17   A case of methemoglobinemia in an infant following the application of an ointment containing 2.5% crude coal tar and 5% benzocaine in a water-soluble base to about half the body surface was reported by Goluboff and MacFadyen [65]. On the fifth day of treatment the infant suddenly became critically ill, cyanotic and anoxic; death appeared imminent. Methylene blue i.v., 1.5–2 ml of 1% solution, brought about a dramatic cure. The clinical diagnosis of methemoglobinemia was confirmed by examination of a blood specimen taken shortly after the methylene blue had been given. Though the child had been treated with several other medicaments as well, the authors believe that the coal tar-benzocaine ointment was the most likely factor to have caused the methemoglobinemia.

Corticosteroids

16.18   It has been amply documented that topically applied glucocorticosteroids are absorbed through the skin and gain access to the systemic circulation [272]. Factors favoring the penetration of corticosteroids have been discussed in Chapter 14. Systemic absorption of topically applied corticosteroids in quantitites sufficient to replace endogenous production is not uncommon. However, iatrogenic Cushing's syndrome resulting from the use of topical steroids is rare. § 16.19 summarizes the relevant data of some of the reported cases. For other case reports see references [274–277].

16.19   **Iatrogenic hypercorticism due to topical corticosteroids.**
Relevant data of 12 cases (Adapted from Pascher, [267])

Age	Diagnosis	Steroid	Occlusion	Therapy	Side effects	Ref.
5 years	chronic eczema	HC ointment 1%	0	16 months	pseudotumor cerebri retarded growth	260
2 months	eczema (generalized)	HC ointment 1%	0	3 months	arrested growth	261
3 weeks	epidermolysis bullosa	HC lotion 0.25%	0	10 days	cushingoid features	262
2 months	eczema (widespread)	betamethasone valerate cream 0.01%	0	2 weeks	failure to thrive	263
18 months	napkin dermatitis	fluocortolone and fluocortolone caproate 0.25%	semi-occlusion (diapers)	14 months	growth inhibition	264
11 weeks	seborrheic dermatitis (disseminated)	betamethasone valerate 0.05%	0	7 weeks	Cushing's syndrome	265
42 years	psoriasis (exfoliative)	betamethasone valerate cream 0.1% diluted 1:8 with bland cream	0	2 years	Cushing's syndrome	266
54 years	mycosis fungoides	betamethasone valerate (vehicle?) 0.1%	0	2½ years	osteoporosis muscle atrophy	268
11 years	epidermolytic hyperkeratosis	triamcinolone acetonide cream 0.05%	0	1 month	cushingoid facies	269

(continued)

16.19 Corticosteroids

(continuation)

Age	Diagnosis	Steroid	Occlusion	Therapy	Side effects	Ref.
8 years	erythroderma ichthysiforme congenita	betamethasone valerate ointment 0.1%	0	$7^1/_2$ years	Cushing's syndrome osteoporosis growth retardation	270
57 years	seborrheic eczema of the face	betamethasone valerate cream 0.1%	0	11 years	Cushing's syndrome glaucoma	273
36 years	psoriasis	desoximethasone cream 0.25%	0	1 year	Cushing's syndrome	271

16.20 Systemic side effects caused by topical corticosteroids occur more frequently in children than in adults [47], which can be accounted for by the relatively large surface area and the increased absorption of drugs through the thin skin in children. Patients with liver disease are more prone to develop systemic side effects due to retardation of the degradation of systemically absorbed drugs [275]. The side effects may remain subclinical [59]. Metabolic indexes of glucocorticoid action may provide useful parameters for assessing systemic absorption of topical glucocorticosteroids [271]. The two main causes of systemic side effects are hypercorticism leading to an iatrogenic Cushing's syndrome and suppression of the hypothalamic-pituitary-adrenal axis [98]. Very potent and readily absorbed corticosteroids may induce these two conditions at the same time.

The iatrogenic Cushing's syndrome includes benign intracranial hypertension, glaucoma, subcapsular cataract, pancreatitis, aseptic necrosis of the bones, panniculitis, obesity, facial rounding, psychiatric symptoms, edema, delayed wound-healing and, to a lesser degree, hypertension, acne, disorders of sexual function, hirsutism, virilism, striae and plethora.

16.21 Skin symptoms of long-term systemic absorption of corticosteroids are:
  – symmetrical steroid striae
  – steroid acne
  – widespread skin atrophy
  – purpura
  – ecchymoses

16.22 It is not easy to provide data on 'safe' doses of topical corticosteroids, but as for the potent corticosteroid clobetasol-17-propionate 0.05% it has been recommended to limit the dosage to 45 g of the 0.05% ointment weekly. Larger doses entail a risk of suppression of the hypothalamic-pituitary-adrenal axis [159]. See also Chapter 19 on side effects of systemic drugs (§ 19.1).

Diethyltoluamide

16.23 Diethyltoluamide has been used as an insect repellent since 1957. It is especially active against mosquitoes, but also repels biting flies, gnats, chiggers, ticks, and other insects. After application, diethyltoluamide remains effective against insects for several hours. Local side effects include contact urticaria (§ 7.5) and irritant reactions with burning, erythema and bullae, sometimes followed by ulceration and scarring [235].

Toxic encephalopathy from topical diethyltoluamide has been reported [236, 237]. In one case the bedding, night clothes, and skin of a $3\frac{1}{2}$-year-old girl were sprayed daily for two weeks with a total amount of 180 ml of a 15% diethyl-toluamide product. Shaking and crying spells, slurred speech and confusion developed. Improvement occurred after vigorous medical treatment that included anti-convulsive therapy. In another report one of two children displaying signs of severe toxic encephalopathy died after prolonged hospitalization. At autopsy, edema of the brain, as well as congestion of the meninges, was found.

Although diethyltoluamide has an overall low incidence of toxic effects, prolonged use in children or application to the antecubital fossa (where most of the irritant reactions have occurred) has been discouraged [235].

Dimethyl sulfoxide

16.24   The toxicology of topical dimethyl sulfoxide (DMSO) has been investigated by Kligman [86]. In this study, 9 ml of 90% diethyl sulfoxide were applied twice daily to the entire trunk of twenty healthy volunteers for three weeks. The following laboratory tests were done: complete bloodcount, urinalysis, blood sedimentation rate, SGOT, BUN and fasting blood sugar determinations. At the end of the study, all laboratory values had remained normal. Except for the appearance of cutaneous signs as erythema, scaling, contact urticaria, stinging and burning sensations, the drug was tolerated well by all but two individuals, who developed systemic symptoms. In one, a toxic reaction developed on the 12th day which was characterized by a diffuse erythematous and scaling rash accompanied by severe abdominal cramps; the other had a similar rash and complained of nausea, chills and chest pains. These signs, however, abated in spite of continued administration of the drug.

16.25   To investigate possible side effects of *chronic* exposure to dimethyl sulfoxide another twenty volunteers were painted with nine ml of 90% dimethyl sulfoxide applied to the entire trunk, once daily for a period of 26 weeks. Neither clinical nor laboratory investigations showed adverse effects of the drug. However, most subjects did experience the well-known DMSO-induced disagreeable oyster-like breath odor, to which they eventually became insensitive. One fatality due to a hypersensitivity reaction has been reported [290].

Dinitrochlorobenzene (DNCB)

16.26   Dinitrochlorobenzene (DNCB), a potent contact allergen, has been used with some succes for the treatment of recalcitrant alopecia areata; today however, its use has been discouraged because suspicion has been aroused that DNCB may be mutagenic. Another drawback for its use is its ability to potentiate epicutaneous sensitization to non-related allergens [222]. DNCB is absorbed in substantial amounts through the skin, and about 50% of the applied dose is ultimately recoverable in the urine [223].

A possible systemic reaction to DNCB has been reported [201]: a 25-year-old man was treated with 0.1% DNCB in an absorbent ointment base for alopecia areata after prior sensitization. After two months of daily applications the patient experienced generalized urticaria, pruritus and dyspepsia; discontinuance of the drug led to cessation of all symptoms, which recurred after reintroduction of DNCB therapy.

16.27 Diphenylpyraline hydrochloride

Diphenylpyraline hydrochloride

16.27 Diphenylpyraline hydrochloride, an antihistamine, has been used topically in Germany for the treatment of eczematous and other itching dermatoses. Symptomatic psychosis apparently due to percutaneous absorption has been observed in 12 patients, 9 of which were children. The amounts of the active drug applied ranged from 225–1350 mg. The first symptoms of intoxication were psychomotoric restlesness in all cases, usually within 24 hours. Other symptoms included disorientation and optic and acoustic hallucinations. Most patients displayed anxiety, which was sometimes converted into agressiveness. After discontinuation of the topical medication all symptoms disappeared within 4 days [215].

Dithranol (cignolin, anthralin)

16.28 Although the topical use of dithranol, which has been used since 1916 for the treatment of psoriasis, may lead to local side effects such as irritant dermatitis, discoloration of the skin and the appendages and, as has recently been reported [36], to contact-allergic reactions, its use is generally considered to be devoid of systemic side effects.

  Gay et al. [57] studied a group of 40 psoriatic patients, treated with dithranol paste or ointment 0.1-0.4%. Creatinine clearance, chemistry profile, complete blood cell count and urinalysis were performed on all patients before treatment and after 1 and 3 months of continuous dithranol therapy. No evidence of systemic toxicity was found.

  No changes in renal function were observed in two dithranol-treated patients with renal disease, which, according to the authors, suggests that even renal disease is not necessarily a contraindication to the use of topically administered dithranol in low concentrations.

  Farber and Harris [45] reported no toxicity in 25 hospitalized patients treated with topical dithranol paste for an average of 11 days. Their toxicity studies included serum electrolytes, total protein and globulin, total bilirubin, alkalic phosphatase, SGOT, blood urea nitrogen, fasting blood glucose and urinalysis.

16.29 Although according to the *Merck Index* [99] application of *chrysarobin,* which is chemically closely related to dithranol, to large areas of skin may lead to percutaneous absorption and 'renal irritation', no cases of renal or hepatic damage due to dithranol have yet been reported. Only one possible case of a systemic side effect of dithranol has been reported [20]: a patient had a fixed drug eruption, which was attributed to percutaneous absorption of dithranol.

Ethyl alcohol

16.30 Twenty-eight children with alcohol intoxication from percutaneous absorption were described by Giménez et al. [60] from Buenos Aires, Argentina. Apparently, in that area it is (or was) a popular procedure to apply alcohol-soaked cloths to the abdomen of babies as a home-remedy for the treatment of disturbances of the gastrointestinal tract such as cramps, pain, vomiting and diarrhea, or because of crying, excitability and irritability.

  The children were of both sexes and ranged in age from 33 months to 1 year (mean: 12 months, 27 days). Alcohol-soaked cloths had been applied on the babies' abdomen under rubber panties, and the number of applications varied from one to three; it was estimated that each application contained approximately 40

180

cc ethanol. Medical consultation took place from 1 to 23 hours after application. Alcoholic breath and abdominal erythema were valuable clues to the diagnosis. Signs and symptoms and their relative frequency are listed in § 16.31.

16.31   **Symptoms of percutaneous alcohol intoxication**

Symptom	No. of patients (n = 28)	%
CNS depression (+ to + + + +)	28	100
abdominal erythema	25	89
alcoholic breath	24	86
miosis	24	86
hypoglycemia	15	54
convulsions	5	18
respiratory depression	5	18
mydriasis	4	14
acidosis	3	11
death	2	7

16.32   These symptoms may be interpreted as a consequence of the alcohol absorption and secondary hypoglycemia. Quantitative determination for alcohol in the blood was made upon admission in 11 cases, with results ranging from 0.6 to 1.49 g%. Of the 2 children who died one was autopsied: the findings were consistent with ethyl alcohol intoxication. As the local population became more aware of the consequences of this practice of topical application of large amounts of alcohol, there was a resultant decrease in the number of cases. More recently a case of acute ethanol intoxication in a preterm infant of 1800 g due to local application of alcohol-imbued compresses on the legs as a treatment for puncture hematomas was reported [291]. Topically applied ethanol in tar gel [294] and beer-containing shampoo [295] has caused antabuse effects in patients on disulfiram for alcoholism, through percutaneous absorption.

Fumaric acid monoethyl ester

16.33   The effect of systemically and/or topically administered fumaric acid monoethyl ester (ethyl fumarate) on psoriasis was studied by Dubiel and Happle [40] in six patients. Two patients who had been treated with locally applied ointments, consisting of 3% or 5% ethyl fumarate in petrolatum, developed symptoms of renal intoxication.

Gentamicin

16.34   Ototoxicity is a well-known hazard of systemic gentamicin administration. However, topical application to large thermal injuries of the skin has similarly caused ototoxic effects, ranging from mild to indeed severe loss of hearing, with an associated decrease of vestibular function [35]. In the two patients described, serum levels of gentamicin measured were 1.0–3.0 µg/ml and 3.3–4.3 µg/ml, respectively.

Drake [39] described a woman who developed tinnitus each time she treated her paronychia with gentamicin sulfate cream 0.1%. Use of gentamicin in ear drops may also be associated with ototoxic adverse reactions [104].

The local adverse reactions to topical use of gentamicin and other aminoglycosides are discussed elsewhere in this book.

Henna dye and p-phenylenediamine

16.35   The use of a henna dye is traditional in Islamic communities. The dye is used on nails, skin and hair by married ladies and traditionally it is also used by the major participants in marriage ceremonies, when the bridegroom and best man also apply henna to their hands.

Henna consists of the dried leaves of *Lawsonia alba* (family Lythraceae), a shrub which is cultivated in North Africa, India and Sri Lanka. The coloring matter, lawsone, is a hydroxynaphthoquinone and this is associated with fats, resin and henna-tanin in the leaf. Dying hair or skin with powdered henna is a somewhat lenghthy procedure, and to speed up this process, Sudanese ladies mix a 'black powder' with henna; this accelerates the fixing process of the dye merely to a matter of minutes. This 'black powder' is paraphenylenediamine. The combination of henna and 'black powder' is particularly toxic and over 20 cases of such toxicity, some fatal, have been noted in Khartoum alone in a 2-year period. Initial symptoms are those of angioneurotic edema with massive edema of the face, lips, glottis, pharynx, neck and bronchi. These occur within hours of the application of the dye-mix to the skin. The symptoms may then progress on the second day to anuria and acute renal failure with death occurring on the third day. Dialysis has helped some patients, but others have died from renal tubular necrosis [230]. Whether this toxicity is due to p-phenylenediamine per se (probably grossly impure) or whether its toxicity is potentiated in its combination with henna powder is unknown. Systemic administration of the 'black powder' leads to similar symptoms, and several deaths due to ingestion with suicidal intent have been reported [231].

Hexachlorophene

16.36   Hexachlorophene (2,2'-methylenebis(3,4,6-trichlorophenol)) has, since 1961, been used extensively in hospital nurseries, mainly for reducing the incidence of staphylococcal infections among the newborns. In addition, it has been an ingredient of many medical preparations, cosmetics and other consumer goods.

Hexachlorophene readily penetrates excoriated or otherwise damaged skin [94], but also has absorption of this antiseptic through intact skin been demonstrated [155, 32, 3]. If hexachlorophene is applied in high concentrations or at frequent intervals to the intact skin, excoriation will result.

16.37   In 1972, in France, accidentally 6.3% of hexachlorophene was added to batches of baby talcum powder [115, 180]. Two hundred-and-four babies fell ill and 36 died owing to respiratory arrest. Symptoms of intoxication included a severe rash in the diaper area, gastro-enteritis, pronounced hyperexcitability and lethargy. In addition, several babies showed hyperesthesia, hypertonicity, opisthotonus, pyramidal tract signs, clonic movement of the extremities and papilledema. High blood levels of hexachlorophene were demonstrated. Distribution of symptoms and signs in 224 hexachlorophene poisoning episodes among 204 children was as follows [180]:

Systemic and skin features:
- Erythema of buttocks   209 (93%)
- Other cutaneous signs   38 (17%)
- Fever   99 (44%)
- Vomiting   77 (34%)
- Refusal of food   75 (33%)
- Diarrhea   65 (29%)

Neurological features:
- Drowsiness   83 (37%)
- Irritability   75 (33%)
- Coma   55 (25%)
- Seizures   39 (17%)
- Babinski signs   24 (11%)
- Decerebration   22 (10%)
- Weakness or paralysis   17 (8%)
- Opisthotonus   9 (4%)

This report was followed by animal experiments with hexachlorophene, confirming a relationship between the drug and morphological and functional disturbances of the nervous system. Consequently, the FDA in 1972 banned all non-prescription use of hexachlorophene, restricting it to prescription use only, as a surgical scrub and handwash product for health care personnel. Hexachlorophene was excluded from cosmetics except as a preservative in levels not exceeding 0.1%.

Neurotoxicity

16.38   Several studies (e.g. by Powell et al. [118], Shuman et al. [133] have confirmed the assumption that hexachlorophene has indeed a high neurotoxic potential. It must be added that only after dermal application to large burned or otherwise damaged skin areas or after the use of high doses on intact skin have symptoms of neurotoxicity been observed.

Hexachlorophene neurotoxicity leads to cerebral edema, affecting exclusively the white matter of the brain and spinal cord, producing a spongiform encephalopathy which transforms the matter into a network of cystic spaces lined by fragments of myelin. There is a degeneration of myelin; nerve cells are unaffected.

This process has been shown to be reversible. The clinical symptoms include nausea, vomiting, spasms, coma and finally apnea and death.

Teratogenicity and carcinogenicity

16.39   There has been concern about possible teratogenicity of hexachlorophene after the report of Halling [70, 71]: Swedish medical personnel apparently had a high number of malformed babies in association with hexachlorophene hand washing during the first trimester of pregnancy. Other authors have also raised suspicion [245, 246]. A detailed study, however, [43] could not confirm this assumption, whereas animal experiments on teratogenicity provide conflicting evidence. As for carcinogenicity, this possible adverse effect of hexachlorophene cannot be assessed on the basis of data currently available [7].

16.40 Hexachlorophene

Contraindications

16.40   Because of the high absorption through damaged skin and the proven neurotoxicity, hexachlorophene is contraindicated for the treatment of burns or application on otherwise damaged skin; premature infants are also at risk. Although it has been stated that hexachlorophene should not be used anymore for routine bathing of babies [155], this point remains controversial [180, 181]. Gluck [247] indicates that there is no evidence that any full-term baby with normal skin, even with the total body washed in the usual manner, has ever shown any untoward effects. However, the prophylactic efficacy of a technique using a 0.5% hexachlorophene powder instead of the usual 3% emulsion has been demonstrated [248], which may indicate that preparations containing a lower hexachlorophene concentration are preferable [182].

For reviews of benefit and risks of hexachlorophene, see also Plueckhahn et al. [116] and Hopkins [79].

4-Homosulfanilamide

16.41   4-Homosulfanilamide (sulfamylon acetate) is a topical sulfonamide which is used for the treatment of large burns. Unfortunately, the drug frequently produces a rash, and is associated with severe pain on application. Sulfamylon as well as para-sulfamoylbenzoic acid, an important metabolite, are carboanhydrase inhibitors. Inhibition of renal carbonic acid anhydrase decreases reabsorption of bicarbonate. Thus, hyperchloremic metabolic acidosis has been observed in patients with extensive burns undergoing topical treatment with 4-homosulfanilamide [111, 212], caused by percutaneous absorption of the drug. Reversible pulmonary complications have been associated with the drug when applied to patients with large burns [176]. It has been suggested that the respiratory failure might be the result of a hypersensitivity reaction, the lung being the shock organ, or the result of high doses of carbonic anhydrase inhibitors formed from the mafenide acetate and its metabolic products.

16.42   Ohlgisser et al. [108] reported methemoglobinemia as a possible side effect of 4-homosulfanilamide in 2 children who were treated with topical 4-homosulfanilamide for extensive burns.

Nowadays, 4-homosulfanilamide has largely been replaced by sulfadiazine silver (see § 16.89).

Iodine

16.43   Alexander [4] reported on a case of fatal dermatitis following the use of a 2.5% solution of resublimated iodine in pure industrial alcohol before a surgical operation. The reaction was thought to be due to idiosyncrasy to iodine.

16.44   Skin disinfection with iodine has caused goiter and hypothyroidism in 5 of 30 newborns under intensive care [22]. See also § 16.73 ff. on povidone-iodine.

Lead

16.45   *Surma* is a topical preparation used in Asian communities in the United Kingdom; it is applied to the eye, apparently for medicinal purposes, and has the appearance

184

of mascara. However, application is not to the outside of the eyelid, but to the conjunctival surface. In addition, it is the custom to apply a small dot of the material on the forehead of a Muslim child to ward off the 'evil eye'.

A case of lead poisoning in a 4-year-old Asian child has been reported [8], which appeared to be attributable to the use of a Surma; this preparation was found to contain 86% lead as lead sulfide. In this case, Surma had been applied to larger areas of the skin, and for prolonged periods of time.

Various Surmas have been investigated by the authors, and 36% of these had lead concentrations in excess of 50%.

Lidocaine

16.46   Lidocaine hydrochloride, an aminoacyl amide, is widely used for both topical and local injection anesthesa; also, topical preparations containing this drug are available for topical anesthesia of irritated or inflamed mucous membranes of the mouth and pharynx. However, when the drug is applied to mucous membranes, blood levels simulate those resulting from intravenous injection [224]. Serum lidocaine concentrations higher than 6 µg/ml are associated with toxicity [225].

In general, the pharmacologic sequence of the signs of toxicity from local anesthetics are central nervous system stimulation, followed by depression, and later inhibition of cardiovascular function. Systemic toxicity from lidocaine viscous applied to the oral cavity in two children has been described [191, 226]. In one, the mother had been applying lidocaine hydrochloride 2% solution to the infant's gums with her finger 5–6 times daily for a week; the child experienced 2 generalized seizures within an hour. Urine examined by thin layer chromatography revealed a large amount of lidocaine, and a blood level of 10 µg/ml was determined [226]. The other child had a seizure after having received 227.8 mg/kg oral viscous lidocaine for stomatitis herpetica over a 24-hour period. In this case, however, ingestion and resorption from the gastrointestinal tract may have contributed to the clinical picture. It has been suggested that for pediatric patients viscous lidocaine should be applied with an oral swab to *individual* lesions, thus limiting buccal absorption by decreasing the surface area exposed to lidocaine [191].

Lindane

16.47   Lindane is the γ-isomer of 1,2,3,4,5,6-hexachlorocyclohexane and is widely used in the treatment of scabies and pediculosis, usually in a lotion containing 1% γ-benzene hexachloride, which is applied to the entire body surface and left on for 24 hours (in cases of scabies). The percutaneous absorption of the drug has been studied by Feldmann and Maibach [48]: after applying lindane in acetone to intact human skin (forearm), at least 9.3% of the substance was found to be absorbed and excreted in the urine during the following five days. There was a marked individual variation relative to transcutaneous lindane absorption in the subjects studied, who were male volunteers.

Ginsburg et al. [61] studied the percutaneous absorption of lindane in children suffering from scabies: mean levels of γ-benzene hexachloride found at 2 and 48 hours after application were 0.015 and 0.006 µg/ml, respectively. These levels tended to be higher in younger and smaller infants and children. In another study [190] plasma lindane levels of 10.3 ± 2.2 ng/ml were determined 3 days after a therapeutic application of 1 % lindane cream.

16.48   Lindane is a potentially toxic agent, and the hazards of excessive industrial exposure and accidental ingestion have been well-documented. Signs and symptoms of intoxication include [140]:

1. *Nervous system disorders:* convulsions, headache, vertigo, mental confusion, dysarthria and death
2. *Gastrointestinal disorders:* nausea, vomiting, diarrhea, stomatitis, intestinal colic, depressed liver function
3. *Miscellaneous:* respiratory failure with cyanosis, blood dyscrasias and hemopoietic depression, altered menses, cardiac arrhythmias, myalgia, blindness.

16.49 Intoxication from *excessive topical therapeutic applications* of lindane has been documented. Six such patients were reported [91]: adverse reactions included seizures (4), nervousness, irritability, anxiety and insomnia (1), and dizziness and amblyopia (1). Seizures after excessive topical application of lindane have been reported by Telch and Jarvis [197].

A 2-month-old male infant was found dead in his crib after excessive application of a 1% lindane lotion [175]. Lindane was identified in the brain at a concentration of 110 ppb. The brain level was three times higher than the levels found in the blood, which may indicate that the drug is concentrated in the central nervous system. The authors admitted that the relationship of the pesticide exposure to the fatal outcome in this case was conjectural.

16.50 The issue of possible toxic adverse reactions *to a single therapeutic application* of lindane, notably central nervous system toxicity, has not been settled yet.

Several poorly documented cases of convulsions following topical treatment with the drug have been reported to the Division of Drug Experience of the United States Food and Drug Administration [46].

Lee and Groth [91] mentioned the case of a 4-year-old boy who started to vomit approximately $8\frac{1}{2}$ hours after total body application of lindane cream, and slowly drifted into unconsciousness. He subsequently had a convulsion and stopped breathing; complete recovery ensued. A 7-year-old boy with tuberous sclerosis had two petit mal seizures within 12 hours after a single total body application of 1% lindane lotion [196].

Pramanik and Hansen [120] reported on a premature, malnourished infant with scabies who developed increased muscle tone, poor orientation to a visual animate stimulus and frequent side-to-side head movements two days after one application of 1% lindane lotion. The patient, who also had a ventriculoseptal defect and was treated for pneumonia and congestive heart failure (which drugs were used?), was diagnosed as having 'clinical seizures'; this latter effect was ascribed to treatment with lindane.

16.51 Most authors seem to agree that the benefits to be derived from the continued use of lindane as a scabicide and pediculicide outweighs the risks involved [140, 194, 195, 239]. Although a potential for adverse reactions from application of lindane preparations therapeutically does exist if the preparations are not used properly, the risk of toxicity appears minimal *when used properly and according to directions* [199]. Continued use of lindane because of its benificial effects, however, does not mean that steps should not be taken to minimize potential risks.

Solomon et al. [140], for example, in their review on lindane toxicity give the following observations and recommendations 'which may have some merit':

1. Lindane should *not* be applied after a hot bath.
2. The regimen of application for 24 hours may be unneccessarily long; 8–12 hours may be sufficient exposure [195].
3. A concentration weaker than 1% may suffice, particularly for badly excoriated patients.

4. Lindane 1% should be used with extreme caution, if at all, in pregnant women, very small infants, and people with massively excoriated skin. Rasmussen [195] does not agree on this point.

5. Lindane treatment should not be repeated within eight days, and then only if active organisms can be demonstrated.

Malathion

16.52   Malathion is used in the treatment of lice, a single application of 0.5% in a solution being customary. Used in this way, it is generally safe, although the same compound has caused fatal poisoning when used as a pesticide in the environment. Ramu et al. [124] reported on 4 children with an intoxication following hair washing with a solution containing malathion (50% in xylene) for the purpose of louse control. One case is described in detail. The patient was in coma and did not respond to painful stimuli. Other symptoms included severe dyspnea, audible extensive moist rales over both lung fields, voluminous frothy saliva and mucus filling the nose, mouth and pharynx, pinpoint pupils not responding to light, excess lacrimation and fasciculation in the upper eye lids, flaccid limbs and absence of tendon reflexes. Hyperglycemia and glucosuria were found in all cases. Their presence may, according to the author, lead to the erroneous diagnosis of diabetic hyperosmolar coma if other symptoms of organophosphate poisoning are overlooked.

In view of the increasing use of malathion for the control of lice it must also be kept in mind that malathion is a weak, but definite sensitizer [102].

Mercury and mercurial compounds

16.53   For several centuries the most popular remedy for syphilis consisted of mercury in the form of an ointment rubbed into the skin. The original preparation was called 'unguentum saracenicum', from its Arabian origin, and contained one-ninth part mercury. If it was used too long or too frequently, the absorption of mercury through the skin led to extensive symptoms of intoxication. These included ulcerations of the jaws, loosening of the teeth, swelling of the gums, ulceration of the tongue, lips and palate, ptyalism, 'salivation', fetid breath, and symptoms of renal intoxication. It has been suggested that, through the centuries, mercury has killed more patients than any other medicament.

16.54   Mercury can be found in three basic states:
1. *Elemental mercury,* as liquid or vapor. This is used in dental fillings.
2. *Inorganic mercury* (mercurous and mercuric salts)
– ammoniated mercury (mercury ammonium chloride)
– mercuric chloride (mercury bichloride, mercury perchloride)
– mercurous chloride (calomel)
Ammoniated mercury may be employed in ointments, used as an antiseptic or ectoparasiticide, in contraceptive jellies, in hemorrhoidal remedies and in 'bleach creams' [25, 169]. When incorporated in ointments this compound dissolves slowly, forming very toxic mercury ions.
Mercurous chloride (calomel) may still be part of laxatives in some countries. It has also been used as diuretic, an antiseptic, and in the treatment of syphilis.
3. *Organic mercury* (in human medicoine: aryl mercurials)
– phenylmercuric acetate
– phenylmercuric nitrate

      – merbromin
      – thiomersal
      – nitromersol.
      These compounds are used for different purposes:
      – as preservatives, e.g. in eyedrops, ointments, vaccines, sera, and other injection liquids
      – as disinfectants
      – in the treatment of infection of the skin, mouth, vagina etc.
      – in contraceptive jellies
      – in hemorrhoidal remedies.

16.55   With a few exceptions, the use of mercury in medicine is considered to be outdated. However, attention should be paid to the possibility of mercurial poisoning even nowadays, as mercury may still be present in many drugs, and in many countries even in over-the-counter remedies, often without mention on the label.

    Although there are considerable differences between various mercurials regarding the rate of absorption through the skin, all mercurial preparations are a potential hazard and may cause intoxication. Metallic mercury is readily absorbed through intact skin; absorption of ammoniated mercury chloride in psoriatic patients was demonstrated by Bork et al. [19].

16.56   Symptoms of chronic mercurial poisoning include [90, 25, 100]:
    – *Nervous system disturbances:* emotional deviations, irritability, hypochondria, psychosis, impaired memory, insomnia, tremors, dysarthria, involuntary movements, vertigo, hypacusis, neuritis optica, mononeuropathy, polyneuropathy, paresthesias of the extremities, headache.
    – *Gastrointestinal disturbances:* anorexia, nausea, vomiting, epigastric pain, diarrhea, constipation, discoloration of the gums and the mucosa of the mouth, stomatitis, ulcerations of the mouth, foetor ex ore.
    – *Cardiovascular symptoms:* hypertension, hypotension, arteritis of the legs.
    – *Blood disorders:* hypochromic anemia, erythrocytosis, lymphocytosis, neutropenia, aplastic anemia.
    – *Skin disorders:* tylotic eczema, dryness of the skin, skin ulcerations, erythroderma.
    – *Renal damage:* nephrotic syndrome.
    – *Disorders of the eye:* corneal opacities and ulcerations, conjunctivitis.
    – *Endocrine abnormalities:* dysmenorrhea, hyperthyroidism.
    – *Miscellaneous:* acrodynia ('pink disease'; see § 16.57), loose teeth.

Acrodynia ('pink disease')

16.57   Topical mercurial-containing remedies such as teething powders, lotions, ointments and napkin rinses have caused acrodynia [34, 41, 166] in children between the ages of 3 months and 8 years.

    This distinctive syndrome usually begins with restlessness and irritability. Other early symptoms include fever, tachycardia and hypotonia. After 2 to 3 weeks one may observe swelling and reddening of the hands and the feet, which are cold to the touch owing to peripheral vasoconstriction. Other dermatological symptoms include skin rashes, usually macular or maculopapular, and the hands and feet may show desquamation.

    The child may complain of burning and itching; the skin is often excoriated. In addition, excessive sweating, diarrhea and renal disturbances may be noticed.

In severe cases, stomatitis with loosening of the teeth and dystrophic changes of the nails and the hair have occurred. The mortality rate is high, 10% of all affected children dying of infections.

After prohibition of mercurial teething powders in 1965 acrodynia has become very rare in Great Britain. Nevertheless, occasionally a new case is reported, as other sources of mercury such as house paint may induce the same syndrome [78].

Case reports

16.58   Young [172] examined 70 psoriatic patients treated with ointment containing ammoniated mercury before, during and after treatment.

Symptoms or signs of mercurial poisoning could be detected in 33 of them; these consisted of:

– albuminuria	11	– conjunctivitis	1
– headache	8	– epistaxis	1
– gingivitis	5	– keratitis	1
– erythroderma	4	– tremor	1
– nausea	2	– neuritis	1
– dizziness	2	– hematological changes	1
– precordial pain	2	– metallic taste in mouth	1
– contact dermatitis	2	– purpura	1

Mercury in dental fillings probably does not contribute much to toxicity, but convincing cases have been reported of mercury amalgam-induced generalized allergic reactions [151, 56].

A case has been reported of a 24-year-old man who, whilst using an ammoniated mercury-containing ointment for his psoriasis, developed a nephrotic syndrome. The predominant lesion was focal membranous glomerulonephritis. As this was thought to be due to mercury, the application was stopped; thereafter, slow, but progressive recovery ensued [134, see also 154]. Nephrotic syndrome due to topical mercury was also reported by Lyons et al. [259].

Stanley-Brown and Frank [141] described a child with an omphalocele treated with merbromin. The patient produced pink urine, and diffuse sclerema and anuria developed. Respiratory arrest occurred on the 5th day and the infant died.

Apparently even nowadays cases of mercury intoxication from use of topical mercurial antiseptics still occur [139]. A premature child had 4 applications of 10% merbromin to an omphalocele; three days later bradycardia developed and the child died [205]. Serum mercury levels were reported as greater than 260 µg/dl (normal $< 10 \,\mu g/dl$).

16.59   In view of the risks of both systemic side effects and contact allergic reactions to mercurials, there hardly seems to be any justification for continuing the use of these drugs in dermatological therapy.

Monobenzone

16.60   Monobenzone (monobenzyl ether of hydroquinone) is used topically by patients with extensive vitiligo to depigment their remaining normally pigmented skin. A patient who had been applying the drug for one year had an anterior linear deposition of pigment in both corneas. Of 15 additional patients with vitiligo, 11 of whom were using monobenzone, acquired conjunctival melanosis in two patients and pingueculae in 3 may have been related to monobenzone use. Light and electron microscopy of one corneal epithelial scraping and 12 conjunctival biopsy specimens revealed pleomorphic, single-membrane-limited intracytoplasmic inclusions within the corneal epithelium and within the epithelium fibrocytes, histiocytes and vascular endothelium of the conjunctiva. The ultrastructural aspects of the inclusions suggested that they are residual bodies containing lipid and lipofuscin [214].

2-Naphthol

16.61   Since its introduction about a century ago, 2-naphthol (β-naphthol) has been used for the treatment of various dermatoses, including psoriasis, scabies, rosacea and acne. Nowadays its use is restricted to acne; however, a considerable proportion of 2-naphthol from peeling paste is absorbed percutaneously, and Harkness and Beveridge [74] reported the isolation from the urine of about 10% of the 2-naphthol applied in such a peeling paste to the skin of a young man. This observation was confirmed by Hemels [76], who showed that on average 5% of a cutaneous dose of 2-naphthol is excreted, mostly in the first 24 hours after application. Also, a brownish-red discoloration of the urine may be noted after systemic or topical administration of this drug. The external application of 2-naphthol ointments has been responsible for systemic side effects, including vomiting and death [110, 99]. Hemels [76] concludes that 2-naphthol-containing pastes should be applied only for short periods of time and to a limited area not exceeding 150 cm^2.

Neomycin

16.62   Not only is ototoxicity a well-known hazard of parenteral neomycin administration, but also has deafness been reported after almost any form of local treatment, including treatment of skin infections and burns, use of neomycin as an intestinal antiseptic or for the control of intestinal infections, application as an aerosol for inhalation, instillation into cavities, irrigation of large wounds and use of neomycin-containing eardrops.

Aerosols

16.63   Already some years ago the Committee on Safety of Medicines in Britain warned about the use of aerosol preparations containing neomycin, after receiving reports of deafness following the use of these preparations in the treatment of extensive skin damage such as burns [55, 6].

Wound treatment

16.64   Acute renal failure and total deafness as a result of intermittent 7-day lavage of a surgical cavity with neomycin in one patient were described by Masur et al. [97]. Peritoneal dialysis promoted complete recovery of the renal function, but the patient remained deaf.

Quante [122] described a case of deafness after treatment of a 2 x 2 cm Pyocyaneus-infected wound with daily neomycin solutions. A total of 30 g was given over a period of 3 months, during which time the patient became deaf.

Already more than 10 years ago a case of progressive auditory impairment leading to almost total deafness after topical irrigation of decubitus ulcers with neomycin was reported by Kelly et al. [84].

For deafness and biochemical imbalance following burns treatment, see Bamford and Jones [10].

Ear drops

16.65   Antibiotic eardrops are widely used in the treatment of aural discharge, and have sometimes been used in cases with perforated tympanic membranes.

In response to a leading article in the *British Medical Journal* on neomycin ototoxicity following the topical use of this antibiotic, Murphy [106], in a letter, stated that he had seen many cases of mixed deafness in children with chronic suppurative otitis media, presumably due to eardrops containing chloramphenicol or neomycin.

Use of eardrops containing neomycin and polymyxin for some days in patients with a perforated tympanic membrane caused ototoxicity in 2 patients in Belgium [63]. Kellerhals [83] reported on an inquiry among the members of an otolaryngological society; this revealed 15 cases of inner ear damage caused by this practice, the frequency of this complication being assessed as one case per 1000-3000 treatments. Eight patients had a total loss of hearing in the affected ear. Neomycin and framycetin were incriminated in 13 cases.

The paper in question concludes that in cases with perforated tympanic membranes one should not use these drops (or also those containing chloramphenicol, colistin and polymyxin) for periods longer than 10 days. The antibiotics concerned may diffuse into the perilymph of the inner ear and attain dangerous levels on continuous use.

Use of neomycin on intact skin

16.66   In a young girl with chronic dermatomyositis approximately 30% of the body surface was treated with an ointment containing 1% neomycin and 11% dimethyl sulfoxide during a period of 3 months. Vertigo, nystagmus and complete loss of hearing occurred [77]. DMSO has probably enhanced percutaneous absorption of neomycin in this case. Though in theory the ototoxic effects may have been due to dimethyl sulfoxide, it was regarded very likely that neomycin was the causative agent (see § 16.24 ff. on dimethyl sulfoxide).

16.67   Application of topical neomycin (and probably other aminoglycosides) should be discouraged for the following reasons:
1. risk of inducing bacterial resistance with an associated risk of cross-resistance with other aminoglycosides, including life-saving drugs such as kanamycin and tobramycin
2. risk of inducing hypersensitivity with an associated risk of cross-allergy with other aminoglycosides
3. risk of systemic eczematous contact-type dermatitis (see § 17.2)
4. potential risk of causing or increasing drug-induced ototoxicity or nephrotoxicity.

Phenol (carbolic acid)

16.68   Phenol is a strong but also a toxic bactericide. It is not used as an antiseptic at the present time, but in dilutions of 0.5-2% it is sometimes prescribed as an antipruritic in the form of various topical medicines. Experimental studies in human volunteers have shown a rise of blood phenol to about 0.4 mg/100 ml after the application of 2% phenol in either calamine lotion or liquid paraffin [130]. Skin absorption of phenol from aqueous solutions was investigated by Baranowska [177]; the concentration of phenol, time of exposure and temperature all influenced the degree of absorption. It was shown that as much as 25% of phenol was absorbed from 2 ml of a solution of 2.5 g phenol/l water applied to the skin of the forearm and left on for 60 minutes. Phenol skin absorption in men from acetone solutions containing ^{14}C-labeled phenol has previously been documented [240].

Case reports

16.69   Phenol-induced ochronosis has been reported in the older literature [241]; the disorder occurred in patients who for many years (10–40) had treated leg ulcers with applications of wet dressings containing phenol in various concentrations. Many patients with phenol ochronosis were noted to have dark urine, much like patients with alkaptonuria. The pigmentation persists for life.

Johnstone [81] reported a fatal reaction in a 22-year-old man who accidentally spilled a bottle of carbolic acid, saturating the right leg, right side of the abdomen and the chest. Fellow employees immediately removed his shirt and threw water over the upper part of his body. The man then walked across the street to a physician's office without difficulty but collapsed and died within 15 minutes of his arrival. Autopsy revealed, in addition to local first and second degree burns, hyperemia and edema of the lower lobes of both lungs, of both kidneys, the pancreas and the spleen. There was no change in the heart or liver.

Cronin and Brauer [30] described a case of fatal poisoning in a 10-year-old boy who was treated for kerosene burns with a preparation called 'Foille', composed of 2.36% phenol, together with traces of a number of other chemicals, in corn oil.

A fatal phenol reaction following the application to wounds was reported by Deichmann [37]. There were symptoms of abdominal pain, dizziness, hemoglobinuria, cyanosis and coma. According to Woolley [168] the *prolonged* use of phenol may produce ochronosis with darkening of the cornea and of the skin of the face and the hands.

Ruedemann and Deichmann [130] reported a case in which repeated applications of 1 or 2% phenol in calamine lotion produced dizziness and collapse in an elderly woman. Serious systemic effects caused by topically applied phenol in 2 newborn infants were reported by Von Hinkel and Kintzel [160]: a 1-day-old child died after the application of 2% phenol to the umbilicus. A marked cyanosis was noted after 6 hours. The other child, 6 days old, developed methemoglobinemia, circulatory failure and cerebral symptoms. Recovery ensued after exchange transfusions.

Phenol face peels

Several cases of acute death and intra- and postoperative complications have been reported after phenol face peels [38]. Laryngeal edema with respiratory stridor, hoarseness, and tachypnea within 24 hours after a chemical face peel has been reported in 3 patients [242], but it was uncertain whether these effects were due to phenol or one of the other constituents of the face peel.

16.70   The toxic dose for adults has been estimated to be 8 to 15 g. In fatal cases, death usually results within 24 hours or less from respiratory failure, but the prognosis is guarded even after this period of time.

Major cardiac arrhythmias were noted by Truppman and Ellerby [153] in 10 out of 43 patients during phenol face peels; 9 of them had no previous ECG abnormalities, but needed intravenous lidocaine and/or propranolol for cardiac rhythm conversion. However, this item is rather controversial, and some authors feel that when the procedure is done in more than one hour, and when the dose applied is carefully monitored, phenol face peels are not risky [243, 244]. *Local* complications of chemical face peeling include [213]: hypopigmentation, hyperpigmentation, phenol bleaching, blotchy pigmentation, demarcation, milia, persistent erythema, skin pore prominence, teleangiectasia and scarring.

p-Phenylenediamine: see under Henna (§ 16.35)

Podophyllum resin

16.71   Podophyllum resin is extracted from the dried rhizome of *Podophyllum peltatum* (mandrake or may apple). It contains numerous lignins and flavonols, including podophyllotoxin and α- and β-peltatins. Podophyllum resin is a powerful skin irritant which is widely used in the local treatment of condylomata acuminata. As a potent antimitotic agent it has been extensively used as a cytotoxic drug. Absorption of podophyllum resin may lead to severe peripheral neuropathy, acute confusional states, vomiting, coma and death.
Podophyllin toxicity from topical application has been reviewed [208].

Case reports

16.72   Grabbe [67] described a girl aged 19, who developed weakness of the legs two days after a single application of a 25% podophyllin solution. On the third day an extensive polyneuritis with absence of reflexes of the extremities could be noted with muscular hypotony and ataxia. On the sixth day she developed a paralytic ileus. The patient recovered after about 10 weeks.
Ward et al. [165] described a black girl aged 18, who became comatose about 24 hours after the application of 25% podophyllin ointment on vulvar warts. She died after eight days.
Schirren [132] observed a man aged 25, whose extensive condylomata acuminata on the prepuce and around the anus were treated with a 16% solution of podophyllin in alcohol. About 2 hours after treatment the patient vomited and became unconscious. A few hours later he showed severe agitation and gross movements of the extremities with stertorous respiration that stopped every 3-4 minutes. There was a marked cyanosis. It must be mentioned that this patient had consumed a large amount of alcohol immediately after the local treatment. This may, according to the author, have increased the absorption of podophyllin.
Cormane [29] examined a girl aged 20, who was treated for an extensive eruption of condylomata acuminata localized on the labia majora, minora and the vaginal mucosa. A 10% podophyllin solution in collodion was applied with a tampon, which was left in place for 6 hours. The patient subsequently developed a temperature which lasted 4 days. About one week after treatment the girl experienced paresthetic sensations in toes and fingers, which was followed by a feeling of weakness in the legs and hands and edema of the legs. This paresis due to a polyneuritis disappeared after about 14 days.
Vomiting and an acute confusional state occurred in one case after the use of podophyllum in the treatment of hairy tongue [75].
Stoehr et al. [142] described a case in which absorption of podophyllin led to bone marrow depression with thrombopenia and leukopenia. In another patient with leukopenia and thrombocytopenia [206] the bone marrow was found to be hypocellular with cytoplasmic vacuolization of myeloid precursors, and showed increased numbers of mitotic figures.
Chamberlain et al. [23] described a case of severe intoxication in a woman in the 32nd week of pregnancy with subsequent delivery of a stillborn infant. According to the authors, podophyllum resin should never be used in pregnancy or in circumstances where the genital warts are either so florid with a large surface area or so hemorrhagic that absorption of the toxic resin is likely.

Teratogenicity from topical application of podophyllum was suspected by Karol et al. [82]. The drug was applied to a woman five times for a duration of 4 hours from the 23rd to the 29th week of her pregnancy. Her baby was noted to have a simian crease on the left hand and a preauricular skin tag. See also Slater et al. [138] and Montaedi et al. [105].

Povidone-iodine

16.73   Povidone-iodine is a water-soluble iodine complex, which is said to retain the non-selective broad-range microbicidal activity of iodine without the undesirable effects of iodine tincture. Betadine products are said to kill both gram-positive and -negative bacteria, including antibiotic-resistant organisms, as well as fungi, viruses, protozoa and yeasts. Apparently povidone-iodine has a more prolonged germicidal action than ordinary iodine solutions, and maintains its effectiveness in the presence of blood, serum and pus.

Several studies have shown that povidone-iodine, or at least iodine, may be absorbed from damaged skin, such as burns, [114, 17, 192, 250], from the vaginal mucosa [162], from the oral mucosa [49], but also from normal skin in children [121, 18].

Effects of thyroid function

16.74   Absorption of povidone-iodine may lead to elevation of iodine blood levels [162], elevation of protein-bound iodine [27], and thyroid function abnormalities [18, 49]; usually there are no clinical manifestations, such as hypothyroidism. However, skin disinfection with *iodine* has caused goiter and hypothyroidism in five of 30 newborns under intensive care [22], and there is concern that absorption of povidone-iodine may give rise to similar adverse reactions. In this regard, children would seem to constitute a high-risk group.

A very rapid absorption of povidone-iodine from the vaginal mucosa, after only two minutes vaginal disinfection, resulting in an increase in serum concentration of total iodine and inorganic iodine up to 5- to 15-fold, has been documented by Vorherr et al. [162].

Etling et al. [44] noted that after vaginal povidone-iodine application during pregnancy, levels of total iodine in amniotic fluid were increased 10 to 150 times over the control values.

As an overload of iodine can suppress thyroid hormonogenesis [22], Vorherr et al. [162] advised not to treat vaginitis in pregnant women with povidone-iodine because of the possible development of iodine-induced goiter and hypothyroidism in the fetus and the newborn. Moreover, Utiger [157] has reported that repeated vaginal application, of povidone-iodine has resulted in goiter and hypothyroidism, with sequelae of airway obstruction, mental and physical retardation, and neurological disturbances. Less dramatic transient hypothyroidism after prenatal and perinatal exposure to povidone-iodine has been noted in a 'significant' number of newborns [202]. The authors suggested not to use iodine in pregnancy or neonatology, when follow-up of the newborn is not guaranteed.

Castaing et al. [21] studied the postnatal iodine overload after cutaneous application of povidone-iodine (0.96% I2) in 11 neonates, of Sterlane (0.03% 2,4,5,7-tetraiodofluorescein) in 20 newborns and of ethanol colored with eosin in 28 neonates. The mean ioduria in the two former groups was significantly higher than that of the control group. There were 12 cases of hypothyroidism among the newborns exposed to the iodine-containing antiseptics, but none in the control group.

According to the authors, postnatal use of iodine preparations in neonates should be avoided.

In one patient with a perineal fistula has prolonged therapy with topical application of povidone-iodine solution and iodoform-impregnated packing strips led to hypothyroidism [119]. Topical povidone-iodine applied to an abdominal wound has also caused transient thyroid suppression [251].

Neutropenia

16.75   A case of neutropenia, presumably due to topical treatment with povidone-iodine was reported by Alvarez [5]: his patient had deep second-degree burns, involving about 50% of the body surface, which were treated with betadine helafoam twice a day.

Renal effects

A 50-year-old woman with chronic renal insufficiency was admitted to hospital for treatment of an extensive decubitus ulcer, gram-negative septicemia and increasing azotemia. The ulcer was packed every 4 hours with PVP-I-soaked gauze. From the 17th day she developed unexplained oliguria, decreasing renal function, hypochloremic metabolic acidosis and cardiovascular instability, which were apparently due to iodide retention (11,200 µg/dl). The authors suggest monitoring serum iodide concentrations if topical povidone-iodine therapy is to be used in patients with renal insufficiency or on large areas of denuded skin [292].

Metabolic acidosis

16.76   Metabolic acidosis was attributed to povidone-iodine in the report of Pietsch and Meakins [114]. Two patients, one with a 75% burn, the second with a 35% burn, were treated topically with povidone-iodine. In both patients severe metabolic acidosis developed, which could not be attributed to sepsis, hypervolemia, renal failure, lactic acidemia, etc. The acidosis associated with the 75% burn required large amounts of sodium bicarbonate to maintain pH at 7.35 and a serum bicarbonate concentration of 15 mmol/l (mEq/l); serum iodine was 48,000 µg/dl (normal 4-8.5 µg/dl). Acidosis in the second patient was not as severe, and serum iodine concentration reached 17,600 µg/dl. Hemodialysis was very effective in reducing serum iodine concentration. According to the authors, the acidosis could have been caused by absorption of the iodine or the acidic povidone-iodine. They suggest that, until the etiology of the acidosis and renal damage is more clear, iodophores should not be used topically for burns greater than 20% of the body surface, or in the presence of renal failure.

Iododerma

16.77   A case of generalized iododerma caused by absorption of povidone-iodine has been described by Bishop and Garcia [17].

Promethazine

16.78   A 16-month-old male (weight 11.5 kg) was treated with 2% promethazine cream for generalized eczema. After approximately 15–20 g of the cream had been applied the child fell asleep; a few hours later he awoke with *abnormal behavior, loss of balance, inability to focus, irritability, drowsiness and failure to recognize his* *mother*. One day later all symptoms had spontaneously disappeared. A diagnosis of promethazine toxicity through percutaneous absorption was made [188].

Known symptoms of promethazine toxicity include disorientation, hallucinations, hyperactivity, convulsions, and coma.

Quinine analogs

16.79   Thrombocytopenia due to quinine analogs, though well known from oral administration, has only rarely been described after topical application.

Case reports

16.80   Khaleeli [85] observed thrombocytopenia in a female patient with extensive bilateral varicose ulcers and myxedema, who was treated with Quinaband-dressings. (Quinaband contains zinc oxide paste 9.25%, gum acacia 18.5%, clioquinol 1%, calamine 5.75%, boric acid 2%, glycerol 27%, propyl hydroxybenzoate 0.0625% and aqua). The patient was hospitalized for surgical treatment of her ulcers. Medication was limited to thyroxine, multivite and ferrous sulfate tablets, and Quinaband dressings were applied to the leg ulcers.

During hospitalization she lapsed into a myxedematous coma. She was treated with triiodothyronine and intravenous hydrocortisone. Because sputum had grown *Staphylococcus aureus*, the patient in addition received intramuscular ampicillin and flucloxacillin. The platelet count dropped from 250x109 to 100x109 and purpura was noted on the chest. She was transfused with 2 units of packed cells but the platelet count continued to fall (to 30x109): hematuria and nose bleeding occurred. Patch tests with Quinaband were negative.

Shortly after discontinuation of the Quinaband application, the patient received 2 units of fresh blood and the platelet count rapidly returned to normal values. Though conclusive evidence is definitely lacking, the author ascribes the thrombocytopenia to the use of Quinaband dressings, and, more specifically, to the clioquinol contained therein.

There can be no doubt, however, that absorption of halogenated hydroxyquinolines does occur: in a child with generalized psoriasis who had received topical treatment with clioquinol-containing ointment, 18.1 mg/100 ml of the conjugated (glucuronic acid) ester of the drug was traced in the urine [72].

Fischer and Hartvig [52] reported on percutaneous absorption of clioquinol: four patients with widespread dermatitis were treated with an ointment containing 3% clioquinol and a corticosteroid. A body area of 40% was treated with 15–20 g of the ointment twice daily. The serum concentration increased to 0.8–1.2 µg/ml within four hours of application, remained constant during treatment, and then fell to zero within four days. Urinary excretion, measured in one case, comprised 15–20 mg conjugated metabolites daily. This topical treatment thus gave about the same urinary excretion as would a daily oral dose of 0.25 g (one tablet) of clioquinol. The authors estimate that 3–4% of the applied clioquinol was absorbed percutaneously.

As chronic oral use of this drug may lead to serious neurological adverse events, concern has been raised about the safety of extensive topical application of clioquinol [73].

An abnormal protein-bound iodine after topical application of clioquinol has been recorded by Upjohn et al. [156].

Systemic side effects of topical clioquinol in a previously sensitized individual were described by Simpson [135]: A woman, known to react to ingested quinine applied 3% clioquinol cream to her submammary region. Twelve hours after the first application she developed a generalized erythema and within hours had bronchospasm which required oral and intravenous steroids.

Resorcinol

16.81   Resorcinol (m-dihydroxybenzene) is used for its keratolytic and 'peeling' properties in the treatment of acne vulgaris; also, it is a constituent for the antifungal Castellani's solution. Formerly, leg ulcers were treated with external application of resorcinol-containing preparations.

Case reports

16.82   Resorcinol can penetrate human skin [227, 228] and an extensive review of the industrial toxicity of resorcinol has been reported [229]. It has been estimated that less than 3% resorcinol in a hydroalcoholic vehicle applied to the skin is absorbed percutaneously (227). Although the drug is chemically unrelated to any of the known groups of antithyroid drugs, resorcinol has an antithyroid activity similar to that of methyl thiouracil. Consequently, several cases of myxedema caused by percutaneous absorption of resorcinol, especially from ulcerated surfaces, have been described [15, 150].

Two cases of resorcinol-induced hypothyroidism were described by Berthezène et al. [15]. All symptoms disappeared after discontinuation of the treatment with resorcinol. The authors assume that resorcinol produced a defect in the organic binding of iodine and in the release of thyroid hormones. This latter effect may be due to a defect in the coupling of iodotyrosines. In the report of Thomas and Gisburn [150] resorcinol-induced myxedema was associated with ochronosis.

Methemoglobinemia in children, caused by the absorption of resorcinol applied to wounds has been reported by Flandin et al. [53] and by Murray [107]. Cunningham [31] reported a case in which the application of an ointment containing 12.5% resorcinol to the napkin area of an infant produced cyanosis, a maculopapular eruption, hemolytic anemia, and hemoglobinuria. In the literature, this author found seven cases of acute poisoning in babies, as a consequence of topical resorcinol application, in some instances to limited areas; five fatalities were recorded.

Wuthrich et al. [170] reported on two young adults who were treated for pustular acne with a peeling paste containing 40% resorcinol. After three to four weeks of treatment with one application daily, adverse reactions were noted consisting of pallor, dizziness, cold sweat, tremors, collapse and violet-black urine.

A case of severe poisoning of a six-week-old infant due to two applications of Castellani's paint (containing basic fuchsin, boric acid, phenol, resorcinol, acetone and alcohol) was described by Lundell and Nordman [95].

Although the use of resorcinol in young children and for leg ulcers should be avoided, topical resorcinol, when used for acne vulgaris, appears to be safe [227].

Salicylic acid

16.83   In 1874, salicylic acid became widely available as the result of its production by a synthetic process. Since that time it has been widely used in dermatology for topical application because of its keratolytic properties.

As early as 1880 Beyer [16, 171] reported the presence of salicylates in the urine following application to the skin. Cases of salicylate poisoning after topical use of salicylic acid have been reported several times. Taylor and Halprin [257] used

16.84   Salicylic acid

6% salicylic acid in a gel base under plastic suit occlusion in adults with extensive psoriasis. During their 5-day study, serum salicylates never exceeded 5 mg/100 ml and no patient developed toxicity. However, toxicity was noted by von Weis and Lever; they found serum salicylate levels ranging from 46–64 mg/100 ml. Salicylic acid therapy for extensive lesions may be especially dangerous for children. An unpublished review [258] revealed 13 deaths associated with the widespread use of salicylic acid preparations, and all but 3 occurred in children. This compound should not be used on large areas (more than 25%) of the skin of a child [258].

16.84   The *signs and symptoms of intoxication* vary according to the level of salicylic acid in the plasma, although considerable differences exist in individual susceptibility [68]. Symptoms may be present with levels of salicylic acid in the plasma as low as 10 mg/100 ml. Ordinarily, symptoms that occur at levels below 35 mg/100 ml are quite mild.

The clinical manifestations of intoxication with salicylic acid include gastrointestinal, respiratory, renal, metabolic, neural and psychic disturbances [161]. The first symptoms are, according to Gorter [66] paleness, fatigue and drowsiness, and a modification of the respiration, which becomes more frequent and at the same time deeper, and can be heard from a distance. Other early signs of intoxication with salicylic acid are nausea, vomiting, changes in the ability to hear, and mental confusion [161]. Several deaths have been recorded, mainly in children.

The treatment of mild to moderate intoxication with salicylic acid consists of discontinuing the salicylic acid ointment, giving large amounts of fluids to promote excretion, and administering sodium bicarbonate, either orally or intravenously, in order to ensure an alkaline pH of the urine [109]. The pH of the urine is a significant factor in the occurrence of intoxication with salicylic acid. In severe renal damage salicylic acid is poorly excreted [69].

Case reports

16.85   In 1952 Young collected 8 fatal cases of salicylate poisoning with symptoms of vomiting, tinnitus, stupor, Cheyne-Stokes respiration and nuchal rigidity.

Von Weiss and Lever [161] reported on 3 adults with extensive psoriasis who were treated with an ointment containing 3% or 6% salicylic acid 6 times daily. Between the second and fourth day, symptoms of salicylism developed in all 3 patients.

The outstanding symptoms were *nausea, dyspnea, decreased ability to hear, confusion* and *hallucinations*.
Other signs included:
– *Gastrointestinal:* vomiting, thirst, anorexia, diarrhea
– *Neural:* headache, dizziness, tinnitus, slurred speech
– *Psychic:* agitation, disorientation, lethargy, delusions, belligerence, retrograde amnesia, depression, feeling of unreality
– *Other:* fever, profuse sweating.
The levels of salicylic acid in the serum ranged from 46 to 64 mg/100 ml.
Within one day after discontinuation of the ointment, the symptoms had largely disappeared. The serum salicylic acid decreased to zero within a few days.

The same authors also recorded 13 deaths resulting from intoxication with salicylic acid following the application of salicylic ointment to the skin, reported in literature up to 1964, and several non-fatal intoxications. The 13 deaths included 3 patients with psoriasis, 5 cases of scabies, 3 of dermatitis, one of lupus vulgaris and one of congenital ichthyosiform erythroderma. Ten of the fatal cases occurred in children, 3 of them being under 3 years of age.

The most dramatic account in the literature is that of 2 plantation workers in

Bougainville, in the Solomon Islands, who were painted twice a day with an alcoholic solution of 20% salicylic acid for tinea imbricata involving about 50% of the body. The victims were comatose within 6 hours and dead within 28 hours [92].

Wechselberg [167] reported a 3-month-old baby with scaly erythroderma treated in a hospital with 1% salicylic acid in soft paraffin. After 10 days the child began to vomit and lose weight. Later hyperpnea developed and an increasing somnolence. When the treatment was stopped the child recovered rapidly.

Recently, a case of salicylic acid intoxication leading to coma in an adult patient with psoriasis, who had been treated with 20% salicylic acid in petrolatum, was described [152].

Lipman et al. [93] summarized the electrolyte changes that occur in salicylate intoxication as follows: 'A hyperpnoea due to the central stimulatory effect of the salicyl radical produces a respiratory loss of carbon dioxide, altering the ratio of carbonic acid to sodium bicarbonate in the direction of increased alkalinity. This then is a state of respiratory alkalosis and represents the first stage of salicylate intoxication. The next stage is a state of compensated acidosis caused by ketosis resulting from altered carbohydrate metabolism and the presence of retained acid anions in the blood and tissue fluids. The final stage is that of decompensated acidosis, with depletion of the alkali reserve, decrease in the blood pH and failure of the respiratory centre in its attempt to achieve compensation.'

Salicylic acid in higher concentrations, combined with ammoniated mercuric chloride ('ammoniated mercury'), can severely irritate the skin because free mercuric chloride is formed.

Selenium sulfide

16.86   Ransone et al. [125] reported a case of *systemic* selenium toxicity in a woman who had been shampooing her hair 2 or 3 times weekly for 8 months with selenium sulfide suspension. One hour after a shampoo the patient noticed a mild non-rhythmical tremor of the arms and hands over a period of 3 or 4 minutes. This was followed by severe perspiration and an increasingly severe generalized tremor. Two hours after the shampoo she noticed a metallic taste in the mouth and others noted that her breath smelled of garlic, though none had been eaten. The tremor lasted for eight hours and was followed by a dull continuous pain in the lower abdomen. For the next three days she felt quite weak, lethargic and anorectic, and occasionally vomited. The patient denied headaches, speech, visual or gait disturbances and skin eruptions except for an excoriated crusted and scaling eruption, 5 by 12 cm, on the scalp.

Sex hormones

Estrogens

16.87   Topical application of estrogen-containing externa may lead to resorption of these hormones and systemic estrogenic effects.

Beas et al. [13] reported on seven children with *Pseudoprecocious puberty* due to an ointment containing estrogens. The common fact found in every patient was the use of the same ointment for treatment or prevention of ammoniacal dermatitis for a period of 2 to 18 months with 2 to ten daily applications. Endocrinological and radiological studies had excluded other possible causes of sexual precocity. The most important clinical signs were: intense pigmentation of the mammillary areola, linea alba of the abdomen and the genitals, mammary enlargement and the presence of pubic hair. Three female patients also had vaginal discharge and bleeding. Estrogenic contamination of the ointment was suspected and confirmed by a biological test of the vaginal opening of castrated female guinea pigs. After discontinuation of the incriminated topical drug all symptomatology progressively disappeared in every patient.

Pseudoprecocious puberty has also been observed in young girls after contact with hair lotions and other substances containing estrogens [14, 88, 123]. Such contact has lead to gynecomastia in young boys [143, 199]. Gynecomastia in a 70-year-old man from exposure to 0.01% dienestrol cream used by his wife for atrophic vaginitis and as a lubricant before intercourse has been reported [189].

Estrogen cream for the treatment of baldness has also caused gynecomastia, which was persistent in the reported case [238]. In adult males both oral and topical administration of estrogens may result first in pigmentation of the areola and then in gynecomastia [12, 62].

Silver nitrate

Case reports

16.88   Ternberg and Luce [148] observed fatal *methemoglobinemia* in a three-year-old girl suffering from extensive burns, involving 82% of the body surface, who was treated with silver nitrate solutions. Two weeks after admission a transient episode of cyanosis was noted, for which no definite diagnosis was established. Ten days later, she became progressively cyanotic, respiratory rate and pulse increased and then the patient became hypothermic and died.

In a post-mortem blood specimen methemoglobin was found to constitute 70% of the hemoglobin. Known causes of methemoglobinemia were excluded. Presumably nitrate had been reduced by *Aerobacter cloacae,* cultured from her wounds, into nitrite, which was absorbed and subsequently caused methemoglobinemia (nitrite is prominent among the agents capable of producing methemoglobin).

Other cases of silver nitrate-induced methemoglobinemia were reported by Cushing and Smith [33], Aberman [1], Strauch et al. [145] and Geffner et al. [202]. It is stated that the appearance of cyanosis in burn patients treated with silver nitrate should suggest the possibility of methemoglobinemia, especially when the cyanosis persists despite oxygen treatment.

Another complication of the use of silver nitrate in the treatment of large burns is *electrolyte disturbance,* especially in children. Due to the hypotonicity of the silver nitrate dressings hyponatremia, hypokalemia and hyperchloremia may develop [42, 28]. Also, loss of other water-soluble minerals and vitamins may occur. Post-mortem examinations of patients treated with silver nitrate have revealed that silver has been deposited in internal organs, showing that absorption of silver from topical preparation does occur [9]. It should be mentioned that the excessive use of silver-containing drugs has led to local and systemic argyria [87] and to renal damage involving the glomeruli with proteinuria [173].

Generalized argyria from uncontrolled silver nitrate application to bleeding gingiva during a period of $2\frac{1}{2}$ years was reported by Marshall and Schneider [96].

Sulfadiazine silver

16.89   Sulfadiazine silver cream is widely used for the topical treatment of burns. Intended primarily for the control of *Pseudomonas* infections, this bactericidal agents acts on the cell membranes and the cell walls of a variety of gram-positive and gram-negative bacteria as well as on yeasts. Its relative freedom from appreciable side effects such as electrolyte and acid-base disturbances, staining and pain on application, has contributed to its popularity. In a series of 314 burn patients treated with sulfadiazine silver the incidence of drug reactions was only 1.3% [113].

Absorption of sulfonamide from burns treated with sulfadiazine silver has been studied [238]. In 3 patients with 17–46% burned surface area, approximately 20–25% of the daily topical dose could be accounted for as conjugated sulfonamide. Unconjugated drug represented from 35%–95% of the total output. Total plasma sulfonamide concentration did not exceed $10 \, \mu g/ml$.

Nephrotic syndrome and leukopenia

16.90   Nephrotic syndrome following topical therapy with this drug has been reported by Owens et al. [112], but this observation has not been confirmed since. Several authors have, however, reported leukopenia during treatment with sulfadiazine silver [24, 80, 54]. This side effect appears to run a typical course: sulfadiazine-induced leukopenia reaches a nadir within 2–4 days of starting therapy, with a characteristic drop in the neutrophil count and a relative increase in the number of band forms. The erythrocyte count is not affected. Two to three days after the onset of leukopenia, the leukocyte count returns to normal levels. Recovery is not affected by the continuation of therapy.

Owing to the circumstances under which topical sulfadiazine therapy is institut-ed (ill patient, septic conditions, additional medication), it is very difficult to prove a causal relationship between the drug and the event. However, there are several arguments in favor of such a relationship [54]: (1) No observations of leukopenia associated with other burn therapies, such as mafenide acetate and silver nitrate soaks, have been reported. (2) Sulfadiazine is absorbed to a considerable extent following the topical administration of sulfadiazine silver (serum levels up to 20 μg/ml). (3) Sulfadiazine is a known cause of leukopenia, agranulocytosis, and oth-er blood dyscrasias. (4) The leukopenic response follows a predictable course. (5) A positive rechallenge has been demonstrated while attempting to reinstitute ther-apy in 2 patients.

Current evidence, therefore, suggests a causal relationship of sulfadiazine silver with leukopenia. The mechanism of this reaction is unknown. Examinations of bone marrow aspirates show hyperplasia with no evidence of maturation arrest. The drug presumably affects the white blood cells peripherally [54].

Sulfur

16.91   Though its efficacy is sometimes questioned, sulfur is still widely used in the treat-ment of acne vulgaris and seborrheic conditions: no toxicity is to be feared from this practice. However, sulfur has been used in the treatment of scabies, and some authors recommend the use of this 'alternative scabicide' in young children, preg-nant patients and in patients with massively excoriated skin, because of the alleged neurotoxic effects of treatment with the most commonly used scabicide, lindane (see § 16.47). It must, therefore, be mentioned that the safety of application of sul-fur-containing topical remedies over large parts of the body has not been estab-lished.

Experimental studies

16.92   The percutaneous absorption of sulfur was studied by Geivitz and Wust [58]: after

201

the application of sulfur in a cream base to the skin of healthy subjects, the substance was traced two hours later in the urine. It was estimated that approximately 1% of the sulfur had been absorbed.

The application of 25% sulfur in petrolatum to abraded guinea pig skin led to total anorexia and paralysis with demonstrable blood levels of hydrogen sulfide in the experiments of Basch [11]. This same author also reported on clinical evidence of poisoning in patients with scabies treated with sulfur ointments, and even noted fatal toxicity in babies after application of sulfur to large areas of the skin.

Tretinoin

16.93   Of 245 patients treated for varying dyskeratotic states (ichthyosis, callosities, palmoplantar keratoderma, acne, and verrucae plantares), 19 (7.8%) had mildly elevated liver function test results of serum transaminase levels, both of which were reversible with cessation of treatment [232]. These changes were seen in patients who had an 'erythematous effect' from treatment.

The significance of the data from this study is unclear. In a multicenter study, 44 patients treated for various keratinizing dermatoses showed no elevation in liver function tests [233]. Physiologic levels of vitamin A have been measured in the dermis after the topical application of tretinoin [234]. Theoretically, increased dermal blood flow (erythema) might lead to the absorption of sufficient amounts of tretinoin to cause temporary alteration in liver function. However, only the one study mentioned above has reported changes in liver function tests, so the risk of liver toxicity from tretinoin that is not in an ointment base, used in a patient who does not have a severe erythematous process, would appear to be negligible [234].

Triclocarban

16.94   Triclocarban (trichlorocarbanilide, TCC) is a bacteriostatic agent used to reduce microbial skin flora, and has been present in antimicrobial toilet soap bars since 1956. Its chemistry and antimicrobial properties have been described by Roman et al. [129].

The percutaneous penetration of TCC has been studied by Scharpf et al. [131]: after a single shower employing a whole body lather with approximately 6 g of soap containing 2% TCC, about 0.23% of the applied dose of TCC was recovered in the feces after six days, and 0.16% of the dose in the urine after two days. At all sampling times blood levels of radioactivity were below the detection limit of 10 parts per billion.

Methemoglobinemia

16.95   In 1962 the Subcommittee on Accidental Poisoning called attention to occurrences of methemoglobinemia in premature and full-term newborn infants whose diapers were autoclaved after a final laundry rinse with triclocarban. Subsequent reports in the pediatric literature confirmed and added to these 'epidemics' of neonatal methemoglobinemia (e.g. Fisch et al. [51]), and suggested that aniline – a well-known cause of methemoglobinemia – resulting from the breakdown of TCC during autoclaving, was absorbed from diapers and other nursery clothing through the skin of the infants.

A more recent report of methemoglobinemia presumably induced by topical TCC was documented by Ponté et al. [117]: Five neonates with methemoglobinemia were seen by the authors. In each case, the family history of methemoglobine-mia was negative; other possible causes, such as drugs, were excluded. A cure was obtained rapidly after injection of methylene blue, completed in some cases by ex-change transfusions; no relapses were noted during the following months. In four cases, TCC-containing solutions had been used during delivery either for antisep-sis of the perineum of the pregnant woman, or by the obstetrician for hand wash-ing. In the fifth case, 2% TCC containing ointment had been applied to the neo-nate's umbilicus.

The authors assume that triclocarban has caused methemoglobinemia in these cases, although they admit that a causative relationship between the drug and the adverse event could not be convincingly demonstrated. Currently, the issue of tri-clocarban and methemoglobinemia is still unsettled.

Triphenylmethane dyes

16.96   Gentian violet and methyl green are triphenylmethane dyes, formerly used for topical antisepsis. A systemic reaction to these drugs in a previously sensitized in-dividual was described by Michel et al. [101]: a woman became cyanosed and then collapsed after the application of a 1% solution of gentian violet and methyl green to a stasis ulcer. An epicutaneous test with the solution was positive.

TRANSDERMAL DRUG DELIVERY

16.97   Percutaneous absorption of skin contactants, usually an undesirable effect, may also be exploited for therapeutic purposes. Classic examples are nitroglycerin and scopolamine. The drug, which is intended to exert a systemic effect, may be ap-plied to the skin in an ointment base, a solution, or in an especially developed 'transdermal drug delivery system'. The transdermal drug delivery system consists in principle of a reservoir with a microporous membrane, which is applied with an adhesive layer to a hairless part of the skin. The drug is presented to the skin in a continuous rate, which is controlled by the semipermeable microporous mem-brane of the reservoir and not by the permeability of the skin. This prevents unin-tended high plasma concentrations of the drugs in patients with unusually perme-able skin.

Clonidine

16.98   Clonidine in a transdermal therapeutic system (clonidine-TTS) has been used for the treatment of mild to moderate hypertension. Systemic side effects reported in 21 patients during stable dose clonidine-TTS treatment were dry mouth (2) and nervousness (1). In 3 patients contact allergy developed. It was not established whether the allergic reaction was due to clonidine or to a condensation product of acetaldehyde and clonidine, which is formed as an impurity during the manu-facture of clonidine-TTS [293].

Glycopyrrolate

16.99   The quaternary ammonium compound glycopyrrolate has been used topically for the treatment of facial gustatory sweating and flushing (Frey syndrome). This syn-drome occurs in 60% of patients after parotidectomy with facial nerve dissection.

Side effects due to the anticholinergic action of glycopyrrollate include blurred vision and dry mouth. The incidence of these side effects is low when compared to topical scopolamine [286].

Nitroglycerin

16.100   Nitroglycerin acts directly on the smooth muscles of both arterial and venous vessels causing relaxation. Sublingual (buccal) administration of nitroglycerin has been the treatment of choice for angina pectoris. Because of its extremely short half-life of 3–5 minutes, nitroglycerin in this way is not suitable for continuous prophylaxis. A disadvantage of *oral* administration is the rapid metabolization to inactive metabolites. A possibility to overcome this 'liver first-pass effect' of oral administration is application to the skin. From industrial use it is known that nitroglycerin easily penetrates the intact epidermis [285]. An oitment formulation of nitroglycerin to be applied under occlusive dressing has been available for many years [279]. However, the dosage for use of the drug is not very accurate, bearing the risk of unnecessarily high plasma concentrations of nitroglycerin. These disadvantages of the ointment have led to the development of several nitroglycerin transdermal delivery systems [287]. Side effects of the nitroglycerin transdermal delivery systems include: headache, pressure feeling in the head, nausea, vomiting, dizziness, tiredness, and black-outs [282]. Gastrointestinal side effects are said to occur very frequently in healthy individuals exposed to the system [287]. Contact allergy to the adhesive [280, 282] has been reported, as has been irritation. Contact allergy to the active drug is not rare (§ 5.42).

Scopolamine

16.101   The use of scopolamine for prevention of motion-sickness is well-established. In tablet or injectable form scopolamine frequently causes (in addition to the intended antiemetic effect) adverse effects due to its anticholinergic action (§ 19.68): dry mouth, hypotension, drowsiness, cycloplegia, bradycardia (low doses), and tachycardia (high doses) [278]. These frequently occurring adverse reactions stimulated the development of a transdermal delivery system.

Side effects of the scopolamine transdermal delivery system include: dry mouth, drowsiness, disturbed concentration, mydriasis (blurred vision), mild hypotension [284]. Incidentally psychotic behavior has been reported [284]. Unilateral mydriasis may have been caused by contamination of the eye [282]. Contact allergy and irritation to the adhesive has been reported, and contact allergy to the active drug may occur. Scopolamine in an ophthalmic preparation has caused erythema multiforme (§ 12.1).

16.102   REFERENCES

1. Aberman, A. (1969): Oxygentension in methemoglobinemia (letter). *New Engl. J. Med., 281,* 1020.
2. Abrams, S. M., Degnan, T. J. and Vinciguerra, V. (1980): Marrow aplasia following topical application of chloramphenicol eye ointment. *Arch. intern. Med., 140,* 576.
3. Alder, V. D., Burman, D., Coroner-Beryl, D. and Gillespie, W. A. (1972): Absorption of hexachlorophene from infant's skin. *Lancet, 2,* 384.
4. Alexander, R. C. (1930): Fatal dermatitis following the use of iodine spirit solution. *Brit. med. J., 2,* 100.
5. Alvarez, E. (1979): Neutropenia in a burned patient being treated topically with povidone-iodine foam. *Plast. reconstr. Surg., 63,* 839.

6. Anonymous (1977): Warning on aerosols containing neomycin. *Lancet, 1,* 1115.
7. Anonymous (1980): Hexachlorophene. *JARC Monographs on the Evaluation of the Carcinogenic Risk of Chemicals to Humans, 20,* 241.
8. Aslam, M., Davis, S. S. and Healy, M. A. (1979): Heavy metals in some Asian medicines and cosmetics. *Publ. Hlth (Lond.), 93,* 274.
9. Bader, K. F. (1966): Organ deposition of silver following silver nitrate therapy of burns. *Plast. reconstr. Surg., 37,* 550.
10. Bamford, M. F. M. and Jones, L. F. (1978): Deafness and biochemical imbalance after burns treatment with topical antibiotics in young children. *Arch. Dis. Childh., 53,* 326.
11. Basch, F. (1926): Über Schwefelwasserstoffvergiftung bei äusserlicher Applikation von elementarem Schwefel in Salbenform. *Arch. exp. Path. Pharm., 111,* 126.
12. Bazex, A., Salvader, R., Dupré, A. and Christol, B. (1967): Gynécomastie et hyperpigmentation aréolaire après oestrogénothérapie locale antiséborrhéque. *Bull. Soc. franç. Derm. Syph., 74,* 466.
13. Beas, F., Vargas, L., Spada, R. P. and Merchak, N. (1969): Pseudoprecocious puberty in infants caused by a dermal ointment containing estrogens. *J. Pediat., 75,* 127.
14. Bertaggia, A. (1968): A case of precocious puberty in a girl following the use of an oestrogen preparation on the skin. *Pediatria (Napoli), 76,* 579.
15. Berthezène, F., Fournier, M., Bernier, E. and Mornex, R. (1973): L'Hypothyroidie induite par la résorcine. *Lyon méd., 230,* 319.
16. Beyer (1880): Cited by Young (1952).
17. Bishop, M. E. and Garcia, R. L. (1978): Iododerma from wound irrigation with povidone-iodine. *J. Amer. med. Ass., 240,* 249.
18. Block, S. H. (1980): Thyroid function abnormalities from the use of topical betadine solution on intact skin of children. *Cutis, 26,* 88.
19. Bork, K., Morsches, B. and Holzmann, H. (1973): Zum Problem der Quecksilber-Resorption aus weisser Präzipitatsalbe. *Arch. derm. Forsch., 248,* 137.
20. Brenn, H. and Röckl, H. (1954): Fixes Exanthem durch perkutane Resorption von Cignolin. *Hautarzt, 5,* 250.
21. Castaing, H., Fournet, J.-P., Léger, F.-A., Kiesgen, F., Piette, C., Dupard, M.-C. and Savoie, J.-C. (1979): Thyroïde du nouveau-né et surcharge en iode après la naissance. *Arch. franç. Pédiat., 36,* 356.
22. Chabrolle, J. P. and Rossier, A. (1978): Goitre and hypothyroidism in the newborn after cutaneous absorption of iodine. *Arch. Dis. Childh., 53,* 495.
23. Chamberlain, M. J., Reynolds, A. L. and Yoeman, W. B. (1972): Toxic effects of podophyllum application in pregnancy. *Brit. med. J., 3,* 391.
24. Chan, C. K., Jarrett, F. and Moylan, J. A. (1976): Acute leukopenia as an allergic reaction to silver sulfadiazine in burn patients. *J. Trauma, 16,* 395.
25. Ciaccio, E. I. (1971): Mercury: therapeutic and toxic aspects. *Semin. Drug Treatm., 1,* 177.
26. Committee on Drugs (1978): Camphor – Who needs it? *Pediatrics, 62,* 404.
27. Connell Jr., J. F. and Rousselot, L. M. (1964): Povidone-iodine, extensive surgical evaluation of a new antiseptic. *Amer. J. Surg., 108,* 849.
28. Connely, D. M. (1970): Silver nitrate – ideal burn wound therapy? *N. Y. St. J. Med., 70,* 1642.
29. Cormane, R. H. (1968): Condylomata acuminata en podophylline. *Ned. T. Geneesk., 112,* 2305.
30. Cronin, T. D. and Brauer, R. O. (1949): Death due to phenol contained in Foille®. *J. Amer. med. Ass., 139,* 777.
31. Cunningham, A. A. (1956): Resorcin poisoning. *Arch. Dis. Childh., 31,* 173.
32. Curley, A., Hawk, R. E., Kimbrough, R. D., Nathenson, G. and Finberg, L. (1971): Dermal absorption of hexachlorophane in infants. *Lancet, 2,* 296.
33. Cushing, A. H. and Smith, S. (1969): Methemoglobinemia with silver nitrate therapy of a burn: Report of a case. *J. Pediat., 74,* 613.
34. Dathan, J. G. and Harvey, C. C. (1965): Pink disease – ten years after. *Brit. med. J., 1,* 1181.
35. Dayal, V. S., Smith, E. L. and McCain, W. G. (1974): Cochlear and vestibular gentamicin toxicity: a clinical study of systemic and topical usage. *Arch. Otolaryng., 100,* 338.
36. De Groot, A. C. and Nater, J. P. (1981): Contact allergy to dithranol. *Contact Dermatitis, 7,* 5.
37. Deichmann, W. B. (1949): Local and systemic effects following skin contact with phenol – a review of the literature. *J. industr. Hyg., 31,* 146.
38. Del Pizzo, A. and Tanski, E. (1980): Chemical face peeling – Malignant therapy for benign disease? (editorial). *Plast. reconstr. Surg., 66,* 121.
39. Drake, T. E. (1974): Reaction to gentamycin sulfate cream. *Arch. Derm., 110,* 638.

40. Dubiel, W. and Happle, R. (1972): Behandlungsversuch mit Fumarsäure mono-äthylester bei Psoriasis vulgaris. *Z. Haut- u. Geschlkr., 47*, 545.

41. Editorial (1963): New source of mercury poisoning. *New Engl. J. Med., 269*, 926.

42. Editorial (1965): Burns and silver nitrate. *J. Amer. med. Ass., 193*, 230.

43. Ericsson, A. and Källen, B. (1978): *Report on a study of deliveries in women employed in medical occupations.* Report to the National Board of Health and Welfare, Sweden, 28 September 1978.

44. Etling, N., Gehin-Fouque, F., Vielh, J. P. et al. (1979): The iodine content of amniotic fluid and placental transfer of iodinated drugs. *Obstet. and Gynec., 53*, 376.

45. Farber, E. M. and Harris, D. R. (1970): Hospital treatment of psoriasis. *Arch. Derm., 101*, 381.

46. FDA Drug Bulletin (1976): Gamma benzene hexachloride (Kwell) and other products alert, *6*, 28.

47. Feiwell, M., James, V. H. T. and Barnett, E. S. (1969): Effect of potent topical steroids on plasma-cortisol levels of infants and children with eczema. *Lancet, 1*, 485.

48. Feldmann, R. J. and Maibach, H. I. (1974): Percutaneous penetration of some pesticides and herbicides in man. *Toxicol. appl. Pharmacol., 28*, 126.

49. Ferguson, M. M., Geddes, D. A. M. and Wray, D. (1978): The effect of a povidone-iodine mouthwash upon thyroid function and plaque accumulation. *Brit. dent. J., 144*, 14.

50. Fink, Th. J. and Gumps, D. W. (1978): Chloramphenicol: an inpatient study of use and abuse. *J. infect. Dis., 138*, 690.

51. Fisch, R. O., Berglund, E. B., Bridge, A. G., Finley, P. R., Quie, P. G. and Raile, R. (1963): Methemoglobinemia in a hospital nursery. *J. Amer. med. Ass., 185*, 760.

52. Fischer, T. and Hartvig, P. (1977): Skin absorption of 8-hydroxyquinolines. *Lancet, 1*, 603.

53. Flandin, C., Rabeau, H. and Ukrainczyk, M. (1953): Intolérance à la résorcine. Test cutané. *Soc. Derm. Syph., 12*, 1804.

54. Fraser, G. L. and Beaulieu, J. T. (1979): Leukopenia secondary to sulfadiazine silver. *J. Amer. med. Ass., 241*, 1928.

55. Friedmann, I. (1977): Aerosols containing neomycin. *Lancet, 1*, 1662.

56. Gasser, F. (1974): Allergien durch zahnärztliche Fremdstoffe. In: *Arzneimittelallergie*, pp. 197-202. Editors: M. Werner and W. Gronemeyer. Gustav Fischer Verlag, Stuttgart.

57. Gay, M. W., Moore, W. J., Morgan, J. M. and Montes, L. F. (1972): Anthralin toxicity. *Arch. Derm., 105*, 213.

58. Geivitz, W. and Wust, H. (1955): Über die Resorption von anorganischen Stoffen durch die menschliche Haut. *Z. ges. exp. Med., 125*, 587.

59. Gill, K. A. and Baxter, D. L. (1964): Plasma cortisol suppression by steroid creams. *Arch. Derm., 89*, 734.

60. Giménez, E. R., Vallejo, N. E., Roy, E., Lis, M., Izurieta, E. M., Rossi, S. and Capuccio, M. (1968): Percutaneous alcohol intoxication. *Clin. Toxicol., 1*, 39.

61. Ginsburg, C. M., Lowry, W. and Reisch, J. S. (1977): Absorption of lindane (gamma benzene hexachloride) in infants and children. *J. Pediat., 91*, 998.

62. Goebel, M. (1969): Mamillenhypertrophie mit Pigmentierung nach lokaler Oestrogentherapie im Kindesalter. *Hautarzt, 20*, 521.

63. Goffinet, M. (1977): A propos de la toxicité cliniquement présumable de certaines gouttes otiques. *Acta oto-rhino-laryng. belg., 31*, 585.

64. Goldbloom, R. B. and Goldbloom, A. (1953): Boric acid poisoning. Report of four cases and a review of 104 cases from the world literature. *J. Pediat., 43*, 631.

65. Goluboff, N. and MacFadyen, D. J. (1955): Methemoglobinemia in an infant. *J. Pediat., 47*, 222.

66. Gorter, E. (1949): On salicylate poisoning in children. *Acta paediat. (Uppsala), 37*, 170.

67. Grabbe, W. (1951): Gefahren bei der Behandlung spitzer Kondylome mit Podophyllin bei gleichzeitiger Neosalvarsan-Therapie. *Hautarzt, 2*, 325.

68. Graham, J. D. P. and Parker, W. A. (1948): Toxic manifestations of sodium salicylate therapy. *Quart. J. Med. (new series), 17*, 153.

69. Gross, H. and Greenberg, L. A. (1948): *Salicylates: Critical Bibliographic Review.* Hillhouse Press, New Haven, Connecticut.

70. Halling, H. (1977): Misstänkt samband mellan hexaklorofenexposition och missbildningsbörd. *Läkartidningen, 74*, 542.

71. Halling, H. (1979): Suspected link between exposure to hexachlorophene and malformed infants. *Ann. N.Y. Acad. Sci., 320*, 426.

72. Hansson, O. (1963): Acrodermatitis enterophatica. *Acta derm.-venereol. (Stockh.), 43*, 465.

73. Hansson, O. (1977): Vioform condemned. *Pediatrics, 60*, 769.

74. Harkness, R. A. and Beveridge, G. W. (1966): Isolation of β-naphthol from urine after its application to skin. *Nature (Lond.), 211*, 413.

75. Hasler, J. F. and Standish, S. M. (1969): Podophyllin treatment of hairy tongue: A warning. *J. Amer. dent. Ass., 78,* 563.

76. Hemels, H. G. W. M. (1972): Percutaneous absorption and distribution of 2-naphthol in man. *Brit. J. Derm., 87,* 614.

77. Herd, J. K., Cramer, A., Hoak, F. C. and Norcross, B. N. (1967): Ototoxicity of topical neomycin augmented by dimethyl sulfoxide. *Pediatrics, 40,* 905.

78. Hirschman, S. Z., Feingold, M. and Boylen, G. (1963): Mercury in house paints as a cause of acrodynia. Effect of therapy with N-acetyl-D,L-penicillamine. *New Engl. J. Med., 269,* 889.

79. Hopkins, J. (1979): Hexachlorophene: more bad news than good. *Food Cosm. Toxicol., 17,* 410.

80. Jarrett, F., Ellerbe, S. and Demling, R. (1978): Acute leukopenia during topical burn therapy with silver sulfadiazine. *Amer. J. Surg., 135,* 818.

81. Johnstone, R. T. (1948): *Occupational Medicine and Industrial Hygiene,* p. 216, C. V. Mosby Co., St. Louis, Mo.

82. Karol, K. D., Conner, Ch. S., Watanabe, A. S. and Murphey, K. J. (1980): Podophyllum: suspected teratogenicity from topical application. *Clin. Toxicol., 16,* 283.

83. Kellerhals, B. (1978): Hörschäden durch ototoxische Ohrtropfen. Ergebnisse einer Umfrage. *HNO (Berl.), 26,* 49.

84. Kelly, D. R., Nilo, E. N. and Berggren, R. B. (1969): Deafness after topical neomycin wound irrigation. *New Engl. J. Med., 280,* 1338.

85. Khaleeli, A. A. (1976): Quinaband-induced thrombocytopenic purpura in a patient with myxoedema. *Brit. med. J., 2,* 562.

86. Kligman, A. M. (1965): Dimethyl Sulfoxide – Part 2. *J. Amer. med. Ass., 193,* 151.

87. Krückemeyer, K. (1972): Argyrosis universalis nach Langzeittherapie mit silberhaltigen Präparaten. *Ärztl. Praxis, 24,* 18.

88. Landolt, R. and Mürset, G. (1968): Vorzeitige Pubertätsmerkmale als Folge unbeabsichtigter Östrogenverabreichung. *Schweiz. med. Wschr., 98,* 638.

89. Leading Article (1966): Boric acid and babies. *Lancet, 2,* 188.

90. Leclercq, A., Melennec, J. and Proteau, J. (1973): Intoxication mercurielle. *Concours méd., 95,* 6055.

91. Lee, B. and Groth, P. (1977): Scabies: Transcutaneous poisoning during treatment. *Pediatrics, 59,* 643.

92. Lindsey, C. P. (1968): Two cases of fatal salicylate poisoning after topical application of an antifungal solution. *Med. J. Aust., 1,* 353.

93. Lipman et al. (1952): Cited by Young (1952).

94. Lockart, J. D. (1972): How toxic is hexachlorophene? *Pediatrics, 50,* 229.

95. Lundell, E. and Nordman, R. (1973): A case of infantile poisoning by topical application of Castellani's solution. *Ann. clin. Res., 5,* 404.

96. Marshall, J. P. and Schneider, R. P. (1977): Systemic argyria secondary to topical silver nitrate. *Arch. Derm., 113,* 1072.

97. Masur, H., Whelton, P. K. and Whelton, A. (1976): Neomycin toxicity revisited. *Arch. Surg., 3,* 822.

98. May, Ph., Stern, E. J., Ryter, R. J., Hirsch, F. S., Michel, B. and Levy, R. P. (1976): Cushing syndrome from percutaneous absorption of triamcinolone cream. *Arch. intern. Med., 136,* 612.

99. Merck Index (1976): Ninth Edition, p. 291. Merck and Co., Inc., Rahway, N.J., U.S.A.

100. Meyboom, R. H. B. (1975): Metals. In: *Meyler's Side Effects of Drugs,* Vol. VIII, pp. 517-522. Editor: M. N. G. Dukes. Excerpta Medica, Amsterdam.

101. Michel, P. J., Buyer, R. and Delorme, G. (1958): Accidents géneraux (cyanose, collapsus cardiovasculaire) par sensibilisation a une solution aqueuse de violet de gentiane et vert de méthyle en applications locales. *Bull. Soc. franç. Derm. Syph., 65,* 183.

102. Milby, T. H. and Epstein, W. L. (1964): Allergic contact sensitivity to malathion. *Arch. environm. Hlth., 9,* 434.

103. Milstone, E. B., McDonald, A. J. and Scholhamer, C. F. (1981): Pseudomembranous colitis after topical application of clindamycin. *Arch. Derm., 117,* 154.

104. Mittelman, H. (1972): Ototoxicity of 'ototopical' antibiotics: past, present, and future. *Trans. Amer. Acad. Ophthal. Otolaryng., 76,* 1432.

105. Montaedi, J. P., Giambrone, J. P., Couley, N. A. and Taefi, P. (1978): Podophyllum poisoning associated with the treatment of condyloma acuminatum. *Amer. J. Obstet. Gynec., 119,* 1130.

106. Murphy, K. W. R. (1970): Deafness after topical neomycin (letter). *Brit. med. J., 2,* 144.

107. Murray, M. C. (1926): An analysis of sixty cases of drug poisoning. *Arch. Pediat., 43,* 193.

108. Ohlgisser, M., Adler, M., Ben-Dov, B., Taitelman, U., Birkhan, H. J. and Bursztein, S. (1978): Methaemoglobinaemia induced by mafenide acetate in children. A report of two cases. *Brit. J. Anaesth., 50,* 299.

207

109. Oliver, T. K. and Dyer, M. E. (1960): Prompt treatment of salicylism with sodium bicarbonate. *Amer. J. Dis. Child., 99,* 553.
110. Osol, A. and Farrar Jr, G. E. (1947): *The Dispensatory of the United States of America,* 24th Edition. Lippincott, Philadelphia.
111. Otten, H. and Plempel, M. (1975): Antibiotika und Chemotherapeutika in Einzeldarstellungen. Chemotherapeutika mit breitem Wirkungsbereich. Sulfonamide, pp. 110-145. In: *Antibiotika-Fibel.* Editors: H. Otten, M. Plempel and W. Siegenthaler. G. Thieme Verlag, Stuttgart.
112. Owens, C. J., Yarbrough, D. R. and Brackett, N. R. (1974): Nephrotic syndrome following topically applied sulfadiazine therapy. *Arch. intern. Med., 134,* 332.
113. Pegg, S. P., Ramsay, K., Meldrum, L. and Laundy, M. (1979): Clinical comparison of maphenide and silver sulphadiazine. *Scand. J. plast. reconstr. Surg., 13,* 95.
114. Pietsch, J. and Meakins, J. L. (1976): Complications of povidone-iodine absorption in topically treated burn patients. *Lancet, 2,* 280.
115. Pines, W. I. (1972): Hexachlorophane: Why FDA concluded that hexachlorophane was too potent and too dangerous to be used as it once was? *FDA Consumer, 6,* 24.
116. Plueckhahn, V. D., Ballard, B. A., Banks, J. M., Collins, R. B. and Flett, P. T. (1978): Hexachlorophene preparations in infant antiseptic skin care: benefit, risks and the future. *Med. J. Aust., 2,* 555.
117. Ponté, C., Richard, J., Bonte, C., Lequien, P. and Lacombe, A. (1974): Méthémoglobinémies chez le nouveau-né. Discussion du rôle étiologique du trichlorcarbanilide. *Ann. Pédiat., 21,* 359.
118. Powell, H., Swarner, O., Gluck, L. and Lamper, P. (1973): Hexachlorophene myelinopathy in premature infants. *J. Pediat., 82,* 976.
119. Prager, E. M. and Gardner, R. E. (1979): Iatrogenic hypothyroidism from topical iodine-containing medication. *West. J. Med., 130,* 553.
120. Pramanik, A. K. and Hansen, R. C. (1979): Transcutaneous gamma benzene hexachloride absorption and toxicity in infants and children. *Arch. Derm., 115,* 1224.
121. Pyati, S., Ramamurthy, R., Krause, M. et al. (1977): Absorption of iodine in the neonate following topical use of povidone-iodine. *J. Pediat., 91,* 825.
122. Quante, M. (1976): Taubheit mit lokaler Neomycinapplikation. *HNO (Berl.), 24,* 127.
123. Ramos, A. S. and Bower, B. F. (1969): Pseudoisosexual precocity due to cosmetics ingestion. *J. Amer. med. Ass., 207,* 369.
124. Ramu, A., Slonim, E. A. and Egal, F. (1973): Hyperglycemia in acute malathion poisoning. *Israel J. med. Sci., 9,* 631 (cited acc. to WHO, VBC/Tox/74.12. p. 24).
125. Ransone, J. W., Scott, N. M. and Knoblock, E. C. (1961): Selenium sulfide intoxication. *New Engl. J. Med., 264,* 384.
126. Omitted.
127. Roemeling, R. V., Hartwich, G. and König, H. (1979): Multilokuläre Krebsentstehung nach Arsentherapie. *Forum clin., 30,* 1928.
128. Rogers, S. C. F., Burrows, D. and Neill, D. (1978): Percutaneous absorption of phenol and methyl alcohol in magenta paint B.P.C. *Brit. J. Derm., 98,* 559.
129. Roman, D. P., Barnett, E. H. and Balske, R. J. (1957): Cutaneous antiseptic activity of 3,4,4`-trichlorocarbanilide. *Proc. sci. Sect. Toilet Goods Ass., 28,* 1213.
130. Ruedemann, R. and Deichmann, W. B. (1953): Blood phenol level after topical application of phenol-containing preparations. *J. Amer. med. Ass., 152,* 506.
131. Scharpf, L. G., Hill, I. D. and Maibach, H. I. (1975): Percutaneous penetration and disposition of triclocarban in man. *Arch. environm. Hlth., 30,* 7.
132. Schirren, C. G. (1966): Schwere Allgemeinvergiftung nach örtlicher Anwendung von Podophyllin-Spiritus bei spitzen Kondylomen. *Hautarzt, 17,* 321.
133. Shuman, R. M., Leech, W. R. and Alvord, E. C. (1974): Neurotoxicity of hexachlorophene in the human. I. A clinicopathologic study of 248 children. *Pediatrics, 54,* 689.
134. Silverberg, D. S., McCall, J. T. and Hunt, J. C. (1967): Nephrotic syndrome with use of ammoniated mercury. *Arch. intern. Med., 120,* 581.
135. Simpson, J. R. (1974): Reversed cross-sensitization between quinine and iodochlohydroxyquinoline. *Contact Dermatitis Newsl., 15,* 431.
136. Skipworth, G. B., Goldstein, N. and McBride, W. P. (1967): Boric acid intoxication from 'medicated talcum powder'. *Arch. Derm. Syph., 95,* 83.
137. Skoglund, R. R., Ware Jr, L. L. and Schanberger, J. E. (1977): Prolonged seizures due to contact and inhalation exposure to camphor. *Clin. Pediatr., 16,* 901.
138. Slater, G. E., Rumack, B. H. and Peterson, R. G. (1978): Podophyllin poisoning – Systemic toxicity following cutaneous application. *Obstet. and Gynec., 52,* 94.

139. Slee, P. H. T. J., Den Ottolander, G. J. and De Wolff, F. A. (1979): A case of merbromin (mercur-ochrome) intoxication possibly resulting in aplastic anemia. *Acta med. scand., 205*, 463.

140. Solomon, L. M., Fahrner, L. and West, D. P. (1977): Gamma benzene hexachloride toxicity. A Review. *Arch. Derm., 113*, 353.

141. Stanley-Brown, E. G. and Frank, J. E. (1971): Mercury poisoning from application to omphalocele (Letter to the Editor). *J. Amer. med. Ass., 216*, 2144.

142. Stoehr, G. P., Petersen, A. L. and Taylor, W. J. (1978): Systemic complications of local podophyllin therapy. *Ann. intern. Med., 89*, 362.

143. Stoppelman, M. R. H. and Van Valkenburg, R. A. (1955): Pigmentaties en gynecomastie ten gevolge van het gebruik van stilboestrol bevattend haarwater bij kinderen. *Ned. T. Geneesk., 99*, 3925.

144. Stoughton, R. B. (1979): Topical antibiotics for acne vulgaris: Current usage. *Arch. Derm., 115*, 486.

145. Strauch, B., Buch, W., Grey, W. and Laub, D. (1969): Successful treatment of methemoglobinemia secondary to silver nitrate therapy. *New Engl. J. Med., 281*, 257.

146. Tan, G. T. (1970): Occupational toxic alopecia due to Borax. *Acta derm.-venereol. (Stockh.), 50*, 55.

147. Tedesco, F. J. (1977): Clindamycin and colitis: A review. *J. infect. Dis., 135* (suppl.), 95.

148. Ternberg, J. L. and Luce, E. (1968): Methemoglobinemia: A complication of the silver nitrate treatment of burns. *Surgery, 63*, 328.

149. *The Merck Index* (1976): Ninth Edition. Merck and Co., Inc., Rahway, N. J., U.S.A.

150. Thomas, A. E. and Gisburn, M. A. (1961): Exogenous ochronosis and myxoedema from resorcinol. *Brit. J. Derm., 73*, 378.

151. Thompson, J. and Russell, J. A. (1970): Dermatitis due to mercury following amalgam dental restorations. *Brit. J. Derm., 82*, 292.

152. Treguer, G., Le Bihan, G., Coloignier, M., Le Roux, P. and Bernard, J. P. (1980): Intoxication salicylée par application locale de vaseline salicylée à 20% chez un psoriasique. *Nouv. Presse Méd., 9*, 192.

153. Truppman, E. S. and Ellerby, J. D. (1979): Major electrocardiographic changes during chemical face peeling. *Plast. reconstr. Surg., 63*, 44.

154. Turk, J. L. and Baker, H. (1968): Nephrotic syndrome due to ammoniated mercury. *Brit. J. Derm., 80*, 623.

155. Tyrala, E. E., Hillman, L. S., Hillman, R. E. and Dodson, W. E. (1977): Clinical pharmacology of hexachlorophene in newborn infants. *J. Pediat., 91*, 481.

156. Upjohn, A. C., Galbraith, H. J. B. and Solomons, B. (1971): Raised serum protein bound iodine after topical clioquinol. *Postgrad. Med., 47*, 515.

157. Utiger, R. D. (1979): Hypothyroidism. In: *Endocrinology*, pp. 471 - 488. Editor: L. J. de Groot. Grune and Stratton Inc., New York.

158. Valdes-Dapena, M. A. and Arey, J. B. (1962): Boric acid poisoning: three fatal cases with pancreatic inclusions and a review of the literature. *J. Pediat., 61*, 531.

159. Van der Harst, L. C. A., Smeenk, G., Burger, P. M., Van der Rhee, H. J. and Polano, M. K. (1978): Waardebepaling en risicoschatting van de uitwendige behandeling met clobetasol-17-propionaat (Dermovate). *Ned. T. Geneesk., 122*, 219.

160. Von Hinkel, G. K. and Kintzel, H. W. (1968): Phenolvergiftungen bei Neugeborenen durch kutane Resorption. *Dtsch. Gesundh.-Wes., 23*, 240.

161. Von Weiss, J. F. and Lever, W. F. (1964): Percutaneous salicylic acid intoxication in psoriasis. *Arch. Derm., 90*, 614.

162. Vorherr, H., Vorherr, U., Mehta, P., Ulrich, J. A. and Messer, R. H. (1980): Vaginal absorption of povidone-iodine. *J. Amer. med. Ass., 244*, 2628.

163. Voron, D. A. (1978): Systemic absorption of topical clindamycin. *Arch. Derm., 114*, 798.

164. Wallerstein, R. O., Condit, P. K., Brown, J. W. and Morrison, F. R. (1969): Statewide study of chloramphenicol-therapy and fatal aplastic anemia. *J. Amer. med. Ass., 208*, 2045.

165. Ward, J. W., Clifford, W. S., Monaco, A. R. and Bickerstaff, H. J. (1954): Fatal systemic poisoning following podophyllin treatment of condyloma acuminatum. *Sth. med. J. (Bgham, Ala.), 47*, 1204.

166. Ward, O. C. and Hingerty, D. (1967): Pink disease from cutaneous absorption of mercury. *J. Irish med. Ass., 60*, 94.

167. Wechselberg, K. (1969): Salizylsäure-Vergiftung durch perkutane Resorption 1%-iger Salizylvaseline. *Anästh. Prax., 4*, 103.

168. Woolley, P. B. (1952): Exogenous ochronosis. *Brit. med. J., 4*, 760.

169. Wüstner, H., Orfanos, C. E., Steinbach, H., Käferstein, H. and Herpers, H. (1975): Nagelverfärbung und Haarausfall. *Dtsch. med. Wschr., 100*, 1694.

170. Wuthrich, B., Zabrodsky, S. and Storck, H. (1972): Percutaneous poisoning by resorcinol, salicylic acid and ammoniated mercury. *Pharm. Acta Helv., 45,* 453.
171. Young, C. J. (1952): Salicylate intoxication from cutaneous absorption of salicylic acid. Citing Beyer (1880) and Lipman et al. (1952). *Sth. med. J. (Bgham, Ala.), 45,* 1075.
172. Young, E. (1960): Ammoniated mercury poisoning. *Brit. J. Derm., 72,* 449.
173. Zech, P., Colon, S., Labeeuw, R., Blanc-Brunat, N., Richard, P. and Porol, M. (1973): Syndrome néphrotique avec dépôt d'argent dans les membranes glomérulaires au cours d'une argyrie. *Nouv. Presse méd., 2,* 161.
174. Weinstein, L. (1975): Antimicrobial agents: Tetracyclines and chloramphenicol. In: *The Pharmacological Basis of Therapeutics, 5th Edition,* Chapter 59, p. 1196. Editors: L. Goodman and A. Gilman. Macmillan Publishing Co., Inc. New York-Toronto-London.

UPDATE – 2nd Edition

175. Davies, J. E., Dedhia, H. V., Morgade, C. et al. (1983): Lindane poisonings. *Arch. Derm., 119,* 142.
176. Albert, Th. A., Lewis, N. S. and Warpeha, R. L. (1982): Late pulmonary complications with use of mafenide acetate. *J. Burn Care Rehabil., 3,* 375.
177. Baranowska-Dutkiewicz, B. (1981): Skin absorption of phenol from aqueous solutions in men. *Int. Arch. occup. environm. Health, 49,* 99.
178. Rubenstein, A. D. and Musher, D. M. (1970): Epidemic boric acid poisoning simulating staphylococcal toxic epidermal necrolysis of the newborn infant: Ritter's disease. *J. Pediat., 77,* 884.
179. Martin-Bouyer, G., Lebreton, R., Toga, M. and Stolley, P. D. (1982): Outbreak of accidental hexachlorophene poisoning in France. *Lancet, 1,* 91.
180. Editorial (1982): Hexachlorophene today. *Lancet, 1,* 87.
181. Goldstein, G. S. (1982): Hexachlorophene poisoning (Letter). *Lancet, 1,* 500.
182. García-Buñuel, L. (1982): Toxicity of hexachlorophene (Letter). *Lancet, 1,* 1190.
183. Fisher, A. A. (1980): Irritant and toxic reactions to phenol in topical medications. *Cutis, 26,* 363.
184. Rubin, M. B. and Pirozzi, D. J. (1973): Contact dermatitis from carbolated vaseline. *Cutis, 12,* 52.
185. Birmingham, B. K., Greene, D. S. and Rhodes, C. T. (1979): Systemic absorption of topical salicylic acid. *Int. J. Derm., 18,* 228.
186. Baer, R. I., Serri, F. and Weissenbach-Vidal, C. (1955): Studies on allergic sensitization to certain topical therapeutic agents. *Arch. Derm., 71,* 19.
187. Andrews, G. C. and Domonkos, A. N. (1971): *Diseases of the Skin,* p. 87. W. B. Saunders, Philadelphia.
188. Bloch, R. and Beysovec, L. (1982): Promethazine toxicity through percutaneous absorption. *Contin. Practice, 9,* 28.
189. DiRaimondo, C. V., Roach, A. C. and Meador, C. K. (1980): Gynecomastia from exposure to vaginal estrogen cream (Letter). *New Engl. J. Med., 302,* 1089.
190. Hosler, J., Tschanz, C., Higuite, C. et al. (1980): Topical application of lindane cream (Kwell) and antipyrine metabolism. *J. invest. Derm., 74,* 51.
191. Giard, M. J., Uden, D. L. and Whitlock, D. J. (1983): Seizures induced by oral viscous lidocaine. *Clin. Pharmacy, 2,* 110.
192. Hunt, J. L., Sato, R., Heck, F. L. and Baxter, C. R. (1980): A critical evaluation of povidone-iodine absorption in thermally injured patients. *J. Trauma, 20,* 127.
193. Delaveau, P. and Freidrich-Noué, P. (1977): Absorption cutanée et élimination urinaire d'une combination sulfadiazine-argent utilisée dans le traitement des brûlures. *Thérapie, 32,* 563.
194. Shacter, B. (1981): Treatment of scabies and pediculosis with lindane preparations: An evaluation. *J. Amer. Acad. Derm., 5,* 517.
195. Rasmussen, J. E. (1981): The problem of lindane. *J. Amer. Acad. Derm., 5,* 507.
196. Matsuoka, L. Y. (1981): Convulsions following application of gamma benzene hexachloride. *J. Amer. Acad. Derm., 5,* 98.
197. Telch, J. and Jarvis, D. A. (1982): Acute intoxication with lindane (gamma benzene hexachloride). *Canad. med. Ass. J., 126,* 662.
198. Schillinger, B. M., Bernstein, M., Goldberg, L. A. and Shalita, A. R. (1982): Boric acid poisoning. *J. Amer. Acad. Derm., 7,* 667.
199. Edidin, D. V. and Levitsky, L. L. (1982): Prepubertal gynecomastia associated with estrogen-containing hair cream. *Amer. J. Dis. Child., 136,* 587.
200. Gabrilove, J. L. and Luria, M. (1978): Persistent gynecomastia resulting from scalp inunction of estradiol: A model for persistent gynecomastia. *Arch. Derm., 114,* 1672.

201. McDaniel, D. H., Blatchley, D. M. and Welton, W. A. (1982): Adverse systemic reaction to dinitrochlorobenzene (Letter). *Arch. Derm., 118,* 371.
202. Geffner, M. E., Powars, D. R. and Choctaw, W. T. (1981): Acquired methemoglobinemia. *West. J. Med., 1347,* 7.
203. Binstock, J. H. (1982): Safety of chemica face peels (Letter). *J. Amer. Acad. Derm., 7,* 137.
204. Barza, M., Goldstein, J. A., Kane, A. et al. (1982) Systemic absorption of clindamycin hydrochloride after topical application. *J. Amer. Acad. Derm., 7,* 208.
205. Clark, J. A., Kasselberg, A. G., Glick, A. D. and O'Neill, J. A. Jr. (1982): Mercury poisoning from merbromin (Mercurochrome^R) therapy of omphalocele. *Clin. Pediat. (Philad), 21,* 445.
206. Leslie, K. O. and Shitamoto, B. (1982): The bone marrow in systemic podophyllin toxicity. *Amer. J. clin. Path., 77,* 478.
207. Von Krogh, G. (1982): Selbstbehandlung von Condylomata acuminata mit 0.5%-iger Podophyllotoxinlösung. *Hautarzt, 33,* 571.
208. Cassidy, D. E., Drewry, J. and Fanning, J. P. (1982): Podophyllum toxicity: a report of a fatal case and a review of the literature. *J. Toxic. clin. Toxic., 19,* 35.
209. Gossweiler, B. (1982): Kampfervergiftungen heute. *Schweiz. Rundschau. Med. (PRAXIS), 71,* 1475.
210. Von Krogh, G. (1982): Podophyllotoxin in serum: absorption subsequent to three-day repeated applications of a 0.5% ethanolic preparation on Condylomata acuminata. *Sex. Transm. Diseases, 9,* 26.
211. Meynadier, J. and Peyron, J.-L. (1982): Résorption transcutanée des médicaments. *Rev. Pract. (Paris), 32,* 41.
212. Liebman, P. R., Kennelly, M. M. and Hirsch, E. F. (1982): Hypercarbia and acidosis associated with carbonic anhydrase inhibition: a hazard of topical mafenide acetate use in renal failure. *Burns, 8,* 395.
213. Litton, C. and Trinidad, G. (1981): Complications of chemical face peeling as evaluated by a questionnaire. *Plast. reconstr. Surg., 67,* 738.
214. Hedges, T. R. III, Kenyon, K. R., Hanninen, L. A. and Mosher, D. B. (1983): Corneal and conjuctival effects of monobenzone in patients with vitiligo. *Arch. Ophthal., 101,* 64.
215. Cammann, R., Hennecke, H. and Beier, R. (1971): Symptomatische Psychosen nach Kolton-Gelee-Applikation. *Psychiat. Neurol. med. Psychol., 23,* 426.
216. Goluboff, N. and MacFayden, D. J. (1955): Methemoglobinemia in an infant. *J. Pediat., 47,* 222.
217. Bloch, A. (1965): More on infantile methemoglobinemia due to benzocaine suppository. *J. Pediat., 67,* 509.
218. Bernstein, B. M. (1952): Cyanosis following the use of anesthesin (Ethyl Aminobenzoate). *Rev. Gastroent., 19,* 411.
219. Steinberg, J. B. and Zepernick, R. G. (1962): Methemoglobinemia during anesthesia. *J. Pediat., 61,* 885.
220. Becker, L. E., Bergstresser, P. R., Whiting, D. A. et al. (1981): Topical clindamycin therapy for acne vulgaris: A cooperative clinical study. *Arch. Derm., 117,* 482.
221. Franz, T. J. (1983): On the bioavailability of topical formulations of clindamycin hydrochloride. *J. Amer. Acad. Derm., 9,* 66.
222. De Groot, A. C., Nater, J. P., Bleumink, E. and de Jong, M. C. J. M. (1981): Does DNCB therapy potentiate epicutaneous sensitization to non-related contact allergens? *Clin. exp. Derm., 6,* 139.
223. Feldman, R. J. and Maibach, H. I. (1970): Absorption of some organic compounds through the skin in man. *J. invest. Derm., 54,* 399.
224. Adriani, J. and Zepernick, R. (1964): Clinical effectiveness of drugs used for topical anesthesia. *J. Amer. Med. Ass., 118,* 711.
225. Seldon, R. and Sasahara, A. A. (1967): Central nervous system toxicity induced by lidocaine. *J. Amer. Med. Ass., 202,* 908.
226. Mofenson, H. C., Caraccio, T. R., Miller, H. and Greensher, J. (1983): Lidocaine toxicity from topical mucosal application. *Clin. Pediat., 22,* 190.
227. Yeung, D., Kantor, S., Nacht, S. and Gans, E. H. (1983): Percutaneous absorption, blood levels and urinary excretion of resorcinol applied topically in humans. *Int. J. Derm., 22,* 321.
228. Roberts, M. S., Anderson, R. S. and Swarbrick, J. (1977): Permeability of human epidermis to phenolic compounds. *J. Pharm. Pharmacol., 29,* 677.
229. Flickinger, C. W. (1976): The benzenediols: A review of the industrial toxicity and current industrial exposure limit. *Amer. Industr. Hyg. Ass. J., 37,* 596.
230. D'Arcy, P. F. (1982): Fatalities with the use of a henna dye. *Pharmacy Int., 3,* 217.
231. El-Ansary, E. H., Ahmed, M. E. K. and Clague, H. W. (1983): Systemic toxicity of para-phenylenediamine. *Lancet, 1,* 1341.

232. Günther, S. and Freitag, F. (1975): Therapeutic value and side-effects of retinoic (vitamin A) acid on human patients and animal experimental investigations on rats. *Derm. Mschr., 161,* 137.
233. Muller, S. A., Belcher, R. W., Esterly, N. B. et al. (1977): Keratinizing dermatoses: Combined data from four centers on short-term topical treatment with tretinoin. *Arch. Derm., 113,* 1052.
234. Thomas, J. R. III and Doyle, J. A. (1981): The therapeutic uses of topical vitamin A acid. *J. Amer. Acad. Derm., 4,* 505.
235. Reuveni, H. and Yagupsky, P. (1982): Diethyltoluamide-containing insect repellent. Adverse effects in worldwide use. *Arch. Derm., 118,* 582.
236. Grybowksy, J., Weinstein, D. and Ordway, N. (1961): Toxic encephalopathy apparently related to the use of an insect repellent. *New. Engl. J. Med., 264,* 289.
237. Zadicoff, C. (1979): Toxic encephalopathy associated with use of insect repellent. *J. Pediat., 95,* 140.
238. Gabrilove, J. L. and Luria, M. (1978): Persistent gynecomastia resulting from scalp inunction of estradiol: A model for persistent gynecomastia. *Arch. Derm., 114,* 1672.
239. Kramer, M. S., Hutchinson, T. A., Rudnick, S. A. et al. (1980): Operational criteria for adverse drug reactions in evaluating suspected toxicity of a popular scabicide. *Clin. Pharmacol. Ther., 27,* 149.
240. Feldman, R. J. and Maibach, H. I. (1970): Absorption of some organic compounds through the skin in man. *J. invest. Derm., 54,* 399.
241. Cullison, D., Abele, D. C. and O'Quinn, J. L. (1983): Localized exogenous ochronosis. Report of a case and review of the literature. *J. Amer. Acad. Derm., 8,* 882.
242. Klein, D. R. and Little, J. H. (1983): Laryngeal edema as a complication of chemical peel. *Plast. reconstr. Surg., 71,* 149.
243. Tromovitch, T. A. (1982): Safety of chemical face peels (Letter). *J. Amer. Acad. Derm., 7,* 137.
244. Baker, T. J. (1979): The voice of polite dissent. *Plast. reconstr. Surg., 63,* 262.
245. Check, W. (1978): New study shows hexachlorophene is teratogenic in humans. *J. Amer. Med. Ass., 240,* 513.
246. Janerich, D. T. (1979): Environmental causes of birth defects. The hexachlorophene issue. *J. Amer. Med. Ass., 241,* 830.
247. Gluck, L. (1980): Hexachlorophene: a useful and lifesaving drug. In: *Controversies in Therapeutics,* p. 436. Ed.: L. Lasagna Saunders, Philadelphia.
248. Plueckhahn, V. D. (1980): Hexachlorophene preparations and the newborn infant. *Aust. Paediat. J., 16,* 40.
249. Stein, K. M., Odom, R. B., Justice, G. R. and Martin, G. C. (1973): Toxic alopecia from ingestion of boric acid. *Arch. Derm., 108,* 95.
250. Hunt, J. L. et al. (1980): The systemic effects of a burn ointment. *Emergency Med., 12,* 159.
251. Lyen, K. R., Finegold, D., Orsini, R. et al. (1982): Transient thyroid suppression associated with topically applied povidone-iodine. *Amer. J. Dis. Child., 136,* 369.
252. Gee, S. (1979): Topical burn agents. *Amer. Pharmacy, 19,* 30.
253. AMA Drug Evaluations (1977). 3d Ed., p. 269. Publishing Sciences Group, Inc., Littleton, MA.
254. Haggerty, R. J. (1962): Blue baby due to methemoglobinemia. *New Engl. J. Med., 267,* 1303.
255. Adriani, J. and Zepernick, R.: Summary of methemoglobinemia: Study of child receiving benzocaine. Letter to the Commissioner in OTC, Volume 060150.
256. Olson, M. L. and McEvoy, G. K. (1981): Methemoglobinemia induced by local anesthetics. *Amer. J. Hosp. Pharm., 38,* 89.
257. Taylor, J. R. and Halprin, K. (1975): Percutaneous absorption of salicylic acid. *Arch. Derm., 106,* 740.
258. United States Department of Health, Education and Welfare, Food and Drug Administration, OTC Antimicrobial II Advisory Panel. Quoted by Rasmussen, J. E. (1979): Percutaneous absorption in children. In: *Year Book of Dermatology, 1979,* p. 28. Ed: R. L. Dobson. Year Book Medical Publishers, Inc., Chicago.
259. Lyons, T. J., Christer, C. N. and Larsen, F. S. (1975): Ammoniated mercury ointment and the nephrotic syndrome. *Minn. Med., 58,* 383.
260. Benson, P. F. and Pharoah, P. O. D. (1960): Benign intracranial hypertension due to adrenal steroid therapy. *Guy's Hosp. Rep., 109,* 202.
261. Fanconi, G. (1962): Hemmung des Wachstums bei einem Säugling durch die zu intensive Anwendung einer 1 %-igen Hydrocortisonsalb auf der Haut bei generalisierten Ekzem. *Helv. Paediat. Acta, 17,* 267.
262. Feinblatt, B. I., Aceto, T. Jr., Bechhorn, G. and Bruck, E. (1966): Percutaneous absorption of hydrocortisone in children. *Amer. J. Dis. Child., 112,* 218.

263. Feiwel, M., James, V. H. T. and Barnett, E. S. (1969): Effect of potent topical steroids on plasma-cortisol levels of infants and children with eczema. *Lancet, 1,* 485.

264. Johns, A. M. and Bower, R. D. (1970): Wasting of napkrin area after repeated use of fluorinated steroid ointment. *Brit. Med. J., 111,* 347.

265. Keipert, J. A. and Kelly, R. (1971): Temporary Cushing's syndrome from percutaneous absorption of betamethasone-17-valerate. *Med. J. Aust., 11,* 542.

266. Kelly, A., Nelson, K., Goodwin, M. and McCluggage, J. (1972): Iatrogenic Cushing's syndrome. *Brit. Med. J., 4,* 114.

267. Pascher, F. (1978): Systemic reactions to topically applied drugs. *Int. J. Derm., 17,* 768.

268. Rimbaud, P., Serre, H., Meynadier, J. and Baumelou, H. (1973): Accidents cortisonique graves a-près corticotherapie locale prolongée pour M. F. avec xanthomatisation des lesions. *Bull. Soc. franç. Derm. Syph., 80,* 176.

269. Schorr, W. F. and Papa, C. M. (1973): Epidermolytic hyperkeratosis. *Arch. Derm., 107,* 556.

270. Vermeer, B. J. and Heremans, G. F. P. (1974): A case of growth retardation and Cushing's syn-drome due to excessive application of betamethasone-17-valerate ointment. *Dermatologica (Basel), 149,* 299.

271. Cook, L. J., Freinkel, R. K., Zugerman, Ch. et al. (1982): Iatrogenic hyperadrenocorticism during topical steroid therapy: assessment of systemic effects by metabolic criteria. *J. Amer. Acad. Derm., 6,* 1054.

272. Feldmann, R. J. and Maibach, H. I. (1965): Penetration of 14C hydrocortisone through normal skin. *Arch. Derm., 91,* 661.

273. Leu, F. (1983): Complications from prolonged topical steroid therapy (Letter to the Editor). *J. Amer. Acad. Derm., 8,* 425.

274. May, P. and Stein, E. J. (1976): Cushing's syndrome from percutaneous absorption of triamcinolone cream. *Arch. intern. Med., 136,* 612.

275. Burton, T. T., Cunliffe, W. J., Holti, G. and Wright, W. (1974): Complications of topical cortico-steroid therapy in patients with liver disease. *Brit. J. Derm., 9 (Suppl. 10),* 22.

276. Staughton, R. C. D. and August, P. (1975): Cushing's syndrome and pituitary adrenal suppression due to clobetasol propionate. *Brit. med., J. 2,* 419.

277. Himathongkam, T., Dasanabhairochana, P., Ninlawan, P. and Sriphrapradang, A. (1978) Florid Cushing's syndrome and hirsutism induced by desoximetasone. *J. Amer. med. Ass., 239,* 430.

278. Brand, J. J. and Whittingham, P. (1970): Intramuscular hyoscine in control of motion-sickness. *Lancet, 2,* 232.

279. Davies, J. A. and Wiesel, B. H. (1955): The treatment of angina pectoris with a nitroglycine oint-ment. *Amer. J. med. Sci., 230,* 259.

280. Garnier, B., Imhof, P., Spinell, F. and Jost, H. (1982): Die Behandlung der Angina Pectoris mit einem neuen transdermalen therapeutischen System von Nitroglycerin unter Praxisbedingungen. *Schweiz. Rundschau Med. (Praxis), 71,* 511.

281. Lepore, F. E. (1982): More on cycloplegia from transdermal scopolamine. *New. Engl. J. Med., 307,* 824.

282. Müller, P., Imhof, P. F., Burkart, F., Chu, L.-C and Gerardin, A. (1982): Human pharmacological studies of a new transdermal system containing nitroglycerin. *Europ. J. clin. Pharmacol., 22,* 473.

283. Osterholm, R. K. and Camoriano, J. (1982): Transdermal scopolamine psychosis. *J. Amer. med. Ass., 247,* 3081.

284. Price, N. M., Schmitt, L. G., McGuire, Ph. D., Shaw, J. E. and Trobough, G. (1980): Transdermal scopolamine in the prevention of motion-sickness at sea. *Clin. Pharmacol. Ther., 29,* 414.

285. Schwartz, A. M. (1946): The cause, relief and prevention of headaches arising from contact with dynamite. *New Engl. J. Med., 235,* 541.

286. Hays, L. L., Novack, A. J. and Worsham, J. C. (1982): The Frey syndrome: A simple, effective treatment. *Otolaryngol. Head Neck Surg., 90,* 419.

287. Olivari, M.-T. and Cohn, J. N. (1983): Cutaneous administration of nitroglycerin: a review. *Phar-macotherapy, 3,* 149.

288. Zackheim, H. S., Epstein, E. H. Jr., McNutt, N. S. et al. (1983): Topical carmustine (BCNU) for mycosis fungoides and related disorders: A 10-year experience. *J. Amer. Acad. Derm., 9,* 363.

289. Zackheim, H. S., Feldman, R. J., Lindsay, C. and Maibach, H. I. (1977): Percutaneous absorption of 1,3-bis(2-chloroethyl)-1-nitrosurea (BCNU, carmustine) in mycosis fungoides. *Brit. J. Derm., 97,* 65.

290. Bennett, C. C. (1980): Dimethyl sulfoxide. *J. Amer. Med. Ass., 244,* 2768.

291. Castot, A., Garnier, R., Lanfranchi, C. et al (1980): Effets systémiques indésirables des médica-ments appliqués sur la peau chez l'enfant. *Thérapie, 35,* 423.

16.102 Systemic side effects

292. Aronoff, G. R., Friedman, S. J., Doedens, P. J. et al (1980): Increased serum iodide concentration from iodine absorption through wounds treated topically with povidone-iodine. *Amer. J. med. Sci., 279*, 173.
293. Boekhorst, J. C. (1983): Allergic contact dermatitis with transdermal clonidine. *Lancet, 2*, 1031.
294. Ellis, C. N., Mitchell, A. J. and Beardsley, G. R. Jr. (1979): Tar gel interaction with disulfiram. *Arch. Derm., 115*, 1367.
295. Stoll, D. and King, L. E. Jr. (1980): Disulfiram – alcohol skin reaction to beer-containing shampoo (Letter). *J. Amer. med. Ass., 244*, 2045.

17. Systemic eczematous contact-type dermatitis medicamentosa

17.1   In patients with a delayed-type hypersensitivity to a certain drug, oral or parenteral administration of this drug or chemically related compounds may lead to the following side effects:

1. Focal flares at sites of previous dermatitis (and sites of patch testing)
2. Dyshidrotic eruptions
3. Generalized eruptions, including generalized urticaria and erythroderma
4. Systemic effects such as nausea, vomiting, generalized itching, fever, headache, diarrhea, hot flush and syncope.

Such reactions were termed 'hämatogenes Kontaktekzem' by Binder [5], and 'endogenic contact eczema' by Pirilä [42]. The title of this chapter is derived from the terminology used by Fisher [15].

These effects may be provoked in some, but not all sensitized subjects; they may be produced not only by the sensitizing drug, but also by chemically related substances.

The most frequent reactions are focal flares at sites of previous dermatitis or occasionally dyshidrotic eruptions, but generalized eruptions may occur, sometimes accompanied by systemic effects. Sometimes reactions are noted within hours after the administration of the allergen, which suggests that both an immediate and a delayed type of hypersensitivity may be involved.

A list of drugs that have caused systemic eczematous contact-type dermatitis, is given in § 17.2.

17.2   **Systemic eczematous contact-type dermatitis medicamentosa**

Delayed-type hypersensitivity to:	Use	Substance that caused the eruption	Comment	Ref.
p-aminobenzoic acid	sunscreen	p-aminobenzoic acid		10
antazoline	antihistamine	pyribenzamine	Both drugs are ethylenediamine derivatives	45
antazoline	antihistamine in eye drops	aminophylline	Antazoline is an ethylenediamine derivative; aminophylline contains ethylenediamine	58
arsphenamine	organic arsenical	neoarsphenamine	Inhalation of neoarsphenamine caused asthma, fever, urticaria and gastrointestinal symptoms	53
balsam Peru	various	orange marmalade, vanilla sugar, fruits and ices		27 42 28

(continued)

17.2   Systemic eczematous contact-type dermatitis

(continuation)

Delayed-type hypersensitivity to:	Use	Substance that caused the eruption	Comment	Ref.
benzocaine	local anesthetic	chlorpropamide	Both drugs are PARA-compounds	59
butylated hydroxyanisole	antioxidant	butylated hydroxyanisole		44 18
butylated hydroxytoluene	antioxidant	butylated hydroxyanisole and butylated hydroxytoluene		44
chloralhydrate	scalp medication, hypnotic	chloral hydrate		2 8
chlorpromazine	sedative	chlorpromazine	Accidental contact in a nurse	40
cinnamon oil	flavor	cinnamon oil	Flare-up of previous eczema of the hands	35
dibucaine	local anesthetic	p-aminophenylsulfamide		46
diphenhydramine hydrochloride	antihistamine	diphenhydramine hydrochloride		57
disulfiram	in cosmetics, foods and rubber industry	disulfiram	One patient had been sensitized by previous disulfiram implants	33 22
ethyl alcohol	antiseptic, in beverages	alcohol		12
ethylenediamine	preservative	aminophylline	Aminophylline is a combination of theophylline and ethylenediamine	43 41 56
ethylenediamine	preservative	piperazine citrate		6 4
formaldehyde	in plastics, textile finishes and antiperspirants	hexamethylene tetramine	Hexamethylene tetramine liberates formaldehyde in an acid medium	49
furazolidine	antimicrobial	furantoin	Accidental contact in food industry	29
glycerol	vehicle ingredient	glycerol		24
halogenated hydroxyquinolines	antiseptics and antifungal drugs	halogenated hydroxyquinolines		48 13 36
mercurials	antiseptics	amalgam filling		30
methyl salicylate	anti-inflammatory drug	acetylsalicylic acid		25
neomycin	antibiotic	neomycin		13
nystatin	antifungal drug	nystatin		9
parabens	preservatives	parabens		1 32

(continued)

(continuation)

Delayed-type hypersensitivity to:	Use	Substance that caused the eruption	Comment	Ref.
penicillin	antibiotic	penicillin	Anaphylaxis may occur	51
peppermint oil	flavor	peppermint oil		11
pheniramine	antihistamine	diphenhydramine		14
phenylbutazone	anti-inflammatory drug	phenylbutazone	Cross-reaction to oxyphenbutazone	52
p-phenylenediamine	various	sulfonamides, procaine	Anaphylactic reactions have occurred	46
piperazine	vermifuge	hydroxyzine, buclizine	Accidental contact in pharmaceutical industry	21 7
pristinamycin	antibiotic	pristinamycin	Anaphylaxis with stupor, vomiting and urticaria occurred	3
procaine	local anaesthetic	procaine		46 20
promethazine	antihistamine	promethazine		47
propylene glycol	vehicle constituent	propylene glycol		24 19 55
quinine	in liquids and hair preparations	quinine		31
sorbic acid	preservative	sorbic acid		63
streptomycin	antibiotic	streptomycin	The drug was administered subcutaneously for desensitization Has caused urticaria also	54
sulfanilamide	chemotherapeutic in vaginal cream	tolbutamide chlorpropamide carbutamide	Tolbutamide, chlorpropamide and carbutamide are sulfonylurea antidiabetic drugs	59 61
sulfonamide	chemotherapeutic	sulfonamides		50 46
tetramethylthiuram disulfide	rubber chemical	tetramethylthiuram disulfide	An oral provocation test was positive. TMTD is also used as antifermentative agent in certain foods	60
thiomersal	antiseptic	thiomersal		37
virginiamycin	antibiotic	virginiamycin		34
vitamin B_1	vitamin	vitamin B_1	Accidental contact	26
vitamin B_{12}	treatment of pernicious anemia	vitamin B_{12}	The patients were sensitized y the cobalt in vitamin B_{12}	16 38
vitamin C	vitamin	vitamin C		39

17.3   Systemic eczematous contact-type dermatitis

17.3   According to Fisher [17, 62] many other substances may or might also induce systemic eczematous contact-type dermatitis after previous sensitization to these or chemically related substances (§ 17.4); however, no case reports were documented.

17.4   **Possibilities for systemic eczematous contact-type dermatitis [17, 62]**

Delayed-type hypersensitivity to:	Use	Drugs that may cause the eruption
p-amino compounds	various	other p-amino compounds, azo-dyes
diphenhydramine	antihistamine	clemastine fumarate, carbinoxamine maleate, dimenhydrinate and doxylamine succinate (all are ethanolamine-antihistamines)
ethanolamine	vehicle constituent	ethanolamine antihistamines (*see under* diphenhydramine)
ethylenediamine	preservative	tripelennamine, promethazine*, phenindamine, methapyrilene, pyrilamine maleate, chlorcyclizine, cyclizine, buclizine, meclizine, hydroxyzine hydrochloride and pamoate
hydrazine hydrobromide (accidental contact)	solder flux	isoniazid, apresoline, phenelzine dihydrogen sulfate
mercurials	antiseptics	mercurial diuretics, calomel, amalgam fillings, cinnabar in tattoos
neomycin	antibiotic	streptomycin, kanamycin, paromomycin, ambutyrosin
procaine	local anesthetic	sulfonamides
promethazine	antihistamine	chlorpromazine, pyribenzamine, phenindamine tartrate
resorcinol	peeling agent	hexylresorcinol
sulfonamides	chemotherapeutics	sulfonamide diuretics, sulfonamide antidiabetics (§ 17.2), sulfonamide sweetening agents
tripelennamine	antihistamine	ethylenediamine tripelennamine methapyrilene pyrilamine maleate

* The study of King and Beck [64] suggests that oral promethazine is safe in ethylenediamine-allergic patients.

17.5   REFERENCES

1. Aeling, J. L. and Nuss, D. D. (1974): Systemic eczematous 'contact type' dermatitis medicamentosa caused by parabens. *Arch. Derm., 110,* 640.
2. Baer, R. L. and Sulzberger, M. B. (1938): Eczematous dermatitis due to chloralhydrate (following both oral administration and topical application). *J. Allergy, 9,* 519.
3. Baes, H. (1974): Allergic contact dermatitis to virginiamycin. *Dermatologica (Basel), 149,* 231.
4. Bernstein, J. E. and Lorincz, A. L. (1979): Ethylenediamine induced exfoliative erythroderma. *Arch. Derm., 112,* 156.

5. Binder, E. (1954): Über das hämatogene Kontaktekzem. *Archive für Derm., 198,* 1.
6. Burry, J. N. (1978): Ethylenediamine sensitivity with a systemic reaction to piperazine citrate. *Contact Dermatitis, 4,* 380.
7. Calas, E., Castelain, P. Y., Blanc, A. and Campana, J. M. (1975): Un nouveau cas de sensibilisation à la pipérazine. *Bull. Soc. franç. Derm. Syph., 82,* 41.
8. Christianson, H. B. and Perry, H. O. (1956): Reactions to chloralhydrate. *Arch. Derm., 74,* 232.
9. Cronin, E. (1980): In: *Contact Dermatitis,* p. 233. Churchill Livingstone, Edinburgh.
10. Curtis, G. H. and Crawford, P. F. (1951): Cutaneous sensitivity to monoglycerol para-aminobenzoate: Cross-sensitization and bilateral eczematization. *Cleveland Clin. Quart., 18,* 35.
11. Dooms-Goossens, A., Degreef, H., Holvoet, C. and Maertens, M. (1977): Turpentine-induced hypersensitivity to peppermint oil. *Contact Dermatitis, 3,* 304.
12. Drevets, C. C. and Seebohm, P. M. (1961): Dermatitis from alcohol. *J. Allergy, 32,* 277.
13. Ekelund, A. G. and Möller, H. (1969): Oral provocation in eczematous contact allergy to neomycin and hydroxyquinolines. *Acta derm.-venereol. (Stockh.), 49,* 422.
14. Epstein, E. (1949): Dermatitis due to antihistamine agents. *J. invest. Derm., 12,* 151.
15. Fisher, A. A. (1966): Systemic eczematous 'contact-type' dermatitis medicamentosa. *Ann. Allergy, 24,* 406.
16. Fisher, A. A. (1972): Contact dermatitis: At home and abroad. *Cutis, 10,* 719.
17. Fisher, A. A. (1973): *Contact Dermatitis,* 2nd Edition, pp. 293-305. Lea and Febiger, Philadelphia.
18. Fisher, A. A. (1975): Contact dermatitis due to food additives. *Cutis, 16,* 961.
19. Fisher, A. A. (1978): Propylene glycol dermatitis. *Cutis, 21,* 166.
20. Fisher, A. A. and Sturm, H. M. (1958): Procaine sensitivity. The relationship of the allergic eczematous contact-type to the urticarial-anaphylactoid variety. *Ann. Allergy, 16,* 593.
21. Fregert, S., cited by Fisher, A. A. (1973): In: *Contact Dermatitis,* 2nd Edition, p. 295. Lea and Febiger, Philadelphia.
22. Goitre, M., Bedello, P. G. and Cane, D. (1981): Allergic dermatitis and oral challenge to tetramethylthiuram disulphide. *Contact Dermatitis, 7,* 272.
23. Hannuksela, M. and Förström, L. (1976): Contact hypersensitivity to glycerol. *Contact Dermatitis, 2,* 291.
24. Hannuksela, M. and Förström, L. (1978): Reactions to peroral propyleneglycol. *Contact Dermatitis, 4,* 41.
25. Hindson, C. (1977): Contact eczema from methylsalicylate reproduced by oral aspirin (acetylsalicylic acid). *Contact Dermatitis, 3,* 348.
26. Hjorth, N. (1958): Contact dermatitis from Vitamin B1 (thiamine). Relapse after ingestion of thiamine. Cross-sensitization to co-carboxylase. *J. invest. Derm., 30,* 261.
27. Hjorth, N. (1961): *Eczematous Allergy to Balsams, Allied Perfumes and Flavoring Agents.* Munkgaard, Copenhagen.
28. Hjorth, N. (1971): Allergy to Balsams. *Spectrum, 8,* 97.
29. Jirásek, L. and Kalensky, J. (1975): Kontakni alergicky ekzém z krmných směsi v živočisné výrobě. *Čs. Derm., 50,* 217.
30. Johnson, H. H., Schonberg, I. L. and Bach, N. F. (1951): Chronic atopic dermatitis with pronounced mercury sensitivity. Partial clearing after extraction of teeth containing mercury amalgam fillings. *Soc. Trans. A.M.A. Arch. Derm., 63,* 279.
31. Klaschka, F. (1964): Zur Kasuistik hochgradiger Chinin-Kontaktallergie. *Derm. Wschr., 149,* 4.
32. Kleinhans, D. and Knoth, W. (1973): Paraben-Kontaktallergie mit enteraler Provokation. *Z. Haut-u. Geschlkr., 48,* 699.
33. Lachapelle, J. M. (1975): Allergic 'contact' dermatitis from disulfiram implants. *Contact Dermatitis, 1,* 218.
34. Lachapelle, J. M. and Lamy, F. (1973): On allergic contact dermatitis to virginiamycin. *Dermatologica (Basel), 146,* 320.
35. Leifer, W. (1951): Contact dermatitis due to cinnamon. *Arch. Derm., 64,* 52.
36. Leifer, W. and Steiner, K. (1951): Studies in sensitization to halogenated hydroxyquinolines and related compounds. *J. invest. Derm., 17,* 233.
37. MacKenzie, D. and Vlahcevic, Z. R. (1979): Adverse reaction to gammaglobulin due to hypersensitivity to thiomersal. *New Engl. J. Med., 290,* 749.
38. Malten, K. E. (1975): Flare reaction due to vitamin B12 in a patient with psoriasis and contact eczema. *Contact Dermatitis, 1,* 325.
39. Metz, J., Hundertmark, U. and Pevny, I. (1980): Vitamin C allergy of the delayed type. *Contact Dermatitis, 6,* 172.
40. Morris-Owen, R. M. (1963): 'Cover-Dose' management of contact sensitivity to chlorpromazine. *Brit. J. Derm., 75,* 167.

17.5 Systemic eczematous contact-type dermatitis

41. Petrozzi, J. W. and Shore, R. N. (1976): Generalized exfoliative dermatitis from ethylenediamine. *Arch. Derm., 112,* 525.
42. Pirilä, V. (1970): Endogenic contact eczema. *Allergie u. Asthma, 16,* 15.
43. Provost, T. T. and Field Jillson, O. (1967): Ethylene diamine contact dermatitis. *Arch. Derm., 96,* 231.
44. Roed-Petersen, J. and Hjorth, N. (1976): Contact dermatitis from antioxidants. *Brit. J. Derm., 94,* 233.
45. Sherman, W. B. and Cooke, R. A. (1950): Dermatitis following the use of pyribenzamine and Antistine. *J. Allergy, 21,* 63.
46. Sidi, E. and Dobkevitch-Morrill, S. (1951): The injection- and ingestion test in cross-sensitization to the ParaGroup. *J. invest. Derm., 16,* 299.
47. Sidi, E., Hincky, M. and Gervais, A. (1955): Allergic sensitization and photosensitization to phenergan cream. *J. invest. Derm., 24,* 345.
48. Skog, E. (1975): Systemic eczematous contact-type dermatitis induced by iodochlorhydroxyquin and chloroquine phosphate. *Contact Dermatitis, 1,* 187.
49. Sulzberger, M. B. (1940): *Dermatologic Allergy,* p. 380. Charles C. Thomas, Springfield, Illinois.
50. Sulzberger, M. B., Kanof, A., Baer, R. L. and Löwenberg, C. (1947): Sensitization by topical application of sulfonamides. *J. Allergy, 18,* 92.
51. Vickers, H. R., Bagratuni, L. and Alexander, S. (1958): Dermatitis caused by penicillin milk. *Lancet, 61,* 351.
52. Vooys, R. Chr. and Van Ketel, W. G. (1977): Allergic drug eruption from pyrazolone compounds. *Contact Dermatitis, 3,* 57.
53. Vuletić, A. (1934): Über Salvarsanüberempfindlichkeit mit akuter Salvarsan-Intoxikation infolge beruflicher Benetzungen der Finger mit Salvarsanlösungen. *Arch. Derm. Syph. (Berl.), 169,* 436.
54. Wilson, H. T. H. (1958): Streptomycin dermatitis in nurses. *Brit. med. J., 1,* 1378.

UPDATE – 2nd Edition

55. Andersen, K.E. and Storrs, F. (1982): Hautreizungen durch Propylenglykol. *Hautarzt, 33,* 12.
56. Neumann, H. (1983): Allergische und toxische Nebenwirkungen von Ethylendiamin. *Allergologie, 6,* 27.
57. Coskey, R.J. (1983): Contact dermatitis caused by diphenhydramine hydrochloride. *J. Amer. Acad Derm., 8,* 204.
58. Berman, B.A. and Ross, R.N. (1983): Ethylenediamine: Systemic eczematous contact-type dermatitis. *Cutis, 31,* 594.
59. Fisher, A.A. (1982): Systemic contact dermatitis from Orinase® and Diabinese® in diabetics with para-amino hypersensitivity. *Cutis, 29,* 551.
60. Goitre, M., Bedello, P.G. and Cane, D. (1981): Allergic dermatitis and oral challenge to tetramethylthiuram disulphide. *Contact Dermatitis, 7,* 273.
61. Angelini, G. and Meneghini, C.L. (1981): Oral tests in contact allergy to para-amino compounds. *Contact Dermatitis, 7,* 311.
62. Fisher, A.A. (1980): The antihistamines. *J. Amer. Acad. Derm., 3,* 303.
63. Röckl, H. and Pevny, I. (1976): *Fortschritte der praktischen Dermatologie und Venereologie.* Springer Verlag, Berlin.
64. King. C.M. and Beck, M. (1983): Oral promethazine hydrochloride in ethylenediamine-sensitive patients. *Contact Dermatitis, 9,* 444.

18. Side effects of photochemotherapy

PUVA THERAPY

18.1 In photochemotherapy, therapeutic advantage is taken of the interaction of a phototoxic drug and light, usually an undesirable effect, for the treatment of cutaneous disorders. Classic examples are the Goeckerman regimen for psoriasis, in which the application of tar preparations (the photosensitizer) is followed by irradiation with ultraviolet B (UVB) [28] and the treatment of vitiligo with psoralens and light. More recently, psoralen and ultraviolet A (PUVA) therapy was introduced for the treatment of various dermatoses, especially psoriasis and mycosis fungoides; other indications have included pustulosis palmoplantaris [131], dyshidrotic eczema [132], urticaria pigmentosa [87], hyperkeratotic dermatitis of the palms [86], alopecia areata [136], atopic eczema [137] and polymorphous light eruption [138]. Various aspects of this form of photochemotherapy have been discussed in detail by Abel and Farber [2].

Although extremely useful in the treatment of psoriasis, it should be appreciated that the risks of long-term PUVA therapy, especially those of carcinogenesis, mutagenesis and cataract formation, have not been fully assessed as yet. Nevertheless, the FDA has approved PUVA therapy for severe psoriasis.

Side effects of PUVA therapy (For reviews, *see* [109, 110, 113])

18.2 Melski et al. [49] provided a report on a large-scale collaborative study in which 1308 patients with psoriasis were treated 2 to 3 times a week with oral 8-methoxy-psoralen (8-MOP) photochemotherapy; 41,000 courses of treatment were analyzed.

The acute side effects observed are summarized in § 18.3. The results are expressed by the authors as a percentage of treatments rather than of patients. Serious acute reactions such as phototoxicity with erythema and blistering, nausea, or pruritus, requiring discontinuation of therapy, were rare. Dizziness, depression and headache were occasional complications of the treatment. The major limiting factor is erythema; however, this is dose-related with respect to both drug and light and is therefore predictable and avoidable.

18.3 **Immediate side effects after PUVA***

Side effect	Percent of treatments	Side effect	Percent of treatments
Erythema/burns – local or diffuse		Nausea after last treatment	3.21
– any grade	9.77	– interfered with activity	0.64
– localized edema or blistering	0.24	– at least 12 hr duration	0.37
– diffuse marked red or edema	1.12	– with vomiting	0.30
– caused missed treatment	1.15	– caused missed treatment	0.08

(continued)

18.3 Immediate side effects after PUVA

(continuation)

Side effect	Percent of treatments	Side effect	Percent of treatments
Pruritus	14.08	Headache	2.00
– generalized	6.43	– continuous	1.25
– interfered with sleep	5.13	– interfered with activity	0.36
– for more than 3 days	5.02	– at least 24 hr duration	0.21
– interfered with activity	1.74	– caused missed treatment	0.02
– caused missed treatment	0.44		
Dizziness	1.52		
– continuous	0.74		
– interfered with activity	0.38		
– at least 8 hr duration	0.29		
– caused missed treatment	0.02		

* Side effects expressed as a percentage of treatments. Neither the major categories nor the subcategories are mutually exclusive. For example, one episode of nausea may cause a missed treatment, result in vomiting, last for more than 12 hr, and interfere with activities.

Cutaneous carcinogenicity

18.4   Potential hazards of PUVA therapy such as cutaneous aging, actinic damage and especially cutaneous carcinogenicity, are major concerns in the appraisal of the safety of this valuable therapeutic modality [22, 110, 113].

Although the oral administration of 8-MOP and subsequent ultraviolet A (UVA) irradiation in therapeutic doses is not followed by an increased tumor incidence in experimental animals [57, 32], it has been shown that topical or intraperitoneal application of psoralens with subsequent UVA irradiation in high doses is carcinogenic in rodents [79].

18.5   One of the major difficulties in determining the oncogenic risks of PUVA in man is the long latency period that is characteristic of the generation of radiation-induced tumors. Several reports are of interest for the discussion of this subject.

Case reports

18.6   Møller and Howitz [52] described a case in which treatment with 8-MOP and sunlight was followed by the development of multiple basal cell carcinomas. However, the patient had been treated with arsenic for vitiligo eight years previously; the development of multiple superficial basal cell carcinomas is a well-known complication of arsenic.

18.7   Four patients receiving long-term PUVA treatment for psoriasis were described by Hofmann et al. [37]. Two developed histologically proven multiple foci of Bowenoid lesions, one developed Bowenoid lesions and Bowen's disease, and in one patient 2 keratoacanthomas were noted to develop. Most lesions occurred on non-sun-exposed but photochemically treated areas. Two patients had a history of arsenic intake.

18.8   In 1979 Stern et al. [72] reported on a 2.1-year prospective study of 1373 patients treated with oral 8-MOP photochemotherapy, the first to implicate PUVA as a (co)carcinogen. Two years later the same group [127] reported on a 4-year-study of 1140 patients (older than 30 years). Data from this study reveal that 73 (6.5%)

had a total of 145 nonmelanoma skin cancers, of which 96 were squamous cell carcinomas. The observed incidence of squamous cell carcinomas was 9.1 times higher than could be expected on the basis of age, sex and geographic location. The frequency of squamous cell carcinomas in patients with a history of cutaneous carcinogens was significantly greater after 80 PUVA treatments, when compared with the frequency of squamous cell carcinoma after fewer than 80 treatments. Unusual features that added to the importance of these findings were the occurrence of squamous cell carcinomas in patients at a younger mean age than those with basal cell carcinomas. Also, the squamous cell carcinomas frequently occurred on relatively non-sun-exposed areas of the body, such as trunk and legs. These data suggest, according to the authors, that PUVA acts as a promotor of squamous cell carcinomas in human subjects previously exposed to cutaneous carcinogens; this effect increases with higher numbers of PUVA treatments.

Especially the reversal of the ratio of squamous cell carcinoma to basal cell carcinoma, squamous cell carcinomas becoming relatively more frequent and occurring on parts of the body not usually exposed to the sun, was considered to reflect the potential (co)carcinogenic properties of PUVA therapy (see also Epstein [19]). It must be mentioned, however, that in an Australian study [129] all observed skin cancers in PUVA-treated psoriatics have been on light-exposed areas; this may suggest that a high exposure to sunlight is also a risk-factor.

18.9   Another large-scale investigation on the development of keratoses and skin tumors in long-term photochemotherapy was reported by Hönigsmann et al. [38]. Four hundred and eighteen patients were treated with oral photochemotherapy up to 5 years, and monitored regularly for the occurrence of precancerous conditions or tumors of the skin. Out of this group, six patients (1.4%) developed actinic keratoses and five (1.2%) epidermal tumors (3 squamous cell carcinomas, 1 basal cell carcinoma, 1 keratoacanthoma) 12 to 53 months after initiation of PUVA therapy. Ten of these eleven patients belonged to a group of 172 individuals with a history of previous exposure to arsenic, ionizing radiation, and/or methotrexate, who were considered to be a risk group.

All of the four carcinoma patients had previously had one or more courses of arsenic therapy. No tumors were observed in the remaining 246 non-risk patients. The mean age of the keratosis-tumor group, and the total cumulative UVA dose were significantly higher than those of the other patients without such skin changes. The observed incidence of epidermal carcinomas in the risk group (2.3%) was considerably higher than the expected age-sex-specific incidence of a randomized population (0.1%), whereas the incidence in the non-risk group (0%) corresponded to the expected rate.

The authors state that 'this study shows that the incidence of non-melanoma skin tumors in long-term PUVA patients without previous medication of arsenic or treatment with ionizing radiation does not differ from the expected incidence in the general population. However, there is an increased incidence of tumors in PUVA patients if certain risk factors are present. The risk factor in our series is previous medication with arsenic.'

18.10   Roenigk and Caro [65] documented a 4-year-follow-up study of 631 patients with psoriasis treated with PUVA therapy. A total of ten basal cell carcinomas and three squamous cell carcinomas developed in ten patients. Most of these malignancies were localized on sun-exposed areas. Actinic keratoses were diagnosed in eight patients. The skin cancer group was on average 14 years older than the group without lesions.

As 7 of the 10 patients with malignancies had previously received ionizing radiation, the authors state that this is an important risk factor. However, it was not evaluated what percentage of the group without malignancies had previously been treated with ionizing radiation. The same goes for previous skin cancer and arsenic exposure ('not significant') whereas skin types and previous chemotherapy were not evaluated.

No control groups of either non-PUVA-treated psoriatics or the general population were used, and the only conclusion the authors draw is that 'although the incidence of skin cancer, locations, and types of tumors seen in the PUVA-48 study would appear to be less alarming than reported by the 16-center study [72], the development of any skin cancer during PUVA should be of concern.'

18.11   Lassus et al. [43] reported a follow-up study on 525 PUVA-treated psoriatics. The mean follow-up period since the beginning of PUVA therapy was 2.1 years (range 1–3.6).

One patient had a basal cell carcinoma, but this had almost certainly been present before the beginning of the PUVA therapy.

Two other patients, both previously treated with methotrexate, developed reversible lesions with Bowenoid histology: they had received high UVA doses. The incidence of skin carcinoma in this series was lower than that in hospitalized psoriatics treated with regimens other than PUVA and was not higher than the incidence in the age-matched general population. The authors consider previous intake of methotrexate to be a risk factor (although the numbers were very small) and suggest that if psoriasis patients are carefully selected, PUVA therapy involves no increased short-time risk of developing skin carcinoma.

18.12   A case of malignant melanoma arising during (uncontrolled) photochemotherapy was described by Forrest and Forrest [25]: A 30-year-old white male was treated for vitiligo with trioxsalen ingested 2 hours before sunbathing. A pigmented lesion appeared on his back 3 weeks later; both the patient and his wife denied the previous existence of a nevus at this site. The patient discontinued the trioxsalen therapy. However, the pigmented lesion continued to grow and the degree of its pigmentation increased. Half a year later, the lesion was excised and turned out to be a superficial spreading melanoma, Clark's level III. An association of the photochemotherapy with the development of this melanoma seems highly unlikely.

18.13   There is evidence from a number of studies suggesting that PUVA is a promotor of epidermal dystrophy, actinic keratoses and skin cancer if certain risk factors are present:
1. Previous intake of arsenic [38]
2. Previous treatment with ionizing radiation [72, 65]
3. History of previous (pre)malignancies [72]
4. (Possibly) previous intake of methotrexate [43, 101, 156]
5. (Possibly) skin types I and II [72].

All such patients should be informed of the possible risks associated with this therapeutic modality. There is a strong relationship between cumulative PUVA dose and the risk of cutaneous carcinoma [127]. Fortunately, to date there are no reports of systemic metastases from squamous cell carcinomas that occurred after PUVA therapy for psoriasis [134]. Whether or not PUVA is also a *primary* carcinogen may not be known until a latency period of 10–20 years or more has elapsed. For this reason, PUVA is a more appropriate treatment of severe psoriasis in patients in the fifth to seventh decade of life than for those in the first two decades. The American Academy of Pediatrics has advised against the use of PUVA therapy in children [135].

18.14   Epidermal dystrophy and actinic keratoses

Epidermal dystrophy is defined as any alteration in cell size or arrangement to a degree not seen in pretreatment control specimens from sunlight-exposed or sunlight-protected clinically uninvolved skin [113]. Epidermal dystrophy, which has histologic features resembling those seen in actinic keratoses, has been reported in association with PUVA therapy by several investigators [37, 96, 122, 139, 140]. No such changes were found in the study of Levin et al. [92]. In a large series [122], epidermal dystrophy was a common occurrence in PUVA-treated patients. In 57% of 107 patients dystrophic changes in keratinocytes were seen, more commonly in patients previously treated with arsenic. Its incidence does not increase with prolonged PUVA therapy [96], but it has been shown that epidermal dystrophy may persist long after cessation of therapy [141].

Abel et al. [96] have noted focal dystrophy of epidermal cells in more than half of 70 patients 1 year or more following the onset of PUVA therapy, in clinically uninvolved skin of sunlight-protected and sunlight-exposed areas. Prior to therapy control biopsies had shown no such changes. Although it is not currently known whether this type of dystrophy is a precursor of keratosis or skin cancer, the possibility that it reflects a precancerous change should be recognized.

In 104 PUVA-treated patients returning for dermatologic follow-up after the first year of therapy, 17 (16.3%) developed actinic keratoses during the course of, or following the cessation of, treatment with PUVA [96]. As in the majority of patients multiple keratoses occurred in sun-exposed areas, it has been suggested that PUVA accelerates or promotes actinically induced lesions.

Mutagenicity

18.15   In vitro observations suggest that non-lethal injury from PUVA may alter the transmission of genetic information during cellular DNA replication. In view of this, Bridges [9] has put the question as to whether one should use a cytotoxic and genotoxic combination of drug and radiation when the condition being treated is a benign one, such as psoriasis.

PUVA has been associated with DNA damage in lymphocytes, but gene mutations have also been found in patients not so treated, which suggests either that psoriasis itself predisposes to mutations, or, more likely, that other treatments which may have been given are (also) mutagenic.

Chromosomal abnormalities were present in a case reported by Wagner et al. [81] on preleukemia in a PUVA-treated psoriatic patient. After 30 weeks of PUVA treatment the patient developed refractory anemia which required several blood transfusions. The bone marrow showed an excess of myeloblasts, abnormal chromosomes and abnormal cultural growth on agar.

Of course, the development of this condition, known as preleukemia, may be coincidental; the suspicion of a causal relationship with PUVA can only be supported by future observations.

Cataract formation

18.16   Experimental studies have clearly shown that animals treated with psoralens in high doses and exposed to ultraviolet light develop cataracts [13, 148]. Therefore, the possible development of cataracts in PUVA-treated patients has always been one of the major concerns regarding the long-term safety of oral photochemotherapy.

8-MOP has been demonstrated in human lenses 12 hours after the ingestion of a single therapeutic dose [149]. From animal studies it has been shown that in the absence of photic stimuli, the 8-MOP will diffuse out of the lens within 24 hours. In the presence of photic stimuli (ambient room light as well as direct UV (360 nm) irradiation) however, there is an enhancement of lenticular fluorescence and phosphorescence. Photoaddition products (at 360 nm) can be generated with tryptophan as well as with lens proteins (*in vitro*) in the presence of 8-MOP and oxygen. Such a reaction *in vivo* would result in permanent retention of the photoproduct within the ocular lens, thus predisposing to cataract formation. Indeed, one such photoproduct has recently been demonstrated in material derived from patients who required cataract surgery after long-term PUVA therapy [102]. These data provide objective evidence that PUVA therapy can generate specific photoproducts within the human ocular lens. These photoproducts have been shown to be associated with experimental PUVA cataracts in rats; this evidence substantiates reports of (presumptive) PUVA cataracts.

Aside from the lens, 8-MOP can be found in other ocular tissues, including the corneal epithelium, the ciliary processes, and the retina (of young animal eyes) after intraperitoneal administration [85]. Because the *mature* ocular lens is an effective filter for UVA radiation in man there can be no photobinding of 8-MOP in the mature retina. However, UVA radiation can penetrate to the retina in aphakic and pseudophakic patients. It has also been suggested that a larger proportion of UVA can penetrate the lens of very young patients [119]. Lerman [85, 119] warns that PUVA therapy in such individuals can result in increasing accumulation of photoproducts in the lens and retina; subtle retinal changes in young children on long-term PUVA might occur, which may be undetectable in standard eye examination [119].

18.17 From the inception of PUVA therapy it has repeatedly been stressed that it is essential to shield the psoralen-photosensitized eye adequately from UVA radiation in order to prevent the development of cataracts. The older recommendations [112] in the section on eye protection of the original PUVA guidelines have recently been revised and published by a subcommittee of the Task Forces of Psoriasis and Photobiology [114]. According to these recommendations, which were reformulated in response to new knowledge of the relationship of PUVA to ocular complications and to advances in optics technology, patients must wear UVA-blocking wraparound glasses on each day of PUVA treatment, from the time of ingestion of the drug. Preferably, these glasses should also be worn on the second day. Of course, while in the PUVA chamber, the eyes must be totally covered with UVA-opaque goggles provided by the PUVA therapist. Environmental sources of UVA have been investigated [159]. With the demonstration of presumed PUVA cataracts patient compliance in wearing their UVA blocking glasses for the advised period of time is essential and this should repeatedly be stressed to the patient. Convenient compliance is much easier with the availability of clear, cosmetically acceptable UVA-blocking spectacles [150]. Unfortunately, many patients are either unwilling or unable to wear such glasses for extended periods, and this poses considerable potential risk of cataracts in PUVA-treated patients.

Clinical studies and case reports

18.18 In the study of Rönnerfält et al. [103] 46 patients with severe psoriasis maintained on long-term PUVA therapy have been followed up for $6^{1}/_{2}$ years after the initiation of treatment. Repeated ophthalmological examinations were performed; no ocular side effects attributed to the photochemotherapy were revealed during this period.

Hammershøy and Jessen [104] examined 96 patients treated with PUVA between 1975 and 1980; no patient developed cataract during the PUVA treatment period and their findings were found to correspond to those in a (control) standard population. However, several cases of cataracts presumably or probably induced by PUVA therapy have been reported [14, 102, 118, 119]. From animal studies it has been reported that the anterior cortical location of punctate lens opacities is characteristic of ocular injury induced by psoralen photosensitization [13]. The first report of a presumptive PUVA cataract was reported in 1980 [14]. Kasick et al. [118] have reported bilateral punctate cortical opacities in two PUVA-treated patients who had normal eye examinations prior to therapy. Lerman [102, 118] has reported additional cases.

Careful monitoring of ocular changes is recommended not only in patients currently receiving photochemotherapy, but also in those who have discontinued PUVA treatment [118].

Other ocular side effects

18.19   Of 15 patients treated with PUVA, 8 were found to have a mild form of photokeratoconjunctivitis [111]. The ocular manifestations included photophobia, conjunctivitis, keratitis and dry eyes. Tear break-up time was reduced significantly immediately after treatment in two patients, but returned to normal 8 hours later. Keratitis may occur when patients neglect to wear their goggles. Visual field defects to PUVA therapy have recently been described in 3 patients [115]. One patient developed nausea and photophobia, with a central scotoma which lasted up to 20 minutes before disappearing to the left of her visual field. These episodes were dose-dependent and reproducible on challenge with an increase in psoralen dosage. Two other patients experienced nausea and tunnel vision lasting for 5 minutes and 8 hours, respectively; in one, attacks of sudden pain in one eye were concomitant. These symptoms were also dose-related [115].

Pigmentary changes

18.20   The diffuse tanning following PUVA therapy indicates that stimulation of melanocytes has occurred. The prolonged nature of PUVA-induced tanning might be attributed in part to a change in the distribution of melanosomes from an aggregated to a large single, dispersed pattern in the keratinocytes. Several other forms of pigment alterations have been described in patients undergoing oral photochemotherapy.

Disseminated small-spotted hyperpigmentation

18.21   Disseminated small-spotted hyperpigmentation [130] appears to be the commonest long-term side effect of PUVA treatment, occurring in more than 20% of patients after 2–3 years of extensive PUVA therapy with more than 100 exposures and a total UVA dose of more than 1000 J/cm^2 [128]. This eruption has been described under various names: lentigo eruptiva [51], freckles [8, 128], disseminated pigmented spots [151], stellate hyperpigmented freckling [90], PUVA-induced pigmented macules [91] and star-like hyperpigmented lentigines [153]. The macules are usually located on the thigh, upper arm, waist and buttocks [154, 155]. Histopathological findings have differed, but Rhodes et al. [91] showed that the pigmented macules are characterized by a lentiginous proliferation of functionally active melanocytes; thus the PUVA-induced macules were rather 'lentigines' than 'freckles' according to current pathologic classification. Dysplastic changes in the melanocytes have been observed [91, 154], and thus, although the significance of these pigment alterations is unknown, a close clinical and histopathological monitoring of PUVA patients for atypical melanocyte lesions has been recommended [91, 154].

Nevus spilus-like hyperpigmentation

18.22   Some authors have described nevus spilus-like hyperpigmentation in PUVA-treated patients [34, 36, 130, 152]. Melanocyte numbers are reportedly normal [34, 36].

Ashen-gray macules

18.23   A male patient treated with PUVA for psoriasis noticed ashen-gray macules up to 1 cm in diameter on the trunk after 130 exposures (total UVA dose 930 J/cm^2). A biopsy revealed large amounts of pigment-containing macrophages (melanophages) in the upper dermis [128]. Berlin blue staining for hemosiderin was negative. Two years after discontinuation of PUVA the macules still persisted. According to the authors, the finding of large amounts of melanophages reflects the greatly increased production of melanin in melanocytes possibly combined with inflammation and a disturbance of the epidermis-dermis junction during PUVA therapy [128].

Mottled hypo- and hyperpigmentation

18.24   Mottled hypo- and hyperpigmentation due to phototoxicity was reported in 13 of 572 patients undergoing PUVA therapy over a long period [117]. The skin in the affected parts of the body appeared dry, glistering and somewhat atrophic. In all patients mottling occurred in skin sites which had been overdosed and had exhibited erythema during the initial treatment phase. Mottling was first noted between 4 weeks and 12 months after the first PUVA exposure. DOPA-preparations revealed increased numbers of melanocytes in hyperpigmented areas, and reduced numbers in hypopigmented areas. In a number of patients the pigmentary changes proved (partially) reversible [117].

Hypo- and depigmentation

18.25   Irreversible hypopigmentation in some PUVA-treated patients has been observed [94]. Increased intracellular lipid deposits were demonstrated, which may precede degeneration of cells; thus overstimulation of melanocytes might explain the irreversible hypopigmentation. Farber et al. [113] have observed a case of extensive depigmentation, resembling vitiligo, appearing during PUVA treatment of psoriasis, and two patients in whom widespread depigmentation developed during PUVA therapy for mycosis fungoides. The depigmentation was not confined to clinically involved areas, nor was it associated with obvious phototoxicity. None of the patients had a history of vitiligo. Three more patients with vitiligo presumably due to PUVA therapy were reported by Todes-Taylor et al. [160].

Pityriasis alba-like hypopigmentation

18.26   Tegner [130] observed hypopigmentation with the clinical appearance of pityriasis alba in 5 patients after prolonged PUVA therapy. Since the clinical picture was identical in all patients, she concluded that this pigmentary change probably represented a side effect of PUVA.

Bullous eruptions

18.27   Two types of bullous eruptions due to PUVA therapy may be distinguished:

1. *A phototoxic eruption*, usually localized on the hands and/or feet. Bullae arise on normal skin; clinically and histologically they resemble bullous pemphigoid, but its characteristic immunofluorescence findings are absent [64, 105, 108, 143, 144].

2. *Bullous pemphigoid.* Coexistence of psoriasis and bullous pemphigoid is well-documented [106, 107]. It has been shown that a variety of cutaneous insults can produce the bullous lesions of pemphigoid, and a number of treatment modalities have been implicated, including dithranol, coal tar, salicylic acid and UVB [107].

    Thomsen and Schmidt [77] were the first to describe bullous pemphigoid in PUVA-treated patients. In one case there was a previous diagnosis of bullous pemphigoid, albeit quiescent at the time of PUVA treatment. It was evident that the photochemotherapy caused the disease to relapse. Subsequently, several authors reported bullous pemphigoid during photochemotherapy [1, 64, 106, 107, 145, 146]. Most patients develop bullous pemphigoid shortly after beginning of PUVA therapy, but delayed onset 4 weeks after discontinuance of photochemotherapy has also been reported [107]. The eruption is sometimes limited to psoriatic lesions; treatment with oral steroids and/or immunosuppressive agents has been necessary in some cases.

    In one report [147] pemphigus foliaceus (Senear-Usher) was seen to exacerbate during PUVA therapy.

Infections

Herpes zoster

18.28   The development of herpes zoster as a complication of PUVA therapy has been reported by Roenigk and Martin [66]. Stüttgen [109] found 8 cases of zoster occurring among 1013 patients treated with PUVA during the first $1^1/_2$ year of therapy.

Herpes simplex

18.29   Herpes simplex and other photosensitive dermatoses may be aggravated or exacerbated by PUVA therapy. A case of Kaposi's varicelliform eruption in a patient with mycosis fungoides during PUVA therapy has been documented by Segal and Watson [70].

Bacterial infections

18.30   Bacterial infections such as folliculitis and erysipelas are said to occur infrequently during PUVA therapy [130].

Other skin disorders

Pustular psoriasis

18.31   Pustular transformation of previously non-pustular psoriasis was reported in 12 of 400 patients in the series described by Langner and Christophers [42]. This

event, the authors postulate, can be linked with an inability of PUVA to completely suppress leukocyte chemotaxis.

The development of pustular psoriasis during PUVA therapy has also been noted by Roenigk and Martin [66].

Lichen planus

18.32   Lichen planus as a possible side effect of PUVA therapy was described by Dupré
et al. [17]: A 62-year-old male suffering from extensive long-standing psoriasis
with joint involvement was treated with photochemotherapy. At the beginning of
the therapy the patient also took pyritinol tablets; previously he had received
chloroquine for five years because of his rheumatism. After three PUVA treatments a lichenoid micropapular eruption developed, which was aggravated by
each subsequent session until it was almost generalized; by that time erythroderma
was noted, which was attributed to photosensitivity. After nine PUVA treatments
the therapy was discontinued and the intake of pyritinol was stopped. Histopathology confirmed the clinical diagnosis of lichen planus. Gradually, the lichenoid
skin eruption improved after discontinuation of PUVA therapy and pyritinol intake.

Lichenoid reactions and photosensitization have been noted with pyritinol before; it is not certain whether the adverse event should be attributed to pyritinol
or to PUVA therapy. The authors hypothesize that pyritinol may have potentiated the effects of PUVA therapy and vice versa; therefore it would seem to be contraindicated, according to these authors, to apply PUVA therapy in patients using
pyritinol.

Scleroderma-like changes

18.33   In two patients treated for vitiligo with PUVA therapy scleroderma-like skin
changes were noted in vitiligo patches after 8 and 16 months of therapy; the patients had received 325.6 J/cm^2 and 683 J/cm^2, respectively. Histopathological examination revealed characteristics of both actinic elastosis and scleroderma. After
cessation of therapy all findings, both clinical and histological, returned to normal
[99].

Granuloma annulare

18.34   The etiology and pathogenesis of annular granuloma is as yet unknown. Dorval
et al. [16] reported a case in which typical granuloma annulare developed in a
psoriatic patient during PUVA treatment. The authors try (somewhat unconvinc-
ingly) to associate these findings.

'Allergic' cutaneous vasculitis

18.35   A 67-year-old woman was being treated with PUVA therapy because of premy-
cotic erythema of one year's standing in patches on the trunk and the extremities.
After the fifth PUVA treatment purpura developed on the legs, first petechial in
appearance, then progressing into a severe necrotic phase. Histopathological examination revealed a typical leukoclastic vasculitis. Later the patient developed
proteinuria and hematuria; a kidney biopsy showed focal necrotizing glomerulonephritis. A spontaneous recovery ensued. The patient had used various drugs,
but the event was most likely due to 8-MOP, as circulating antibodies to this drug
could be demonstrated [4].

Seborrheic dermatitis of the face

18.36   Seborrheic dermatitis of the face was observed in 28 of 347 patients on PUVA therapy for psoriasis. Most patients had never previously noted any facial rash. The dermatitis always started after discontinuation of the PUVA therapy, the latency time ranging from a few days to a couple of weeks. When patients with induced seborrheic dermatitis were given a new PUVA series, the facial rash again cleared up but recurred soon after discontinuation of treatment.

The author hypothesizes that PUVA treatment means both an acitvation and a therapy of a latent seborrheic dermatitis. The clinical appearance of the dermatitis would then respresent a rebound phenomenon due to withdrawal of the PUVA treatment. Of the postulated causes of seborrheic dermatitis, sebaceous gland dysfunction is most favored; PUVA treatment has been shown to cause a marked increase in the total lipid, and the induced dermatitis may be connected with this [123].

Acne

18.37   A case of acneiform eruption induced by PUVA treatment has been described by Jones and Bleehen [40].

According to the authors, this is due to the hot and humid atmosphere in the enclosed cabinets in which patients undergoing PUVA treatment are usually irradiated.

Acneiform exanthema has also also been observed by Hofmann et al. [36].

Disseminated superficial actinic porokeratosis

18.38   Disseminated superficial actinic porokeratosis is a rare dominant autosomal dermatosis, of which some sporadic cases are recorded.

Reymond et al. [63] have described a 67-year-old female patient with psoriasis, who developed lesions essentially localized on the anterior surface of both legs, clinically and histologically designated as superficial actinic porokeratosis; she had been treated with 8-MOP photochemotherapy, 8-MOP being administered both orally and (on the legs) topically. There was no family history of this dermatosis. The authors state that this entity might be expected as a side effect of PUVA therapy; typical lesions have been experimentally provoked with prolonged artificial UV light [11].

Systemic lupus erythematosus

18.39   Systemic lupus erythematosus (SLE) developed in a 23-year-old woman with psoriasis during PUVA therapy. She displayed a typical facial rash, hair loss, photosensitivity, arthralgia with pain on joint movements, renal and CNS involvement, splenomegaly and leukopenia. Serum antinuclear antibodies were present in high titer, and hypocomplementemia developed. Kidney and skin biopsy specimens were consistent with SLE [21]. Although the authors admit that the association of psoriasis and SLE in this case may have been coincidental, they argue that the appearance of SLE shortly after the onset of PUVA treatment suggests that ultraviolet A or photoactivated psoralen may have played a role in the development of this connective tissue disease.

In the investigation reported by Bjellerup et al. [7], circulating antinuclear antibodies (ANA) developed in 7 of 34 patients during PUVA therapy. Only 3 patients had these antibodies prior to treatment. Titers were low and the patients had no other signs of connective tissue disorders. Antibodies to native DNA were negative.

231

At 14 centers, 1023 patients had two or more ANA determinations. There was no statistically significant increase of positive ANA's following PUVA therapy [73]. These authors point out that psoralen-DNA photoproducts are antigenic and may give rise to antinuclear antibodies, which may be detected only when using a tissue substrate irradiated with UVA in the presence of psoralens.

Contact allergy

18.40   Cases of contact allergy to 8-MOP have been described by Weissmann et al. [82] and Saihan [68].

Photoallergic dermatitis

18.41   A case of photoallergic dermatitis to 8-MOP has been described by Plewig et al. [60]: A 36-year-old woman with psoriasis developed generalized photoallergic dermatitis to 8-MOP after 16 uneventful courses of PUVA. The diagnosis of photoallergy was confirmed by re-exposure, phototests using both topical and oral 8-MOP with a new high-intensity light apparatus for the delivery of UVA, and histological studies. Photoallergy occurred only with UVA, but not with either UVB or UVC.

Three cases of photoallergy to topically applied 8-MOP were documented by Fulton and Willis [27].

Prolonged phototoxicity

18.42   Stüttgen [109] has reported that up to 4–6 weeks after 8-MOP has been discontinued, it is possible to provoke a phototoxic reaction to sunbathing.

This author has seen erythroderma-like eruptions following exposure to subtropical sun after discontinuance of PUVA-therapy.

Hair

Hypertrichosis

18.43   Hypertrichosis as a side effect of psoralen photochemotherapy has been reported by Hofmann et al. [36], Elliott [18], Singh and Lal [71] and Tegner [130]. Rampen [158] reported moderate to severe hypertrichosis in 11/14 (79%) of patients on PUVA therapy; especially the face and extremities were affected. Excessive hair growth started within 6–12 weeks after commencement of PUVA. According to the author the hair growth is most likely to be attributed to the psoralens, although UVA light may play a potentiating role [158].

Hirsutism

18.44   Whereas hypertrichosis following photochemotherapy with oral psoralens has been reported by several authors (see § 18.43), there is only one documented case of hirsutism [33]:

A 31-year-old female patient with psoriasis was treated with PUVA. There were no signs of hypertrichosis or hirsutism at the beginning of the therapy. Seventy days after the first treatment (having received a total dose of 171.5 J/cm^2) the patient noticed increased hair growth on her face. Four weeks later, she had abnormal hair growth on the cheeks, chin, upper lip, lower back and buttocks, designated as hirsutism Grade III according to Baron [3]; no signs of virilization were present. Hormonal causes for hirsutism were excluded.

The authors consider this to be a case of iatrogenic hirsutism caused by PUVA therapy; they hypothesize that the photosensitizing agents change the metabolism of androgens in the skin.

Nails

Nail pigmentation

18.45   Naik and Singh [54] reported on nail pigmentation that developed in four patients while on oral 8-MOP photochemotherapy for vitiligo. Although other possible causes for this phenomenon were not excluded, the authors believed this pigmentation to be attributable to 8-MOP. The same authors treated 10 psoriatic patients with PUVASOL (8-MOP and sunlight exposure) and observed hyperpigmentation of the nail plates in three. The hyperpigmentation started about one month after beginning of treatment, starting proximally and spreading distally to involve the entire nail plate [100]. After cessation of therapy the pigmentation disappeared (in one patient observed after two months). The adverse effect was ascribed to increased melanogenesis.

Photo-onycholysis

18.46   Zala et al. [84] described two patients who had developed photo-onycholysis from orally administered 8-MOP and exposure to sunlight. One of these patients had taken 8-MOP for vitiligo, the other for cosmetic reasons. Histological examination of the nail bed showed edema of the extracellular spaces and deposits of an unidentified crystalline substance. Numerous multinuclear cells were evident in the epithelium; globular keratohyaline granules were seen in some of the malpighian layer cells. An intraepithelial cyst-like degeneration was present in the upper malpighian layers.

Other cases of photo-onycholysis induced by PUVA therapy have been described by Orlonne and Baran [55], Rau et al. [62], Briffa and Warin [10] and Tegner [130].

Subungual bleeding

18.47   Subungual bleeding due to PUVA therapy has been described by Hofmann et al. [37] and Tegner [130].

Cardiovascular effects

Cardiovascular stress

18.48   According to established guidelines [19], one of the relative contraindications of PUVA treatment is for 'patients with severe cardiovascular disease who may not be able to tolerate the stress of PUVA treatment'. In the investigation of Ciafone et al. [12], oral PUVA therapy in a treatment enclosure (mean duration 19.3 minutes) resulted in ambient temperatures of 39.2°C ± 2.1°C and skin temperatures of 38.2°C ± 1.4°C in 17 patients. In the upright position, the heart rate rose by 30.8% to 114.4 ± 25.2 beats per minute, and the authors warned that PUVA therapy is thus associated with a definite cardiovascular stress when the box-type of therapeutic unit is used. However, Chappe et al. [98] concluded from their study that PUVA therapy is a safe method of treatment, since their patients, including those with cardiovascular disease and hypertension, tolerated the stress of PUVA therapy well. The study group of these investigators consisted of 40 patients, of which 6 had cardiovascular disease; 16 had documented hypertension. The following parameters were monitored: standing brachial artery blood pressure immediately before and after PUVA, taken in the same arm by the same observer; 12-lead electrocardiograms in 22 patients immediately before and after PUVA; heart rate and rhythm of all patients while standing in the phototherapy cabinet, using standard Holter monitoring technic (modified leads V_1 and V_5). The patients were closely observed during treatment, and any subjective symptoms were recorded. Electrocardiograms showed no significant changes after PUVA; Holter monitoring revealed no significant arrhythmias other than recorded before therapy. All patients had an increase in heart rate, the mean increase being 20 beats per minute (22%). There were no significant changes in the systolic or diastolic blood pressure. Subjective symptoms of dizziness occurred in 6 patients: in 3 of them this did not interfere with treatment but in 3 others dizziness required interruption of treatment. In these cases dizziness was ascribed to anxiety and hyperventilation (2) and influenza (1). In general, patients tolerated the stress of standing in a warm phototherapy cabinet well, and therefore PUVA therapy was considered to be a safe method (in their group) by the investigators. Nevertheless, they also state that it would be desirable to use cardiac monitoring, including electrocardiogram and arterial blood pressure, when treating patients with significant heart disease, in whom a rise in heart rate might present a significant stress.

Temporal arteritis

18.49   Temporal arteritis in a 75-year-old male developed after three weeks of photochemotherapy with oral trioxsalen and subsequent exposure to sunlight [47]. This disease has not been reported before in connection with photochemotherapy and must probably be regarded as coincidental.

Liver disease

Hepatitis

18.50   The incidence of psoralen hepatotoxicity, if any, has been debated and certain literature is frequently cited [24, 78]. Slight and transient elevations of liver enzymes during PUVA treatment have been reported, but were usually attributable to pre-existing liver injury caused by intake of alcohol or other drugs. Liver damage is not considered to be a contraindication to the use of PUVA [20].

Case reports

18.51   Up to now, in only two reports could hepatotoxicity be clearly attributed to PUVA therapy, or rather to oral 8-MOP. Bjellerup et al. [6] presented a case of liver damage due to 8-MOP. The reaction manifested itself by elevated serum alanine-aminotransferase and serum aspartate-aminotransferase; it was provoked by PUVA on 3 occasions. During the last such episode, the liver enzymes were elevated after a test dose of 40 mg 8-MOP, without irradiation. The liver damage seemed to be of the hepatocellular type; unfortunately, no liver biopsy was available. The authors reporting the case believe this side effect to be allergic in nature.

The other report on hepatotoxicity of PUVA was published by Pariser and Wyles [56]. A 59-year-old white nurse with long-standing psoriasis, who had a damaged liver from methotrexate, developed a toxic hepatitis while on oral 8-

MOP photochemotherapy. Fever and marked elevation of the liver enzymes occurred after the fifteenth PUVA treatment; spontaneous recovery ensued within
5 days after stopping PUVA. One week later, following the next PUVA treatment,
the same toxic hepatitis developed and again spontaneously resolved. Topical 8-
MOP followed by UVA did *not* produce this reaction.

Tegner [130] reports liver damage in two patients, but no details are mentioned.

Renal disease

Glomerulonephritis

18.52   Dahl [15] reported an increase in serum creatinine to abnormal values in 12 of
106 patients treated with PUVA therapy. A renal biopsy showed uncharacteristic
glomerulonephritis in one of them.

Miscellaneous

Skin pain

18.53   Severe skin pain lasting for up to 2 months occurred in 8 of 210 psoriatic patients
treated with PUVA [76]. The pain generally started 4-8 weeks after the initial dose,
in 5 about one week after discontinuation of the treatment. In others the pain
started 1-2 hours after PUVA therapy, and the treatment had to be discontinued.
The reaction was described as a prickling, burning pain, usually coming in bouts,
and confined to limited areas 'deep under the skin'. Neither analgesics, antihistamines, topical steroids nor local anesthetics could alleviate the pain.

Miller and Munro [50] reported on skin pain in 3 patients while on PUVA therapy. All 3 patients described this unpleasant sensation as a 'deep itch with a marked burning character', which began after 3, 6 and 8 weeks of therapy, respectively,
and only after the psoriasis had shown marked improvement. In 2 of the 3 the
symptoms were paroxysmal but not obviously precipitated by any particular action. Although generalized, the pain tended to be worse on the buttocks in each
case. In one patient PUVA treatment was stopped, but the symptoms were still
present after 6 months despite various attempts to treat them. Tegner [130] reported severe skin pain in 5% of her patients. The pathophysiological mechanism remains obscure, though some form of neuritis has been suggested as the cause.

Effects on Langerhans cells (LC)

18.54   ATPase-stained LC have been shown to disappear during PUVA treatment [116].
Friedmann et al. [89] have studied the effects of PUVA therapy in psoriatic patients on LC using both ATP-ase staining of epidermal biopsies obtained from
suction blisters and electron microscopy on blister tops. Langerhans cells lost
ATPase activity before they disappeared by ultrastructural criteria: 90% of
ATPase-stained cells had disappeared after 7 treatments (2 weeks), whereas it was
only after 15 treatments (5 weeks) that they were seen to be reduced on electron
microscopy. Their numbers remained low throughout the course of treatment, but
they had returned to normal by 3 weeks after cessation of therapy. It was shown
that these effects were due to PUVA potentiated by 8-MOP. Disappearance of
LC may cause or contribute to changes in delayed cutaneous hypersensitivity,
which reportedly is reduced in psoriatic patients undergoing oral photochemotherapy [88] (§ 18.57).

18.55 Miscellaneous

Effects on delayed cutaneous hypersensitivity

18.55   Several investigators have shown that PUVA reduced delayed hypersensitivity to 2,4-dinitrochlorobenzene (DNCB) in patients with psoriasis [75, 88, 133]. PUVA suppresses both induction and expression of delayed cutaneous hypersensitivity by systemic as well as local actions, but the major effect is local inhibition of induction [88]; reduction of the numbers of Langerhans cells, which are required for the induction of contact hypersensitivity is probably a major factor for the latter.

The pathological consequences of impairment of immunity by PUVA are uncertain. However, it has been shown that DNCB responsiveness is reduced in patients with cancer, and a possible role of impaired immunity in the cutaneous carcinogenicity of PUVA has been suggested [75]. On the other hand, Moss et al. [88] argue that treatment with conventional therapy (tar, UVB and anthralin) has also reduced DNCB responsiveness [133], and that these forms of treatment have proved safe over many years of use.

Inadequate or uncontrolled application of photochemotherapy

18.56   Fritsch [26] discussed the danger of uncontrolled use of 8-MOP. He described 2 patients who painted their skin with 8-MOP and went out into the sun. This resulted in an extensive erythematous and bullous dermatitis. Other accidents listed are mistakes in the dose of UV light, and accidental contact with 8-MOP (e.g. by hospital personnel).

Miscellaneous

18.57   Several histological studies on the skin during and after photochemotherapy have been performed. Findings have included amyloid deposition [93], selective accumulation of lipid within melanocytes [94], an increase in melanin pigmentation, mucin accumulation, and changes in the elastic tissue in the dermis. Other studies indicate that patients with psoriasis treated with large cumulative doses of UVA resulting in evidence of cutaneous damage have a decrease in circulating T-lymphocytes and a decreased response of their lymphocytes to mitogen [120]. It has also been found that the proportion of T4-positive (helper/inducer) lymphocytes was reduced in PUVA-treated patients [121]. Possible induction of ANA-formation has been investigated [95], and the effect of UV-light and 5-S-cysteinyl-dopa was reported recently [130].

PUVA treatment has also been shown to elevate the level of serum interferon in psoriatic patients [157]. These findings are not discussed here, as they are considered to fall outside the scope of this book.

ONCOGENIC EFFECTS OF THE GOECKERMAN REGIMEN

Tar

18.58   Coal tar ointments have been used for many decades in the treatment of various dermatoses, especially eczematous dermatitis and psoriasis. Crude coal tar, a heterogeneous mixture of 10,000 different compounds of which 400 have been identified, has the known dermatological effects of being antipruritic, antibacterial, keratoclastic and photosensitizing [53].

The carcinogenic effects of coal tar, particularly of the benzpyrene constituent, have been well documented in laboratory animals [35]. Concentrations that are used clinically can cause benign as well as malignant neoplasms in animals [61]. Moreover, workers in the coal tar industry have an increased risk of developing malignancies, particularly non-melanoma skin cancers [29]. There is concern that prolonged topical application of tar preparations might induce skin cancers [83]. Also, urine extracts prepared from patients undergoing Goeckerman therapy have been shown to contain (unidentified) materials, which are mutagenic in the Ames assay [125]. It has previously been established that as little as 100 µg of crude coal tar is mutagenic in this test [124].

Case studies

18.59   In a review of the world literature up to 1967, made at that time by Greither et al. [30], a total of 13 cases of skin cancer were reported, all probably induced by prolonged application of therapeutic tar preparations. The most frequent sites of the cancers were the genital areas and the adjacent skin. In nine of the cases there was a history of prolonged self-medication, ranging from three months to 34 years.

One case was reported in detail by Rook et al. [67], who commented on the rarity of carcinomas induced by therapeutical application of tar, as contrasted with the frequency of occupational tar cancer.

A more recent survey of the literature was documented by Zackheim [83]; this did not contain essentially new evidence on this score.

Although several case reports have suggested an association between tar exposure and cutaneous carcinomas, no study has been able to document an increased risk of cutaneous carcinomas in patients treated with these externa. At present, therapy with tar preparations would hardly seem to endanger patients thus treated with regard to the development of skin cancers [61, 5].

Tar + ultraviolet light

18.60   Adequate evidence exists to support the statement that sunlight is a causal factor in human skin cancer [80, 142]. Artificial light in the UVB range has been shown to induce cutaneous tumors in albino and hairless mice [31]. Ultraviolet radiation potentiates the carcinogenic effect of topical coal tar in animals [23].

The successful treatment of psoriasis by the application of crude coal tar and subsequent exposure to ultraviolet light was first reported by Goeckerman in 1925 [28]. Although the action spectrum of coal tar lies within the long-wave ultraviolet range (UVA, 400 to 320 nm), studies have shown that exposure to erythemal radiation (UVB, 320 to 280 nm) is more effective in this regimen [58]. Therefore, the 'Goeckerman regimen' commonly employed for the treatment of psoriasis, consists of topical tar preparations (1–5%), followed by short-wave (UVB) radiation.

The question as to whether or not the Goeckerman therapy increases the risk of cutaneous carcinomas has always been a matter of dispute.

Case studies

18.61   Earlier studies have failed to document an increased risk of cutaneous carcinomas in patients treated for psoriasis with tar and artificial ultraviolet radiation [39].

Several new reports are of interest: Maughan et al. [48] reported on a 25-year follow-up study of 305 patients with atopic dermatitis or neurodermatitis, who had been hospitalized and treated with coal tar ointments and ultraviolet light at the Mayo Clinic from 1950 through 1954; information concerning the development of malignancies of the skin or other cancers since the initial treatment was gained either by follow-up questionnaire or telephone. Of the 305 patients with adequate follow-up, thirteen reported that skin cancer had developed; eight patients had basal cell carcinomas, one had a squamous cell carcinoma, two had an unknown variety of skin malignancy (biopsy specimens not available and therefore regarded as 'presumed skin cancers'), and two had malignant melanoma. Ten of eleven non-melanoma skin cancers were localized to sun-exposed areas.

The number of patients with atopic dermatitis in whom skin cancer developed, was compared with the anticipated values of occurrence calculated from data of the Third National Cancer Survey for non-melanoma skin cancer [69]; the incidence in this study was not significantly increased. A total of 8 non-cutaneous malignancies was noted in the Mayo group, which does not differ appreciably from values reported elsewhere.

Comparison with the general population, as has been done in this study, is not ideal, but seems to be valid, since Kaaber [41] has shown that the incidence of skin cancer in patients with atopic dermatitis is similar to that in the general population.

Those patients in whom skin cancers developed did not receive tar products for any longer period of time during their hospitalization than did those without skin cancers, nor were they hospitalized more frequently. They also did not receive any more coal tar than the others, and many had received even less. The authors state that 'Our study provides some reassurance that the clinical use of coal tar products has not significantly altered the frequency of neoplasms from the natural course'.

A similar study of the long-term effects of tar and/or ultraviolet radiation on the incidence of cutaneous neoplasms in psoriatics was reported by Pittelkow et al. [59]: A 25-year follow-up of 280 psoriasis patients treated with the Goeckerman regimen, revealed twenty patients with a total of thirty-three skin cancers. There were twenty-two basal cell carcinomas, seven squamous cell carcinomas, three of 'unknown variety', and one melanoma. The vast majority of these cancers occurred on exposed areas of the skin. Prior to initial treatment, 9% had a history of premalignant skin diseases (radiodermatitis, actinic dermatitis, and arsenical keratoses) and 70% received ionizing radiation, arsenic, methotrexate, or prolonged UV radiation. Two major risk factors were noted for the cancer patients: history of precancerous dermatitis and previous treatment with ionizing radiation.

Just as in the study of Maughan et al. [48] on patients with dermatitis, there was no more cancer in this group of psoriatics treated with tar and ultraviolet light than would be expected in a normal population, considering sex, age and geographic distribution [69].

Stern et al. [74] conducted a case-control study, consisting of 59 skin cancer patients with severe psoriasis, to evaluate the effect of treatment with tar and/or artificial UV radiation on the risk of developing cutaneous carcinoma.

Using 924 unmatched controls, the crude rate of skin cancer was estimated to be 2.4 fold for patients *with high exposure* to tar and ultraviolet radiation compared with those *lacking high exposure*. When using a control series of 126 patients matched for age, skin type, region of residence, sex, history of exposure to ionizing radiation, and number of PUVA treatments, a stronger association (relative rate = 4.7, 95% confidence limits = 2.2 to 10.0) was observed. The rate of cutaneous carcinoma for subjects exposed to ultraviolet radiation or tar was significantly increased *only* for patients with histories of *very high* exposure. A separate analysis of patients, who were moderately exposed to either of these agents, showed that they had insignificant increases in their risk of developing cutaneous carcinoma, suggesting a dose-response relation between exposure and risk. Although the increased risk of skin carcinoma for patients with psoriasis, who have had very high exposures to tar or ultraviolet radiation is an argument in favor of continued careful surveillance for the early detection of tumors among patients with psoriasis on long-term tar and UV light therapy, it is not a contraindication to the use of these agents, considering the extremely limited morbidity from skin cancer.

18.62   At present, the Goeckerman regimen may be considered as a safe therapeutic approach to psoriasis, although it must be kept in mind that patients with very high exposure to tar and/or ultraviolet light may have a slightly increased risk of developing cutaneous carcinomas.

18.63   REFERENCES

1. Abel, E. A. and Bennett, A. (1979): Bullous pemphigoid. Occurrence in psoriasis treated with psoralens plus long-wave ultra violet radiation. *Arch. Derm., 115,* 988.
2. Abel, E. A. and Farber, E. M. (1980): Photochemotherapy. In: *Recent Advances in Dermatology, Vol. 5,* pp. 259-284. Editors: A. Rook and J. Savin. Churchill Livingstone, Edinburgh.
3. Baron, J. (1974): Diagnostik und Therapie des Hirsutismus. *Zbl. Gynäk., 96,* 129.
4. Barrière, H., Bureau, B. and Planchon, B. (1981): Purpura par sensibilisation au (8 MOP) au cours d'une puvathérapie. *Nouv. Presse Méd., 10,* 337.
5. Bickers, D. R. (1981): The carcinogenicity and mutagenicity of therapeutic coal tar – a perspective (Editorial). *J. invest. Derm., 77,* 173.
6. Bjellerup, M., Bruze, M., Hansson, A., Krook, G. and Ljunggren, B. (1979): Liver injury following administration of 8-methoxypsoralen during PUVA therapy. *Acta derm.-venereol. (Stockh.), 59,* 371.
7. Bjellerup, M., Bruze, M., Forsgren, A., Krook, G. and Ljunggren, B. (1979): Antinuclear antibodies during PUVA therapy. *Acta derm.-venereol. (Stockh.), 59,* 73.
8. Bleehen, S. S. (1978): Freckles induced by PUVA treatment. *Brit. J. Derm., 99, Suppl. 16,* 20.
9. Bridges, B. A. (1978): PUVA and carcinogenicity. *Clin. exp. Derm., 3,* 349.
10. Briffa, D. V. and Warin, A. P. (1977): Photo-onycholysis caused by photochemotherapy. *Brit. med. J., 2,* 1150.
11. Chernosky, M. E. and Anderson, D. E. (1969): Disseminated superficial actinic porokeratosis. Clinical studies and experimental production of lesions. *Arch. Derm., 99,* 401.
12. Ciafone, R. A., Rhodes, A. R., Audley, M., Freedberg, I. M. and Abelmann, W. H. (1980): The cardiovascular stress of photochemotherapy (PUVA). *J. Amer. Acad. Derm., 3,* 499.
13. Cloud, T. M., Hakim, R. and Griffin, A. C. (1961): Photosensitization of the eye with methoxsalen. II. Chronic effects. *Arch. Ophthal., 6,* 689.
14. Cyrlin, M. N., Pedvis-Leftick, A. and Sugar, W. (1980): Cataract formation in association with ultraviolet photosensitivity. *Ann. Ophthal., 12,* 786.
15. Dahl, K. B. (1979): Fotokemoterapi af psoriasis med psoralen og langbolget ultraviolet lys (PUVA). *Ugeskr. Laeg., 141,* 1975.
16. Dorval, J. C., Leroy, J. P. and Massé, R. (1979): Granulomes annulaires disséminés après Puva thérapie. *Ann. Derm. Vénéréol. (Paris), 106,* 79.
17. Dupré, A., Carrère, S., Launais, B. and Bonafé, J. L. (1980): Lichen plan avec photosensibilisation après pyritinol et PUVA-thérapie. *Ann. Derm. Vénéréol. (Paris), 107,* 557.
18. Elliott, J. A. (1959): Clinical experiences with methoxsalen in the treatment of vitiligo. *J. invest. Derm., 32,* 311.
19. Epstein, J. P. (1979): Risks and benefits of the treatment of psoriasis. *New Engl. J. Med., 300,* 852.
20. Epstein, J. H. et al. (1979): Current status of oral PUVA therapy for psoriasis. *J. Amer. Acad. Derm., 1,* 107.
21. Eyanson, S., Greist, M. C., Brandt, K. D. and Skinner, B. (1979): Systemic lupus erythematodes. Association with psoralen-ultraviolet, a treatment of psoriasis. *Arch. Derm., 115,* 54.
22. Farber, E. M., Abel, E. A. and Schaefer, H. (1978): PUVA appraisal. *Brit. J. Derm., 99,* 715.
23. Findlay, G. M. (1928): Ultraviolet light and skin cancer. *Lancet, 2,* 1070.
24. Fitzpatrick, T. B., Imbrie, J. D. and Labby, D. (1958): Effect of methoxsalen on liver function. *J. Amer. med. Ass., 167,* 1586.
25. Forrest, J. B. and Forrest, H. J. (1980): Case report on malignant melanoma arising during drug therapy for vitiligo. *J. Surg. Oncol., 13,* 337.
26. Fritsch, P. (1977): Gefahren unsachgemässer und unkontrollierter Anwendung von Psoralen. *Z. Hautkr., 52,* 1058.

239

27. Fulton, J. E. and Willis, I. (1968): Photoallergy to methoxsalen. *Arch. Derm.*, *98*, 445.
28. Goeckerman, W. H. (1925): Treatment of psoriasis. *Northw. Med. (Seattle)*, *24*, 229.
29. Götz, H. (1976): Tar keratosis. In: *Cancer of the Skin: Biology-Diagnosis-Management. Vol. 1*, pp. 492-523. Editors: R. Andrate, S. L. Gumport, G. L. Popkin et al. W. B. Saunders Co., Philadelphia.
30. Greither, A., Gisbertz, C. and Ippen, H. (1967): Teerbehandlung und Krebs. *Z. Haut- u. Geschlkr.*, *42*, 631.
31. Griffin, A. C., Dolman, V. S., Bohlke, E. F., Bouvart, P. and Tatum, E. (1955): The effect of visible light on the carcinogenicity of ultraviolet light. *Cancer Res.*, *15*, 523.
32. Griffin, A. C., Hakim, R. E. and Knox, J. (1959): The wavelength effect upon erythemal and carcinogenic response in psoralen-treated mice. *J. invest. Derm.*, *31*, 289.
33. Heise, H., Geidel, H. and Valerius, B. (1980): Hirsutismus als seltene Komplikation der PUVA-Therapie. *Derm. Mschr.*, *166*, 611.
34. Helland, S. and Bang, G. (1980): Nevus spilus-like hyperpigmentation in psoriatic lesions during PUVA therapy. *Acta derm.-venereol. (Stockh.)*, *60*, 81.
35. Hirohata, T., Masuda, Y., Horie, A. and Masanori, K. (1973): Carcinogenicity of tar-containing skin drugs: animal experiment and chemical analysis. *Gann*, *64*, 323.
36. Hofmann, C., Plewig, G. and Braun-Falco, O. (1977): Ungewöhnliche Nebenwirkungen bei oraler Photochemotherapie (PUVA Therapie) der Psoriasis. *Hautarzt*, *28*, 583.
37. Hofmann, C., Plewig, G. and Braun-Falco, O. (1979): Bowenoid lesions, Bowen's disease and keratoacanthomas in long-term PUVA-treated patients. *Brit. J. Derm.*, *101*, 685.
38. Hönigsmann, H., Wolff, K., Gschnait, F., Brenner, W. and Jaschke, E. (1980): Keratoses and non-melanoma skin tumors in long-term photochemotherapy (PUVA). *J. Amer. Acad. Derm.*, *3*, 406.
39. Jacobs, P. H., Farber, E. M. and Hall, M. L. (1977): Psoriasis and skin cancer. In: *Psoriasis: Proceedings of the Second International Symposium*, pp. 350-352. Editors: E. M. Farber, A. Cox, P. Jacobs et al. Yorke Medical Books, New Jersey.
40. Jones, C. and Bleehen, S. S. (1977): Acne induced by PUVA treatment. *Brit. med. J.*, *2*, 866.
41. Kaaber, K. (1976): Occurrence of malignant neoplasms in patients with atopic dermatitis. *Acta derm.-venereol. (Stockh.)*, *56*, 445.
42. Langner, A. and Christophers, E. (1977): Leukocyte chemotaxis after in vitro treatment with 8-methoxypsoralen and UVA. *Arch. derm. Res.*, *260*, 51.
43. Lassus, A., Reunala, J., Idänpää-Heikkilä, J., Juvakoski, T. and Salo, O. (1981): PUVA treatment and skin cancer: a follow-up study. *Acta derm.-venereol. (Stockh.)*, *61*, 141.
44. Omitted.
45. Lerman, S., Jocoy, M. and Borkman, R. F. (1977): Photosensitization of the lens by 8-methoxypsoralen. *Invest. Ophthal. vis. Sci.*, *16*, 1065.
46. Lerman, S., Megaw, J. and Willis, I. (1980): The photoreaction of 8-MOP with tryptophan and lens proteins. *Photochem. Photobiol.*, *31*, 235.
47. Mahakrishnan, A. and Shesan Narayanan, G. V. (1981): Temporal arteritis following trimethoxypsoralen therapy. *Indian J. Derm. Venereol. Leprol.*, *47*, 53.
48. Maughan, W. Z., Muller, S. A., Perry, H. A., Pittelkow, M. R. and O'Brien, P. C. (1980): Incidence of skin cancers in patients with atopic dermatitis treated with coal tar. *J. Amer. Acad. Derm.*, *3*, 612.
49. Melski, J. W., Tanenbaum, L., Parrish, J. A., Fitzpatrick, T. B., Bleich, H. L. et al. (1977): Oral methoxsalen photochemotherapy for the treatment of psoriasis: a cooperative clinical trial. *J. invest. Derm.*, *68*, 328.
50. Miller, J. and Munro, D. D. (1980): Severe skin pain following PUVA. *Acta derm.-venereol. (Stockh.)*, *60*, 187.
51. Molin, L., Thomsen, K., Volden, G. and Groth, O. (1980): Photochemotherapy (PUVA) in the pretumour stage of mycosis fungoides: a report from the Scandinavian mycosis fungoides study group. *Acta derm.-venereol. (Stockh.)*, *61*, 47.
52. Møller, R. and Howitz, J. (1976): Methoxsalen and multiple basal cell carcinomas. *Arch. Derm.*, *112*, 1613.
53. Muller, S. A. and Kierland, R. R. (1964): Crude coal tar in dermatologic therapy. *Mayo Clin. Proc.*, *39*, 275.
54. Naik, R. P. C. and Singh, G. (1979): Nail pigmentation due to oral 8-methoxypsoralen. *Brit. J. Derm.*, *100*, 229.
55. Orlonne, J. P. and Baran, R. (1978): Photo-onycholyse induite par la photochimiothérapie orale. *Ann. Derm. Vénéréol. (Paris)*, *105*, 887.
56. Pariser, D. M. and Wyles, R. J. (1980): Toxic hepatitis from oral methoxsalen photochemotherapy (PUVA). *J. Amer. Acad. Derm.*, *3*, 248.

57. Pathak, M. A., Daniels Jr., F., Hopkins, C. E. and Fitzpatrick, T. B. (1959): Ultraviolet carcinogenesis in albino and pigmented mice receiving furocoumarins: Psoralen and 8-methoxypsoralen. *Nature (Lond.), 183,* 728.

58. Petrozzi, J. W., Barton, J. O., Kaidbey, K. H. and Kligman, A. M. (1978): Updating the Goeckerman regimen for psoriasis. *Brit. J. Derm., 98,* 437.

59. Pittelkow, M. R., Perry, H. O., Muller, S. A., Maughan, W. Z. and O'Brien, P. C. (1980): Skin cancer in patients with psoriasis treated with coal tar. *Arch. Derm., 117,* 465.

60. Plewig, G., Hofmann, C. and Braun-Falco, O. (1978): Photoallergic dermatitis from 8-methoxypsoralen. *Arch. derm. Res., 261,* 201.

61. Rasmussen, J. E. (1978): The crudeness of coal tar. *Progr. Derm., 12,* 23.

62. Rau, R. C., Flowers, F. P. and Barrett, J. L. (1978): Photo-onycholysis secondary to psoralen use. *Arch. Derm., 114,* 448.

63. Reymond, J. L., Beani, J. C. and Amblard, P. (1980): Superficial actinic porokeratosis in a patient undergoing long-term PUVA therapy. *Acta derm.-venereol. (Stockh.), 60,* 539.

64. Robinson, J. K., Baughman, R. D. and Provost, T. T. (1978): Bullous pemphigoid induced by PUVA therapy. *Brit. J. Derm., 99,* 709.

65. Roenigk, H. H. and Caro, W. A. (1981): Skin cancer in the PUVA-48 cooperative study. *J. Amer. Acad. Derm., 4,* 319.

66. Roenigk, H. H. and Martin, J. S. (1977): Photochemotherapy for psoriasis. *Arch. Derm., 113,* 1667.

67. Rook, A. J., Gresham, G. A. and Davis, R. A. (1956): Squamous epithelioma possibly induced by the therapeutic application of tar. *Brit. J. Cancer, 10,* 17.

68. Saihan, E. M. (1979): Contact allergy to 8-methoxypsoralen. *Brit. med. J., 2,* 20.

69. Scotto, J., Kopf, A. W. and Urbach, F. (1974): Non-melanoma skin cancer among Caucasians in four areas of the United States. *Cancer, 34,* 1333.

70. Segal, R. J. and Watson, W. (1978): Kaposi's varicelliform eruption in mycosis fungoides. *Arch. Derm., 114,* 1067.

71. Singh, F. and Lal, S. (1967): Hypertrichosis and hyperpigmentation with systemic psoralen treatment. *Brit. J. Derm., 79,* 501.

72. Stern, R. S., Thibodeau, L. A., Kleinerman, R. A., Parrish, J. A. and Fitzpatrick, T. B. (1979): Risk of cutaneous carcinoma in patients treated with oral methoxsalen photochemotherapy for psoriasis. *New Engl. J. Med., 300,* 809.

73. Stern, R. S., Morison, W. L., Thibodeau, L. A., Kleinerman, R. A., Parrish, J. A., Geer, D. E. and Fitzpatrick, T. B. (1979): Antinuclear antibodies and oral methoxsalen photochemotherapy (PUVA) for psoriasis. *Arch. Derm., 115,* 1320.

74. Stern, R. S., Zierler, S. and Parrish, J. A. (1980): Skin carcinoma in patients with psoriasis treated with topical tar and artificial ultraviolet radiation. *Lancet, 1,* 732.

75. Strauss, G. H., Bridges, B. A., Greaves, M., Vella Briffa, D., Hall Smith, P. and Price, M. (1980): Methoxsalen photochemotherapy. *Lancet, 2,* 1134.

76. Tegner, A. (1979): Severe skin pain after PUVA treatment. *Acta derm.-venereol. (Stockh.), 59,* 467.

77. Thomsen, K. and Schmidt, H. (1976): PUVA-induced bullous pemphigoid. *Brit. J. Derm., 95,* 568.

78. Tucker, H. H. (1959): Clinical and laboratory tolerance studies in volunteers given oral methoxsalen. *J. invest. Derm., 32,* 277.

79. Urbach, F. (1959): Modification of ultraviolet carcinogenesis by photoactive agents: preliminary report. *J. invest. Derm., 32,* 373.

80. Urbach, F., Epstein, J. H. and Forbes, P. D. (1974): Ultraviolet carcinogenesis: experimental, global and genetic aspects. In: *Sunlight and Man, Normal and Abnormal Photobiologic Responses,* p. 259. Editors: M. A. Pathak, L. C. Harber, M. Seiji and A. Kukita. University of Tokyo Press, Tokyo.

81. Wagner, J., Manthorpe, R., Philip, P. and Frost, F. (1978): Preleukemia (haemopoietic dysplasia) developing in a patient with psoriasis treated with 8-methoxypsoralen and ultraviolet light. *Scand. J. Haemat., 21,* 299.

82. Weissmann, I., Wagner, G. and Plewig, G. (1980): Contact allergy to 8-methoxypsoralen. *Brit. J. Derm., 102,* 113.

83. Zackheim, H. S. (1978): Should therapeutic coal-tar preparations be available over the counter? *Arch. Derm., 114,* 125.

84. Zala, L., Omar, A. and Krebs, A. (1977): Photo-onycholysis induced by 8-methoxypsoralen. *Dermatologica (Basel), 154,* 203.

18.63 Side effects of photochemotherapy

UPDATE – 2nd Edition

85. Lerman, S., Megaw, J.M., Gardner, K.H. and Drake, L. (1983): Ocular and cutaneous manifestations of PUVA therapy – a review. *J. Toxicol.-Cut. ocul. Toxicol., 1,* 257.
86. Mobacken, H., Rosén, K. and Swanbeck, G. (1983): Oral psoralen photochemotherapy (PUVA) of hyperkeratotic dermatitis of the palms. *Brit. J. Derm., 109,* 205.
87. Vella Briffa, D., Eady, R.A.J., James, M.P. et al. (1983): Photochemotherapy (PUVA) in the treatment of urticaria pigmentosa. *Brit. J. Derm., 109,* 67.
88. Moss, C., Friedmann, P.S. and Shuster, S. (1982): How does PUVA inhibit delayed cutaneous hypersensitivity? *Brit. J. Derm., 107,* 511.
89. Friedmann, P.S., Ford, G., Ross, J. and Diffey, B.L. (1983): Reappearance of epidermal Langerhans cells after PUVA therapy. *Brit. J. Derm., 109,* 301.
90. Miller, R.A. (1982): Psoralens and UV-A-induced stellate hyperpigmented freckling. *Arch. Derm., 118,* 619.
91. Rhodes, A.R., Harrist, T.J. and Momtaz, T. K. (1983): The PUVA-induced pigmented macule: A lentiginous proliferation of large, sometimes cytologically atypical, melanocytes. *J. Amer. Acad. Derm., 9,* 47.
92. Levin, D.L., Roenigk, H.H. Jr., Caro, W.A. and Lyons, M. (1982): Histologic, immunofluorescent, and antinuclear antibody findings in PUVA-treated patients. *J. Amer. Acad. Derm., 6,* 328.
93. Greene, I. and Cox, A.J. (1979): Amyloid deposition after psoriasis therapy with psoralen and longwave ultraviolet light. *Arch. Derm., 115,* 1200.
94. Schuler, G., Hönigsmann, H., Jaschke, E. and Wolff, K. (1982): Selective accumulation of lipid within melanocytes during photochemotherapy (PUVA) of psoriasis. *Brit. J. Derm., 107,* 173.
95. Stern, R.S., Morison, W.L., Thibodeau, L.A. et al. (1979): Antinuclear antibodies and oral methoxsalen photochemotherapy (PUVA) for psoriasis. *Arch. Derm., 115,* 1320.
96. Abel, E.A., Cox, A.J. and Farber, E.M. (1982): Epidermal dystrophy and actinic keratoses in psoriasis patients following oral psoralen photochemotherapy (PUVA). *J. Amer. Acad. Derm., 7,* 333.
97. Halprin, K.M., Comerford, M. and Taylor, J.R. (1982): Cancer in patients with psoriasis. *J. Amer. Acad. Derm., 7,* 633.
98. Chappe, S.G., Roenigk, H.H. Jr., Miller, A.J. et al. (1981): The effects of photochemotherapy on the cardiovascular system. *J. Amer. Acad. Derm., 4,* 561.
99. Thürlimann, W. and Harms, M. (1982): Sklerodermiforme Veränderungen nach PUVA-Therapie bei Vitiligo. *Dermatologica (Basel), 164,* 305.
100. Naik, R.P.C. and Parameswara, Y.R. (1982): 8-Methoxypsoralen-induced nail pigmentation. *Int. J. Derm., 21,* 275.
101. Fitzsimons, C.P., Long, J. and MacKie, R.M. (1983): Synergistic carcinogenic potential of methotrexate and PUVA in psoriasis (Letter). *Lancet, 1,* 235.
102. Lerman, S., Megaw, J. and Gardner, K. (1982): Psoralen-long-wave ultraviolet therapy and human cataractogenesis. *Invest. Ophthalmol. vis. Sci., 23,* 801.
103. Rönnerfält, L., Lydahl, E., Wennersten, G. et al. (1982): Ophthalmological study of patients undergoing long-term PUVA therapy. *Acta derm.-venereol. (Stockh.)., 62,* 501.
104. Hammershøy, O. and Jessen, F. (1982): A retrospective study of cataract formation in 96 patients treated with PUVA. *Acta derm.-venereol. (Stockh.), 62,* 444.
105. Pullmann, H., Trost, Th. and Witte, U. (1982): Akrale Blasenbildung unter PUVA-Therapie. *Z. Hautkr., 57,* 288.
106. Brun, P. and Baran, R. (1982): Pemphigoïde bulleuse induite par la photochimiothérapie du psoriasis. *Ann. Derm. Vénéréol. (Paris), 109,* 461.
107. Albergo, R.P. and Gilgor, R.S. (1982): Delayed onset of bullous pemphigoid after PUVA and sunlight treatment of psoriasis. *Cutis, 30,* 621.
108. Marsch, W.Ch. and Stüttgen, G. (1982): Ultrastruktur der 'akrobullösen Dermatose' PUVA-therapierter Psoriatiker. *Z. Hautkr., 57,* 1811.
109. Stüttgen, G. (1982): The risk of photochemotherapy. *Int. J. Derm., 21,* 198.
110. Bickers, D.R. (1983): Position paper - PUVA therapy. *J. Amer. Acad. Derm., 8,* 265.
111. Backman, H.A. (1982): The effects of PUVA on the eye. *Amer. J. Optom. Physiol. Optics, 59,* 86.
112. Epstein, J.H., Farber, E.M. (co-chairman), Nall M.L. (ed) and 27 compilers (1979): Current status of oral PUVA therapy for psoriasis. *J. Amer. Acad. Derm., 1,* 107.
113. Farber, E.M. Abel, E.A. and Cox, A.J. (1983): Long-term risks of psoralen and UV-A therapy for psoriasis. *Arch. Derm., 119,* 426.
114. Farber, E.M., Epstein, J.H. (co-chairman), Nall, M.L. (Ed.) and 41 compilers (1982): Current status of oral PUVA therapy for psoriasis: Eye protection revisions. *J. Amer. Acad. Derm., 6,* 851.

115. Fenton, D.A. and Wilkinson, J.D. (1983): Dose-related visual-field defects in patients receiving PUVA therapy. *Lancet, 1,* 1106.

116. Friedmann, P.S. (1981): Disappearance of epidermal Langerhans cells during PUVA therapy. *Brit. J. Derm., 105,* 219.

117. Gschnait, F., Wolff, K., Hönigsmann, H. et al. (1980): Long-term photochemotherapy: histopathological and immunofluorescence observations in 243 patients. *Brit. J. Derm., 103,* 11.

118. Kasick, J.M., Berlin, A.J., Berfeld, W, et al. (1982): Development of cataracts with photochemotherapy. In: *Proceedings of the Third International Symposium on Psoriasis,* pp. 467-468. Eds.: E.M. Farber and A.J. Cox. Grune & Stratton Inc., New York.

119. Lerman, S. (1982): Ocular phototoxicity and psoralen plus ultraviolet radiation (320-400 nm) therapy: An experimental and clinical evaluation. *J. nat. Cancer Inst., 69,* 287.

120. Morison, W.L., Wimberly, J., Parrish, J.A. and Bloch, K.J. (1983): Abnormal lymphocyte function following long-term PUVA therapy for psoriasis. *Brit. J. Derm., 108,* 445.

121. Mosciki, R.A., Morison, W.L., Parrish, J.A., et al. (1983): Reduction of the fraction of circulating helper-inducer T-cells identified by monoclonal antibodies in psoriatic patients treated with long-term psoralen ultraviolet-A radiation (PUVA). *J. invest. Derm.* in press.

122. Niemi, K.M., Niemi, A.J., Juvakoski, T. et al. (1982): Epidermal dystrophy in psoriasis patients with or without PUVA and with or without previous arsenic treatment. In: *Proceedings of the Third International Symposium on Psoriasis,* pp. 449-450. Eds.: E.M. Farber and A.J. Cox. Grune & Stratton Inc., New York.

123. Tegner, E. (1983): Seborrhoeic dermatitis of the face induced by PUVA treatment. *Acta derm.-venereol. (Stockh.), 63,* 335.

124. Saperstein, M.D. and Wheeler, L.A. (1979): Mutagenicity of coal tar preparations used in the treatment of psoriasis. *Toxicol. Lett., 3,* 325.

125. Wheeler, L.A., Saperstein, M.D. and Lowe, N.J. (1981): Mutagenicity of urine from psoriatic patients undergoing treatment with coal tar and light *J. invest. Derm., 77,* 181.

126. Bickers, D.R. (1981): The carcinogenicity and mutagenicity of therapeutic tar – a perspective (Editorial). *J. invest. Derm., 77,* 173.

127. Stern, R.S., Parrish, J.A., Bleich, H.L. and Fitzpatrick, T.B. (1981): PUVA (psoralen and ultraviolet A) and squamous cell carcinoma in patients with psoriasis. *J. invest Derm., 76,* 311.

128. Kanerva, L., Laurahanta, J., Niemi, K.M. et al. (1983): Persistent ashen-gray maculae and freckles induced by long-term PUVA treatment. *Dermatologica (Basel), 166,* 281.

129. Lobel, E., Paver, K., King, R. et al. (1981): The relationship of skin cancer to PUVA therapy in Australia. *Aust. J. Derm., 22,* 100.

130. Tegner, A. (1983): Observations on PUVA-treatment of psoriasis and on 5-S-cysteinyldopa after exposure to UV light. *Acta derm.-venereol. (Stockholm), Suppl.,* 107.

131. Murray, D., Corbett, M.F. and Warin, A.P. (1980): A controlled trial of photochemotherapy for persistent palmoplantar pustulosis. *Brit. J. Derm. 102,* 659.

132. LeVine, M.J., Parrish, J.A. and Fitzpatrick, T.B. (1981): Oral methoxsalen photochemotherapy (PUVA) of dyshidrotic eczema. *Acta derm.-venereol. (Stockh.), 61,* 570.

133. Moss, C., Friedmann, P.S. and Shuster, S. (1981): Impaired contact hypersensitivity in untreated psoriasis and the effects of photochemotherapy and dithranol/UV-B. *Brit. J. Derm., 105,* 503.

134. Stern, R.S. (1982): Carcinogenic risks of psoriasis therapy. In: *Proceedings of the Third International Symposium on Psoriasis.* Eds.: E.M. Farber and A.J. Cox. Grune & Stratton Inc., New York.

135. Segal, S., Cohen, S.N., Freeman, J. et al. (1978): A caution. *Amer. Acad. Pediat., 62,* 253.

136. Lassus, A., Kianto, U., Johansson, E. and Juvakoski, T. (1980): PUVA treatment for alopecia areata. *Dermatologica (Basel), 161,* 298.

137. Morison, W.L., Parrish, J.A. and Fitzpatrick, T.B. (1978): Oral psoralen photochemotherapy of atopic eczema. *Brit. J. Derm., 98,* 25.

138. Gschnait, F., Hönigsmann, H., Brenner, W. et al. (1978): Induction of UV-light tolerance by PUVA in patients with polymorphous light eruption. *Brit. J. Derm., 99,* 293.

139. Cox, A.J. and Abel, E.A. (1979): Epidermal dystrophy: Occurrence after psoriasis therapy with psoralen and long-wave ultraviolet light. *Arch. Derm., 115,* 567.

140. Gschnait, F., Wolff, K., Hönigsmann, H. et al. (1980): Long-term photochemotherapy: Histopathological and immunofluorescence observations in 243 patients. *Brit. J. Derm., 103,* 11.

141. Ingraham, D., Bergfeld, W., Balin, P. et al. (1982): Histopathologic changes in the skin after prolonged PUVA therapy and after discontinuance of PUVA therapy. In: *Psoriasis: Third International Symposium on Psoriasis,* pp. 457-458. Eds.: E.M. Farber and A.J. Cox. Grune & Stratton Inc., New York.

142. Epstein, J.H. (1978): Photocarcinogenesis: A review. *Nat. Cancer Inst. Monogr. 50,* 13.

143. Heidbreder, G. (1980): Lokalisierte Blasen bei Fotochemotherapie - eine akrobullöse Fotoderma-tose. *Z. Hautkr., 55,* 84.

144. McGibbon, D.H. and Vella-Briffa, D. (1978): Histologic features of PUVA-induced bullae in pso-riatic skin. *Clin. exp. Derm., 3,* 371.

145. Crickx, B., Girouin, D., diCrescenzo, M.C. and Hewitt, J. (1979): Psoriasis et pemphigoïde bulleuse. *Journées derm. Paris,* March 1979, p. 56.

146. Gissler, K. and Lischka, G. (1978): PUVA induziertes bullöses Pemphigoid bei Psoriasis vulgaris. *Akta Derm., 4,* 47.

147. Grupper, C., Bernejo, D., Durepaire, R. and Berretti, B. (1977): Pemphigus séborrhéique de Senear-Usher compliquant un psoriasis. Rôle aggravant de la PUVA thérapie. *Journées derm. Paris,* March 9-10, p. 77.

148. Freeman, R.G. and Troll, D. (1969): Photosensitization of the eye by 8-methoxypsoralen. *J. invest. Derm., 53,* 449.

149. Lerman, S., Megaw, J. and Willis, I. (1980): Potential ocular complications of PUVA therapy and their prevention. *J. invest. Derm., 74,* 197.

150. Davey, J.B., Diffey, B.L. and Miller, J.A. (1981): Eye protection in psoralen photochemotherapy. *Brit. J. Derm., 104,* 295.

151. Szekeres, E., Török, L. and Szücs, M. (1981): Auftreten disseminierter hyperpigmentierter Flecke unter PUVA-Behandlung. *Hautarzt, 32,* 33.

152. Skogh, M. and Moi, H. (1978): Naevus-spilus-artige Hyperpigmentierung bei Psoriasis. *Hautarzt, 29,* 607.

153. Konrad, K., Gschnait, F. and Wolff, K. (1977): Ultrastructure of poikiloderma-like pigmentary changes after repeated experimental PUVA-overdosage. *J. cutan. Pathol., 4,* 219.

154. Kanerva, L., Niemi, K.-M. and Lassus, A. (1981): Hyperpigmentation and hypopigmentation of the skin after long term PUVA therapy. *J. cutan. Pathol., 8,* 199.

155. Kanerva, L., Lauharanta, J., Niemi, K.-M. et al. (1982): *Fine Structure of Freckles Induced by Long Term PUVA Treatment of Psoriasis.* XVI Int. Congr. Dermatology, Tokyo. Abstr. 582, pp. 408-409.

156. MacKie, R.M. and Fitzsimons, C.P. (1983): Risk of carcinogenicity in patients with psoriasis treat-ed with methotrexate or PUVA singly or in combination. *J. Amer. Acad. Derm., 9,* 467.

157. Diezel, W., Waschke, S.R. and Sönnichsen, N. (1983): Detection of interferon in the sera of patients with psoriasis, and its enhancement by PUVA treatment *Brit. J. Derm., 109,* 549.

158. Rampen, F.H.J. (1983): A neglected side effect of PUVA therapy: hypertrichosis (Netherlands Soci-ety Proceedings). *Brit. J. Derm., 109,* 481.

159. Morison, W.L. and Strickland, P.T. (1983): Environmental UVA radiation and eye protection dur-ing PUVA therapy. *J. Amer. Acad. Derm., 9,* 522.

160. Todes-Taylor, N., Abel, E.A. and Cox, A.J. (1983): The occurrence of vitiligo after psoralens and ultraviolet A therapy. *J. Amer. Acad. Derm., 9,* 526.

19. Side effects of systemic drugs used in dermatology

CORTICOSTEROIDS

19.1   Corticosteroids are used in dermatology in four ways: orally, parenterally, topically and intralesionally; the side effects of *topical* steroids are discussed in Chapter 14. Unless a rapid effect is needed, or practical circumstances make this impossible, the corticosteroids are usually given by mouth.

19.2   The main dermatological uses of oral or parenteral corticosteroids are the following [9]:
    – As a short-time 'cover' for acute and severe reactions running a defined course, e.g. erythema exsudativum multiforme, acute urticaria of known cause, severe drug eruptions and, rarely, acute contact sensitivities.
    – For certain allergic or anaphylactic reactions carrying danger to life, e.g. anaphylactic shock, multiple bee or wasp stings, poisonous bites (sometimes).
    – In severe or generalized immunological disorders, e.g. systemic lupus erythematosus, active dermatomyositis and pyoderma gangrenosum.
    – In certain generalized vascular disorders of supposed immunological origin, e.g. polyarteritis nodosa, temporal arteritis, Wegener's granulomatosis, thrombocytopenic purpura and some cases of allergic vasculitis where vital organs are involved.
    – For certain chronic disorders otherwise fatal or disabling, e.g. pemphigus, pemphigoid, mucous membrane pemphigoid (some cases) and exfoliative dermatitis.
    – In some miscellaneous conditions such as epidermolysis bullosa in childhood and persistent aphthosis accompanied by severe pain.
    – In sarcoidosis, when the posterior uveal tract is involved or when progressive pulmonary or renal disease is present.
    – *Relative indications:* severe lichen planus, reticuloses, severe eczema, Reiter's disease, Sjögren's syndrome. Occasionally severe acne and hidradenitis suppurativa.

19.3   The value of the corticosteroids in dermatology need not be stressed; however, side effects are numerous and often quite serious, and therefore systemic corticosteroids should only be prescribed after careful consideration of alternative means of treatment. The metabolic, anti-immunologic and anti-inflammatory effects of systemic steroid therapy are listed in § 19.4.

19.4   **Metabolic, anti-immunologic and anti-inflammatory effects of systemic steroid therapy**

Metabolic effects:
– increases gluconeogenesis in liver
– increases synthesis of specific liver enzymes
– increases synthesis of RNA in liver

- decreases peripheral protein synthesis
- decreases synthesis of nucleic acids in most tissues
- increases activity of lipolytic enzymes
- decreases long chain fatty acid synthesis
- decreases calcium absorption from the gastrointestinal tract (anti-Vitamin D effect)
- produces osteoporosis and osteomalacia
- tends to lead to peptic ulceration in gastrointestinal tract
- maintains peripheral vascular responsiveness to endogenous vasoconstrictors like nor-epinephrine
- maintains normal internal water distribution

Anti-immunologic effects:
- *the afferent limb* (macrophage processing of antigen)
- suppresses phagocytic activity of macrophages
- slows down intracellular digestion
- inhibits diapedesis of mononuclear cells (decreasing influx of macrophages to the site of injury)
- *the central limb* (leading to sensitized T- and B-cells)
- lymphocytolytic
- prevents formation of the mature sensitized lymphocyte (low doses affect T-cells; higher doses required to affect B-cells)
- *the efferent limb* (sensitized T- and B-lymphocytes versus antigen)
- suppresses cell mediated immunity; decreases active RNA and protein synthesis necessary for lymphocyte activity; directly antagonizes lymphokines such as MIF
- suppresses humoral immunity – primary response more affected than anamnestic response; increases immunoglobulin catabolism; diminishes Arthus reaction because of diminished release of lysosomal enzymes; inhibits subfractions of complement

Anti-inflammatory effects:
- stabilizes lysosomal and other biomembranes, therefore decreases enzymatic degradation of tissues; affects cleavage of complement components to active subfractions; decreases disruption of mast cells and consequent release of vasoactive amines
- decreases the margination and sticking of polymorphs to vascular endothelium
- inhibits NADH oxidase activity necessary for killing of ingested bacteria in polymorphs
- decreases vascular permeability
- diminishes release of mediators of inflammation such as histamine
- decreases fibroblastic activity; therefore decreases granulation tissue production

There are several preparations available for parenteral and oral use; for routine oral use, prednisolone or prednisone (which is inactive, but is converted to prednisolone in the liver) is advisable. The comparative potency of the glucocorticosteroids is listed in § 19.5 [4]:

19.5   Comparative potency of glucocorticosteroids

Compound (or its ester)	Glucocorticoid potency*	Mineralocorticoid potency	Equivalent dose
HYDROCORTISONE	1.0	+ +	20.0 mg
betamethasone	30	0	0.6 mg
cortisone	0.8	+ +	25.0 mg
dexamethasone	30	0	0.75 mg
fluprednisolone	10	0	1.5 mg
meprednisone	5	0	4.0 mg
methylprednisolone	5	0	4.0 mg

(continued)

(continuation)

Compound (or its ester)	Glucocorticoid potency*	Mineralocorticoid potency	Equivalent dose
paramethasone	10	0	2.0 mg
prednisolone	4	+	5.0 mg
prednisone	4	+	5.0 mg
triamcinolone	5	0	4.0 mg

* As compared to hydrocortisone (expressed on a mg/mg basis).

Side effects

19.6   Unwanted effects of the glucocorticosteroids can apparently be prevented to some extent by giving them in a single dosis in the morning, preferably on alternate days [69].

19.7   Side effects of orally administered corticosteroids include [e.g. 61, 69, 23]:
– Iatrogenic Cushing's syndrome: benign intracranial hypertension, glaucoma, subcapsular cataract, pancreatitis, aseptic necrosis of the bones, panniculitis, obesity, facial rounding, psychiatric symptoms, edema, delayed wound healing and, to a lesser degree, hypertension, acne, disorders of sexual function, hirsutism, virilism, striae of the skin, plethora.
– Pituitary-adrenal suppression [26], leading to atrophy of the adrenal cortex; this may induce 'withdrawal reactions' when the steroid therapy is terminated. Symptoms include: headache, nausea, dizziness, anorexia, weakness, emotional changes, lethargy, fever and death [69].
– Central nervous system derangement: cerebral atrophy, manifestation of latent epilepsy, various behavioral and personality changes ranging from nervousness, insomnia, euphoria or mood swings to psychotic episodes [198].
– Skin disorders: hirsutism, striae, atrophic changes, ecchymoses, acne, infections of the skin, erythematous rash (rare [120]), perioral dermatitis [224].
– Inhibition of immune responses: aggravation of tuberculosis, fungal and candidal infections; increased risk of bacterial and viral infection.
– Osteoporosis, leading to fractures, vertebral compression fractures, aseptic bone necrosis [225].
– Ophthalmological changes: cataract, glaucoma, exophthalmus (rare).
– Retardation of growth in children.
– Hematological changes: leukocytosis, thrombocytosis, polycythemia (very rare), increase in hemoglobin, depression of the lymphocyte count, changes in blood coagulation leading to thrombosis.
– Metabolic changes: 'steroid diabetes', hypertriglyceridemia with milky plasma.
– Gastrointestinal disturbances: peptic ulceration (not proven), pancreatitis, derangements of pancreatic secretion, perforation of the colon [169].
– Changes in mineral and fluid balance (in steroids with marked mineralocorticoid activity): salt and water retention, increase in calcium and phosphorus excretion (may lead to tetany).
– Urinary calculi formation.
– Disorders of menstruation.
– Muscular atrophy and fibrosis.
– Cardiac myopathy, arrhythmias and cardiac arrest secondary to hypokalemia.
– Nocturia.
– Allergic reactions, including urticaria (very rare after oral administration).

247

19.8   Intralesional corticosteroid therapy

- Pathological changes in thyroid function (rare).
- Reduced sperm count and motility (?).

Intralesional corticosteroid therapy

19.8   Indications for intralesional corticosteroid therapy include alopecia areata, keloids, lichen ruber obtusus, acne cystica and necrobiosis lipoidica.

Systemic side effects

19.9   Systemic side effects of intralesional corticosteroid therapy are usually related to suppression of the adrenal glands [103]. Severe cramps in the back, shoulders and legs immediately following intralesional injection of corticosteroids and lasting for about half an hour have been reported by Shelmire [119]. This side effect was attributed by the author to injection of crystals into a small vein.

Local side effects

19.10   The local side effects of intralesional corticosteroids include [105]:
- Depigmentation (leucoderma)
- Cutaneous atrophy, sometimes with striae
- Necrosis
- Local erythema, appearing after 12 hours and lasting for about 36 hours [36]
- Calcinosis cutis [7]
- Linear atrophy along lymphatic vessels [67]
- Amaurosis? [11]

CYTOSTATIC AND IMMUNOSUPPRESSIVE DRUGS

19.11   Cytostatic drugs may be divided into four groups:
1. Antimetabolites
- *folic acid antagonists:* methotrexate
- *purine analogs:* azathioprine, mercaptopurine, mycophenolic acid
- *pyrimidine analogs:* azarabine, fluorouracil
2. Alkylating agents
- *nitrogen mustards:* chlorambucil, melphalan, cyclophosphamide
- *alkyl sulphonates:* busulfan
- *ethylenimine derivatives:* triethylenemelamine
- *nitrosoureas:* carmustine, lomustine
- *triazines:* dacarbazine
3. Natural products
- *alkaloids:* colchicine, vincristine, vinblastine
- *enzymes:* L-asparaginase
- *antibiotics:* bleomycin, actinomycin D
4. Miscellaneous agents
- procarbazine
- hydroxyurea
- radioactive isotopes

Use of cytostatics in dermatology

19.12   The following drugs are used in dermatological practice [10]:

Cyclophosphamide: pemphigus vulgaris, bullous pemphigoid, Wegener's granulomatosis, systemic lupus erythematosus, polymyositis, mycosis fungoides, histiocytosis-X

Chlorambucil: mycosis fungoides, Behçet's disease, systemic lupus erythematosus, Wegener's granulomatosis, steroid-resistant sarcoidosis, Sézary syndrome

Dacarbazine: metastatic malignant melanoma

Methotrexate: psoriasis, Reiter's disease, pityriasis rubra pilaris, ichthyosiform erythroderma, keratoacanthoma, pemphigus vulgaris, pemphigus foliaceus, bullous pemphigoid, corticosteroid-resistant dermatomyositis (for methotrexate guidelines in psoriasis, see [180])

Azarabine: mycosis fungoides, psoriasis

Azathioprine: psoriasis, psoriatic arthropathy, pemphigus vulgaris, bullous pemphigoid, systemic lupus erythematosus, dermatomyositis, Wegener's granulomatosis, pityriasis rubra pilaris

Mycophenolic acid: psoriasis

Bleomycin: squamous cell carcinoma of the skin, mycosis fungoides, intralesionally for intractable virus warts

Hydroxyurea: psoriasis

Most of the available cytostatics are active against rapidly growing tumors and they damage those normal tissues which are mitotically most active, namely the bone marrow, the digestive tract, the germinative epithelium and the active cells of the hair follicle. Most of the direct toxic effects therefore are localized in these organ systems. A distinction must be made between acute and long-term effects.

Acute effects

19.13   These are due to the direct toxic effects of the cytostatics on the tissues comprising rapidly dividing cells: bone marrow depression, alopecia, gastrointestinal bleeding, nausea, vomiting, impairment of gonadal function.

Long-term effects

19.14   It is becoming increasingly clear that patients who have been treated with intensive chemotherapeutic regimens, are more prone to develop second malignancies [132]. Notable examples are patients with Hodgkin's disease, in whom a definite increase in the risk of acute myeloblastic leukemia is now recognized [46]. However, in many other malignant conditions as well, secondary malignancies are being reported with increasing frequency after the prolonged therapy with cytostatics.

19.15   Cytostatics

Side effects

19.15   A number of side effects are common to many cytostatics:
- Bone marrow depression: leukopenia, thrombocytopenia, anemia, morphological alterations in hematopoietic cells
- Gastrointestinal tract disturbances: nausea, vomiting, diarrhea, anorexia, glossitis, gingivitis, ulcerating enteritis, gastritis
- Alopecia
- Infections, especially with *Pseudomonas* and opportunistic organisms such as fungi, viruses and parasitic disease
- Teratogenicity, when administered in the first trimester of pregnancy
- Induction of second malignancies
- Growth retardation in children
- Uric acid nephropathy in the treatment of lymphomas and leukemias
- Hyperkalemia due to the sudden lysis of large volumes of tumor tissue
- Gonadal dysfunction, eventually leading to sterility.

19.16   The side effects of individual cytostatics include:

Cyclophosphamide:
- sterile cystitis, fibrosis of the bladder
- blurred vision (rare) [199]
- interstitial pneumonia (rare) [199]
- myocardial necrosis (rare)
- Graves' disease (one report)
- myxedema (one report)
- pigmentation of the nails [117] and skin

Chlorambucil:
- allergic urticarial skin rash (one report, Knisley et al. [68])
- interstitial pulmonary fibrosis (rare) [199]
- focal seizures
- peripheral neuropathy (rare)

Dacarbazine
- photosensitivity [144, 185]
- facial flushing [186]
- paresthesia [186]

Methotrexate:
- hepatic damage leading to cirrhosis [96, 106, 223]
- photosensitivity and reactivation of sunburn reaction [173, 179]
- neurological symptoms, when administered intrathecally
- interstitial pneumonia [83, 199]
- nephrotoxicity [35]
- toxic epidermal necrolysis [161], skin necrosis [164]
- conjunctivitis [199]

Azarabine:
- neurotoxicity
- thromboembolism

Azathioprine:
- pancreatitis

– cholestatic jaundice (rare)
– acneiform eruption [324]

Bleomycin:
– (often fatal) interstitial pneumonia [199]
– mental disturbances
– drug fever
– skin disorders: swelling of the skin and joints, hyperkeratosis, pigmentation, blisters, scleroderma-like changes [66].

Hydroxyurea:
– strong teratogenicity
– hyperpigmentation
– hepatitis (rare)
– 'influenza-like' reaction

ANTIBIOTICS AND CHEMOTHERAPEUTICS

Penicillins

19.17   Penicillins are bactericidal antibiotics; they are virtually non-toxic in man and may also be given to pregnant women and children. Various newer semisynthetic penicillins have a broad spectrum activity (e.g. amino- and amidopenicillins, carbenicillin, ticarcillin and the ureidopenicillins) or are penicillinase-resistant (e.g. isoxazolyl-penicillins, nafcillin and methicillin).
Penicillin is the drug of choice for infections due to *Streptococcus pneumoniae* and Group A *Streptococcus pyogenes;* many staphylococci are resistant. *Treponema pallidum* and almost all strains of corynebacteria are fully sensitive.

Indications

19.18   Dermatological indications for the use of oral or parenteral penicillin preparations include:
– Pyodermas caused by sensitive organisms
– Erysipelas
– Erysipeloid
– Syphilis
– Gonorrhea
– Acrodermatitis chronica atrophicans
– Fusospirochaetal infections.
Penicillin has also been used for the treatment of:
– Cold urticaria
– Erythema chronicum migrans
– Morphea

Side effects

19.19   The side effects of penicillins include:

Hypersensitivity reactions [22, 200]

Type 1 reactions: Anaphylactic shock [59, 121], urticaria and angioneurotic edema, allergic rhinitis and bronchial asthma

Type 2 reactions:	Hemolytic anemia, agranulocytosis (see below), thrombocytopenia
Type 3 reactions:	Drug fever, vasculitis allergica, Arthus phenomenon, serum sickness syndrome (fever, exanthema, arthritis, lymphadenitis, leukopenia)
Type 4 reactions:	See the paragraph on contact allergy to antibiotics (§ 5.25)

Many other side effects of penicillins may also be due to hypersensitivity, but classification is usually impossible.

Skin rashes [74, 8]: macular and maculopapular rashes, fixed drug eruptions, vesicular and bullous eruptions. Lyell syndrome [108, 140], exfoliative dermatitis, erythema-multiforme-like eruptions, vascular purpura, pemphigus vulgaris [234]

Gastrointestinal disturbances: diarrhea with nausea and sometimes vomiting, pseudomembranous colitis [201], acute hemorrhagic diarrhea (rare)

Allergic nephropathy, especially interstitial nephritis (with many penicillins, but especially with methicillin) [235]

Neurological symptoms after high intravenous doses: myoclonic jerks, seizures, hyperreflexia, coma [236]

Jarisch-Herxheimer reaction after the start of syphilis treatment [80]: this may comprise fever, chills, headache, joint pains, jaundice, aggravation of the syphilitic symptoms, aneurysma aortae, acute coronary occlusion, neuritis optica, epileptic fits

Hematological disorders (all rare): hemolytic anemia, thrombocytopenia (methicillin), neutropenia/agranulocytosis (semisynthetic penicillinase-resistant compounds) [202], hemolytic uremic syndrome

Hepatitis and intrahepatic cholestasis (very rare, mainly oxacillin)

Transient eosinophilic pulmonary infiltrate (rare), respiratory distress syndrome

Alterations of electrolyte balance after administration of high doses of the potassium or sodium salts of benzylpenicillin

Side effects of depot-preparations:
- embolic-toxic reactions, comprising fear of death, confusion, acoustic and visual hallucinations, generalized seizures and twitches of the extremities, and possibly palpitations and cyanosis
- painful swelling at the injection site
- occlusion and thrombosis after intra-arterial injection
- infantile quadriceps femoris contracture after repeated intramuscular injections into the thighs.

Tetracyclines

19.20   The tetracyclines are closely related antibiotics with similar pharmacological properties and side effects. They are bacteriostatic against many gram-positive and -negative bacteria and are also active against rickettsiae, *Mycoplasma, Chlamydia,* as well as amebae.

The absorption of tetracycline is impaired by the simultaneous taking of milk, aluminium-, calcium- or magnesium-salts or iron preparations; doxycycline and minocycline absorption is not interfered with by food intake.

Apart from skin infections with streptococci and staphylococci, dermatological indications for its use include acne, rosacea, erythrasma, erythema chronicum migrans and lymphogranuloma venereum.

19.21   Side effects reported include:

Gastrointestinal disturbances: nausea, vomiting, epigastric burning, black hairy tongue, stomatitis, rashes in and around the mouth, esophageal ulcers

Skin rashes: photosensitivity, photo-onycholysis [110, 143, 203], urticaria, fixed drug eruption, lichenoid eruptions, EEM-like eruptions, acneiform rashes [12], maculopapular rashes, fever and skin hemorrhage [116], systemic eczematous contact-type dermatitis medicamentosa [118], lupus erythematosus-like eruptions and drug-induced SLE [25], skin pigmentation (minocycline [85, 146, 151, 159]), fixed drug eruption (minocycline) [227]

Monilial infections of the vulva and vagina

Discoloration of the teeth (yellow, greyish-brown or brown) in patients who receive tetracyclines during mineralization of the deciduous or permanent teeth, i.e. before the age of eight or during intrauterine life; yellow nail pigmentation [56].

Deterioration of pre-existing renal disease (doxycycline excepted)

Vestibular symptoms, especially with minocycline [52, 294]

Deposition in bone; uncertain whether this has pathological implications [152]

Anaphylactoid reactions, including shock, asthma [31], allergic edema and exanthema [2]

Benign intracranial hypertension [177], especially in combination with vitamin A orally

Diabetes insipidus-like syndrome

Decreased efficacy of oral contraceptives (?) [147]

Anemia, neutropenia, thrombocytopenia and aplastic anemia (extremely rare)

Tetracycline-associated fatty liver (nowadays very rare)

Erythromycin

19.22   This antibiotic of the macrolide group is a very useful drug for the outpatient treatment of staphylococcal and streptococcal pyodermas; it may also be used for atypical mycobacterial infections. Particular dermatological uses are for erythrasma and acne.

Erythromycin may be considered to be a very safe antibiotic, virtually the only serious side effect being hepatotoxicity from the use of its estolate ester [205, 325].

19.23   Side effects reported include [86]:
- Gastrointestinal disturbances: nausea, vomiting, cramps, diarrhea, abdominal pain, rectal irritation, pseudo membranous colitis (rare [41])
- Cholestasis
- Transient elevations of the transaminases SGOT and SGPT
- Bacterial resistance with cross-resistance to the lincomycins
- Transient perceptive deafness after high parenteral doses [175, 176]

19.24   Co-trimoxazole

- Hypersensitivity reactions: maculopapular rashes, pruritus, urticaria, angioneurotic edema, anaphylaxis, fixed drug eruption (all very rare)
- Acute respiratory distress (rare [1])

Co-trimoxazole

19.24   Co-trimoxazole is a combination of sulfamethoxazole and trimethoprim; it has a bactericidal effect on a wide range of gram-positive and -negative organisms. The drug is used primarily for urinary tract and respiratory tract infections. Dermatological indications for its use include acne, gonorrhea and infections with atypical mycobacteria.

Co-trimoxazole is usually well-tolerated, though skin rashes may occur in a high percentage of patients treated. Overall, the adverse reactions are similar to those of a sulfonamide of low toxicity; however, in contrast to the sulfonamides, renal damage is rare.

19.25   Side effects of co-trimoxazole include [14, 64, 54, 111, 206]:
- Skin disorders: maculopapular rashes, toxic epidermal necrolysis (rare), Stevens-Johnson syndrome (rare [13, 15]), fixed drug eruption (trimethoprim) [208]
- Gastrointestinal disturbances: nausea, vomiting, loss of appetite, pseudomembranous colitis (very rare)
- Drug fever
- Mild leukopenia (in up to 10% of patients), mild thrombocytopenia (common), megaloblastic anemia (very rare), aplastic anemia (very rare), pancytopenia (very rare), agranulocytosis (rare)
- Crystalluria and renal insufficiency (very rare), hemolytic uremic syndrome (very rare)
- Multi-system toxicity, probably of allergic origin (very rare)
- Impairment of male fertility (?)
- Intrahepatic cholestasis [207]

Clindamycin

19.26   The semisynthetic lincomycin derivative clindamycin acts against gram-positive cocci including some penicillin-resistant staphylococci; it is very active against bacteroides. Clindamycin is a very effective drug for the treatment of acne [126]; however, in view of its toxicity, especially regarding pseudomembranous colitis, other, safer drugs should always be considered first.

19.27   Side effects of orally administered clindamycin include:
- Diarrhea, varying from mildly loose bowels to life-threatening pseudomembranous colitis [128, 5]
- Esophageal ulcers
- Maculopapular and pruritic eruptions (10% of all cases)
- Superinfections with resistant strains of Proteus, Pseudomonas and Staphylococci
- Stevens-Johnson syndrome (one case [84])
- Anaphylaxis (one case [79])
- Granulocytopenia (?), thrombocytopenia (?)

Spectinomycin

19.28   Spectinomycin is used in dermatology for the treatment of gonorrhea, especially in those forms complicated by multiple antibiotic resistance [104]. Although it belongs to the group of aminoglycosides, spectinomycin lacks the broad toxicological spectrum of these antibiotics. In fact, its tolerance in the treatment of gonorrhea (one dose, 3.2 g) is excellent.

19.29   Virtually the only side effects reported are pain and induration at the injection site; allergic reactions seem to occur, but are very rare.

H_1 AND H_2 HISTAMINE ANTAGONISTS

19.30   Antihistamines are classified according to their histamine-blocking actions as H_1 and H_2 antagonists. H_2 antagonists are mainly used for the treatment of gastric and duodenal ulcers; cimetidine may be useful for some cases of intractable urticaria. The older antihistamines are nowadays referred to as H_1 antagonists.

The nucleus of the typical antihistamine structure is $-CH_2-CH_2-N=$, which is present in the histamine molecule as well. The antihistamines antagonize most of the pharmacological effects of histamine, those on the H_1 receptors on blood vessels and smooth muscles. In addition, the H_1 antagonists have varying anticholinergic, anti-adrenaline and anti-serotonin effects.

Classification

19.31   The antihistamines comprise a large number of different chemical compounds, which can be classified into the following main groups:
1. Ethylenediamines
2. Alkylamines
3. Ethanolamines
4. Piperazines
5. Phenothiazines.
For the classification of individual H_1 antagonists, see § 5.27. Azatadine, cyproheptadine and thiazinamium do not fit into any of the groups listed above.

Indications

19.32   The major dermatological indications for the use of antihistamines are urticaria and angioneurotic edema. Unfortunately, as these affections are caused not only by histamine, but by a variety of other vasoactive amines as well, antihistamines may fail to prevent attacks. One of the major side effects, namely drowsiness, is often used to advantage for therapeutic purposes; thus, some H_1 antagonists, especially the phenothiazines, have become much-used sedatives. The newer H_1 antagonist terfenadine probably causes little or no sedation.

Side effects

19.33   For several reasons, the assessment of side effects of the individual antihistamines is rather difficult. Therefore, the side effects mentioned below will deal with H_1 antagonists as a group; well-documented particular side effects of individual drugs will be mentioned separately.

It is estimated that some 20–50% of all patients taking antihistamines experience some adverse reaction.

19.34   Side effects reported include:
- Central nervous system depression (especially by the phenothiazines)
- Central nervous system stimulation, especially in children: insomnia, irritability, tremor, nightmares, hallucinations
- Facial dyskinesia
- Anticholinergic effects: dryness of the mouth and oropharynx, blurred vision, constipation, nasal stuffiness, urinary retention (see also § 19.67)
- Gastrointestinal disturbances: nausea, vomiting, epigastric pain, diarrhea, and constipation
- Sensitization in cases of topical use (see § 5.26)
- Lowering of sperm counts (reversible)
- Tachycardia and hypertension (infrequent)
- Anaphylactoid reactions (rare)
- Cholestatic jaundice (rare)
- Blood dyscrasias (rare): agranulocytosis, thrombocytopenia, aplastic anemia, hemolytic anemia
- Hyperpyrexia (rare)
- Hypoglycemia (?)
- Carcinogenicity (?), teratogenicity (?).

19.35   Documented side effects of individual drugs include:

Cinnarizine:	improvement of peripheral blood flow
Cyproheptadine:	stimulation of appetite, inhibition of lactation
Dimenhydrinate:	impairment of color discrimination, night vision and reaction time
Methapyrilene:	carcinogenicity (?)
Phenothiazines:	worsening of asthma, skin pigmentation [51]
Thiazinamium:	attacks of epigastric and sternal pain.

Cimetidine

19.36   Cimetidine is an H₂ antagonist used for the treatment of gastric and duodenal ulcers. In dermatology, cases of chronic therapy-resistant urticaria and/or angioneurotic edema may respond favorably to this compound; combination with a traditional H₁ receptor antagonist may be beneficial. A more recently developed H₂ receptor antagonist, ranitidine, which is a less likely cause of interactions with other drugs, is not (yet) discussed in this book, as the limited use in dermatological practice does not warrant its inclusion.

Side effects

19.37   Of 9907 patients treated with cimetidine, adverse effects were reported by 442 (4.4%) [43].

19.38   Side effects of cimetidine include [19, 33, 114]:
- Nervous system disturbances [229, 230]: mental confusion (especially in the elderly patient), emotional upset, drowsiness, depression, disorientation, agitation, hallucinations, delirium, psychosis [209], brain stem dysfunction: slurred speech, dysarthria, diplopia, pyramidal symptoms.

- Gastrointestinal disturbances: nausea, abdominal pain, discomfort, meteorism, diarrhea, constipation, paralytic ileus, perforation of peptic ulcers, erosive gastritis and/or duodenitis, malabsorption syndrome, ileus, malignant changes in peptic ulcers (?), pancreatitis (rare), hepatitis (rare)
- Skin and appendages: urticaria [29], Quincke's edema [24], Stevens-Johnson syndrome [3], exfoliative dermatitis [137], worsening of psoriasis [138], transient alopecia [211], erythema multiforme [213], asteatotic dermatitis [214], pruritus [233], erythema annulare centrifugum [231], seborrheic dermatitis [232]
- Cardiovascular disturbances: deep vein thrombosis (?), bradycardia and other cardiac arrhythmias, cardiac arrest, leucocytoclastic vasculitis
- Endocrine disorders: gynecomastia, impotence and impairment of spermatogenesis
- Blood disorders (uncommon) [229]: leukopenia, thrombocytopenia, autoimmune hemolytic anemia, agranulocytosis [210]
- Miscellaneous: impaired glucose tolerance (rare), pyrexia (rare), renal damage (rare), joint pain [212], muscular pain [212], renal dysfunction, polymyositis, inflammatory urethritis

ANTIFUNGAL DRUGS

Griseofulvin

19.39   Side effects of the oral use of this fungistatic drug include (e.g. Götz and Reichenberger [48]):
- Gastrointestinal disturbances: nausea, diarrhea, anorexia, vomiting, abdominal cramps
- Nervous system disturbances: fatigue, dizziness, drowsiness, confusion, depression, irritability, insomnia, headache (up to 50%), impaired coordination, visual disturbances, peripheral neuritis
- Various types of skin rashes, including cutaneous vasculitis [77], Stevens-Johnson syndrome [237]
- Photosensitivity, fixed drug eruptions and angioneurotic edema, porphyria-like eruption
- Drug-induced systemic lupus erythematosus [135]
- (usually mild) Blood disorders, including leukopenia (rare)
- Liver damage [122]
- Interferes with porphyrin metabolism [122]
- Oral symptoms: angular stomatitis, disturbances of taste, glossodynia, black hairy tongue
- Serum-sickness-like syndromes (rare)
- Albuminuria (rare)
- Estrogen-type effects in children, including gynecomastia

Ketoconazole

19.40   Ketoconazole [75, 250, 254, 270, 271] is a new oral antifungal agent with a broad spectrum of activity against superficial and deep mycoses. Ketoconazole is an imidazole like miconazole and clotrimazole, but distinguishes itself from other imidazoles by the presence of a piperazine ring. Adverse effects to the drug are frequent, but usually minor. However, in 1% of patients treated with ketoconazole side effects were serious enough to lead to discontinuation of the drug [250]. The most frequently observed adverse effects (3–10%) are nausea and vomiting [270].

The most notable adverse effects reported to date are gynecomastia, elevations of hepatic enzyme levels, and manifest hepatitis. Drug resistance has been reported [253, 272], but later disputed [269]. Side effects of ketoconazole include:
- Cardiovascular: epistaxis
- Nervous system: pruritus, headache, dizziness, somnolence, insomnia, fever and chills, nervousness
- Endocrine, metabolic [274]: DeFelice et al. [251] were the first to observe that gynecomastia occurs in some males treated with ketoconazole. In this report, there appeared to be no abnormal endocrine function associated with ketoconazole administration, and the process appeared not to be dose-related. However, depressed serum [264, 273] and saliva [264] testosterone levels have been observed, especially at high doses. Also, impotence [268] and loss of libido [274] have been ascribed to ketoconazole. Gynecomastia appears to be common in male patients on 800 mg ketoconazole or more per day [274]. Another endocrine effect, blocking the response of the adrenal gland to ACTH has been documented [273]. This effect is dose-related; however, there does not appear to be a clinical problem with adrenal dysfunction at dosages as high as 1600 mg per day [274].
- Alterations of triglycerides [276], transient hypocholesterolemia [263, 275].
- Hematological: reversible thrombocytopenia [261]
- Liver: during ketoconazole treatment silent as well as symptomatic hepatic reactions have been reported. The silent reaction (transient asymptomatic elevations of the SGOT, SGPT, 5'-nucleotidase and alkaline phosphatase) may occur at any time during ketoconazole treatment [253, 256, 262, 265]. A liver biopsy may show mild acute hepatitis consistent with either toxic or viral hepatitis [258]. A small number of patients may develop symptomatic hepatic reactions [252, 257, 266]. A patient history of hepatitis, idiosyncratic reaction or long-term use of griseofulvin appear to be predisposing factors. Up to February 1983, 96 patients with symptomatic hepatic reactions have been reported to the manufacturer, an estimated incidence of 1 in 10,000/13,000 [255]. Symptomatic hepatic reactions have occurred mainly during the first few months of treatment [254]. The development of hepatitis is not dose-related and is apparently caused by an idiosyncratic effect of ketoconazole [255]. A few patients have died from ketoconazole-hepatitis [254]. In spite of the low incidence of these adverse effects liver enzymes should be monitored carefully during ketoconazole treatment. Liver function tests before and periodically during treatment are mandatory. In the event of abnormal values the immediate withdrawal of the drug and consideration of liver biopsy is suggested [262]
- Gastrointestinal: nausea and vomiting (3–10%), diarrhea, abdominal pain, constipation
- Skin and appendages: generalized erythematous eruption [249, 267], exfoliative erythroderma [259], morbilliform eruption [268]
- Special senses: photophobia [256, 260], transient visual blurring [249]
- Second generation effects: ketoconazole should not be used in pregnancy.

Nystatin

19.41   This antibiotic is used topically and orally for the treatment of *Candida albicans* infections. It is not absorbed from the gut and is therefore only of value in intestinal infections, when administered orally; however, it is often useful in combination with topical therapy in cases of perianal or inguinal candidiasis, where the gastrointestinal tract may be a source of infection of the skin.

Nystatin is nearly always well tolerated; nausea, vomiting and diarrhea have been described, but may have been due to the disease for which the therapy was instituted. Fixed drug eruptions [99] and pustular reactions [102] have rarely been reported. Topical nystatin has very rarely caused contact allergy (see § 5.32).

19.42   Other antifungal drugs for systemic use include amphotericin B, clotrimazole, miconazole and flucytosine, which are effective in generalized candidiasis. Their systemic use in dermatology is limited; evaluation of their side effects, therefore, falls outside the scope of this book.

ANTIPROTOZOAL DRUGS

Metronidazole and tinidazole

19.43   Metronidazole is used for the treatment of *Trichomonas vaginalis* infections; it is bactericidal for many anaerobic bacteria including *Bacteroides*.

Metronidazole has also been effective in the treatment of rosacea [191, 192]. This drug is generally well tolerated, but mild gastrointestinal intolerance does not infrequently occur. Tinidazole, a related nitroimidazole compound, appears to have a similar pattern of adverse reactions.

19.44   Side effects include [21, 107, 17, 42, 215, 216]:
   - Gastrointestinal disturbances: nausea, vomiting, diarrhea, abdominal pain, anorexia, bad taste, furring of the tongue, pseudomembranous colitis (?) [184]
   - Nervous system disturbances (mostly with high-dose therapy): peripheral polyneuritis, headache, dizziness, ataxia, depression, epileptiform insults (rare), paraesthesiae (rare), vertigo
   - Alcohol intolerance (disulfiram-like)
   - Transient leukopenia and neutropenia [183]
   - Hepatotoxicity (?) [226]
   - Urethral discomfort, darkening of the urine
   - Skin rashes, including fixed drug eruption, pityriasis rosea-like rash and urticaria
   - Serum-sickness-like reaction [142]
   - Carcinogenicity (?, unlikely) [217].

DRUGS USED IN LEPROSY

Dapsone (4,4-diaminodiphenylsulfone, DDS)

19.45   The two major indications for treatment with dapsone are leprosy and dermatitis herpetiformis Dühring; in recent years, dapsone has also been used for other dermatological affections such as bullous dermatoses [154], pustular eruptions [154], various forms of vasculitis, acne conglobata, facial granuloma [182], verrucous pyoderma [181] and lupus erythematosus [70, 113]. For other indications of its use, see Tomecki and Catalano [130], and Barranco [155].

Dapsone always induces subclinical hemolysis and shortens red cell life, but clinical hemolytic anemia is uncommon.

Side effects

19.46   The most frequently encountered side effects are nausea, vomiting, loss of appetite and skin rashes [218].

19.47 Dapsone

19.47   In leprosy, dapsone may induce the so-called 'reactional states' [60]:

Type 1 reaction: This reaction may occur in tuberculoid and borderline leprosy, less commonly in subpolar lepromatous leprosy; it is due to a rapid change in cell-mediated immunity. Apart from exacerbation of the skin lesions and neurological symptoms including nerve swelling and pain, the 'sulfone syndrome' may comprise fever, queasiness, exfoliative dermatitis, lymphadenopathy, jaundice with liver necrosis, methemoglobinemia and anemia [130]. The dapsone syndrome has also been observed in patients treated with DDS for other indications [165].

Type 2 reaction: This reaction, seen exclusively in lepromatous leprosy, is an immune-complex syndrome and is characterized by one or more of the following: erythema nodosum leprosum, intermittent fever, nerve swelling and pain, myositis, iridocyclitis, epistaxis, glottic edema, dactylitis, lymphadenitis, epididymo-orchitis, edema of the face, hands and feet, and mental depression [60]. This type of reaction may also be precipitated by a number of other factors including emotional stress, pregnancy and protective immunization.

19.48   Other side effects of dapsone include [50]:
- CNS disturbances: headache, insomnia, nervousness, reversible peripheral neuropathy, psychic depression (rare), irritability, agitation and hostility [228]
- Gastrointestinal symptoms: nausea, vomiting, loss of appetite
- Tachycardia from (relative) overdosage
- Hemolysis and methemoglobinemia (frequent)
- Pruritus and exanthemas (common)
- Hepatitis with jaundice (rare)
- Renal papillary necrosis (very rare)
- Mononucleosis-like states leading to death
- Hypoalbuminemia.

An extensive list of references is provided by Tomecki and Catalano [130].

Clofazimine (Lamprene)

19.49   Clofazimine is a phendimetrazine-tartrate derivative, which is the best alternative drug for sulfone-resistant leprosy; it also has anti-inflammatory properties and may therefore prevent the development of erythema nodosum leprosum (Type 2 reaction).

Clofazimine is also a tuberculostatic drug, and has been used for the treatment of Buruli ulcer caused by *M. ulcerans,* pyoderma gangrenosum [88], and discoid lupus erythematosus [193].

A detailed review of adverse reactions to clofazimine has been presented by Yawalkar and Vischer [139].

19.50   Side effects include:

Skin disorders: Reversible red discoloration of the skin, later becoming brown (especially on the exposed parts). Discoloration of sweat, hair, sputum, urine and feces; phototoxicity, pruritus, ichthyosis, xeroderma, acneiform eruptions, nonspecific rashes.

Gastrointestinal disorders: Early symptoms, shortly after introduction of the drug: nausea, vomiting, abdominal pain. Late symptoms, after months or years of high doses: persistent diarrhea, abdominal pain and loss of weight, splenic infarction [170].

Ocular changes: Conjunctival pigmentation, corneal streaks.

DRUGS USED IN TUBERCULOSIS

19.51 The most commonly used drugs in tuberculosis are isoniazid, ethambutol, rifampicin, p-aminosalicylic acid and streptomycin.

Adverse reactions of antituberculosis drugs have been reviewed [166, 219, 220]. All the main antituberculosis drugs can cause or contribute to cutaneous and generalized hypersensitivity reactions and hepatitis. The drugs which most commonly cause such hypersensitivity reactions are streptomycin, p-aminosalicylic acid and its salts, and thiacetazone. The clinical manifestations of hypersensitivity are diverse, but the most common features are rash and fever. The rash is usually erythematous and itchy, and may be macular or papular. Generalized reactions may also include periorbital swelling, conjunctivitis, and systemic symptoms and signs such as rigors, malaise, vomiting, aching limbs, headache, generalized lymphadenopathy, albuminuria, hepatosplenomegaly and occasionally transient jaundice.

All the antituberculosis drugs can cause hepatitis [158]. Adverse effects to individual drugs used for the treatment of tuberculosis are discussed in the following paragraphs. For adverse effects of antituberculosis drugs not discussed here, *see* [158].

Ethambutol

19.52 This drug has a low incidence of side effects; these include [136, 158]:
- Gastrointestinal disturbances: vomiting, loss of appetite and abdominal pain
- Ocular effects (2–3% of patients treated) [87]: diminution of color vision and visual acuity, tired eyes, spots in the visual fields, difficulties in reading, restricted visual fields, central scrotoma, retrobulbar neuritis, irreversible optic atrophy (rare), hemorrhages and retinal defects, open-angle glaucoma
- Headache, mental confusion and dizziness
- Increase in serum uric acid (due to decreased renal excretion), only very seldom leading to gouty arthritis
- Jaundice and non-icteric liver disturbances (rare)
- Polyneuritis (very rare)
- Exanthemas, vasculitis (very rare)
- Drug fever, joint pains (very rare)
- Nephrotoxicity (very rare).

Isoniazid

19.53 Side effects of isoniazid are found only in 1% of patients treated with low doses of up to 5 mg/kg/day; higher doses in adults may result in an adverse reaction incidence of up to 20%. The most frequent side effects involve the liver and peripheral and central nervous system; they have become rarer and milder since the routine addition of pyridoxine to isoniazid. Diabetics, patients with hepatic insufficiency, hyperthyroidism and epilepsy as well as alcoholics and pregnant women are more prone to display side effects to the drug.

19.54 Side effects of isoniazid include [45, 158]:
- Nervous system disturbances: polyneuritis (1–2%), headache, drowsiness, vertigo, retrobulbar neuritis, convulsions, disturbances in color vision, mental disturbances (rare), optic nerve neuritis (very rare)
- Gastrointestinal disturbances: anorexia, nausea, upper abdominal pain, hemorrhage (rare)

- Various forms of liver toxicity [49]
- Skin disorders [32]: pruritus, urticaria, Quincke's edema, exanthema, purpura, aggravation of existing eczema, pellagra-like symptoms (before pyridoxine was routinely administered), allergic reaction in connection with foods [131], Stevens-Johnson syndrome (one case [16]), toxic epidermal necrolysis Lyell [89], aggravation of pre-existing SLE and SLE-like syndrome [45]
- Drug fever
- Vasculitis in various organs
- Antinuclear antibodies and positive LE-cell phenomenon
- Rheumatic syndrome with pain and stiffness in the joints of the hands, wrists, elbows and other joints
- Glomerulonephritis (rare) and renal insufficiency (rare)
- Asthmatic symptoms (very rare) and rhinitis (rare)
- Leukopenia (very rare)
- Keratitis (rare)
- Pubertas praecox (very rare)
- Cushingoid symptoms (very rare)
- Gynecomastia, menstrual disturbances, amenorrhea (very rare)
- Acute abdomen (one report).

Rifampicin

19.55   Side effects of this drug, which is also used in the treatment of leprosy, include [44, 158, 221]:
- Gastrointestinal disturbances: stomach pain, loss of appetite, nausea, vomiting, meteorism, diarrhea (rare), pseudomembranous colitis
- Acne [95], exanthema, pruritus, urticaria (up to 5%), pemphigus-like rash (one report [40]), redness and watering of the eyes
- Liver dysfunctions as shown by laboratory tests (2–10%), hepatitis (rare)
- The 'flu syndrome' (up to 20%): this is characterized by fever, headache, chills, bone and muscle pain, starting 1–2 hours after each dose and lasting for up to eight hours
- Stimulation/inhibition of the menstrual bleeding, impairment of the efficacy of hormonal contraceptives
- Shock
- Myopathy (very rare)
- Acute renal insufficiency (uncommon); urine may be colored red
- Headache and dizziness (rare)
- Rhinitis and respiratory problems resembling bronchial asthma (rare), sometimes accompanied by a fall in blood pressure and shock
- Hematological disorders (rare): thrombocytopenic purpura, leukopenia, hemolytic anemia (rare)
- Pancreatitis (very rare)
- Osteomalacia (very rare)
- Teratogenesis (?)

ANTIMALARIALS

Chloroquine and hydroxychloroquine

19.56   Side effects of chloroquine and hydroxychloroquine [163] at the doses prescribed for antimalarial treatment and prophylaxis are few; most of the side effects discussed below relate to the prolonged use of large doses for rheumatoid arthritis and discoid lupus erythematosus. In dermatology, these antiprotozoals are used mainly for discoid lupus erythematosus, polymorphic light eruption [148] and sarcoidosis. They are a possible alternative for venesection in porphyria cutanea tarda, although large doses may produce liver damage in patients with PCT [163].

An excellent review of various aspects of the use of antimalarials has been published [163]. For other useful review papers, see [127] and [167]. The most serious side effect no doubt is retinopathy, which is often irreversible and may lead to blindness [30]. Ocular toxicity seems to be less prevalent with *hydroxy*chloroquine [149] than with chloroquine. For a review of 'antimalarials and ophthalmologic safety', *see* [168] and [222]. Daily doses of chloroquine less than 250 mg and hydroxychloroquine less than 400 mg are considered to be safe [168], even after prolonged periods of time.

19.57   Other side effects include [127, 163]:
- Various psychiatric disorders [47]
- Nervous system disorders: EEG changes, vertigo, nervousness, tinnitus, irritability, neuromyopathy, extrapyramidal involuntary movements, peripheral neuritis and neuromyopathy (rare), sweating, headache, insomnia, grand mal seizures
- Gastrointestinal discomfort and diarrhea (common), anorexia, nausea, vomiting (very common)
- Dermatological side effects: photosensitivity, exacerbation of porphyria cutanea tarda [129], exacerbation of psoriasis, various skin rashes [78] including maculopapular/morbilliform eruptions, erythema annulare centrifugum, palmar squamous cell carcinomas, lichenoid eruptions, exfoliative erythroderma, urticaria, fixed drug eruption, pigmentation and depigmentation (25%), bleaching of the hair (achromotrichia), toxic epidermal necrolysis (one report [62]), pruritus
- Neutropenia, agranulocytosis, aplastic anemia (very rare)
- Stomatitis and oral pigmentation (uncommon)
- Diplopia, loss of accommodation, keratopathy (usually reversible)
- Tinnitus and nerve deafness (both rare)
- Renal: hemoglobinuria, renal insufficiency
- Teratogenicity: deafness, mental retardation and convulsions.

ORAL RETINOIDS

19.58   The antikeratinizing activity of vitamin A has led to research on the effects of this vitamin, its metabolites, and synthetic retinoid derivatives on diseases such as acne, psoriasis, ichthyosis, lichen ruber planus, Darier's disease, and pityriasis rubra pilaris. Four retinoids – retinol (vitamin A), tretinoin (retinoic acid), etretinate (Ro/10-9359, Tigason®) and isotretinoin (13-*cis*-retinoic acid, Accutane®) – have been administered orally for therapeutic purposes. In addition to their well-known action on keratinizing epithelia, retinoids have some other actions, which may have significant clinical implications:
1. Anti-inflammatory activity [301] Oral retinoids influence dermal components such as cutaneous capillaries and dermal inflammatory cells. On this basis, they act as an anti-inflammatory drug. In particular, they reduce the elevated skin temperature, inhibit the motility of neutrophils and eosinophils and their migration into the epidermis, decrease DNA synthesis of human lymphocytes by blocking their response to lectins, and stimulate Langerhans cells, monocytes and macrophages in various *in vivo* and *in vitro* models. This would suggest that oral retin-

oids may benefit patients suffering from skin diseases with dermal inflammatory involvement, regardless of their particular etiology [301]

2. Effects on tumors [302, 318, 319] Several retinoids have been used with some success in the treatment and prevention of tumors such as basal cell carcinomas, keratoacanthomas, and melanomas. The exact mechanisms of action have not been conclusively determined. The antineoplastic activity may involve effects via cytosol-binding proteins, inhibition of ornithine decarboxylase activity, and effects on the immune system [302, 303]

3. Effects on cell-mediated immunity There is evidence that vitamin A and the retinoids may act on the immune system. Reactions to recall antigens have been shown to be increased after 4 weeks treatment with etretinate. DNCB reactivity also significantly increased in 23 non-psoriatic patients after retinoid therapy. These results indicate that etretinate may stimulate cell-mediated immunity [285].

Vitamin A (retinol)

19.59   Although not entirely abated, oral vitamin A has been largely replaced by other oral retinoids with a higher therapeutic activity and less toxicity. Nevertheless, it is important to note symptoms and signs of acute and chronic vitamin A intoxication, as the specter of adverse effects from retinoids will resemble those of vitamin A intoxication.

§ 19.60 and § 19.61 list the clinical and laboratory findings in acute and chronic vitamin A intoxication. These are arranged in order of decreasing frequency [291]. In *acute* vitamin A intoxication symptoms of the central nervous system are more prominent, with gastrointestinal symptoms on the second place. In *chronic* vitamin A intoxication cutaneous problems are most prominent, followed by abnormalities of the mucous membranes and pain and tenderness of the bones.

19.60   **Findings in acute vitamin A intoxication arranged in order of decreasing frequency [291]**

Clinical findings
Increased cerebrospinal fluid pressure
    infants and children: pseudotumor cerebri and cranial hyperostosis
    adolescents and adults: headache, predominantly occipital
Anorexia, nausea, vomiting
Scaling of the skin, dry mucous membranes, cheilitis, hair loss
Fatigue, lassitude, vertigo, somnolence, etc.
Hemorrhages: formation of petechiae; epistaxis
Edema
Tenderness of the long bones
Hepatomegaly and splenomegaly

Laboratory findings
Vitamin A plasma levels increased
Calcium increased
Alkaline phosphatase increased
SGOT and SGPT increased

Findings in chronic hypervitaminosis A arranged in order of decreasing frequency [291]

Clinical findings
Scaling skin, erythema, pruritus, disturbed hair growth
Dry mucous membranes, cheilitis, angular stomatitis, gingivitis, glossitis
Pain and tenderness of the bones; restricted movement
Occipital headache
Hyperirritability; sleep disturbance
Papillary edema; diplopia
Anorexia and loss of weight
Hepatomegaly, sometimes with splenomegaly
Edema and swelling
Fatigue, lassitude, occasionally somnolence
Hemorrhages, epistaxis, increased menstrual bleeding

Laboratory findings
Radiologically detectable bone changes in children
Increased serum alkaline phosphatase, hypercalcemia
Increased cerebrospinal fluid pressure
Disturbed blood clotting (hypoprothrombinemia)

Etretinate

19.62   Etretinate (Tigason®, Ro/10-9359, ethyl-(*all-trans*)-9-(4-methoxy-2,3,6-trimethyl-phenyl)-3,7-dimethyl-2,4,6,8-nonatetraenoate) [71, 94, 97, 283, 311] has a profound effect on proliferation and differentiation of keratinocytes. The efficacy of etretinate in dermatoses partly or mainly characterized by disturbances in keratinization has been well established. Major indications for its use include (various forms of) psoriasis, Darier's disease, pityriasis rubra pilaris, (various forms of) ichthyosis and lichen ruber planus, but many other dermatoses have been successfully treated with this aromatic retinoid.

Following oral administration etretinate undergoes significant first-pass biodegradation to its corresponding carboxylic acid. The acid appears rapidly in the circulation, often earlier than the parent drug, and its plasma concentration is usually comparable to, or greater than that of the parent etretinate. The apparent elimination rates of drug and metabolite are similar (6–13 hours) following a single dose, suggesting that metabolic elimination may be formation-rate limited [277]. Storage of etretinate and metabolites during maintenance therapy is supposed to occur in the liver and/or fat, as significant serum levels of the main metabolites of etretinate are found for prolonged periods (6–12 months) after cessation of the therapy.

Adverse reactions

19.63   The adverse effects of etretinate are essentially similar to those of other retinoids, but central nervous system effects are not prominent with etretinate. Side effects of etretinate are dose-related and usually reversible. The cutaneous adverse effects are its most prominent features; serious alopecia and paronychia may necessitate discontinuance of therapy. Adverse reactions to etretinate include [71, 94, 97, 283, 311]:

– Nervous system: sweating (either diffuse or at palms and soles), thirst, headache, drowsiness, fatigue

– Endocrine, metabolic: Increases in serum lipid levels have been reported in patients during treatment with etretinate. Serum triglyceride, cholesterol and high-density lipoprotein cholesterol (HDLC) were investigated in 21 patients treated with etretinate for psoriasis [280]. Elevation out of the normal range occurred in 77% of patients for serum triglycerides and in 25% for serum cholesterol, whereas mean HDLC-levels did not change. After 8 weeks all levels had returned to normal, although in some patients cholesterol remained 20% over the pretreatment values. The mechanisms for the etretinate-induced lipid elevations are unknown. Patients with increased tendency to develop hypertriglyceridemia include those with diabetes mellitus, obesity, increased alcohol intake, and family history.

– Mineral and fluid balance: generalized edema (rare) [293, 299]

– Hematological: monocytosis [300], leukopenia (?)

– Liver [286, 283, 311]: A transient, slight elevation of SGOT, SGPT, and/or serum bilirubin may occur in some patients on etretinate therapy [282, 300], which is reversible upon cessation of therapy and usually has no clinical implications. However, in 1978 chronic agressive hepatitis was mentioned as a possible complication in 2 patients treated with etretinate [284], and since then other cases of hepatitis presumably due to etretinate have been documented [282, 307, 309] although other hepatotoxic factors may have played a role [322]. The histological studies of Glazer et al. [286] seem to indicate that most patients with a past history of liver problems are able to tolerate exposure, although some have shown increasing abnormalities in the biopsies. On the other hand, Fontan et al. [283], reviewing the subject of etretinate-induced hepatic changes, warn that plethorics, alcoholics, and patients who have been treated with methotrexate, are at greater risk of developing serious liver injury

– Gastrointestinal: anorexia, loss or stimulation of appetite, vomiting, stomach pain

– Skin and appendages: erythema and desquamation, especially palms and soles, thinning of the skin, petechiae especially at the extremities, burning, itching, cheilitis with or without rhagades, dryness of nasal and oral mucosae, mucosal erosions, conjunctivitis, paronychia, thinning of hair, nail disorders [294], rosacea-like eruption (uncommon) [278], epistaxis, oiliness of the hair, alopecia areata (?), pyogenic granulomata (?) [323]

– Musculoskeletal symptoms: bone pain, arthralgia

– Miscellaneous: earache [289], excessive cerumen production [292]

– Use in pregnancy: Etretinate is teratogenic and women of childbearing age should receive adequate contraceptives when using etretinate. In view of the half-life of elimination of 80–100 days, contraception should be continued accordingly (12 months or longer) after cessation of therapy.

Isotretinoin (13-*cis*-retinoic acid)

19.64   Although isotretinoin [303, 313, 320] may be useful for the treatment of keratinizing disorders, its main indication is for severe nodulocystic acne. The exact mechanism of action of isotretinoin in the treatment of acne is not fully understood, but appears to include inhibition of sebaceous gland function and follicular keratinization. Isotretinoin reduces the size of sebaceous glands and inhibits sebum production. In large doses isotretinoin reduces the concentration of *P. acnes* on the surface of the skin. The reduction of the bacterial flora probably does not result from a direct effect of the drug on the bacteria, but from a drug-induced reduction in sebum production. In patients with cystic acne prolonged remissions frequently occur following discontinuance of isotretinoin. The pharmacokinetics of this oral retinoid have been reviewed [277, 303, 313].

Adverse reactions

19.65   One or more side effects from isotretinoin can be expected to occur in almost every patient [303, 313, 320]. They are, in general, somewhat predictable, resembling in type, though not in incidence, those of the parent compound's syndrome of chronic hypervitaminosis A. The frequency and severity of adverse reactions to isotretinoin are generally dose-related [288], with more pronounced effects occurring at dosages greater than 1 mg/kg/day. Adverse effects usually subside with a reduction in dosage, and are reversible following discontinuance of therapy. Adverse mucocutaneous affects are seen very frequently during therapy with isotretinoin. Adverse reactions to isotretinoin include:
– Respiratory: respiratory infections (?) [314]
– Nervous system: lethargy, fatigue, headache, paresthesias (?) [314], dizziness (?) [314], depressive symptoms [287, 316]
– Endocrine, metabolic: hypertriglyceridemia occurs in about 25% of patients receiving isotretinoin. Blood lipid concentrations should be monitored. Decreases in serum high-density lipoprotein (HDL) occur in 15% of patients, and increases in serum cholesterol concentration in 7%. These effects are reversible upon discontinuance of isotretinoin. Patients with increased tendency to develop hypertriglyceridemia include those with diabetes mellitus, obesity, increased alcohol intake, and family history. The consequences of hypertriglyceridemia are not well understood, but it may increase the patient's cardiovascular risk status [288, 295]. Even with low doses of isotretinoin triglyceride concentrations will rise in a high percentage of patients [315]. An obese male patient with Darier's disease developed elevated triglycerides and subsequently eruptive xanthomas [279]. Increases in fasting serum glucose concentrations have been reported [314]. Thyroxine concentrations and free thyroxine index have sometimes fallen during treatment, but remained within the reference range [295]
– Mineral and fluid balance: edema (?) [314]
– Hematological: increased erythrocyte sedimentation rate (40%), decreased hemoglobin concentration and hematocrit, decreased erythrocyte and leukocyte counts, increased platelet counts (10–20%)
– Liver: minimal transient increases in serum concentrations of alkaline phosphatase, SGOT, and SGPT occur in 10% of patients
– Gastrointestinal: anorexia, nausea, vomiting, increased appetite, thirst, weight loss (?), [379], gastrointestinal bleeding (?) [379], acute hemorrhagic pancreatitis (1 case). Gastrointestinal symptoms occur in 20% of patients treated with isotretinoin
– Urinary system: proteinuria, hematuria, nonspecific urogenital findings (all ??) [314]. Abnormalities in urinary protein [288], inflammation of the urethral meatus (rare) [320]
– Skin and appendages: cheilitis (90%!), xerosis, xerostomia, dry nose, facial rash, epistaxis, pruritus (all about 25%); temporary thinning of the hair, palmoplantar desquamation, skin fragility, infections of the skin, brittle nails, photosensitivity [296], occur in 5–10% of patients. Paronychia [310], hypo/hyperpigmentation (?) [314], urticaria (?) [314], bruising (?) [314], exuberant granulation tissue (uncommon) [320], flare-up of cystic acne [321]
– Eyes: conjunctivitis and irritation of the eyes may occur in about 40% of patients [297]. Isotretinoin probably causes a decrease in tearfilm breakup-time [281]. Patients wearing contact lenses may experience intolerance to their lenses. Corneal opacities have been observed in some patients with disorders of keratinization [317]

– Musculoskeletal effects: Bone or joint pain, generalized muscle ache, and stiffness occur in 15% of patients receiving isotretinoin. Skeletal abnormalities have occurred in several patients with disorders of keratinization who were treated with isotretinoin for more than two years. Hyperostosis [312] with spine degeneration occurred in several adults, and radiographic findings suggestive of possible premature closure of the epiphyses occurred in some children [298]. An ossification disorder resembling diffuse idiopathic skeletal hyperostosis was found in 4 patients on long-term high-dose isotretinoin therapy for ichthyosis [304]

– Use in pregnancy: Isotretinoin may cause fetal harm when administered to pregnant women. Women of childbearing age should be instructed to use an effective form of contraception during isotretinoin therapy and at least one menstrual cycle after discontinuance.

Tretinoin

19.66 Tretinoin (retinoic acid) is not widely used as an oral drug, as it has been shown to be less effective and more toxic than isotretinoin and etretinate. Tretinoin has its widest use as a topical therapeutic agent, especially for acne and ichthyosis.

In the investigation of Stuttgen [308] 30 patients were given 50–100 mg/day of oral tretinoin for 4 weeks. Increases in SGOT, SGPT and alkaline phosphatase were each noted in 1 patient (of 11 investigated). Adverse reactions to tretinoin in these patients included:

cheilitis	(80%)
xerosis/inflammation	(50%)
pruritus	(23%)
thinning of hair	(10%)
dry mucous membranes	(30%)
epistaxis, petechiae	(17%)
headache	(80%)
lethargy, fatigue	(43%)
psychological changes	(10%)
visual disturbances	(30%)
bulb pressure increased (eye)	(11%)
anorexia	(30%)
nausea, vomiting	(30%)

Propantheline

19.67 Propantheline is a synthetic quaternary ammonium compound which has anticholinergic properties; it is used in dermatology in the treatment of hyperhydrosis. The bioavailability of the oral form is poor and variable, which may account for the persistent doubt as to the incidence of adverse reactions. All anticholinergic effects may occur, but central nervous and ocular adverse reactions are relatively slight.

19.68 Typical anticholinergic effects are:
– Decreased saliva secretion and dry mouth
– Decreased nasal, bronchial and lacrimal secretion, with irritation of the mucosae
– Ocular effects: paralysis of accommodation, pupillary dilatation, photophobia, increase of intra-ocular pressure

- Central nervous symptoms: confusion, excitement, hallucinations, sedation, tachypnoe
- Decrease of bladder tone and speed micturition, sometimes resulting in acute urinary retention
- Delayed gastric emptying, constipation
- Tachycardia with palpitations, dysrhythmias
- Hyperpyrexia due to blocking of eccrine sweating.

Symptoms of poisoning with anticholinergic agents have been reviewed by Shader and Greenblatt [141].

Colchicine

19.69 Colchicine is an anti-inflammatory agent which has long been used in the treatment of gouty arthritis; in dermatology it has been reported useful in treating necrotizing vasculitis [55], Behçet's disease [90], dermatitis herpetiformis [194], pustulosis palmoplantaris [195], scleroderma [196] and Sweet's syndrome [150]. For other indications, *see* [157]. The incidence of toxic reactions is high and an (accidental) overdosage may be fatal [93, 197].

19.70 Side effects reported include:
- Gastrointestinal disturbances: nausea, vomiting, abdominal pain, distension, diarrhea, malabsorption (with chronic use)
- Thrombocytopenia, leukopenia, agranulocytosis, megaloblastic anemia (rare)
- Myopathy, peripheral neuritis, muscular weakness
- Azoospermia, amenorrhea (rare)
- Alopecia [53]
- Burning of the throat and skin.

D-Penicillamine

19.71 D-Penicillamine (D-β,β-dimethylcysteine) [162] is a sulfhydryl aminoacid which may be synthesized or prepared by the hydrolytic degradation of penicillin. Penicillamine has been used in the treatment of lead poisoning, because it is an effective chelator of heavy metals. Due to its cupruretic effect, penicillamine has been efficacious in Wilson's disease. Its ability to solubilize cystine has led to its use in the treatment of cystinuria and associated nephrolithiasis. In both rheumatoid arthritis and primary biliary cirrhosis, the efficacy of penicillamine is probably due to its effect on immunoglobulins and immune complexes. It has also been useful in the treatment of progressive systemic sclerosis, morphea, disorders of keratin formation, and chronic liver disease. In these disorders, the mechanism of action of penicillamine has not been clearly elucidated.

19.72 Adverse reactions to oral administration of penicillamine are reported to occur in 30% of patients treated or even more; the most frequent ones are localized to the gastrointestinal tract and the skin. Side effects of penicillamine include [82, 58, 124, 65]:
- Gastrointestinal disturbances: anorexia, nausea, vomiting, diarrhea (common), aphthous stomatitis, temporary taste derangement (very common), hepatic toxicity [160], pancreatitis (rare)
- Skin and appendages: maculopapular and urticarial rashes, both localized and generalized, allergic reactions with pruritus, edema, eosinophilia and lymphadenopathy

- Late reactions (due to the interaction of penicillamine with the connective tissue constituents and their precursors) include: wrinkling and thinning of the skin (penicillamine dermopathy), friability, traumatic purpura, bullae, pigmented hypertrophic scars, milia, cutis hyperelastica, perforating elastoma [153].
  Other skin manifestations include: pemphigus-like conditions [166, 171, 178], systemic lupus erythematosus [162, 187], discoid lupus erythematosus [20], Lyell's syndrome [57], hirsutism, dermatomyositis [123], lichen planus [133, 145, 163, 174, 188], yellow nail syndrome [81], psoriasiform dermatitis and alopecia [189], onychopathy [190].
- Urinary system: proteinuria (15%), membranous glomerulonephritis, nephrotic syndrome, Goodpasture's syndrome (rare)
- Hematological: various blood dyscrasias (although uncommon, fatalities due to penicillamine are usually due to blood dyscrasias), leukemia (?)
- Nervous system: exacerbation of neurological symptoms in Wilson's disease, ptosis, strabism, peripheral neuropathy, nerve paresis (all rare), migraine-like headaches
- Miscellaneous: myasthenia with or without thyroid dysfunction, bronchospasm (uncommon), bronchiolitis obliterans (sometimes fatal), thrombotic thrombocytopenic purpura (very rare), liver damage, osteopathy, polymyositis, polyarthritis, gigantism of the breasts, Sjögren's syndrome, thyroiditis (very rare), retinal detachment (very rare).

Acyclovir

19.73   Acyclovir (9-[(2-hydroxyethoxy)methyl]guanine) is an acyclic nucleoside analog of guanoside which is a new potent and selective antiviral agent. It has been found to have strong *in vitro* antiviral activity against herpes viruses. The selective activity of acyclovir for cells infected with herpes viruses is due to the production of 2 unique herpes-specific enzymes, an isofunctional deoxynucleoside kinase and a herpes-specific DNA polymerase.

In man, acyclovir has been found to exert a beneficial effect in the prophylaxis and treatment of selected herpes virus infections when used intravenously [248], orally [246], and topically [247]. After oral administration absorption of acyclovir is slow, variable, and incomplete. The estimated total bioavailability in man is believed to be between 15% and 30%, and it appears that the bioavailability decreases with increasing dose. The drug is distributed in all tissues and enters the cerebrospinal fluid, saliva and vaginal excretions at concentrations inhibitory to herpes simplex virus. Acyclovir is eliminated mainly via the kidney.

A review of the clinical pharmacokinetics of acyclovir has been published [241].

Side effects

19.74   Acyclovir seems to have a large therapeutic index, toxicity to date having been minor. Intravenous injection has caused local irritation and phlebitis [240], which may be related to the high pH of the infusion fluid, or may sometimes be due to extravasation of the drug. Of 96 patients treated with intravenous acyclovir for various virus infections 3 experienced pain at the site of drug infusion. Ten patients complained of nausea, and an erythematous and urticarial rash developed in one [238]. Acyclovir uncommonly causes a reversible elevation in serum creatinine. This may be due to cristallization of the drug in the renal tubules or collecting ducts [239, 240]. The development of renal dysfunction appears to be related to the method of administration. It is more likely to occur if acyclovir is administered as a bolus injection rather than in a 1-hour infusion. In patients suffering from renal insufficiency dosage modifications are necessary to maintain an effective plasma acyclovir level without concomitant drug accumulation. Acyclovir has been reported to cause an elevation of the liver transaminases (SGOT, SGPT) [240, 243], but the clinical significance of these findings has not yet been established. Central nervous system disturbances (delirium, tremor, and abnormal EEG) have been reported in patients treated with acyclovir [245], but these effects tend to occur in extremely complicated cases and a causal relationship with the drug has not been proven. In one patient suffering from herpes zoster and treated with aciclovir progressive bilateral amaurosis developed. Autopsy revealed as possibly drug-related necrotizing vasculitis of the left optic nerve at the chiasm [244]. Thus far, bone marrow toxicity at clinical relevant concentrations has not been reported [242].

19.75   REFERENCES

1. Abramov, L. A., Yust, I. C. et al. (1978): Acute respiratory distress caused by erythromycin hypersensitivity. *Arch. intern. Med., 138,* 1157.
2. Ad Hoc Committee on the use of antibiotics in dermatology (1975): Systemic antibiotics for treatment of acne vulgaris. *Arch. Derm., 111,* 1630.
3. Ahmed, A. H., McCarthy, D. G., Sharma, S. K. and Masawe, A. E. J. (1978): Stevens-Johnson syndrome during treatment with cimetidine. *Lancet, 1,* 433.
4. Anonymous (1977): *AMA Drug Evaluations.* PSG Publishing Co., Inc., Littleton, Mass.
5. Anonymous (1979): *Antibiotic Induced Colitis.* Adverse Reactions Series (Committee on Safety of Medicines), No. 17, June.
6. Omitted.
7. Baden, H. P. and Bonaz, L. C. (1967): Calcinosis cutis following intralesional injection of triamcinolone hexacetonide. *Arch. Derm., 96,* 689.
8. Baer, R. L. and Harris, H. (1967): Types of cutaneous reactions to drugs. Importance in recognition of adverse reactions. *J. Amer. med. Ass., 202,* 710.
9. Baker, H. (1979): Systemic Therapy. In: *Textbook of Dermatology, Vol. II, third Edition,* pp. 2262-2263. Editors: A. Rook, D. S. Wilkinson and F. J. G. Ebling. Blackwell Scientific Publications, Oxford.
10. Baker, H. (1979): Systemic therapy. In: *Textbook of Dermatology, Vol. II, third Edition,* pp. 2285-2286. Editors: A. Rook, D. S. Wilkinson and F. J. G. Ebling. Blackwell Scientific Publications, Oxford.
11. Baran, M. L. R. (1964): Le risque d'amaurose au cours du traitement local des alopécies par corticothérapie injectable. *Bull. Soc. franç. Derm. Syph., 71,* 25.
12. Bean, S. F. (1971): Acneiform eruption from tetracycline. *Brit. J. Derm., 85,* 585.
13. Beck, M. H. and Portnoy, B. (1979): Severe erythema multiforme complicated by fatal gastro-intestinal involvement following co-trimoxazole therapy. *Clin. exp. Derm., 4,* 201.
14. Bernstein, L. S. (1975): Adverse reactions to trimethoprim-sulphamethoxazole, with particular reference to long-term therapy. *Canad. med. Ass. J., 112,* 96.
15. Bernstein, L. S. and Cooper, J. (1978): Co-trimoxazole and Stevens-Johnson syndrome. *Lancet, 1,* 988.
16. Bomb, B. S., Purohit, S. D. and Bedi, H. K. (1976): Stevens-Johnson syndrome caused by isoniazid. *Tubercle (Lond.), 57,* 229.
17. Brogden, R. N., Heel, R. C., Speight, T. M. and Avery, G. S. (1978): Metronidazole in anaerobic infections. A review of its activity, pharmacokinetics and therapeutic use. *Drugs, 16,* 387.
18. Omitted.
19. Burland, W. L., Hunt, R. H., Mills, J. G. and Milton-Thompson, G. J. (1979): 1970-1979 Cimetidine. *J. Pharmacother., 24,* 40.
20. Burns, D. A. and Sarkany, I. (1979): Penicillamine-induced discoid lupus erythematosus. *Clin. exp. Derm., 4,* 389.
21. Catterall, R. D. (1977): Fifteen years' experience with metronidazole. In: *Proceedings International Metronidazole Conference Quebec, Vol. 1,* pp. 106-111.
22. Coombs, R. R. A. and Gell, P. G. H. (1968): Classification of allergic reactions responsible for clinical hypersensitivity and disease. In: *Clinical Aspects of Immunology, 2nd Ed.,* pp. 575-596. Editors: P. G. H. Gell and R. R. A. Coombs. Blackwell Scientific Publications, Oxford.

23. David, D. S., Gricco, M. H. and Cushman Jr., P. (1970): Adrenal glucocorticoids after twenty years. *J. chron. Dis., 22,* 637.
24. Delaunois, L. (1979): Hypersensitivity to cimetidine. *New Engl. J. Med., 300,* 1216.
25. Domz, C. A., McNamara, D. H. and Holzapfer, H. F. (1959): Tetracycline provocation on lupus erythematosus. *Ann. intern. Med., 50,* 1217.
26. Downie, W. W., Dixon, J. S., Lowe, J. R., Rhind, V. M., Leatham, P. A. and Pickup, M. E. (1978): Adrenocortical suppression by synthetic corticosteroid drugs: a comparative study of prednisolone and betamethasone. *Brit. J. clin. Pharm., 6,* 397.
27. Omitted.
28. Omitted.
29. Editorial (1979): Cimetidine and giant urticaria. *Ann. intern. Med., 91,* 128.
30. Elman, A., Gullberg, R., Nilsson, E., Rendahl, I. and Wachtmeister, L. (1976): Chloroquine retinopathy in patients with rheumatoid arthritis. *Scand. J. Rheumatol., 5,* 161.
31. Fanning, W. L. and Gump, D. W. (1976): Distressing side-effects of minocycline hydrochloride. *Arch. intern. Med., 136,* 761.
32. Feldmann, H. U. and Barleben, P. (1977): Medikamentenbedingte Hautausschläge. *Medizin (Erlangen), 5,* 75.
33. Finkelstein, W. and Isselbacher, K. J. (1978): Cimetidine. *New Engl. J. Med., 299,* 992.
34. Omitted.
35. Fox, R. M. (1979): Methotrexate nephrotoxicity. *Clin. exp. Pharmacol. Physiol.,* Suppl. 5, 43.
36. Françon, F. (1968): Accidents cutanés et souscutanés par le Tédarol en injections locales. *Méd. et Hyg. (Genève), 26,* 480.
37. Omitted
38. Omitted.
39. Omitted.
40. Gange, R. W., Rhodes, E. L., Edwards, C. O. and Powell, M. E. A. (1976): Pemphigus induced by rifampicin. *Brit. J. Derm., 95,* 445.
41. Gantz, N. M., Zawacki, J. K. and Dickerson, J. (1979): Pseudomembranous colitis associated with erythromycin. *Ann. intern. Med., 91,* 866.
42. George, R. H. (1979): Metronidazole – an assessment. *Prescr. J., 19,* 118.
43. Gifford, L. M., Aeugle, M. E., Myerson, R. M. and Tannenbaum, P. J. (1980): Cimetidine postmarket, outpatient surveillance program. *J. Amer. med. Ass., 243,* 1532.
44. Girling, D. J. and Hitze, K. L. (1979): Adverse reactions to rifampicin. *Bull. Wld Hlth Org., 57,* 45.
45. Goldman, A. L. and Braman, S. S. (1972): Isoniazid, a review with emphasis on adverse effects. *Chest, 62,* 71.
46. Gonzalez, F., Trujillo, J. M. and Alexanian, R. (1977): Acute leukaemia and multiple myeloma. *Ann. intern. Med., 86,* 440.
47. Good, M. I. and Shader, R. I. (1977): Behavioral toxicity and equivocal suicide associated with chloroquine and its derivatives. *Amer. J. Psychiat., 134,* 798.
48. Götz, H. and Reichenberger, M. (1972): Ergebnisse einer Fragebogenaktion bei 1670 Dermatologen der Bundesrepublik Deutschland über Nebenwirkungen bei der Griseofulvin-Therapie. *Hautarzt, 11,* 485.
49. Graham, W. G. B. and Dundas, G. R. (1979): Isoniazid-related liver disease. *J. Amer. Med. Ass., 242,* 353.
50. Graham Jr., W. R. (1975): Adverse effects of dapsone. *Int. J. Derm., 14,* 494.
51. Greiner, A. C. and Berry, K. (1964): Skin pigmentation and corneal and lens opacities with prolonged chlorpromazine therapy. *Canad. med. Ass. J., 90,* 663.
52. Gump, D. W., Ashikaga, T., Fink, Th. J. and Radin, A. M. (1977): Side effects of minocycline: different dosage regimes. *Antimicrob. Agents Chemother., 12,* 642.
53. Harms, M. (1980): Haarausfall und Haarveränderungen nach Kolchizintherapie. *Hautarzt, 31,* 161.
54. Havas, L., Fernex, M. and Lenox-Smith, I. (1973): The clinical efficacy and tolerance of co-trimoxazole. *Clin. Trials J., 3,* 81.
55. Hazen, P. G. and Michel, B. (1979): Management of necrotizing vasculitis with colchicine. *Arch. Derm., 115,* 1303.
56. Hendricks, A. A. (1980): Yellow lunulae with fluorescence after tetracycline therapy. *Arch. Derm., 116,* 438.
57. Hennemann, H. H., Hubertus, H. and Stocker, W. G. (1975): Schwere Nebenwirkungen bei der Therapie mit D-Penizillamin. *Dtsch. med. Wschr., 100,* 1634.

58. Hill, H. F. H. (1979): Penicillamine in rheumatoid arthritis: adverse effects. *Scand. J. Rheumatol.*, *Suppl. 28*, 94.

59. Idsøe, O., Guthe, T., Willcox, R. R. and De Weck, A. L. (1969): Art und Ausmass der Penizillinnebenwirkungen unter besonderer Berücksichtigung von 151 Todesfällen nach anaphylaktischem Schock. *Schweiz. med. Wschr., 99*, 1190 and 1221.

60. Jopling, W. H. and Harman, R. R. M. (1979): Leprosy. In: *Textbook of Dermatology, Vol. I, third Edition*, pp. 749-766. Editors: A. Rook, D. S. Wilkinson and F. J. G. Ebling. Blackwell Scientific Publications, Oxford.

61. Kaiser, H. (1977): *Cortisonderivate in Klinik und Praxis, 7th Edition*. G. Thieme Verlag, Stuttgart.

62. Kanwar, A. J. and Singh, O. B. (1976): Toxic epidermal necrolysis drug induced. *Indian J. Derm., 21*, 73.

63. Omitted.

64. Kasanen, A., Anttila, M., Elfving, R., Kahela, P., Saarimaa, H., Sundquist, H., Tikkanen, R. and Toivanen, P. (1978): Trimethoprim. *Ann. clin. Res., 10*, Suppl. 22.

65. Kean, W. F., Dwosh, I. L., Anastassiades, T. P., Ford, P. M. and Garfield, K. H. (1980): The toxicity pattern of d-penicillamine therapy. *Arthr. and Rheum., 23*, 158.

66. Kiefer, O. (1973): Über die Nebenwirkungen der Bleomycintherapie auf der Haut. *Dermatologica (Basel), 146*, 229.

67. Kikuchi, J. and Horikawa, S. (1974): Perilymphatic atrophy of the skin, a side effect of topical corticosteroid injection therapy. *Arch. Derm., 109*, 558.

68. Knisley, R. E., Settipane, G. A. and Albala, M. M. (1971): Unusual reaction to chlorambucil in a patient with chronic lymphocytic leukaemia. *Arch. Derm., 104*, 77.

69. Labhart, A. and Martz, G. (1978): Grundzüge der Hormontherapie nicht-endokriner Krankheiten. In: *Klinik der inneren Sekretion*, Chapter XX, p. 1037. Springer-Verlag, Berlin.

70. Lang, P. G. (1979): Sulfones and sulfonamides in dermatology today. *J. Amer. Acad. Derm., 1*, 479.

71. Lassus, A. (1980): Systemic treatment of psoriasis with an oral retinoic acid derivative (Ro 10-9359). *Brit. J. Derm., 102*, 195.

72. Omitted.

73. Lever, W. F. (1979): Pemphigus and pemphigoid. *J. Amer. Acad. Derm., 1*, 2.

74. Levine, H. B. (1972): Skin rashes with penicillin-therapy: Current management. *New Engl. J. Med., 286*, 42.

75. Levine, H. B. (1982): *Ketoconazole in the Management of Fungal Disease*. Editor: H. B. Levine. Adis Press, Balgowla, Australia.

76. Omitted.

77. Livingood, C. S., Stewart, R. H. and Webster, S. B. (1970): Cutaneous vasculitis caused by griseofulvin. *Cutis, 6*, 1346.

78. Lloyd, K. M. (1968): Figurate erythema due to antimalarial therapy. *Cutis, 4*, 67.

79. Lochmann, O., Kohout, P. and Vymola, F. (1977): Anaphylactic shock following the administration of clindamycin. *J. Hyg. Epidemiol. Microbiol., 21*, 441.

80. Lomholt, G. (1979): Syphilis, Yaws and Pinta. In: *Textbook of Dermatology, Vol. I, third Edition*, p. 733. Editors: A. Rook, D. S. Wilkinson and F. J. G. Ebling. Blackwell Scientific Publications, Oxford.

81. Lubach, D. and Marghescu, S. (1979): Yellow-Nail-Syndrom durch d-Penizillamin. *Hautarzt, 30*, 547.

82. Lyle, W. H. (1979): Penicillamine. *Clin. rheum. Dis., 5*, 569.

83. Manni, J. J. and Van Den Brock, P. (1977): Pulmonary complications of methotrexate therapy. *Clin. Otolaryngol., 2*, 131.

84. Maulide, I. and Villar, T. G. (1974): Therapeutic trial with clindamycin in non-tuberculosis infections of the respiratory tract. *Pneumologia (Lisbon), 5*, 79.

85. McGrae, J. and Zelickson, A. S. (1980): Skin pigmentation secondary to minocycline therapy. *Arch. Derm., 116*, 1262.

86. Meade, R. H. III (1979): Drug therapy reviews: Antimicrobial spectrum, pharmacology and therapeutic use of erythromycin and its derivatives. *Amer. J. Hosp. Pharm., 36*, 1185.

87. Mellin, K.-B. and Waubke, Th. N. (1978): Schäden am Auge durch Ethambutol. *Münch. med. Wschr., 120*, 995.

88. Michaëlsson, G., Molin, L., Öhman, S., Gip, L., Lindström, B., Skogh, M. and Trolin, I. (1976): Clofazimine, a new agent for the treatment of pyoderma gangrenosum. *Arch. Derm., 112*, 344.

89. Mital, O. P., Singh, R. P., Katiyar, S. K. and Mehrotra, R. K. (1976): Toxic epidermal necrolysis due to isoniazid. *Indian J. Tuberc., 23*, 32.

90.   Miyachi, Y., Taniguchi, S., Ozaki, M. and Horio, T. (1981): Colchicine in the treatment of the cutaneous manifestations of Behçet's disease. *Brit. J. Derm., 104*, 67.

91.   Moulopoulou-Karakitsou, K., Mavrikakis, M. and Anastasiou-Nana, M. (1981): An unusual adverse reaction to Ro 10-9359. *Brit. J. Derm., 104*, 709.

92.   Omitted.

93.   Naidius, R. M. et al. (1977): Colchicine toxicity. *Arch. intern. Med., 137*, 394.

94.   Notowicz, A., Vermeiden, I. and Stolz, E. (1980): Aromatisch retinoid in de dermatologie. *Ned. T. Geneesk., 124*, 1284.

95.   Nwokolo, U.   91974): Acneiform lesions in combined rifampicin treatment in Africans. *Brit. med. J., 3*, 473.

96.   Nyfors, A. (1980): Methotrexate therapy of psoriasis. Effect and side effects with particular reference to hepatic changes. A survey. *Dan. med. Bull., 27*, 74.

97.   Orfanos, C. E. (1980): Oral retinoids – present status. *Brit. J. Derm., 103*, 473.

98.   Omitted.

99.   Pareek, S. S. (1980): Nystatin-induced fixed eruption. *Brit. J. Derm., 103*, 679.

100.   Omitted.

101.   Omitted.

102.   Petrozzi, J. W. and Witkowski, J. A. (1971): Acrodermatitis perstans. *Arch. Derm., 103*, 442.

103.   Potter, R. A. (1971): Intralesional triamcinolone and adrenal suppression in acne vulgaris. *J. invest. Derm., 57*, 364.

104.   Raab, W. (1975): Spectinomycin. Indikationen und unerwünschte Wirkungen. *Schweiz. med. Wschr., 105*, 1116.

105.   Rimbaud, P., Meynadier, J., Guilhou, J. J. and Meynadier, J. (1974): Complications dermatologiques locales secondaires aux injections cortisonées. *Nouv. Presse méd., 3*, 665.

106.   Robinson, J. K., Baughman, R. D., Auerbach, R. and Cimis, R. J. (1980): Methotrexate hepatotoxicity in psoriasis. *Arch. Derm., 116*, 413.

107.   Roe, F. J. C. (1977): Metronidazole: Review of uses and toxicity. *J. antimicrob. Chemother., 3*, 205.

108.   Rosenthal, A. L., Binnick, S., Panzer, P. and Pirozzi, D. J. (1979): Drug-induced toxic epidermal necrolysis in children. *Cutis, 24*, 437.

109.   Omitted.

110.   Rothstein, M. S. (1977): Onycholysis through phototoxicity. *Arch. Derm., 113*, 520.

111.   Rubin, R. H. and Schwartz, N. (1980): Trimethoprim-sulfamethoxazole. *New Engl. J. Med., 303*, 426.

112.   Omitted.

113.   Ruzicka, T. and Goerz, G. (1981): Dapsone in the treatment of lupus erythematosus. *Brit. J. Derm., 104*, 53.

114.   Scharschmidt, B. (1979): Cimetidine. *West. J. Med., 131*, 417.

115.   Omitted.

116.   Schindel, L. E. (1965): Clinical side-effects of the tetracyclines. *Antibiot. et Chemother. (Basel), 13*, 300.

117.   Sham, P. C., Rao, K. R. P. and Patel, A. R. (1978): Cyclophosphamide-induced nailpigmentation. *Brit. J. Derm., 98*, 675.

118.   Shelley, W. B. and Heaton, C. L. (1973): Minocycline sensitivity. *J. Amer. med. Ass., 224*, 125.

119.   Shelmire, D. (1968): Reaction to intralesional triamcinolone. *Cutis, 4*, 71.

120.   Shimegi, F., Tanaka, M. and Ohtsuka, (1978): A case of sensitization to oral corticosteroids. *J. Derm. (Tokyo), 5*, 231.

121.   Simmonds, J., Hodges, S., Nicol, F. and Barnett, D. (1978): Anaphylaxis after oral penicillin. *Lancet, 2*, 1404.

122.   Simon, N., Berko, G., Polay, A. and Kocsis, G. (1971): Der Einfluss der Griseofulvin-Therapie auf die Leberfunktion und den Porphyrin-Stoffwechsel. *Arch. derm. Forsch., 241*, 148.

123.   Simpson, N. B. and Golding, J. R. (1980): Dermatomyositis induced by penicillamin. *Acta derm.-venereol. (Stockh.), 59*, 543.

124.   Stein, H. B., Patterson, C. A., Offer, R. C., Atkins, C. J., Teufel, A. and Robinson, H. S. (1980): Adverse effects of d-penicillamine in rheumatoid arthritis. *Ann. intern. Med., 92*, 24.

125.   Omitted.

126.   Tan, S. G. and Cunliffe, W. J. (1976): The unwanted effects of clindamycin in acne. *Brit. J. Derm., 94*, 313.

127.   Tanenbaum, L. and Tuffanelli, D. L. (1980): Antimalarial agents. *Arch. Derm., 116*, 587.

128.   Tedesco, F. J. (1977): Clindamycin and colitis. A review. *J. infect. Dis., Suppl. 135*, 95.

129. Thornsvard, C. T., Guider, G. A. and Kimball, D. B. (1976): An unusual reaction to chloroquine-primaquine. *J. Amer. med. Ass., 235,* 1719.
130. Tomecki, K. and Catalano, C. J. (1981): Dapsone hypersensitivity. *Arch. Derm., 117,* 38.
131. Uragoda, C. G. and Kottegoda, S. R. (1977): Adverse reactions to isoniazid on ingestion of fish with a high histamine content. *Tubercle (London), 58,* 83.
132. Valagussa, P., Kenda, R., Fossam Bellani, F., Franchi, F., Banfi, A., Rilke, F. and Bonadonna, G. (1979): Incidence of second malignancies in Hodgkin's disease after various forms of treatment. *Proceedings of the Fifteenth Meeting of the American Society of Clinical Oncology, 20,* abstract 285, p. 360.
133. Van der Staak, W. J. B. M., Cotton, D. W. K., Jonckheer-Venneste, M. M. H. and Boerbooms, A. M. T. H. (1975): Lichenoid eruption following penicillamine. *Dermatologica (Basel), 150,* 372.
134. Omitted.
135. Watsky, M. S. and Lynfield, Y. L. (1976): Lupus erythematosus exacerbated by griseofulvin. *Cutis, 17,* 361.
136. Weinstein, L. (1975): Antimicrobial agents. Drugs used in the chemotherapy of tuberculosis and leprosy. In: *The Pharmacological Basis of Therapeutics, 5th Edition,* pp. 1201-1223. Editors: L.S. Goodman and A. Gilman. Macmillan Publishing Co., New York.
137. Yantis, P. L., Bridges, M. E. and Pittmann, F. E. (1980): Cimetidine-induced exfoliative dermatitis. *Dig. Dis. Sci., 25,* 73.
138. Yates, V. M. and Kerr, R. E. I. (1980): Cimetidine and thrombocytopenia. *Brit. med. J., 1,* 1453.
139. Yawalkar, S. J. and Vischer, W. (1979): Lamprene (clofazimine) in leprosy. *Leprosy Rev., 50,* 135.
140. Zucker, G. and Stiller, D. (1978): Zur immunologischen In-vitro-Diagnostik des Lyell-Syndroms. *Derm. Mschr., 164,* 521.
141. Shader, R. I. and Greenblatt, D. J. (1971): Uses and toxicity of belladonna alkaloids and synthetic anticholinesterases. *Semin. Psychiat., 3,* 449.

UPDATE – 2nd Edition

142. Weart, C. W. and Hyman, L. C. (1983): Serum sickness associated with metronidazole. *Sth. med. J., 76,* 410.
143. Jeanmougin, M., Morel, P. and Civatte, J. (1982): Photo-onycholyse induite par la doxycycline. *Ann. Derm. Vénéréol. (Paris), 109,* 165.
144. Yung, C. W., Winston, E. M. and Lorincz, A. L. (1981): Dacarbazine-induced photosensitivity reaction. *J. Amer. Acad. Derm., 4,* 541.
145. Powell, F. C., Rogers, R. S. III. and Dickson, E. R. (1982): Lichen planus, primary biliary cirrhosis and penicillamine (Letter). *Brit. J. Derm., 107,* 616.
146. Ridgway, H. A., Sonnex, T. S., Kennedy, C. T. C. et al. (1982): Hyperpigmentation associated with oral minocycline. *Brit. J. Derm., 107,* 95.
147. Hudson, C. P. and Callen, J. P. (1982): The tetracycline-oral contraceptive controversy. *J. Amer. Acad. Derm., 6,* 269.
148. Corbett, M. F., Hawk, J. L. M., Herxheimer, A. and Magnus, I.A. (1982): Controlled therapeutic trials in polymorphic light eruption. *Brit. J. Derm., 107,* 571.
149. Tobin, D. R., Krohel, G. B. and Rynes, R. I. (1982): Hydroxychloroquine. Seven-year experience. *Arch. Ophthal., 100,* 81.
150. Suehisa, S., Tagami, H., Inoue, F. et al. (1983): Colchicine in the treatment of acute febrile neutrophilic dermatosis (Sweet's syndrome). *Brit. J. Derm., 108,* 99.
151. White, S. W. and Besanceney, C. (1983): Systemic pigmentation from tetracycline and minocycline therapy (Letter). *Arch. Derm., 119,* 1.
152. Oklund, S. A. and Prolo, D. J. (1981): The significane of yellow bone. *J. Amer. med. Ass., 246,* 761.
153. Barr, R. J., Siegel, J. M. and Graham, J. H. (1980): Elastosis perforans serpiginosa associated with morphea. *J. Amer. Acad. Derm., 3,* 19.
154. Piamphongsant, Th. (1982): Dapsone for the treatment of vesiculobullous and pustular diseases. *Int. J. Derm., 21,* 512.
155. Barranco, V. P. (1982): Dapsone - other indications. *Int. J. Derm., 21,* 513.
156. Granstein, R. D. and Sober, A. J. (1981): Drug- and heavy metal-induced hyperpigmentation. *J. Amer. Acad. Derm., 5,* 1.
157. Malkinson, F. D. (1982): Colchicine - New uses of an old, old drug (Editorial). *Arch. Derm., 118,* 453.

158.   Girling, D. J. (1982): Adverse effects of antituberculosis drugs. *Drugs, 23,* 56.
159.   Leroy, J. -P., Dorval, J. -C., DeWitte, J. -D. et al. (1981): Deux cas de pigmentation cutanée au cours de traitements par la minocycline. *Ann. Derm. Vénéréol. (Paris), 108,* 871.
160.   Wozel, G. and Julius, U. (1982): Ikterus durch D-Penizillamin und hormonale Kontrazeption bei progressiver Sklerodermie. *Dtsch. Z. Verdau.-u. Stoffwechselkr., 42,* 85.
161.   Reed, K. M. and Sober, A. J. (1983): Methotrexate-induced necrolysis. *J. Amer. Acad. Derm., 8,* 677.
162.   Levy, R. S., Fisher, M. and Alter, J. N. (1983): Penicillamine: Review and cutaneous manifestations. *J. Amer. Acad. Derm., 8,* 548.
163.   Isaacson, D., Elgart, M. and Turner, M. L. (1982): Anti-malarials in dermatology. *Int. J. Derm., 21,* 379.
164.   Lawrence, C. M. and Dahl, M. G. C. (1982): Cutaneous necrosis associated with methotrexate treatment for psoriasis. *Brit. J. Derm., 107, (Suppl. 22),* 24.
165.   Kromann, N. P., Vilhelmsen, R. and Stahl, D. (1982): The dapsone syndrome. *Arch. Derm., 118,* 531.
166.   Troy, J. L., Silvers, D.N., Grossman, M.E. and Jaffe, I.A. (1981): Penicillamine - associated pemphigus: Is it really pemphigus? *J. Amer. Acad. Derm., 4,* 547.
167.   Koranda, F. C. (1981): Antimalarials. *J. Amer. Acad. Derm., 4,* 650.
168.   Olansky, A. J. (1982): Antimalarials and ophthalmologic safety. *J. Amer. Acad. Derm., 6,* 19.
169.   Webb, P. K., Conant, M. A. and Maibach, H.I. (1982): Perforation of the colon in high-dose corticosteroid therapy of pemphigus. *J. Amer. Acad. Derm., 6,* 1040.
170.   McDougall, A. C., Horsfall, W. R., Hede, J. E. and Chaplin, A. J. (1980): Splenic infarction and tissue accumulation of crystals associated with the use of clofazimine (Lamprene; B 663) in the treatment of pyoderma gangrenosum. *Brit. J. Derm., 102,* 227.
171.   Matkaluk, R. M. and Bailin, P. L. (1981): Penicillamine-induced pemphigus foliaceus. *Arch. Derm., 117,* 156.
172.   Seehafer, J. R., Rogers, R. S. III, Fleming, C. R. and Dickson, E. R. (1981): Lichen planus-like lesions caused by penicillamine in primary biliary cirrhosis. *Arch. Derm., 117,* 140.
173.   Korossy, K. S. and Hood, A. F. (1981): Methotrexate reactivation of sunburn reaction. *Arch. Derm., 117,* 310.
174.   Van Hecke, E., Kint, A. and Temmerman, L. (1981): A lichenoid eruption induced by penicillamine. *Arch. Derm., 117,* 676.
175.   Eckman, M. R., Johnson, T. and Riess, R. (1975): Partial deafness after erythromycin. *New Engl. J. Med., 292,* 649.
176.   Quinnan, G. V. and McCabe, W. R. (1978): Ototoxicity of erythromycin. *Lancet, 1,* 1160.
177.   Walters, B. N. and Gubbay, S. S. (1981): Tetracycline and benign intracranial hypertension: Report of five cases. *Brit. med. J., 282,* 19.
178.   Yung, C. W. and Hambrick, G. W. Jr. (1982): D-Penicillamine-induced pemphigus syndrome. *J. Amer. Acad. Derm., 6,* 317.
179.   Armstrong, R. B. and Poh-Fitzpatrick, M. B. (1982): Methotrexate and ultraviolet radiation. *Arch. Derm., 118,* 177.
180.   Roenigk, H. H., Auerbach, R., Maibach, H. I. and Weinstein, G. D. (1982): Methotrexate guidelines-revised. *J. Amer. Acad. Derm., 6,* 145.
181.   Person, J. R. and Schwartz, J. H. (1982): Dapsone-responsive, non-infectious verrucous pyoderma. *Arch. Derm., 118,* 336.
182.   Guill, A. and Aton, J. K. (1982): Facial granuloma responsive to dapsone therapy. *Arch. Derm., 118,* 332.
183.   Goldman, P. (1980): Metronidazole. *New Engl. J. Med., 303,* 1212.
184.   Saginur, R., Hawley, C. R. and Bartlett, J.G. (1980): Colitis associated with metronidazole therapy. *J. infect. Dis., 141,* 772.
185.   Kunze, J., Roeber, H. and Kollakowski, M. (1979): Phototoxic dermatitis with DTIC treatment. *Z. Hautkr., 55,* 100.
186.   *AMA Drug Evaluations, Ed. 3.* (1977), p. 1124. Publishing Sciences Group, Inc., Littleton, U.S.A.
187.   Walshe, J. M. (1981): Penicillamine and the SLE syndrome. *J. Rheumat., 8, (Suppl. 7),* 155.
188.   Graham-Brown, R. A. C., Sarkany, I. and Sherlock, S. (1982): Lichen planus and primary biliary cirrhosis. *Brit. J. Derm., 106,* 699.
189.   Sternlieb, I., Fisher, M. and Scheinberg, I. H. (1981): Penicillamine-induced skin lesions. *J. Rheumat., 8, (Suppl. 7),* 149.
190.   Thivolet, J., Perrot, H. and Francois, R. (1967): Glossite, stomatite, et onychopathie provoquée par la penicillamine. *Bull. Soc. franç. Derm. Syph., 75,* 61.

191. Saihan, E. and Burton, J. (1980): A double-blind trial of metronidazole versus oxytetracycline therapy for rosacea. *Brit. J. Derm., 102,* 443.

192. Schirner, A. and Haneke, E. (1981): Rosacea and metronidazole. *Acta Derm., 7,* 27.

193. Mackey, J. P. and Barnes, J. (1974): Clofazimine in the treatment of discoid lupus erythematosus. *Brit. J. Derm., 91,* 93.

194. Silvers, D. N., Juhlin, E. A., Berczeller, P.H. et al. (1980): Treatment of dermatitis herpetiformis with colchicine. *Arch. Derm., 116,* 1373.

195. Takigawa, M., Miyachi, Y., Uehara, M. and Tagami, H. (1982): Treatment of pustulosis palmaris et plantaris with oral doses of colchicine. *Arch. Derm., 118,* 458.

196. Alarcón-Segovia, D., Ramos-Niembro, F., deKasep, G.I. et al. (1979): Long-term evaluation of colchicine in the treatment of scleroderma. *J. Rheumat., 6,* 705.

197. Stapczynski, J. S., Rothstein, R. J., Goye, W. A. et al. (1981): Colchicine overdose: Report of two cases and review of the literature. *Ann. emerg. Med., 10,* 364.

198. Ling, M. H. M., Perry, P.J. and Tsuang, M. T. (1981): Side effects of corticosteroid therapy. Psychiatric aspects. *Arch. gen. Psychiat., 38,* 471.

199. Wierzba, K., Wańkowicz, B., Piekarczyk, A. and Danysz, A. (1983): Cytostatic and immunosuppressive drugs. In: *Side effects of Drugs, Annual 7* (Ed. M. N. G. Dukes), Chapter 47, pp 425-450. Excerpta Medica, Amsterdam.

200. Erffmeyer, J. E. (1981): Adverse reactions to penicillin. *Ann. Allergy, 47,* 288.

201. Bartlett, J. G. (1981): Antimicrobial agents implicated in Clostridium difficile toxin-associated diarrhea or colitis. *Johns Hopk. med. J., 149,* 6.

202. Neftel, K. A., Wälti, M., Spengler, H. et al. (1981): Neutropenia after penicillins: toxic or immune-mediated? *Klin. Wschr., 59,* 877.

203. Kestel, J. (1981): Photo-onycholysis from minocycline. *York med. J., 28,* 53.

204. Garnier, R., Gastot, A., Louboutin, Ph. et al. (1981): Intolérance à la minocycline. A propos d'une épidémie de troubles vestibulaires. *Thérapie, 35,* 313.

205. Anonymous (1982): Erythromycin estolate to remain on market. *FDA Drug Bull., 12,* 14.

206. Lawson, D. H. and Paice, J. B. (1982): Cotrimoxazole. *Rev. infect. Dis., 4,* 429.

207. Døssing, M. and Andreasen, P. B. (1982): Drug-induced liver disease in Denmark. *Scand. J. Gastroenterol., 17,* 205.

208. Gibson, J. R. (1982): Skin eruptions after trimethoprim. *Brit. med. J., 284,* 1529.

209. Weddington, W. W., Muelling, A. E. and Moosa, H. H. (1982): Adverse neuropsychiatric reactions to cimetidine. *Psychosomatics, 23,* 49.

210. Selker, H. P., Rosenbloom, B. E. and Weinstein, I. M. (1981): Cimetidine and cytopenia. *West. J. Med., 135,* 330.

211. Vircburger, M. I., Prelevéc, G. M., Brkic, S. et al. (1981): Transitory alopecia and hypergonadotrophic hypogonadism during cimetidine treatment. *Lancet, 1,* 1160.

212. Committee on Safety of Medicines (1981): Cimetidine and arthropathy. *Committ. Safety Med. Bull., 7.*

213. Bjaeldager, P. A. L. (1981): Erythema multiforme som sandsynlig bivirkning til cimetidinbehandling. *Ugeskr. Laeg., 143,* 1406.

214. Greist, M. C. and Epinette, W. W. (1982): Cimetidine-induced xerosis and asteatotic dermatitis. *Arch. Derm., 118,* 253.

215. Stranz, M. H. and Bradley, W. E. (1982): Metronidazole. *Drug. Intell. clin. Pharm., 15,* 838.

216. Molavi, A., LeFrock, J. L. and Prince, R. A. (1982): Metronidazole. *Med. Clin. N. Amer., 66,* 121.

217. Bostofte, E., Føge Bak, J. and Høier, R. (1981): Metronidazole, eventuelle karcinogene og mutagene effekt. *Ugeskr. Laeg., 143,* 2211.

218. Editorial (1981): Adverse reactions to dapsone. *Lancet, 2,* 184.

219. Yoshikawa, T. T. and Fujita, N. K. (1982): Antituberculous drugs. *Med. Clin. N. Amer., 66,* 209.

220. Desmukh, P. A., Parekh, K. J., Kundra, N. and Shaw, T. (1982): Drug toxicity in tuberculosis. *Ind. J. Tuberc., 26,* 84.

221. Farr, B. and Mandell, G. L. (1982): Rifampin. *Med. Clin. N. Amer., 66,* 157.

222. Marks, J. S. (1982): Chloroquine retinopathy. Is there a safe daily dose? *Ann. Rheum. Dis., 41,* 52.

223. Thiers, B. H. (1981): Hazards of therapy. *J. Amer. Acad. Derm., 4,* 495.

224. Adams, S. J., Davison, A. M., Cunliffe, W. J. and Giles, G. R. (1982): Perioral dermatitis in renal transplant recipients maintained on corticosteroids and immunosuppressive therapy. *Brit. J. Derm., 106,* 589.

225. Baylink, D. J. (1983): Glucocorticoid-induced osteoporosis. *New. Engl. J. Med., 309,* 306.

226. Appleby, D. H. and Vogtland, H. D. (1983): Suspected metronidazole hepatotoxicity. *Clin. Pharmacy, 2,* 373.

227.   LePaw, M. I. (1983): Fixed drug eruption due to minocycline – report of one case (Letter). *J. Amer. Acad. Derm., 8,* 263.

228.   Fine, J. -D., Katz, S. I., Donahue, M. J. and Hendricks, A.A. (1983): Psychiatric reaction to dapsone and sulfapyridine (Letter). *J. Amer. Acad. Derm., 9,* 274.

229.   Lavarenne, J. and Moreau, Ch. (1980): Pharmacovigilance. Les effets indésirables de la cimetidine. Travail coopératif des Centres de Pharmacovigilance hospitalière. Bilan des observations et confrontation aux données de la littérature. *Thérapie, 35,* 83.

230.   Russell, W. L. and Lopez, L. M. (1980): Cimetidine-induced mental status changes: Case report and literature review. *Amer. J. Hosp. Pharm., 37,* 1667.

231.   Merrett, A. C., Marks, R. and Dudley, F. J. (1981): Cimetidine-induced erythema annulare centrifugum: no cross-reactions with ranitidine. *Brit. med. J., 283,* 698.

232.   Kanwar, A. J., Majid, A., Garg, M. P. and Singh, G. (1981): Seborrheic dermatitis-like eruption caused by cimetidine. *Arch. Derm., 117,* 65.

233.   Taillandier, J., Bussone, A. and Manigand, G. (1981): Prurit par la cimétidine. *Nouv. Press. Méd., 10,* 258.

234.   Fellner, M. J. and Mark, A. S. (1980): Penicillin- and ampicillin-induced pemphigus vulgaris. *Int. J. Derm., 20,* 392.

235.   Appel, G.B. (1980): A decade of penicillin related acute interstitial nephritis - more questions than answers. *Clin. Nephrol., 13,* 151.

236.   Nicholls, P. J. (1980): Neurotoxicity of penicillin. *J. antimicrob. Chemother., 6,* 161.

237.   Walinga, H. and van Bengen, L. (1981): Syndroom van Stevens-Johnson na gebruik van griseofulvine. *Ned. T. Geneesk., 125,* 759.

238.   Balfour, H. H., Bean, B., Sachs, G. W. et al. (1981): Acyclovir, an effective antiviral. *Minn. Med., 29,* 739.

239.   Brigden, D., Rosling, A. E. and Woods, N. C. (1982): Renal function after acyclovir intravenous injection. *Amer. J. Med., 73, (Suppl.),* 182.

240.   Keeney, R. E., Kirk, L. E. and Brigden, D. (1982): Acyclovir tolerance in humans. *Amer. J. Med., 73, (Suppl.),* 176.

241.   Laskin, O. L. (1983): Clinical pharmacokinetics of acyclovir. *Clin. Pharmacokin., 8,* 187.

242.   Laskin, O. L., Saral, R., Burns, W. H. et al. (1982): Acyclovir concentrations and tolerance during repetitive administration for 18 days. *Amer. J. Med., 73, (Suppl.),* 221.

243.   Van der Meer, J. W. M. and Versteeg, J. (1982): Acyclovir in severe herpes virus infections. *Amer. J. Med., 73, (Suppl.),* 271.

244.   Von Schulthess, G. K. and Sauter, Chr. (1981): Acyclovir and herpes zoster. *New Engl. J. Med., 305,* 1349.

245.   Wade, J. C., Hintz, M., McGuffin, R. W. et al. (1982): Treatment of cytomegalovirus pneumonia with high-dose acyclovir. *Amer. J. Med., 73, (Suppl.),* 249.

246.   Bryson, Y. J., Dillon, M., Lovett, M. et al. (1983): Treatment of first episodes of genital herpes simplex virus infection with oral acyclovir. *New Engl. Med., 308,* 916.

247.   Fiddian, A. P. and Ivanyi, L. (1983): Topical acyclovir in the management of recurrent herpes labialis. *Brit. J. Derm., 109,* 321.

248.   Mindel, A., Adler, M. W., Sutherland, S. and Fiddian, A. P. (1982): Intravenous acyclovir treatment for primary genital herpes. *Lancet, 1,* 697.

249.   Cox, F. W., Stiller, R. L., South, D. A. and Stevens, D. A. (1982): Oral ketoconazole for dermatophyte infections. *J. Amer. Acad. Derm., 6,* 455.

250.   Editorial (1982): Ketoconazole. *Arch. Derm., 118,* 217.

251.   DeFelice, R., Johnson, D. G. and Galgiani, J. N. (1981): Gynecomastia with ketoconazole. *Antimicrob. Agents Chemother., 19,* 1073.

252.   Heiberg, J. K. and Svejgaard. E. (1981): Toxic hepatitis during ketoconazole treatment. *Brit. Med. J., 283,* 827.

253.   Horsburgh, C. R. Jr., Kirkpatrick, C. H. and Teutsch, C. B. (1982): Ketoconazole and the liver. *Lancet, 1,* 860.

254.   Janssen, P. A. J. and Symoens, J. E. (1983): Hepatic reactions during ketoconazole treatment. *Amer. J. Med., 74, (Suppl.),* 80.

255.   Janssen, P. A. J., Cauwenbergh, G. and Middag-Broekman, J. H. F. F. (1983): *Hepatitis tijdens een Behandeling met Ketoconazol (Nizoral). Een Overzicht van Alle tot Februari 1983 Gemelde Gevallen.* Research News, Janssen Pharmaceutica B.V., Goirle.

256.   Jones, H. E., Simpson, J. G. and Artis, W. M. (1981): Oral ketoconazole, an effective and safe treatment for dermatophytosis. *Arch. Derm., 117,* 129.

257. Macnair, A. L., Gascoigne, E., Heap, J. et al. (1982): Hepatitis and ketoconazole therapy. *Brit. Med. J., 283,* 1058.
258. Peterson, E. A., Alling, D. W. and Kirkpatrick, C. H. (1980): Treatment of chronic mucocutaneous candidiasis with ketoconazole. *Ann. intern. Med., 93,* 791.
259. Rand, R., Sober, A. J. and Olmstead, P. M. (1983): Ketoconazole therapy and exfoliative erythroderma. *Arch. Derm., 119,* 97.
260. Robertson, M. H., Rich, P., Parker, F. and Hanifin, J. M. (1982): Ketoconazole in griseofulvin-resistant dermatophytosis. *J. Amer. Acad. Derm., 6,* 224.
261. Rogers, S. (1981): *Double-blind Comparison of Ketoconazole and Griseofulvin in the Treatment of Dermatophyte Infections.* 21st Interscience Conference on Antimicrobial Agents and Chemotherapy, Chicago. American Society for Microbiology, 1981.
262. Rollman, O. and Lööf, L. (1983): Hepatic toxicity of ketoconazole. *Brit. J. Derm., 107,* 376.
263. Rosenblatt, H. M., Byrne, W., Ament, M. E., et al. (1980): Successful treatment of chronic mucocutaneous candidiasis with ketoconazole. *J. Pediat., 97,* 657.
264. Schürmeyer, Th. and Nieschlag, E. (1982): Ketoconazole-induced drop in serum and saliva testosterone. *Lancet, 2,* 1098.
265. Strauss, J. S. (1982): Ketoconazole and the liver. *J. Amer. Acad. Derm., 6,* 546.
266. Tkach, J. R. and Rinaldi, M. G. (1982): Severe hepatitis associated with ketoconazole therapy for chronic mucocutaneous candidiasis. *Cutis, 29,* 482.
267. Van Ketel, W. G. (1983): An allergic reaction probably caused by ketoconazole. *Contact Dermatitis, 9,* 313.
268. Stern, R. S. (1982): Ketoconazole: Assessing its risks. *J. Amer. Acad. Derm., 6,* 544.
269. Levine, H. B. (1982): Resistance to ketoconazole (Letter to the Editor). *Lancet, 2,* 211.
270. Hume, A. L. and Kerkering, Th. M. (1983): Ketoconazole. *Drug Intell. Clin. Pharmacy, 17,* 169.
271. Meinhof, W. (1983): Ketoconazol – Wende in der antimykotischen Therapie? *Hautarzt, 34,* 155.
272. Horsburgh, C. R. Jr. and Kirkpatrick, C. H. (1983): Therapy of chronic muco-cutaneous candidiasis with ketoconazole: experience with twenty-one patients. *Amer. J. Med., 74, (Suppl.)* 23.
273. Stevens, D. A., Stiller, R. L., Williams, P. L. and Sugar, A. M. (1983): Experience with ketoconazole in three major manifestations of progressive coccidioidomycosis. *Amer. J. Med., 74, (Suppl.),* 58.
274. Graybill, J. R. (1983): Summary: potential and problems with ketoconazole. *Amer. J. Med., 74, (Suppl.),* 86.
275. Graybill, J. R., Lundberg, D. and Donavan, W. (1980): Treatment of coccidioidomycosis with ketoconazole: clinical and laboratory studies of 18 patients. *Rev. Infect. Dis., 2,* 661.
276. Restrepto, A., Stevens, D. A. and Gomez, I. (1980): Ketoconazole: a new drug for the treatment of paracoccidioidomycosis. *Rev. Infect. Dis., 2,* 633.
277. Brazzell, R. K. and Colburn, W. A. (1982): Pharmacokinetics of the retinoids isotretinoin and etretinate. *J. Amer. Acad. Derm., 6,* 643.
278. Crivellato, E. (1982): A rosacea-like eruption induced by Tigason (RO 10-9359) treatment. *Acta derm.-venereol. (Stockh.), 62,* 450.
279. Dicken, C. H. and Connolly, S. M. (1980): Eruptive xanthomas associated with isotretinoin. *Arch. Derm., 116,* 951.
280. Ellis, Ch. N., Swanson, N. A., Grekin, R. C. et al. (1982): Etretinate therapy causes increases in lipid levels in patients with psoriasis. *Arch. Derm., 118,* 559.
281. Ensink, B. W. and van Voorst Vader, P. C. (1983): Ophthalmological side-effects of 13-cis-retinoid therapy. (Letter to the Editor) *Brit. J. Derm., 108,* 627.
282. Foged, E. K. and Jacobsen, F. K. (1982): Side-effects due to RO 10-9359 (Tigason). *Dermatologica (Basel), 164,* 365.
283. Fontan, B., Bonafé, J. L. and Moatti, J.-P. (1983): Tolerance du rétinoïde aromatique (RO 10-9359, étrétinate). *Ann. Derm.-vénéréol. (Paris), 110,* 23.
284. Fredriksson, T. (1978): Oral treatment of psoriasis and pustulosis palmoplantaris with RO 10-9359. *Dermatologica (Basel), 157, (Suppl. 1),* 13.
285. Fulton, R. A., Souteyrand, P. and Thivolet, J. (1982): Influence of retinoid RO 10-9359 on cell-mediated immunity in vivo. *Dermatologica (Basel), 165,* 568.
286. Glazer, S. D., Roenigk, H. H. Jr., Yokoo, H. and Sparberg, M. (1982): A study of potential hepatotoxicity of etretinate used in the treatment of psoriasis. *J. Amer. Acad. Derm., 6,* 683.
287. Hazen, P. G., Carney, J. F., Walker, A. E. and Stewart, J. J. (1983): Depression - a side-effect of 13-*cis*-retinoic acid therapy (Letter to the Editor). *J. Amer. Acad. Derm., 9,* 278.
288. Jones, D. H., King, K., Miller, A. J. and Cunliffe, W. J. (1983): A dose-response study of 13-*cis*-retinoic acid in acne vulgaris. *Brit. J. Derm., 108,* 333.

289. Juhlin, L. (1983): Ear ache during etretinate treatment. *Acta derm.-venereol. (Stockh.)*, *63*, 181.
290. King, K., Jones, D. H., Daltrey, D. C. and Cunliffe, W. J. (1982): A double-blind study of the effects of 13-cis-retinoic acid on acne, sebum excretion rate and microbial population. *Brit. J. Derm.*, *107*, 583.
291. Korner, W. F. and Vollm, J. (1975): New aspects of the tolerance of retinol in humans. *Int. J. Vitam. Nutr. Res.*, *45*, 363.
292. Kramer, M. (1982): Excessive cerumen production due to the aromatic retinoid Tigason in a patient with Darier's disease. *Acta derm.-venereol. (Stockh.)*, *62*, 267.
293. Lauharanta, J. (1982): Oedema, a rare adverse reaction to etretinate (Tigason). *Brit. J. Derm.*, *106*, 251.
294. Lindskov, R. (1982): Soft nails after treatment with aromatic retinoids. *Arch. Derm.*, *118*, 535.
295. Lyons, F., Laker, M. F., Marsden, J. R. et al. (1982): Effect of oral 13-cis-retinoic acid on serum lipids. *Brit. J. Derm.*, *107*, 591.
296. McCormack, L. S. and Turner, M. L. C. (1983): Photosensitivity and isotretinoin therapy (Letter to the Editor). *J. Amer. Acad. Derm.*, *9*, 273.
297. Milson, J., Jones, D. H., King, K. and Cunliffe, W. J. (1982): Ophthalmological effects of 13-cis-retinoic acid therapy for acne vulgaris. *Brit. J. Derm.*, *107*, 491.
298. Milstone, L. M., McGuire, J. and Ablow, R. C. (1982): Premature epiphyseal closure in a child receiving oral 13-*cis*-retinoic acid. *J. Amer. Acad. Derm.*, *7*, 663.
299. Moulopoulou-Karakitsou, K., Mavrikakis, M. and Anastasiou-Nana, M. (1981): An unusual adverse reaction to RO 10-9359. *Brit. J. Derm.*, *104*, 709.
300. Orfanos, C. E., Mahrle, G., Goerz, G., et al. (1979): Laboratory investigations in patients with generalized psoriasis under oral retinoid treatment. *Dermatologica (Basel)*, *159*, 62.
301. Orfanos, C. E. and Bauer, R. (1983): Evidence for anti-inflammatory activities of oral synthetic retinoids: experimental findings and clinical experience. *Brit. J. Derm.*, *109*, *(Suppl. 25)*, 55.
302. Peck, G. L., Gross, E. G., Butkus, D. and DiGiovanna, J. J. (1982): Chemoprevention of basal cell carcinoma with isotretinoin. *J. Amer. Acad. Derm.*, *6*, 815.
303. Perry, M. D. and McEvoy, G. K. (1983): Isotretinoin: new therapy for severe acne. *Clin. Pharmacy*, *2*, 12.
304. Pittsley, R. A. and Yoder, F. W. (1983): Retinoid hyperostosis: Skeletal toxicity associated with long-term administration of 13-*cis*-retinoic acid for refractory ichthyosis. *New Engl. J. Med.*, *308*, 1012.
305. Pochi, P. E. (1982): Oral retinoids in dermatology. *Arch. Derm.*, *118*, 57.
306. Van der Rhee, H. J., Tijssen, J. G. P., Herrmann, W. A. et al. (1980): Combined treatment of psoriasis with a new aromatic retinoid (Tigason) in low dosage orally and triamcinolone acetonide cream topically: a double-blind study. *Br. J. Derm.*, *102*, 203.
307. Van Voorst Vader, P. C., Houthoff, H. J., Eggink, H. F. and Gips, C. H. (1983): Etretinate (Tigason) hepatitis in 2 patients. *Dermatologica (Basel)*, in press.
308. Stuttgen, G. (1975): Oral vitamin A acid therapy. *Acta derm.-venereol. (Stockh.)*, *55*, *(Suppl. 74)*, 174.
309. Thune, P. and Mörk, N. J. (1980): A case of centrilobular toxic necrosis of the liver due to aromatic retinoid - Tigason (RO 10-9359). *Dermatologica (Basel)*, *160*, 405.
310. Voorhees, J. J. and Orfanos, C. E. (1981): Oral retinoids. *Arch. Derm.*, *117*, 418.
311. Windhorst, D. B. and Nigra, Th. (1982): General clinical toxicology of oral retinoids. J. Amer. Acad. Derm., 6, 675.
312. Yoder, F. W. (1983): Isotretinoin: a word of caution. *J. Amer. med. Ass.*, *249*, 350.
313. Rumsfield, J. A., West, D. P., Ted Tse, C. S. et al (1983): Isotretinoin in severe recalcitrant cystic acne: a review. *Drug Intell. clin. Pham.*, *17*, 329.
314. Roche Laboratories (1982). *Accutane Package Insert*. Nutley, N. J.
315. Marsden, J. R., Shuster, S. and Laker, M. F. (1983): Isotretinoin and serum lipids (Letter to the Editor). *Lancet 1*, 134.
316. Meyskens, F. L. Jr. (1982): Short clinical reports. *J. Amer. Acad. Derm.*, *6*, 732.
317. Weiss, J., Degnan, M., Leupold, R. and Lumpkin, L. R. (1981): Bilateral corneal opacities. Occurrence in a patient treated with oral isotretinoin. *Arch. Derm.*, *117*, 182.
318. Moon, R. C. and McCormick, D. L. (1982): Inhibition of chemical carcinogenesis by retinoids. *J. Amer. Acad. Derm.*, *6*, 809.
319. Meyskens, F. L. Jr. (1982): Studies of retinoids in the prevention and treatment of cancer. *J. Amer. Acad. Derm.*, *6*, 824.
320. Shalita, A. R., Cunningham, W. J., Leyden, J. J. et al. (1983): Isotretinoin treatment of acne and related disorders: An update. *J. Amer. Acad. Derm.*, *9*, 629.

321. Katz, R. A., Jorgensen, H. and Nigra, T. P. (1983): Flare of cystic acne from oral isotretinoin (Letter to the Editor). *J. Amer. Acad. Derm., 8,* 132.

322. Beck, H. T. and Foged, E. K. (1983): Toxic hepatitis due to combination therapy with methotrexate and etretinate in psoriasis. *Dermatologica (Basel), 167,* 94.

323. Williamson, D. M. and Greenwood, R. (1983): Multiple pyogenic granulomata occurring during etretinate therapy (Letter to the Editor). *Brit. J. Derm., 109,* 615.

324. Schmoeckel, C. and von Liebe, V. (1983): Acneiform eruption due to azathioprine. *Hautarzt, 34,* 413.

325. Straughan, J. L. and Anderson, R. (1983): Erythromycin - three decades later. *S. Afr. med. J., 64,* 197.

20. Side effects of cosmetics: introduction

COSMETICS: WHAT THEY DO

20.1   Cosmetics are used by millions of consumers with one or more of the following intentions:
- for the daily care and hygiene of the body: soap, shampoo, toothpaste, moisturizing and cleansing cream
- to beautify: makeup, hair color, permanent wave
- to obtain a good and fresh smell: deodorant, perfume, aftershave, mouth freshener
- for protection: sunscreen, barrier cream.

RISK INCREASING FACTORS FOR ADVERSE SKIN REACTIONS

20.2   Cosmetics are used on the skin and may therefore initiate adverse skin reactions. The incidence of adverse reactions is influenced by the following factors:
- The intensity of skin contact. The intensity is low for rinse-off products like shampoos, and for this reason rinse-off products will not cause much trouble. The intensity and duration of skin contact for stay-on products is much greater. Examples are moisturizing and cleansing creams, deodorants and antiperspirants. These products indeed do cause more skin reactions (see § 20.17).
- The site of application. The area around the eyes in particular is more sensitive than other parts of the skin; eye make-up products can therefore be expected to cause a certain amount of adverse effects.
- The pH of the product. Highly alkaline products, such as depilatories and hair straightening agents, which have a pH of 12 or more, are high-risk cosmetics (see § 20.18). Because of this alkalinicity these products should not be used 'as such' for patch testing.
- High contents of volatile ingredients, such as water, ethanol, and aerosol propellants in stay-on products may be hidden risk-increasing factors for side effects. One should keep in mind that the concentration of an antimicrobial, for example, may increase 2–5 fold if and when the volatile ingredients evaporate. This might happen in poorly formulated skin creams (facial, hand, body creams), in deodorants and antiperspirants.

NATURE OF SIDE EFFECTS

20.3   Side effects from cosmetics are mainly skin reactions (irritation, allergy, phototoxicity, photoallergy), but other organs may also be involved. Some examples are:
- Eye irritation is often reported from shampoos or foam baths, when they accidentally come into the eyes. Some face or eye creams, when applied near the eyes, may be lacrimatory. This is caused by several lacrimatory volatile perfume

ingredients, such as benzyl acetate and benzyl alcohol; such compounds are extensively used for perfuming facial creams.
- Bubble baths may cause urinary tract irritation, especially in children.
- Respiratory complaints may result from the use of cosmetics, e.g. when aerosol hairsprays or aerosol deodorants are used in badly ventilated rooms.
- More difficult to assess, but extremely important are the *long-term toxic effects* of cosmetics: blood and organ damage, embryotoxicity and teratogenicity, estrogenicity, mutagenicity and carcinogenicity. Only prospective studies can provide adequate data to investigate such possibilities.

INCIDENCE OF SIDE EFFECTS

20.4 The actual incidence of side effects of cosmetics is difficult to assess because:
1. Only a minority of the cases is seen by a dermatologist, and relatively few cases are fully investigated. Most consumers reacting unfavorably to a particular cosmetic merely stop using it, without consulting their doctor.
2. Data on the incidence of adverse reactions to cosmetics provided by recent important reports differ considerably.

20.5 The results of the following studies may illustrate the latter problem:

I. **The FDA pilot study (Westat report)** among 10,000 US families.
With regard to this study it must be pointed out that the limited period (3 months) may have influenced the reliability of the results. In one month 290 untoward experiences were related to the use of 428,801 person-brand used cosmetics. This is an incidence of *680 experiences per million cosmetic units*.
If 15% of the experiences one considered to be 'severe' or 'moderate' (as was assessed in this report), the incidence of such reactions is *100 experiences per million cosmetic units*. An estimated 2.2% of the experiences were graded 'severe'. If only severe experiences are considered the incidence would be *15 experiences per million cosmetic units*.

II. **The US manufacturers' file** (1975).
The incidence of side effects is calculated from the following data: during a period of 18 months 8,399 experiences were reported, and 4.263 millions of cosmetic units were estimated to be distributed. The calculated incidence is *2 experiences per million cosmetic units*.

III. **The Dutch Government (or Enschede) file** (1979).
The Dutch Government Food Inspection Service in Enschede recorded 207 experiences in 1979. The estimated market volume for cosmetics in the Netherlands is 68.5 million units. (Only the value is known: 685 million guilders; the average value is estimated at 10 guilders per unit.) The incidence of side effects is then calculated to be *3 experiences per million cosmetic units*. The real figure however, probably lies between 5–10 severe experiences per million cosmetic units.

INCIDENCE OF SIDE EFFECTS FROM THE VARIOUS COSMETIC PRODUCT CATEGORIES

20.6 Eight studies on the incidence of cosmetic-related side effects will be briefly discussed. Though each of the studies has its own character and special aspects, they fortunately all have specified the different product categories for the reported

20.7   Cosmetic product categories

cases. This has permitted the composition of § 20.17 on the 'top six' of adverse reactions-causing cosmetic products, and § 20.18 on the 'risk index' of each individual category of cosmetic products.

US manufacturer's file – 1975 [1] (FDA's Voluntary Cosmetic Regulatory Program)

20.7   Under the FDA's Voluntary Cosmetic Regulatory Program more than 100 cosmetic firms have submitted 8399 product experiences in the 18 month period of January 1974 to June 1975, during which period 4263 million cosmetic units were estimated to have been distributed. FDA has tabulated for each product category the number of untoward experiences, the estimated number of units distributed and the number of experiences per million units distributed.

The 'Top-6' of adverse reactions-causing products in this study were (see § 20.17):

Hair color and bleach	17.4%	
Face care (moisturizing-cleansing cream)	13.5%	
Eye make-up	11.1%	of a total of 8399
Deodorant-antiperspirant	8.6%	
Face make-up	6.8%	
Hair conditioner	4.3%	

US hospitals' file - 1977 [2] (NEISS report)

20.8   Cosmetic-related injuries treated in US hospital emergency rooms were filed through the National Electronic Injury Surveillance System (NEISS). The results for the Federal Year 1977 were:

Total number of injuries: 1079; from misuse (ingestion, inhalation): 381; from normal use: 698.
Specification of the 698 injuries from normal use:

Contact dermatitis	47%	
Eye injury	45%	
Foreign body injury	21%	of a total of 698
Contusions, abrasions	16%	
Chemical burns	9%	

The 'Top-6' of adverse reactions-causing products were (see § 20.17):

Hair color and bleach	15%	
Face care (moisturizing-cleansing cream)	13.5%	
Feminine hygiene cosmetics	13.4%	of a total of 698
Eye make-up	12.4%	
Nail cosmetics	10.3%	
Soap	9.5%	

FDA-pilot study – 1974 [3] (Westat report)

20.9   The FDA-pilot study was a 3-month study among 10,000 US families (35,000 persons) that were recruited by Westat, Inc. all over the USA; they were instructed to report on cosmetic usage patterns and perceived injuries. These injuries were verified by project dermatologists concerning their relation to cosmetics, and the severity of the injury was assessed; furthermore, the patients were examined for signs of atopic conditions. The results were tabulated in product categories. A total of 589 adverse reactions were noted, which were graded as 'mild', 'moderate' or 'severe'.

505 (85.7%)   **Mild** (symptoms described were of minor irritant type; no loss of time from normal activities; symptoms would not require medication or a medical evaluation; symptoms were of fleeting nature).

63 (10.7%)   **Moderate** (symptoms considered to be rather annoying to the patient; could have caused loss of time from normal activities; subject may have sought advice from physician; symptoms persisted for prolonged period of time)

13 (2.2%)   **Severe** (symptoms may have been of systemic nature and were painful to the patient; would cause loss of time from normal activities; symptoms were of such a degree of severity that subject would have been well advised to seek medical evaluation; symptoms persisted for prolonged period of time)

8 (1.4%)   were not determined.

The 'Top-6 of adverse reactions-causing products in this study were (see § 20.17):

Deodorant-antiperspirant	30.9%	
Soap	12.6%	
Face care (moisturizing-cleansing cream)	9.0%	of a total of 589
Eye make-up	6.8%	
Hairspray, setting lotion	4.9%	
Bath foam and oil	4.2%	

Spanish study – 1983 [4]

20.10   Of 58,128 patients attending 2 dermatological clinics in Barcelona, Spain, 5539 (9.52%) were patch-tested. Of these, 460 (8.31%) were considered to have positive tests related to cosmetics; cosmetic allergy was suspected in less than half of the patients. Occupational sensitization to cosmetics accounted for approximately a quarter of the total (24.35%). Positive patch tests were noted in 210 cosmetic products.

The 'Top-6' of adverse reactions-causing products in this study were (see § 20.17):

Nail polish	24.1%	
Cologne	19.5%	
Cream	11.8%	of a total of 210
Make-up	10.8%	
Pre- and after-shave	5.6%	
Cleansing milk	5.1%	

Other cosmetics accounted for 5% or less.

Dutch Government file - 1979 (Food Inspection Service, Cosmetic Department, Enschede, The Netherlands)

20.11   The reporting system for cosmetic-related experiences in the Netherlands (14 million inhabitants) has been optimized since 1977 as a result of frequent contact between the Dutch Study Group of Occupational Dermatology, consumers' organizations, and organizations of beauticians and hairdressers. The Enschede Laboratory serves as a central point, and results are summarized in annual reports.

285

20.11   Cosmetic product categories

The annual number of cosmetic-related experiences and their sources for the period of 1978-1980 are as follows:

Year:	Total no. reports	Source		
		Dermatologists	Other physicians	Consumers, beauticians and others
1978	188	83	63	42
1979	202	113	76	13
1980	153	80	31	42

The 'Top-6' of adverse reactions-causing products in the year 1979 in this study were (see § 20.17):

Face care (moisturizing-cleansing cream)	16.7%	
Eye make-up	15.3%	
Hand and body lotion	11.3%	of a total of 202
Shampoo	9.8%	
Deodorant/antiperspirant	7.8%	
Face make-up	4.9%	

British Consumers' report – 1979 [5] (Consumers' Association)

20.12   The Association has interviewed 11,062 adults all over the UK, of which 1047 persons (12%) reported an adverse reaction related to cosmetics in the preceding 12 months. These persons were sent inquiries for details. From the answers received the incidence of experiences could be calculated for each product category.

The 'Top-6' of adverse reactions-causing products in this study were (see § 20.17):

Deodorant-antiperspirant	25%	
Eye make-up	14%	
Soap	12%	of a total of 626
Face care (moisturizing-cleansing cream)	7%	
Perfume	5%	
Aftershave	5%	

Strassburg study 1973–1980 [7]

20.13   In a 7-year-period, patch testing with cosmetic products showed 96 positive reactions in 91 patients (85 female, 6 male).

The 'Top-6' of adverse reactions causing products in this study were (see § 20.17):

Face care (moisturing and cleansing cream)	31.2%	
Nail polish	20.8%	
Eye and face make-up	10.4%	
Hair colors	10.4%	of a total of 96
Deodorants	8.3%	
Depilatories	5.2%	

NACDG 1977–1980 [6]

20.14 During the 40 months of this study, 11 dermatologists of the North American Contact Dermatitis Group (NACDG) identified 487 cases of cosmetic-related contact dermatitis. These represent 6% of the patients (8093) tested for contact dermatitis and approximately 0.3% of the total estimated number of patients seen by the participating dermatologists. In only about half of the cases did the patients or investigators suspect that the clinically examined cutaneous reaction may have been caused by a cosmetic. Sensitization to a cosmetic product was seen in 80% of all cases, irritation in 16%, whereas less than 2% of the reactions were caused by phototoxicity or photoallergy. 'Other' cutaneous reactions (not specified) accounted for 2% of cases.

Fragrances, preservatives, lanolin and lanolin derivatives, p-phenylenediamine, and propyleneglycol were the most commonly identified causative agents.

The 'Top-6' of adverse reactions-causing products in this study were:

Skin care products	26%	
Hair preparations (colors excluded)	16%	
Facial make-up products	12%	of a total of 499*
Nail preparations	8%	
Fragrance products	7%	
Personal cleanliness products	7%	

* Because some cutaneous reactions were caused by more than one product, the total of 499 exceeds the number of cosmetic-related cases.

'Top-6' adverse reactions-causing cosmetics

20.15 Cosmetics with untoward side effects mentioned most frequently in 7 of the preceding 8 reports are listed in § 20.17. The results of the NACDG are not included, as the product categories used by these investigators differ from those mentioned in § 20.17.

Risk grading

20.16 The data for the *incidence of side effects* are nor directly correlated to the actual risk of a product. Risk grading is only possible if the number of cosmetic units involved has also been counted or estimated in the reports. This is the case in two reports only. The results of risk grading are summarized in § 20.18.

The *risk index* is defined as the number of cosmetic units that caused one untoward cosmetic experience. Risk grading (high-, medium- and low-risk cosmetics) is based on these calculated risk indices. Some striking discrepancies are shown in § 20.18, for example:
– Eye make-up: high incidence of reports (Top-6), but only 'medium-risk' cosmetic
– Depilatory: low incidence of reports, but graded as 'high-risk' cosmetic.
– An example of a cosmetic product with a high incidence of untoward experiences and also a 'high-risk' product is a deodorant-antiperspirant.

Detailed risk indices for each product category are presented in the next chapter.

20.17   'Top-6' of adverse reactions-causing cosmetics

Cosmetic	Report						
	A	B	C	D	E	F	G
Hair							
Shampoo	–	–	–	–	●(10)	–	–
Hair conditioner	●(4)	–	–	–	–	–	–
Hair spray, setting lotion	–	–	●(5)	–	–	–	–
Permanent wave	–	–	–	–	–	–	–
Hair straigthener	–	–	–	–	–	–	–
Hair color, bleach	●(17)	●(15)	–	–	–	–	●(10)
Hair dressing, growth promotion	–	–	–	–	–	–	–
Face, mouth							
Face care, moisturizing and cleansing creams	●(14)	●(14)	●(9)	●(17)	●(17)	●(7)	●(31)
Face mask	–	–	–	–	–	–	–
Face: anti-acne	–	–	–	–	–	–	–
Face: skin bleach	–	–	⋅	–	–	–	–
Face: make-up	●(7)	–	–	●(11)	●(5)	–	●(10)
Eye make up	●(11)	●(2)	●(7)	–	●(15)	●(14)	●(10)
Lipstick	–	–	–	–	–	–	–
Toothpaste	–	–	–	–	–	–	–
Mouth freshener	–	–	–	–	–	–	–
Aftershave	–	–	–	●(6)	–	●(5)	–
Other shaving aids	–	–	–	–	–	–	–
Body – parts of the body							
Hand and body lotion	–	–	–	–	●(11)	–	–
Body talc	–	–	–	–	–	–	–
Deodorant-antiperspirant	●(9)	–	●(31)	●(5)	●(8)	●(25)	●(8)
Feminine hygiene cosmetics	–	●(13)	–	–	–	–	–
Soap	–	●(10)	●(13)	–	–	●(12)	–
Bath foams – oils	–	–	●(4)	–	–	–	–
Perfume, colognes	–	–	–	●(19)	–	●(5)	–
Sun cosmetics	–	–	–	–	–	–	–
Depilatories	–	–	–	–	–	–	●(5)
Nail cosmetics	–	●(10)	–	●(24)	–	–	●(21)
Foot cosmetics	–	–	–	–	–	–	–

A: US manufacturers' file   1975   (18 mths)   8399 experiences - FDA's Voluntary Cosmetic Regulatory Program
B: US hospitals' file   1977   (12 mths)   698 experiences - Neiss report
C: FDA pilot study   1974   (3 mths)   589 experiences - Westat report
D: Spanish study   1983   210 experiences - Barcelona Clinics
E: Dutch file   1979   (12 mths)   202 experiences - Enschede food Inspection Service
F: British Consumers' report   1979   (12 mths)   626 experiences - Consumers' Association
G: Strassburg Study   1973–1980   96 experiences

● Indicates this cosmetic to belong to the 'Top-6'.
( ) Indicates the % of the total number of experiences reported in each particular study.

20.18   Risk index of cosmetic products

Average risk index*	500,000 A	1500 B
Hair		
Shampoo	L	L
Hair conditioner	L	L
Hair spray, setting lotion	L	**H** (700)
Permanent wave	M	L
Hair straightener	**H** (87,000)	L
Hair color, bleach	M	**H** (800)
Hair dressing, growth promotion	L	L
Face, mouth		
Face, moisturizing-cleansing cream	M	**H** (800)
Face mask	M	–
Face: anti-acne	M	M
Face: skin bleach	**H** (55,000)	–
Face: make-up	M	M
Eye make-up	M	M
Lipstick	M	M
Toothpaste	L	L
Mouth freshener	L	L
Aftershave	L	L
Other shaving aids	L	L
Body – parts of the body		
Hand and body lotion	M	L
Body talc	L	M
Deodorant-antiperspirant	M	**H** (250)
Feminine hygiene cosmetics	M	M
Soap	L	M
Bath foam – Oil	M	H (800)
Perfume, cologne	L	M
Sun cosmetics	M	L
Depilatories	**H** (26,000)	**H**(250)
Nail cosmetics	L	M
Foot cosmetics	L	L

A: From US manufacturers' file - 1975 (18 month period: FDA's Voluntary Cosmetic Regulation
       Program)
       Risk grading:
       L(ow)   = more than 750,000 units per experience
       M(edium)   = 100,000–750,000 units per experience
       H(igh)   = less than 100,000 units per experience
B: From FDA pilot study (1974: Westat report) among 10,000 US families.
       Only for the month September.
       Risk grading:
       L(ow)   = more than 4000 units per experience
       M(edium)   = 1000-4000 units per experience
       H(igh)   = less than 1000 units per experience.

H ( ) indicates high-risk cosmetics, with the number of cosmetic units to cause one adverse reaction.

* Risk index = number of cosmetic units to cause one adverse reaction.

Product formulas

20.19   Cosmetics are complicated mixtures of chemical compounds. It has been estimated that there are more than 3000 cosmetic ingredients (Estrin 1977), and more
than 3000 perfume ingredients (Arctander 1960, 1969).

Though the rational approach of formulation is fairly logical and simple the
abundant availability of ingredients has created endless varieties in cosmetic formulations. An illustrative example is moisturizing cream (§ 20.20).

20.20   Moisturizing cream

Ingredient class:	Estimated number of available compounds
Lipid	500
Surfactant; emulsifier	1000
Polyol; humectant	20
Thickener	30
Moisturizing agent	50
Antioxidant	40
Preservative	150
Color	500
Perfume	3500
Total	5790

20.21   Nearly 6000 ingredients can be chosen to formulate a moisturizing cream (day or
night cream); hence it follows that patch testing with standard cosmetic batteries
is hardly sufficient in cases of suspected contact allergy to such cosmetics.

The ingredients of the formulas have to be tested separately. However, the
knowledge of a cosmetic formula is often hidden by trade secrecy. Until 1979 it
was very difficult to obtain the necessary information about formulas from the
manufacturers. The introduction of mandatory ingredients labelling in the USA
(since April 15th, 1977) has been a great improvement indeed (though these regu-
lations were actually enforced by consumers' demands).

The situation in the EEC countries is – up to the present date – less satisfying.
Formula information can only be obtained in cases of medical necessity according
to Article 7.3 of the *EEC-Cosmetic Directive* (document 76/768/EEC), which states that:

*'A member State may require for purposes of prompt and appropriate medical
treatment in the event of difficulties that adequate and sufficient information regarding substances contained in cosmetic products is made available to the compe-
tent authority, which shall ensure that this information is used only for the purpose
of such treatment.'*

However, with the introduction of mandatory ingredients labelling for cosmetics in the USA, another problem has arisen, namely the nomenclature of cosmetic
ingredients. Standardization work has been undertaken by the US Cosmetic Toiletry and Fragrance Association (CTFA), which resulted in the *'CTFA Cosmetic
Ingredients Dictionary'* (Editor: N. Estrin; 1st edition 1973, 2nd edition 1977, 3rd
edition 1982, CTFA Inc., Washington DC). Throughout this part of the book the
nomenclature of the 2nd edition of the CTFA Cosmetic Ingredients Dictionary
has been used. In some instances other references have been used:
– Colors (§ 27.9-27.11):
Color index numbers according to the *'Colour Index', 3rd edition*. Society of Dy-
ers and Colourists, Bradford, U.K. (1971).

- Perfume materials (§ 27.7):
  RIFM names (Research Institute of Fragrance Materials), as published by D. Opdyke in *Food and Cosmetic Toxicology, 11-18* (1973-1980).
- UV absorbers (§ 27.13):
  EEC Draft List for UV-absorbers (November 1980).
- Preservatives (§ 27.5):
  EEC Draft List for Preservatives (November 1980).

20.22   REFERENCES

1. *Tabulation of Cosmetic Product Experience Report,* submitted to the Food and Drug Administration under Voluntary Cosmetic Regulatory Program (Jan. 1974 – June 1975). Food & Drug Administration, Division of Cosmetic Technology, 200 'C' street SW, Washington DC 20204, USA.
2. *Cosmetic-related injuries: A MODS study of NEISS data, July 1th 1977 to June 30th 1978.* National Technical Information Service, US Department of Commerce, Springfield, VA 22161, USA.
3. *(PB-242 480) An investigation of Consumers' perception of adverse reactions to cosmetic products.* Westat Inc., Prepared for Food and Drug Administration, June 1975. National Technical Information Service US Department of Commerce, Springfield, VA 22161, USA.
4. Romaguera, C., Camarasa, J. M. G., Alomar, A. and Grimalt, F. (1983): Patch tests with allergens related to cosmetics. *Contact Dermatitis, 9,* 167.
5. *Reactions of the skin to cosmetic and toiletry products* (1979): Consumers' Association, 14 Buckingham Street, London WC2.

UPDATE–2nd Edition

6. Eiermann, H. J., Larsen, W., Maibach, H. I. and Taylor, J. S. (1982): Prospective study of cosmetic reactions: 1977-1980. *J. Amer. Acad. Derm., 6,* 909.
7. Ngangu, Z., Samsoen, M. and Foussereau, J. (1983): Einige Aspekte zur Kosmetika-Allergie in Straßburg. *Dermatosen Beruf Umw., 31,* 126.

21. Patch testing with cosmetic preparations

21.1   Ideally, when a cosmetic is suspected of having caused a contact allergic reaction, all ingredients should be tested separately, in a suitable patch testing vehicle and at an adequate concentration. Unfortunately, this procedure is rarely performed, as such an analysis to determine the actual cause of sensitivity poses several practical difficulties, all of which make the investigation very laborious:
1. Unlike in the United States, in many countries the cosmetic industry is not committed to declare the ingredients on cosmetic products labels. Most companies require an individual request to be written for each product, before providing ingredient information for their products (if at all!).
2. Patients often use several cosmetic preparations, and it is frequently impossible to decide which one of these has caused the adverse reaction.
3. Cosmetics are often composed of numerous ingredients.
4. Many, if not most of the cosmetic ingredients have no published documentation as to proper non-irritating patch test concentrations. Serial dilutions and control tests must then be performed.

21.2   For the above reasons, the cosmetic as such is usually used for patch testing. However, there are several pitfalls to this procedure:
1. False positive reactions may be noted, as many cosmetics act as weak irritants when tested under occlusion; such reactions are sometimes hard to distinguish from weak allergic reactions. Irritant reactions are frequently seen with testing of cosmetics that contain volatile chemicals (which may be irritants), such as hair lacquers, liquid mascaras, and nail lacquers. It is advisable to allow such cosmetics to dry on the skin, before they are covered with patch testers.
2. False negative reactions frequently occur, because the concentration of the sensitizer in the cosmetic may be too low to elicit a positive patch test reaction. This is seen especially in cases of contact allergy to preservatives and fragrance materials.
3. Patch testing under occlusion with undiluted cosmetics may (rarely) carry the risk of sensitizing the patient, as has been noted with hair dyes.

21.3   When patch testing with a cosmetic yields a weak positive reaction, the patch test should be repeated; weak irritant reactions are less likely to be reproducible than allergic ones.

Sometimes an open test may be helpful: the cosmetic is applied 2-3 times daily to the same area of one forearm for 2 days, and subsequently the reaction is recorded. Whereas a positive open test indicates the patch test reaction to be allergic in nature, a negative result does not exclude the possibility of a cosmetic allergy.

The patient should then be instructed to use the cosmetic as she/he would normally have done, and reappear for clinical examination. Nevertheless, confirmation of contact allergy by patch testing with the ingredients of the cosmetic separately is always advisable, if not mandatory. A. guideline to the testing of cosmetics is provided in § 21.4 (adapted from Cronin [6] and Fregert and Hjorth [10]).

21.4   **Patch testing with cosmetics**

antiperspirant	as is
cold wave	2% aqua
deodorant	as is
eye cream	as is
eyeliner	as is
eyeshadow	as is
face cream	as is
face powder	as is
feminine hygiene spray	as is
hair bleach	the ingredients separately
hair cream	as is
hair dye	10% aqua
hair lacquer	as is (should be allowed to dry before occlusion)
hair lotion	as is and 50% o.o./alc.
hair spray	as is
hand lotion	as is and 50% pet.
lipstick	as is
mascara	as is (liquid mascara should be allowed to dry before occlusion)
nail varnish	10% and 50% o.o./acet. (when tested pure, should be allowed to dry before occlusion)
perfume	as is (i.e. 10% in alc.)
rouge	as is
shaving preparations*	2% aqua (closed test), 5% aqua (open test)
shampoo*	2% aqua (closed test), 5% aqua (open test)
soap*	2% aqua (closed test), 5% aqua (open test)
sunscreen	as is
toilet water	as is (i.e. 1% perfume in alc.)
toothpaste*	2% aqua (closed test) 5% aqua (open test)

When photoallergy is suspected, photopatch tests are indicated.

* Patch tests with dilutions of shaving preparations, soap, shampoo and toothpaste are of doubtful value. The ingredients (especially preservatives and fragrance materials) should be tested separately.

21.5   Many ingredients of cosmetic preparations are also used in non-cosmetic topical preparations. Only those compounds that have caused side effects *as incorporated in cosmetic products* will be listed in this part of the book. An exception is made for plant products used for cosmetics; the side effects mentioned usually do not relate to the use of these compounds in cosmetics (with the exception of fragrances). For ingredients of cosmetics that have caused adverse reactions *in non-cosmetic topical preparations only*, the reader is referred to Chapter 4.

293

21.6   Literature for cosmetic formulation

21.6   Tabulation of relevant literature for cosmetic formulation

1. Alexander, P. (1966): Hand preparations. Part 1: Formulation of nail varnishes. *Manuf. Chem. and Aerosol News, June*, p. 37.
2. Arctander, S. (1960): *Perfume and Flavor Materials of Natural Origin: 300 materials.* S. Arctander, P.O. Box 114, Elizabeth NJ 07207, USA
3. Arctander, S. (1969): *Perfume and Flavor Chemicals, I and II: 3100 Chemicals.* S. Arctander, P.O. Box 114, Elizabeth NJ 07207, USA.
4. Balsam, M. S. and Sagarin E. (1972): *Cosmetics Science and Technology.* Wiley Interscience, New York.
5. *Cosmetics and Toiletries:* Documentary/Formulary issues: Sun products (*91*, March 1976); Shaving products (*91*, July 1976); Hair dyes (*91*, December 1976); Moisturizing and emolliency (*93*, March/April 1978); Hair treatment products (*94*, March/April 1979); Bath products (*94*, July 1979); Creams and Lotions (*95*, March/April 1980). Allured Publishing Corporation, Wheaton, ILL 60187, USA.
6. Cronin, E. (1980): Cosmetics. In: *Contact Dermatitis.* Churchill Livingstone, London.
7. De Navarre, M. G. (1975): *The Chemistry and Manufacture of Cosmetics, 2nd edition, Vols. I-IV.* Continental Press, Orlando, USA.
8. *EEC List for Permitted Colours* (EEC-cosmetic directive, 27 July 1976) and the EEC draft lists (November 1981) of permitted preservatives and UV-absorbers.
9. Estrin, N. CTFA (U.S. Cosmetics and Toiletries Fragrance Association) *Cosmetic Ingredients Dictionary.* 1st edition 1973; 2nd edition 1977. CTFA, Washington DC, USA.
10. Fregert, S. and Hjorth, N. (1979): The principal irritants and sensitizers. In: *Textbook of Dermatology*, 3rd Edition, pp. 443-484. Editors: A. Rook, D. S. Wilkinson and F. J. G. Ebling. Blackwell Scientific Publications, Oxford.
11. Isihara, M. (1975): The composition of hair preparations and their skin hazards. In: *Biology and Disease of the Hair*, p. 602-629. Editors: T. Kobori and W. Montagna. University Park Press, Tokyo, London.
12. Jellinek, J. S. (1970): *Formulation and Function of Cosmetics.* John Wiley & Sons, Inc., New York.
13. Nowak, G.A. (1975): *Die Kosmetischen Präparate*, 2nd edition. Ziolkowsky Verlag, Augsburg.
14. Opdyke, D. (1973-1981): RIFM monographs published in Food and Cosmetic Toxicology: (1973): *11*, p. 95, 477, 855, 1011; (1974): *12*, p. 385, 517, 703, 807; (1975): *13*, p. 91, 449, 545, 683; (1976): *14*, p. 307, 443, 601, 663; (1977): *15*, p. 611; (1978): *16*, p.637; (1979): *17*, p. 241, 357, 509, 695; (1980): *18*, p. 649; (1981): *19*, p. 97, 237.

22. Hair cosmetics

SHAMPOO AND ANTI-DANDRUFF SHAMPOO

22.1   A shampoo cleans the hair by removing dirt, excessive fat and scaling by means of surfactants. It should not clean too much and should leave sufficient natural sebum on the hair. The shampoo-washed hair must be well-manageable (in wet as well as in dry condition), easily set in style and not dull in appearance. When a shampoo accidentally comes into contact with the eye, the product should not sting.

A shampoo has a very short contact time with the skin of the scalp and is generally diluted several times with water; it is washed off thoroughly after use. Because of this, no serious side effects are to be expected. In general, most complaints relate to itching or stinging of the eyes after accidental contact with the shampoo.

22.2   A typical **shampoo** formula is:

Ingredients:		*Example*
50–70%	water	*water*
7–15%	anionic surfactant (principal)	*TEA lauryl sulfate*
3– 5%	foam builder	*lauramide DEA*
0.5– 1%	thickener	*sodium chloride*
ca 1%	additive for pearlescent appearance	*PEG-8 distearate*
ca 2%	conditioner	*quaternium-19*
ca 0.2%	preservatives	*formaldehyde*
ca 0.005%	color	*CI 19140*
ca 0.5%	perfume	*perfume*

22.3   **Anti-dandruff shampoos** are shampoos to which 1–2% active ingredients have been added. The following anti-dandruff agents are mentioned in the literature:

captan
coal tar
climbazol
piroctone olamine
pyrithione disulfide Mg-sulfate
salicylic acid

selenium sulfide (sold as drug)
sodium pyrithione
sulfur (colloidal)
undecylamide DEA/MEA
zinc pyrithione

Quaternary ammonium compounds (e.g. alkyldimethylbenzylammonium chloride) are sometimes used as anti-dandruff agents, but their efficacy is rather doubtful.

22.4   **Incidence of side effects: Shampoos** (see § 20.17)

		% of total	
US manufacturers' file:		2.6	(220/8399)
US hospitals' file:		5.2	(36/698)
FDA pilot study:		4.1	(24/589)*
Spanish study:		4.1	(8/210)**
Dutch file:		9.9	(20/202)***
British consumers' report:		3.0	(19/626)
Strassburg study:		0	(0/96)

*0 severe   **reactions to soap included
 4 moderate   ***mostly eye stinging and itching
20 mild

22.5   **Risk index: Shampoos** (see § 20.18)

Shampoos including anti-dandruff shampoos are graded as *low risk* cosmetics according to:
US manufacturers' file (at 1 experience per 788,000 estimated units distributed).
FDA pilot study (at 1 experience per 4,000 person-brand used cosmetics).

22.6   Patch testing with shampoos undiluted may cause mild irritant false positive reactions. They may be tested as 5% aqueous solutions (open test) or as 2% aqueous solutions (closed test). It is, however, possible that the resulting dilution of the offending agent in the shampoo causes a false negative patch test reaction. Patch tests with the separate ingredients, properly diluted, are therefore necessary.
Side effects of shampoo ingredients are listed in § 22.7 and § 22.8.

22.7   **Contact allergy to ingredients of shampoos**

Ingredient	Use	Patch test conc. & vehicle (§ 5.2)	Cross-reactions (§ 5.5)	Comment	Ref.
captan				*See under* chlormercapto-dicarboximide	
carbon tetrachloride	solvent for fat	10% o.o.		No controls tested	46
chlormercaptodi-carboximide (captan)	anti-dandruff agent	0.25% pet.		*Photoallergy* (§ 6.5) For patch testing, *see* § 27.5.5 *under* captan	19
cocobetaine	amphoteric detergent	2% aqua		cocamidopropyl betaine (Tegobetaine®)	61
formaldehyde	preservative	2% aqua		*See also* § 5.7, § 24.12, § 24.13 *and* § 25.53	6 49 1
miranols (imidazole derivatives)	amphoteric surfactants	1% aqua		Testing with miranols in 3% conc. may sensitize	56
perfume (?)		1% o.o.			44
selenium sulfide	anti-dandruff agent	2% aqua		Contact allergy not proven	18

(continued)

(continuation)

Ingredient	Use	Patch test conc. & vehicle (§ 5.2)	Cross-reactions (§ 5.5)	Comment	Ref.
sodium laureth sulfate	in dish-washing liquids and possibly also in shampoos (amphoteric surfactant)	1% aqua		Contained allergic reactions caused by an impurity, i.e. sultones	12 53
sodium lauryl ether sulfate	detergent	2% aqua			61
zinc pyrithione	anti-dandruff agent	1% aq. susp. 1–5% pet.	possibly piperazine, ethylene diamine and hydroxyzine	*See also* § 5.7 *and* § 22.8	38 59

22.8   Other adverse reactions to ingredients of shampoos

Ingredient	Use	Side effect	Comment	Ref.
cetrimonium bromide	hair conditioner	matting of the hair (bird's nest hair), irritant dermatitis	*See* § 5.7 *under* quaternary ammonium compounds	16
cinnamon oil (10% alc.)	fragrance	contact urticaria *See* § 7.5	Also present in toothpastes (§ 13.3)	45
ethyl alcohol in a beer-containing shampoo	fragrance enhancer	antabuse effect in a patient taking disulfiram for alcoholism	A similar reaction has been noted due to alcohol in tar gel (§ 16.31)	74
medicated shampoos		wash the color out of dyed hair		52
selenium sulfide	anti-dandruff agent	irritant dermatitis, reversible hair loss and oiliness of the scalp, systemic toxicity	*See* § 2.4 *See* § 12.1 *See* § 16.86	
shampoo ingredient, not specified	shampoo	contact urticaria	*See* § 7.7	74
sorbic acid	preservative	contact urticaria	*See* § 7.5	45
surfactant in shampoo		irritant dermatitis in subjects employed in shampoo manufacture; also in hairdressers		51 3
zinc pyrithione	anti-dandruff agent	postinflammatory hyper- and hypopigmentation; photosensitization and actinic reticuloid	*See* § 22.7	38 59

AFTER-SHAMPOO RINSES OR HAIR CONDITIONERS

22.9   Shampooed hair (in particular when slightly damaged by repeated coloring, bleaching or waving) is often in a bad condition. If such (wet) hair is treated with an after-shampoo rinse, significant improvement may be obtained: better luster and feel, good combability and ease of styling. It has been assumed that the presence of many negatively charged sites on the hair surface is the cause of the bad condition. The active after-shampoo ingredients are large positively charged (cationic) molecules that neutralize the anionic sites.

In several shampoos conditioning agents are formulated; in these cases the use of an after-shampoo rinse is not necessary. Such 'conditioning' shampoos must be formulated carefully, as incompatibility of the anionic principal surfactant and the cationic conditioner will result in inactivation of the conditioning properties.

22.10   The most important hair conditioning agents are:
– Quaternary ammonium compounds (see § 27.11.3)
– Amphoteric surfactants (see § 27.11.5)
– Amine oxides (see § 27.11)
– Hydrolyzed animal protein.

22.11   A typical formula of an **aftershampoo rinse** is:

Ingredients:		*Example:*
ca 93%	water	*water*
2–5%	hair conditioning agent	*stearalkoniumchloride*
		lauramine oxide
ca 2%	lipid	*cetyl alcohol*
		glyceryl stearate
ca 0.5%	thickener	*carbomer-934*
ca 0.2%	perfume	*perfume*
ca 0.05%	color	*CI 45170*

22.12   **Incidence of the side effects: After-shampoo rinses** (see § 20.17)

	% of total	
US manufacturers' file:	3.9	(328/8399)
US hospitals' file:	0	(0/698)
FDA pilot study:	0.3	(2/589)*
Spanish study:	1	(2/210)
Dutch file:	0	(0/202)
British consumers' report:	no data available	
Strassburg study:	0	(0/96)

*0 severe
 0 moderate
 2 mild

22.13   **Risk index: Aftershampoo rinses** (see § 20.18)

Aftershampoo rinses are graded as *low risk* cosmetics according to:
US manufacturers' file (at 1 experience per 794,000 estimated units distributed)
FDA pilot study (at 1 experience per more than 5000 person-brand used cosmetics)

HAIR COLORS

22.14   There are 5 types of hair colors, each with a specific composition and action mechanism. Therefore, when an adverse reaction from a hair color is suspected, it is important to find out which type of product is used by the patient.

22.15   **1. Hair restorers** are hair dressings which gradually (after several days) darken grey hair to a brownish-black color. The active ingredient is (ca 1%) lead acetate and colloidal sulfur or sodium thiosulfate, which forms black lead sulfide on the hair surface. For toxicological and/or regulatory reasons lead acetate had been replaced by bismuth citrate in some countries, but unfortunately this gives less satisfactory results.

22.16   A typical **hair restorer** formula is:

Ingredients:		Example:
0–10%	water	water
ca 10%	polyol	glycerol
70–80%	lipid	petrolatum, lanolin
0–1%	surfactant	ceteth-20
ca 2%	active ingredients	lead acetate, sulfur (colloidal)
ca 0.5%	perfume	perfume

22.17   **2. Vegetable hair dyes:** in particular henna, the powdered leaves of *Lawsonia alba*. The active ingredient is 2-hydroxy-1,4-naphthoquinone (lawson), which colors the hair in approximately one hour. It can be applied as an aqueous (hot water) paste of the dried leaves, but the long reaction is not very convenient. The color obtained is reddish. Other vegetable materials which can be used are indigo leaves, chamomile flowers, and powdered walnuts. Synthetic Lawson, which is commercially available, or other naphthoquinones may be added to enhance the coloring power. Henna extracts mixed with ordinary shampoo bases are also available.

22.18   **3. Temporary dyes** (washable after one shampooing) are particularly applied in *hair color setting lotions*.

22.19   **4. Semi-permanent dyes** (which will withstand 4-5 shampooings) are formulated in shampoo bases. Direct colors used are of small molecular size, which facilitates the penetration of the dye into the hair cortex. Some of these dye ingredients are also used in the *permanent* type (§ 22.22).

22.20   A typical formula of a **semi-permanent hair color shampoo is:**:

Ingredients:		Example:
70%	water	water
ca 10%	principle surfactant	sodium laureth sulfate
ca 1%	thickener	carbomer-914
ca 0.2%	preservatives	bromonitropropanediol
1–3%	semi-permanent hair colors	HC Blue 1, HC Red 3, 2-nitro-p-phenylenediamine

22.21 Hair colors

22.21   Examples of hair colors which are used as **semi-permanent hair colors** are (see also § 27.10):

Aminonitrophenols (several isomers)
Disperse Blue 1
Disperse Violet 4 and 8
HC Blue 1-2-3
HC Orange 1
HC Red 1-3-6
HC Yellow 2-3-4-5
Nitrophenylene diamines (several isomers)

22.22   **5. Oxidation hair colors** or **Permanent hair colors:** This is the most important type. It is easily applied and the colors will withstand more than 10 shampooings, because the color is formed within the hair cortex. Oxidation hair colors are easily recognized.

The two separate parts should be mixed just before use. One part is a mixture of the color intermediates and the other is a hydrogen peroxide solution or a peroxide powder in a shampoo or a viscous lotion base. The mixture should be immediately applied to the hair after mixing. Two different reactions occur in the mixture: the hydrogen peroxide bleaches the original hair melanin (the bleached hair permits better coloring), the other reaction is a comlex (new) color formation (for a part within the hair cortex by the hydrogen peroxide and the color intermediates). After 15 minutes, when sufficient new color has formed, the product is washed off.

22.23   A typical formula is:

Color shampoo of intermediates (Part I)

Ingredients:		*Example:*
ca 70%	water	*water*
ca 10%	surfactant	*TEA lauryl sulfat*
ca 1%	thickener	*carbomer-914*
0.5–4%	hair color (intermediates)	*toluene-2,5-diamine,*
		m-aminophenol,
		4-methoxy-m-phenylene diamine,
		resorcinol
ca 1%	antioxidant: stabilizer	*erythorbic acid, sodium sulfite*
ca 1%	ammonia	*ammonia*

Hydrogen peroxide lotion (Part II)

Ingredients:		*Example:*
ca 85%	water	*water*
ca 5%	lipid	*cetyl alcohol*
ca 2%	surfactant: nonionic	*ceteth-20*
3–5%	hydrogen peroxide	*hydrogen peroxide*
ca 1–2%	stabilizer and pH adjacent agent	*EDTA, phenacetine, potassium phosphate*

22.24   Examples of color intermediates (See § 27.11) are:

Aromatic diamines:
meta- and para-phenylene diamines (PPD & MPD)
meta- and para-toluene diamines (25TDA, 24TDA)
methoxyphenylene diamines (4MMPD & 5MPPD) = diaminoanisoles,
diaminophenols

Aminophenols:
ortho- meta- and para-aminophenol (OAP, MAP, PAP)

Nitro-compounds:
nitrophenylene diamines (2NPPD & 4NOPD)
aminonitrophenols (several isomers)
picramic acid

Polyphenols:
dihydroxybenzenes (3 isomers: resorcinol, pyrocatechine, hydroquinone)
trihydroxybenzenes (2 isomers: pyrogallol, phloroglucinol)
1-naphtol and 1,5-naphthalenediol.

22.25   **Incidence of side effects: Hair colors** (see § 20.17)

	% of total	
US manufacturers' file:	14.9	(1178/8399)
US hospitals' file:	0	(104/698)
FDA pilot study:	1.9	(11/589)*
Spanish study:	5.1	(10/210)
Dutch file:	4.0	(8/202)
British consumers' report:	2.0	(13/626)
Strassburg study:	10.4	(10/96)

*0 severe
 2 moderate
 9 mild

22.26   **Risk index: Hair colors** (see § 20.18)

Risk grading according to:
US manufacturers' file: *medium risk* (at 1 experience per 198,000 estimated units distributed)
FDA pilot study: *high risk* (at 1 experience per 800 (!) person-brand used cosmetics).

The allergenicity of hair dyed with p-phenylenediamine

22.27   Some investigations indicate that p-phenylenediamine-sensitive individuals can come in intimate contact with hairs or furs colored with this dye, without risking an allergic contact dermatitis. Once the p-phenylene diamine is oxidized, which happens very rapidly in the hair, the resultant p-benzoquinone-diamine that is formed is not allergenic [20].
          This statement however is only valid when the hair has been correctly dyed. Un-reacted not fully oxidized dye (because of inadequate mixing or rinsing after dye-

301

ing) may result in residues of unreacted p-phenylenediamine remaining in the hair [57,24] which are then capable of inducing contact-allergic reactions in sensitized individuals.

Tabulation of side effects to hair color ingredients

Side effects of ingredients of hair colors are tabulated in § 22.28 (contact allergy) and § 22.29 (other side effects).

22.28   Contact allergy to ingredients of hair colors

Ingredient	Patch test conc. & vehicle (§ 5.2)	Cross-reactions (§ 5.5)	Comment	Ref.
m-aminophenol	2% pet.	related compounds		4
p-aminophenol	2% pet.	related compounds	Ortho- and paraaminophenol patch-testing may sensitize	4 47
henna (dried leaves of *Lawsonia alba*, containing 2-hydroxy-1,4-naphthoquinone = lawson)	prick test with 1% aqua 10 mg henna powder in 100 ml aqua, ether and ethanol		Immediate-type reaction: sneezing, facial swelling, urticaria, asthma [68] Causes brown discoloration of the nails and skin (§ 10.1) Has caused systemic side effects (§ 16.35) *See also* § 5.39	13 68
lead acetate	1% aqua		The reported case may have been due to patch-test sensitization	64
2-nitro-p-phenylene-diamine	1–2% pet.			41
p-phenylenediamine	2% pet.		Has caused photosensitivity (§ 5.5); purpuric eruption (§ 12.1) Has caused systemic side effects (§ 16.35) *See also* § 22.29	29 14 42 57
N-phenyl-p-phenylene-diamine (p-amino-diphenylamine)	0.25–2% pet.	4-isopropylamino-diphenylamine and other related compounds, diphenylamine [60]		4 48
resorcinol	2% pet.		*See also* § 5.38 *and* § 22.65	4
toluene-2,4-diamine	1% pet	related compounds	*See* § 22.29	4
toluene-2,5-diamine	2% pet.	related compounds	*See* § 22.29	4 14 35

See for cross-sensitivity between para-dyes and certain antihistamines MacKie and MacKie [34].

22.29   **Other side effects of ingredients of hair colors**

Ingredient	Side effect	
4-amino-2-nitrophenol	mutagenic (?)	28
4-methoxy-m-phenylenediamine	mutagenic(?), carcinogenic(?)	28
4-nitro-o-phenylenediamine	mutagenic(?), carcinogenic(?)	28
2-nitro-p-phenylenediamine	mutagenic(?), carcinogenic(?)	28
m-phenylenediamine	mutagenic(?), carcinogenic (?)	28
p-phenylenediamine	systemic absorption with darkening of	37
	the urine	36
	vertigo, anemia, gastritis, exfoliative dermatitis and death	73
	chromosomal damage(?)	32
	mutagenic(?)	28
	aplastic anemia(?)	55
	immediate-type hypersensitivity with edema and difficulty in breathing	9
toluene-2,4-diamine	mutagenic(?), carcinogenic(?)	28
toluene-2,5-diamine	mutagenic(?)	28

Presently no definite evidence exists that hair dyes are carcinogenic in people using them.

Percutaneous penetration of hair dyes under usage conditions has been reported [72]: diaminoanisole (0.015%), p-phenylenediamine (0.14%) and HC Blue 1 (0.09%).

PERMANENT WAVE

22.30   Permanent waving of hair is performed nowadays without the application of heat (cold wave). For cold wave a dual solution is needed, the components of which are used separately and succesively:

1. An alkaline thioglycolate solution of pH 8-10 (*Waving fluid*)
2. An acid hydrogen peroxide solution (*Fixation* or *Neutralization Fluid*).

The hair is pretreated with an alkaline shampoo to make the hair surface more permeable to the waving fluid. The hair is then set in curls and wetted with the waving fluid. The alkaline reaction swells the hair to almost 150% of its original size, which promotes the action of the thioglycolate. Even the strong S–S bridges of the keratin filaments are broken. This treatment lasts for 10–20 minutes.

The thioglycolate solution is subsequently removed thoroughly with the aid of a towel, while the hair is still in curls. The second fluid is then applied to the hair. The acid reaction stops the action of residual thioglycolate, and the hydrogen peroxide restores the S–S bridges. As this happens in the curly state of the hair, the curl becomes permanent. The fixation takes about 15 minutes.

22.31   A typical formula for a **waving fluid** is:

Ingredients:		*Example:*
ca 90%	water	*water*
5–11%	thioglycolic acid	*thioglycolic acid*
ca 1%	cloudifier	*styrene/acrylate copolymer, laureth-20, carbomer-941*
ca 0.05%	color	*CI 45170*
ca 0.1%	perfume	*perfume*
	ammonia, sufficient for a pH of 8.5	*ammonia*

22.32 Permanent wave

22.32 The thioglycolate solution can also be applied as an aerosol foam. The following is a typical formula for an **aerosol waving fluid:**

Ingredients:		*Example:*
ca 80%	water	*water*
ca 5%	propellant	*butane, isobutane*
ca 10%	MEA-thioglycolate	*MEA-thioglycolate*
ca 5%	lipid	*dibutyl phthalate*
ca 1%	surfactant	*laureth-20*
ca 0.1%	perfume	*perfume*

22.33 A typical formula for the **fixation fluid** is:

Ingredients:		*Example:*
ca 95%	water	*water*
ca 4%	hydrogen peroxide	*hydrogen peroxide*
0.1%	stabilizer for hydrogen peroxide	*phenacetine*
ca 0.5%	citric acid	*citric acid*
ca 1%	cloudifier	*styrene/acrylate copolymer, laureth-20, Carbomer-941*
ca 0.05%	color	*CI 40850*

22.34 Allergic reactions to thioglycolic acid, its salts and to other ingredients of these preparations are rare. In most cases reactions are of an irritant nature and are caused by the alkaline character of the solution [5].

In case of a suspected allergic reaction, other cosmetic materials such as setting materials, coloring agents, perfumes etc. should be investigated as a possible cause.

22.35 **Incidence of side effects: permanent wave cosmetics** (see § 20.17)

	% of total	
US manufacturers' file:	1.7	(144/8399)
US hospitals' file:	5.2	(36/698)**
FDA pilot study:	0.5	(3/589)*
Spanish study:	0	(0/210)
Dutch file:	2.5	(5/202)
British consumers' report:	no data available	
Strassburg study:	0	(0/96)

*0 severe   **includes hair
 2 moderate   straightener
 1 mild

22.36 *Risk index:* **Ingredients of permanent wave cosmetics** (see § 20.18)
Risk grading according to:
US manufacturers' file: *Medium risk* (at 1 experience per 341.000 estimated units distributed)
FDA-pilot study: *low risk* (at 1 experience per more than 5000 person-brand used cosmetics)

Tabulation of side effects

Side effects of ingredients of permanent wave cosmetics are tabulated in § 22.65 (contact allergy) and § 22.66 (other side effects).

HAIRSPRAY AND HAIRSETTING LOTIONS

22.37   Styled hair can be kept in place by applying a film polymer around the hair filament. A few flushes of an aerosol hairspray is a very convenient and popular way to perform this operation. A pump spray, in which no propellant gases are used, does not give equally satisfactory results.

22.38   A typical formula for a **hairspray** is:

Ingredients:		*Example:*
2–4%	filmpolymer	*PVM/VA copolymer*
ca 0.5%	polymer neutralizer	*aminopropanediol (APD)*
0–0.1%	plasticizer (lipid)	*lanolin oil*
30–40%	solvent	*ethanol, methylene chloride*
ca 0.5%	perfume	*perfume*
40–70%	propellant	*chlorofluorocarbon 11 and 12*

One should be aware that the volatile propellants evaporate almost immediately; consequently, the concentration in which the ingredients reach the skin is much higher than indicated above.

22.39   A **setting lotion** is a non-aerolized solution of film polymers. It is applied to wet (but towel-dry) hair, before it is being set in style. A special type of a setting lotion is a *'föhn' lotion*, designed for use with an electric hair-dryer and which has basically the same composition, but contains more volatile solvents like ethanol.

22.40   An important modification of the setting lotion is the *'color setting lotion'*, which is a normal setting lotion with additional (direct) colors.

A typical formula for **hair color setting lotion** is:

Ingredients:		*Example:*
30–50%	water	*water*
30–50%	ethanol	*ethanol*
2–4%	film polymer	*quaternium-40, vinyl acetate/crotonates polymer*
0–0.5%	polymer neutralizer	*aminomethyl propanediol (AMPD)*
0–0.1%	plasticizer (lipid)	*dibutyl phthalate*
ca 0.5%	perfume	*perfume*
0–0.2%	preservative	*propyl paraben*
0.1%	colors	*CI 42595 (methylviolet), CI 42510 (basic violet 14)*

NB: Preservatives are necessary when the content of ethanol is lower than 30%.

22.41 **Incidence of side effects: Hairspray and setting lotions** (see § 20.17)

	% of total	
US manufacturers' file:	2.0	(167/8399)
US hospitals' file:	2.9	(20/698)
FDA pilot study:	4.9	(29/589)*
Spanish study:	0	(0/210)
Dutch file:	1.5	(3/202)
British consumers' report:	no data available	
Strassburg study:	3.1	(3/96)

*2 severe
3 moderate
22 mild
2 not recorded

22.42 **Risk index: Hairspray and setting lotions** (see § 20.18)

Risk grading according to:
US manufacturers' file: *low risk* (at 1 experience per 1,163,000 estimated units distributed)
FDA pilot study: *high risk* (at 1 experience per 700 person-brand used cosmetics)

Side effects

For side effects of ingredients of hair-spray and hair-setting lotions see § 22.65 and § 22.66.

HAIR BLEACH

22.43 There are two types of hair bleaches: one is based on the action of hydrogen peroxide or a 'per-salt', and the second is based on zinc formaldehyde sulfoxylate; the latter is used mainly to bleach artificially colored hair.

The type based on hydrogen peroxide is most frequently used. Home bleaches often contain multiple separated packages per unit, to assure stability of the hydrogen peroxide. The various components are mixed just before use, and this will result in an viscous paste which is easily applied to the hair. After 10-40 minutes, depending on the desired degree of bleaching, the paste is rinsed off thoroughly to avoid traces of the peroxide being left on the hair, which can cause brittleness.

22.44 A typical 3-parts **home bleach** is as follows (1 + 2 + 3 to be mixed just before use):

Cream with hydrogen peroxide (Part I):

ca 60%		*water*
ca 5%	lipid	*glyceryl stearate*
ca 2%	emulsifier	*PEG-100 stearate*
ca 0.5%	stabilizer	*phenacetine*
ca 0.1%	stabilizer	*ethylenediamine tetra-acetate*
ca 1%	acid agent	*phosphoric acid*
5–8%	bleaching agent	*hydrogen peroxide*

'Oily' liquid (so-called 'bleach base') (Part II):

ca 80%		*water*
ca 1%	foam builder	*oleamide DEA*
ca 2%	emulsifier	*nonoxynol-10*
5–10%	emulsifier	*ammonium oleate*
ca 1%	alkaline agent	*ammonia*
ca 0.01%		*color*

Powder, containing a 'booster', to increase bleaching power (Part III):

ca 20%	*sodium persulfate*
ca 75%	*magnesium carbonate*
ca 5%	*sodium lauryl sulfate*

Frequent bleaching with hydrogen peroxide will cause increased brittleness of the hair.

22.45   The second type of hair bleach, used to bleach artificially colored hair, contains 5–7% zinc formaldehydesulfoxylate (Rongalit®) which is a condensation product of two bleaching agents: formaldehyde and sodium sulfite.
    The Dutch file of 1975 mentioned a serious skin reaction after the use of such a bleaching agent.

22.46   **Incidence of side effects: Hair bleaches** (see § 20.17)

	% of total	
US manufacturers' file:	1.7	(141/8399)
US hospitals' file:	no data available	
FDA pilot study:	no data available	
Spanish study:	0	(0/210)
Dutch file:	0	(0/202)
British consumers' report:	no data available	
Strassburg study:	0	(0/96)

22.47   **Risk index: Hair bleaches** (see § 20.18)

Hair bleaches are graded as *medium-risk* cosmetics according to the following report:
US manufacturers' file (at 1 experience per 355,000 estimated units distributed.)

Tabulation of side effects

Side effects of ingredients of hair bleaches are tabulated in § 22.65 (contact allergy) and § 22.66 (other side effects).

HAIR DRESSING

22.48   The 'classic' hair care consists of a daily application of a hair dressing, which is mainly an oil as such, or an emulsion of an oil with water.

22.49 A typical formula for a **hair dressing** (non-aqueous type) is:

Ingredients:		*Example:*
ca 99%	lipid	*petrolatum, lanolin oil*
ca 1%	perfume	*perfume*
ca 0.01%	color	*CI 75810 (chlorophyllin-copper)*

22.50 A typical formula for a **hair dressing emulsion** is:

Ingredients:		*Example:*
ca 20%	water	*water*
ca 80%	lipid	*mineral oil, beeswax*
ca 2%	surfactant	*sodium borate* (reacts with beeswax to a soap emulsifier)
ca 0.5%	perfume	*perfume*

Anti-dandruff hair dressings are formulated by addition of approx. 0.1% of an anti-dandruff agent (e.g. zinc pyrithione).
Coloring hair dressings have been mentioned under *hair restorers* (§ 22.15).

22.51 **Incidence of side effects: Hair dressings – including hair growth promoters –** (see § 20.17)

	% of total	
US manufacturers' file:	0.6	(49/8399)
US hospitals' file:	1.6	(11/698)
FDA pilot study:	0.3	(2/589)*
Spanish study:	0	(0/210)
Dutch file:	1.0	(2/202)
British consumers' report:	no data available	
Strassburg study:	0	(0/96)

*0 severe
 0 moderate
 2 mild

22.52 **Risk index: Hair dressings - including hair growth promoters** (see § 20.18)

Hair dressings and hair growth promoters are graded as *low-risk* cosmetics according to the following reports:
US manufacturers' file (at 1 experience per 1,500,000 estimated units distributed).
FDA pilot study (at 1 experience per more than 5000 person-brand used cosmetics).

Tabulation of side effects

Side effects of ingredients of hair dressings are tabulated in § 22.65 and § 22.66.

HAIR STRAIGHTENER (HAIR RELAXER)

22.53   Straightening curly hair is performed in 3 consecutive steps: (1) the hair is wetted with the straightening fluid for approximately 15 minutes; (2) the hair is subsequently straightened by intermittent combing with a special comb for approximately 15–20 minutes, followed by (3) rinsing off with plenty of water, and neutralizing with neutralizing liquid for 3–5 minutes.
Usually, a dual solution is used:
1. The straightening fluid, based on one of the three following agents: sodium (potassium) hydroxide, sodium bisulfite or ammonium thioglycolate.
2. The neutralizing fluid, using special neutralizers for each type:
   For sodium hydroxide: a non-alkaline shampoo is sufficient.
   For sodium bisulfite: sodium bicarbonate.
   For ammonium thioglycolate: hydrogen peroxide.

   N.B. The thioglycolate solution is basically similar to the permanent wave fluid and neutralizer.

22.54   A typical formula for the **sodium hydroxide hair straightener** is:

Ingredients:		*Example:*
ca 65%	water	*water*
ca 2%	sodium hydroxyde	*sodium hydroxide*
25–30%	lipid	*cetyl alcohol, mineral oil, petrolatum*
ca 4%	surfactant	*sodium lauryl sulfate*

22.55   A typical formula for a **sulfite hair straightener** is:

Ingredients:		*Example:*
70–80%	water	*water*
ca. 8–9%	sodium bisulfite	*sodium bisulfite*
ca 25%	gelling agent	*poloxamer 407*

22.56   A typical formula for a **thioglycolate hair relaxer** is:

ca 95%	water	
6–8%	ammonium thioglycolate	

22.57   **Incidence of side effects: Hair straighteners** (see § 20.17)

	% of total	
US manufacturers' file:	3.0	(248/8399)
US hospitals' file:	no data available	
FDA pilot study:	0	(0/589)*
Spanish study:	0	(0/210)
Dutch file:	0	(0/202)
British consumers' report:	no data available	
Strassburg study:	0	(0/96)

22.58   **Risk index: Hair straighteners** (see § 20.18)

Risk grading according to:
US manufacturers' file: *high risk* (at 1 experience per 87,000 estimated units distributed)
FDA pilot study: *low risk* (at 1 experience per more than 5000 person-brand used cosmetics)

Tabulation of side effects

Side effects of hair straighteners are tabulated in § 22.65 and 22.66.

HAIR GROWTH PROMOTION

22.59   In spite of the lack of any scientific proof for remedies to cure baldness, to promote hair growth or to prevent hair loss, these products are still on the market. Many of the active ingredients are rubefacients, which promote blood circulation nearby the hair follicles.

22.60   The following 'active' ingredients are mentioned in an OTC-proposed monograph (*Fed. Reg., Vol. 45, No. 218,* November 7, 1980):

allantoin	lanolin
amino acids	lauric DEA
ammonium lauryl sulfate	olive oil
ascorbic acid	polyethylene glycol (PEG)
benzethonium chloride	polysorbate 80
benzoic acid	propylene glycol
dichlorophene	proteins
estradiol	tar
eucalyptus oil	tetracaine hydrochloride
hormones	vitamins
isopropylalcohol	wheat germ oil

22.61   Other 'active' ingredients mentioned in the literature are:

aloe	methyl salicylate
androgenic hormones	nicotinamide
benzyl nicotinate	nicotinic acid
cantharidine	panthenol
capsicum oleoresin	pilocarpine
cinchona extract	quinine
diethyl stilbestrol (DES)	resorcinol
estrogenic hormones	salicylic acid
methyl nicotinate	

22.62 A typical formula for a **hair tonic** is:

Ingredients:		*Example:*
ca 70%	water	*water*
ca 20%	solvent	*isopropanol*
ca 1–2%	active ingredients	*cantharidine, quinine tincture, panthenol*
0–0.02%	color	*CI 19140*
ca 0.1%	perfume	*perfume*

22.63 **Incidence of side effects** (§ 20.17): see *hair dressing*

22.64 **Risk index** (§ 20.18): hair growth promoters are graded a *low-risk* cosmetics (see *hair dressing*).

Side effects

Side effects of hair cosmetics (shampoos and colors excluded) are tabulated in § 22.65 (contact allergy) and § 22.66 (other side effects).

22.65 **Contact allergy to ingredients of hair preparations (shampoos and colors excluded)**

Ingredient	Cosmetic	Patch test conc. & vehicle (§5.2)	Cross-reactions (§5.5)	Comment	Ref.
ammonium persulfate (bleaching agent)	hair bleach	1–2.5% pet. 1% aqua		Contact allergy has caused sneezing and rhinitis in an Latopic individual For rashes amongst workers employed in the manufacture of persulfates *See* [62] *See also* § 22.66	21 58
ammonium thioglycolate (hair waving agent)	permanent wave	2% aqua		Has also caused irritant dermatitis. *See also* § 22.66	50 17
benzoin (resin)	hair lacquer	2–10% pet. 10% alc.		Also contact allergy to benzoin in rose water For cross-references, *see under* compound tincture of benzoin	66
colophony and maleic anhydride (resins)	hair lacquer	colophony 20% pet. maleic anhydride?			69 70
compound tincture of benzoin (fragrance)	permanent wave	2–10% pet./alc.		*See also* § 5.39, § 25.9, § 23.47 *and* § 26.3 *under* Styrax benzoin	25
dye	colored hair setting lotion	0.1% pet.		Dye possibly a 'polyamino anthraquinone'	40
fenticlor (antidandruff agent)	hair cream	1–10% pet.		Caused *photosensitivity* in the reported case *See also* § 6.5 *and* § 25.53	2

(continued)

311

22.65   Ingredients of hair preparations

(continuation)

Ingredient	Cosmetic	Patch test conc. & vehicle (§5.2)	Cross-reactions (§5.5)	Comment	Ref.
hinokitiol (β-thujaplicin) (hair growth stimulator)	hair liquid	0.1% alc.		Mainly used in Japan	63
Ineral®* (formaldehyde cyanoguanide and polyvinyl pyrrolidine solution) (hair film polymer)	hair strengthener	10% aqua/pet.		Has caused irritant dermatitis; nail dystrophy with onycholysis (§ 22.66)	7 33 30 31
maleic anhydride				*See under* colophony	
petrolatum (highly refined) (hair dressing)	hair tonic	7% in alc. 30%		No controls tested The patient did *not* react to crude liquid petrolatum Contact allergy not proven *See also* § 5.22	39
pyridoxine 3,4-dioctanoate (antiseborrheic drug)	hair liquid	1% pet.	pyridoxine hydrochloride		63
resorcinol (hair growth promoter)	hair tonic	5% alc. (?)	hexylresorcinol	Contact allergy not proven *See also* § 5.38 *and* § 22.28	54
sulfonated castor oil (hair dressing)	hair conditioner spray	pure?		Repeated insult patch tests were positive in 10% of normal volunteers	65
thioglycerol (depilatory)	depilating cream	1-2.5% pet.			23
thioglycerol (1,2-dithioglycerol) (hair waving agent)	permanent wave	10% aqua	BAL	Has also caused irritant dermatitis	17 8
thioxolone	'hair product'	1 and 2% pet.		Also used in anti-acne products (§ 5.38)	11

* The product 'Ineral' has been reformulated: the active ingredient in current use is dihydroxymethyl-1,3-thione-2-imid-azolidine (DHMTI) (See *EEC Cosmetic Directive 1976* in Annex IV, No. 26): this product polymerizes spontaneously in acid medium when applied to the hair or nails.

22.66   Other side effects of hair preparations (shampoos and colors excluded)

Ingredient	Cosmetic	Side effect	Ref.
aerosol propellants (fluoroalkane gases)	hair spray	cardiac arrhythmias 'sudden sniffing death'	43
ammonium persulfate	hair bleach	immediate-type hypersensitivity: – contact urticaria – headache and drowsiness – respiratory symptoms	21 10
ammonium thioglycolate	permanent wave	respiratory symptoms due to immediate-type allergy	26
estrogens	hair tonic/cream	systemic side effects *See* § 16.87	

(continued)

(continuation)

Ingredient	Cosmetic	Side effect	Ref.
ethanol	hair spray	bronchoconstriction *See also under* perfume	71
ethylene diamine	hair spray	respiratory symptoms due to immediate-type allergy	26
fixation fluid for permanent wave		contact urticaria; causative ingredient not specified *See* § 7.6	
hair bleach		contact urticaria; causative ingredient not specified. *See* § 7.6. *See also under* ammonium persulfate	
hair spray		contact urticaria: causative ingredient not specified *See* § 7.6	
hexamethylene tetramine	hair spray	respiratory symptoms due to immediate-type allergy	26
Ineral® (see § 22.65)	hair strengthener	irritant deermatitis, (reversible) nail dystrophy with onycholysis	31 33 7
monoethanolamine	hairsetting lotion	respiratory symptoms due to immediate-type allergy	26
perfume (?)	hair spray	alteration of pulmonary function in persons with preexisting disease such as asthma [67] and healthy individuals [71]	67 71
permanent wave fluid		contact urticaria; causative ingredient not specified *See* § 7.6	
phenolic derivatives	hair tonic	pigmentation of palms, temples and hair margins	22
polyvinylpyrrolidine (PVP)	hair setting preparation	thesaurosis in the lung	27
thioglycolate solution	permanent wave	nickel release from nickel-plated clips due to the alkalinicity of the solution	15

22.67   REFERENCES

1. Ancona-Alayon, A., Jiminez-Castilla, J. L., Gomez-Alvarez, E. M. (1976): Dermatitis from epoxy resin and formaldehyde in shampoo packers, *Contact Dermatitis, 2,* 356.
2. Beer, W. E. (1970): Sensitivity to fentichlor. *Contact Dermatitis Newsl., 8,* 188.
3. Black, M. M. and Russell, B. F. (1973): Shampoo dermatitis in apprentice hairdressers. *J. Soc. Occ. Med., 23,* 120.
4. Borelli, S. (1958): Die Verträglichkeit gebräuchlicher Haarfärbungspräparate, Farbstoffgrundsubstanzen und verwandter chemischer Verbindungen. *Hautarzt, 9,* 19.
5. Borelli, S. and Manok, M. (1961): Ergebnisse von Untersuchungen bei Berufsanfängern im Friseurgewerbe. *Berufsdermatosen, 9,* 271.
6. Bork, K., Heise, D. and Rosinus, A. (1979): Formaldehyd in Haarshampoos. *Beruf u. Umwelt, 27,* 10.

7.   Bourgeois-Spinasse, J. and Grupper, M. Ch. (1971): Insuffisance des tests prophétiques, nouvelles méthodes d'investigation allergique. *Bull. Soc. franç. Derm. Syph., 78*, 571.
8.   Burckhardt, W. (1953): Coiffeurekzem verursacht durch ein neues Kaltdauerwellenwasser. *Dermatologica (Basel), 107*, 253.
9.   Calnan, C. D. (1967): Hair dye reaction. *Contact Dermatitis Newsl., 1*, 16.
10. Calnan, C. D. and Shuster, S. (1963): Reactions to ammonium persulphate. *Arch. Derm, 88*, 812.
11. Camarasa, J. G. (1981): Contact dermatitis to thioxolone. *Contact Dermatitis, 7*, 213.
12. Conner, D. S., Ritz, H. L., Ampulsti, R. S., Kowollik, H. G., Lim, P., Thomas, D. W. and Parkhurst, R. (1975): Identification of sultones as the sensitizers in alkylethoxysulfate. *Fette, Seifen, Anstrichm., 72*, 25.
13. Cronin, E. (1979): Immediate-type hypersensitivity to henna. *Contact Dematitis, 5*, 198.
14. Cronin, E. (1980): Cosmetics. In: *Contact Dermatitis*, pp. 93-170. Churchill Livingstone, Edinburgh.
15. Dahlquist, I., Fregert, S. and Grauberger, B. (1979): Release of nickel from plated utensils in permanent wave liquids. *Contact Dermatitis, 5*, 52.
16. Dawber, R. P. R. and Calnan, C. D. (1976): Bird's nest hair. Matting of scalp hair due to shampooing. *J. Clin. exp. Derm., 1*, 155.
17. Downing, J. G. (1951): Dangers involved in dyes, cosmetics and permanent wave solutions applied to hair and scalp. *Arch. Derm. 63*, 561.
18. Eisenberg, B. C. (1955): Contact dermatitis from selenium sulfide shampoo. *Arch. Derm., 72*, 71.
19. Epstein, S. (1968): Photoallergic contact dermatitis; report of a case due to Dangard. *Cutis (N.Y.), 4*, 856.
20. Fisher, A. A. (1975): Is hair dyed with PPD allergenic? *Contact Dermatitis, 1*, 266.
21. Fisher, A. A. and Dooms-Goossens, A. (1976): Persulphate hair bleach reactions. *Arch. Derm., 112*, 1407.
22. Forman, L. (1975): Pigmentation of the palms and scalp probably due to proprietary hair tonics containing various phenols and phenolic derivatives. *Brit. J. Derm., 93*, 718.
23. Foussereau, J. and Benezra, Cl. (1970): *Les Eczémas Allergiques Professionels*, p. 385. Masson et Cie, Paris.
24. Foussereau, J., Reuter, G. and Petitjean, J. (1980): Is hair dyed with PPD-like dyes allergenic? *Contact Dermatitis, 6*, 143.
25. Garnier, G. (1955): Dermatitis bullosa due to wave set containing tincture of benzoin. *Bull. Soc. franç. derm. Syph., 57*, 397.
26. Gelfand, H. H. (1963): Respiratory allergy due to chemical compounds encountered in the rubber, lacquer, shellac and beauty culture industries. *J. Allergy, 34*, 374.
27. Gowdy, J. M. and Wagstoff, M. J. (1972): Pulmonary infiltration due to aerosol thesaurosis. *Arch. environm. Hlth., 25*, 101.
28. Hanlon, J. (1978): Tint of suspicion. *New Scientist, May 11*, 352.
29. Hindson, C. (1975): o-Nitro-paraphenylenediamine in hair dye - an unusual dental hazard. *Contact Dermatitis, 1*, 333.
30. Hjorth, N. (1973): Occupational dermatitis from Ineral (new formula). *Contact Dermatitis Newsl. 13*, 385.
31. Hjorth, N. and Niordson, A. M. (1972): Occupational dermatitis with onycholysis in hairdressers. *Contact Dermatitis Newsl., 11*, 254.
32. Kirkland, D. J., Lawler, S. D. and Venitt, S. (1978): Chromosomal damage and hair dyes. *Lancet, 2*, 124.
33. Lépine, M. J. and Fachot, M. L. (1971): Dermatite allergique des mains des coiffeurs par un nouveau produit capillaire: l'Ineral. *Bull. Derm. Syph., 78*, 150.
34. MacKie, B. S. and MacKie, L. E. (1964): Cross-sensitisation in dermatitis due to hair dyes. *Aust. J. Derm., 7*, 189.
35. Magnusson, B. (1974): The allergenicity of paraphenylenediamine versus that of paratoluenediamine. *Contact Dermatitis Newsl., 15*, 432.
36. Maibach, H. I., Leaffer, M. A. and Skinner, W. A. (1975): Percutaneous penetration following use of hair dyes. *Arch. Derm., 111*, 1444.
37. Marshall, S. and Palmer, W. S. (1973): Dark urine after hair colouring. *J. Amer. med. Ass., 226*, 1010.
38. Muston, H. L., Messenger, A. G. and Byrne, J. P. H. (1979): Contact dermatitis from zinc pyrithione, an anti-dandruff agent. *Contact Dermatitis, 5*, 276.
39. Niles, H. D. (1941): Dermatitis of hands caused by liquid petrolatum in a proprietary hair tonic. *Arch. Derm. Syph., 43*, 689.
40. Osmundsen, P. E. (1975): Contact dermatitis from a hair dye. *Contact Dermatitis, 1*, 186.

41. Pasricha, J. S., Gupta, R. and Panjwani, S. (1980): Contact dermatitis to Henna (Lawsonia). *Contact Dermatitis, 6,* 288.

42. Rajka, G. and Blohm, S. G. (1970): The allergenicity of paraphenylenediamine. *Acta derm.-venereol. (Stockh.), 50,* 51.

43. Reinhardt, C. F., Azar, A., Maxfield, E., Smith, P. E. and Mullin, L. S. (1971): Cardiac arrhythmias and aerosol sniffing. *Arch. environm. Hlth, 22,* 265.

44. Ridley, C. M. (1978): Perfume in shampoo dermatitis. *Contact Dermatitis, 4,* 170.

45. Rietschel, R. L. (1978): Contact urticaria from synthetic cassia oil and sorbic acid limited to the face. *Contact Dermatitis, 4,* 347.

46. Romaguera, C. and Grimalt, F. (1980): Sensitization to benzoyl peroxide, retinoic acid and carbonte-trachloride. *Contact Dermatitis, 6,* 442.

47. Rudzki, E., Napriórkowska, T. and Grzywa, Z. (1980): Active sensitization to ortho- and para-aminophenol with negative patch test to meta-aminophenol. *Contact Dermatitis, 6,* 501.

48. Schønning, L. and Hjorth, N. (1969): Cross sensitisation between hair dyes and rubber chemicals. *Berufsdermatosen, 17,* 100.

49. Schorr, W. F. (1971): Formaldehyde in shampoos and toiletries. *Contact Dermatitis Newsl. 9,* 220.

50. Schulz, K. H. (1961): Durch Thioglykolsäurederivate ausgelöste Kontaktekzeme im Friseurberuf. *Berufsdermatosen, 9,* 244.

51. Sheffrin, S. (1974): Shampoo dermatitis. *J. Soc. Occ. Med., 24,* 31.

52. Spoor, H. J. (1977): Shampoos and hair dyes. *Cutis, 20,* 189.

53. Sylvest, B., Hjorth, N. and Magnusson, B. (1975): Laurylether sulphate dermatitis in Denmark. *Contact Dermatitis, 1,* 359.

54. Templeton, H. J. (1940): Cheilitis and dermatitis from resorcinol and a derivative. *Arch. Derm. Syph., 42,* 138.

55. Toghill, P. J. and Wilcox, R. G. (1976): Aplastic anaemia and hair dye. *Brit. med. J., 4,* 502.

56. Verbov, J. L. (1969): Contact dermatitis from Miranols. *Trans. St. John's Hosp. derm. Soc. (Lond.), 55,* 192.

57. Warin, A. P. (1976): Contact dermatitis to partner's hair dye. *Clin. exp. Derm. 1,* 283.

58. Widström, L. (1977): Allergic reactions to ammonium persulphate in hair bleach. *Contact Dermatitis, 3,* 343.

59. Yates, V. M. and Finn, O. A. (1980): Contactallergic sensitivity to zinc pyrithione followed by the photosensitivity dermatitis and actinic reticuloid. *Contact Dermatitis, 6,* 349.

60. Calnan, C. D. (1978): Diphenylamine. *Contact Dermatitis, 4,* 301.

UPDATE – 2nd Edition

61. Van Haute, N. and Dooms-Goossens, A. (1983): Shampoo dermatitis due to cocobetaine and sodium lauryl ether sulphate. *Contact Dermatitis, 9,* 169.

62. White, I. R., Catchpole, H. E. and Rycroft, R. J. G. (1982): Rashes amongst persulphate workers. *Contact Dermatitis, 8,* 168.

63. Fujita, M. and Aoki, T. (1983): Allergic contact dermatitis to pyridoxine ester and hinokitiol. *Contact Dermatitis, 9,* 61.

64. Edwards, E. K. Jr. and Edwards, E. K. (1982): Allergic contact dermatitis to lead acetate in a hair dye. *Cutis, 30,* 629.

65. Fisher, L. B. and Berman, B. (1982): Contact allergy to sulfonated castor oil. *Contact Dermatitis, 8,* 339.

66. Garnier, M. G. (1950): Dermite bulleuse par un fixateur d'ondulations. *Bull. Soc. franc. Derm. Syph., 57,* 397.

67. Schleuter, D. P., Soto, R. J., Baretta, E. D. et al. (1979): Airway response to hair spray in normal subjects and subjects with hyperreactive airways. *Chest, 75,* 544.

68. Starr, J. C., Yunginger, J. and Brahser, G. W. (1982): Immediate type I asthmatic response to henna following occupational exposure in hairdressers. *Ann. Allergy, 48,* 98.

69. Schwartz, L. (1943): An outbreak of dermatitis from hair lacquer. *Publ. Hlth Rep., 58,* 1623.

70. Ginsburg, L. and Ellis, F. A. (1944): Hair lacquer pad dermatitis. *Arch. Derm. Syph., 49,* 198.

71. Zuskin, E., Bouhuys, A. and Beck, G. (1978): Hair sprays and lung function (Letter). *Lancet, 2,* 1203.

72. Maibach, H. I. and Wolfram, L. J. (1981): Percutaneous penetration of hair dyes. *J. Soc. cosmet. Chem., 32,* 223.

73. D'Arcy, P. F. (1982): Fatalities with the use of a henna dye. *Pharm. Int., 3,* 217.

74. Stoll, D. and King, L. E. Jr. (1980): Disulfiram-alcohol skin reaction to beer-containing shampoo (Letter). *J. Amer. med. Ass., 244,* 2045.

23. Face cosmetics

FACE CREAM (MOISTURIZING CREAM)

23.1 For facial care creams, lotions and milks are used, which are sold under various names: cold cream, emollient cream, day cream, night cream, moisturizing cream, vanishing cream, etc. They all have the same basic formulation of emulsions, and they will therefore all be considered here as moisturizing cream/milk.

23.2 A typical basic formula for a **moisturizing cream/milk/lotion** is as follows:

Ingredients:		Example:
20–90%	water	water
1– 5%	polyol	sorbitol
10–80%	lipid	stearic acid, cetearyl alcohol, squalane
2– 5%	surfactant	polysorbate 40, TEA-oleate
0– 5%	special moisturizer	polyamino-sugar condensate
ca 0.3%	preservative	methyl and propyl paraben, DMDM-hydantoin
ca 0.2%	perfume	perfume

23.3 As many possibilities exist for the choice of the functional ingredients, endless variations can be made (see § 20.20).

For all these emulsions the water/lipid ratio determines the result. Ratios of 7–9 make fluid products (milks/lotions). Most oil-in-water creams have ratios of 1–2: they are the most popular types. The 'oily' water-in-oil creams have ratios of 0.5–1.

For many (often expensive) moisturizing creams a large variety of 'special moisturizers' is commercially available (see § 23.4).

23.4 **'Moisturizers' in face creams (moisturizing creams)**

Name	Synonym (®)
– animal protein derivative	Hydropro 220, Polypeptide AAS, Crotein ACS
– collagen	
– elastin	
– estradiol (hormone)	
– estrogen (hormone)	
– estron (hormone)	

(continued)

(continuation)

	Synonym (®)
– ethisteron (hormone)	
– hydrolyzed animal protein	Peptein 2000, Lexein X250, Crotein SPA, Crotein SPO, Albanil, Polypeptide 10-12-40, Chempro 41CG, Lanasan CL, Nutrilan H and L, Protein WSP X250 and WSP X1000
– hydrolyzed milk protein	Edamin S, Hy case SF
– mixture of glycerin, sodium lactate, TEA lactate, serine, lactic acid, urea, sorbitol, lauryl diethylene diaminoglycine, lauryl aminopropylglycine, allantoin	Hydroviton
– mixture of hexylene glycol, glucose, fructose, sucrose, urea, dextrin, alanine, glutamic acid, aspartic acid	Hygroplex HHG
– mixture of urea, collagen, sodium lactate, sodium PCA	Lactil
– orotic acid (uracil-4-carboxylic acid)	
– placental extract (human or animal)	
– polyamino-sugar condensate	Aqualizer EJ (to be tested 10% aqua; CIR, 1981)
– pregnenolone acetate	
– royal jelly	
– sodium lactate (including lactic acid and sarcolactic acid)	
– sodium polyhydroxycarboxylate	Hydagen
– sodium pyrrolidone carboxylic acid (sodium PCA)	Ajidew (to be tested 30% aqua acc. to Ajinomoto Inc.)
– triethanolamine pyrrolidone carboxylate (TEA-PCA)	
– urea	

23.5   Incidence of side effects: Moisturizing creams (see § 20.17)

	% of total	
US manufacturers' file:	12.3	(1029/8399)
US hospitals' file:	3.2	(22/698)
FDA pilot study:	5.6	(33/589)*
Spanish study:	11.8	(23/210)
Dutch file:	16.8	(34/202)
British consumers' report:	7.0	(44/626)
Strassburg study:	31.3	(30/96)**

*2 severe   ** including 'milks'
 5 moderate
24 mild
 2 not determined

317

23.6 Moisturizing creams

23.6   **Risk index: Moisturizing creams** (see § 20.18)
Risk grading according to:
US manufacturers' file: *medium risk* (at 1 experience per 221,000 estimated units distributed).
FDA pilot study: *high risk* (at 1 experience per 800 (!) person-brand used cosmetics).

Tabulation of side effects

Side effects of ingredients of moisturizing creams are tabulated in § 23.47.

CLEANSING LOTION

23.7   Cleansing milks/lotions are used to aid cleansing the face with a tissue, in order to remove excessive fat, make-up residues and dirt. The cleansing agents in these products are always oils and surfactants. The formulas of cleansing lotion and moisturizing cream bases are the same.

23.8   The following is a typical formula for **cleansing milk (emulsion type):**

Ingredients:		*Example:*
60–80%	water	*water*
ca 2%	polyol	*propylene glycol*
20–30%	lipid	*mineral oil, isopropyl myristate*
2– 8%	surfactants	*sodium lauryl sulfate*
ca 0.3%	preservative	*bromonitropropanediol*
ca 0.2%	perfume	*perfume*

Almond meal and pumice may also be incorporated as extra cleansing aids.

23.9   The concentration of surfactants in cleansing products may be high. Cleansing milk should not be patch-tested undiluted. A 5–10 fold dilution with water is necessary to avoid irritant reactions.

23.10   **Incidence of side effects: Cleansing lotion** (see § 20.17)

	% of total	
US manufacturers' file:	3.2	(267/8399)
US hospitals' file:	no data available	
FDA pilot study:	3.4	(20/589)*
Spanish study:	5.1	(10/210)
Dutch file:	2.0	(2/202)
British consumers' report:	no data available	
Strassburg study:	31.3	(30/96)**

*0 severe   ** including creams
 2 moderate
18 mild

23.11   **Risk index: Cleansing lotion** (see § 20.18)

Risk grading-according to:

US manufacturers' file: *medium risk* (at 1 experience per 200,000 estimated units distributed)
FDA pilot study: *low risk* (at 1 experience per more than 5000 person-brand used cosmetics)

Tabulation of side effects

Side effects of ingredients of cleansing lotions are tabulated in § 23.47.

FACIAL MAKE-UP

23.12   There are make-up products for the entire facial area and the neck, and products for the cheeks only (rouge); the basic formula for both products is the same. The functional part is always a **color pigment mixture** of the following composition:

20–80% *talc* as the powder base
ca 10% *kaolin* or *rice starch* for adsorption of fat
ca 5% *zinc stearate* for improving skin adherence
ca 2% *magnesium carbonate* as carrier for perfume
 0–10% *titanium dioxide* to increase covering power
10–70% colored pigments to obtain the desired tint, e.g.
        – brown: *iron oxide* (CI 77491)
        – red: *Brilliant Lake Red R* (CI 15800)
                     carmine (CI 75470)
                     many other red pigments (see § 27.10)
        – pearlescent *titanated mica*
          pigments   *bismuth oxychloride coated mica*
                      silk powder

23.13   Facial make-up products are available in various forms: as a loose powder, compact powder, cream make-up, and fluid make-up. The following typical formulas will illustrate the various products.

Face powder (loose)

ca 99%	color pigment mixture	see § 23.12
ca 1%	(fused) silica, to improve 'free flow'	

Compact face powder or compact rouge

95%	color pigment mixture	see § 23.12
ca 5%	lipid, as binder	*acetylated lanolin*
0–0.3%	preservative	*methyl paraben*

23.13   Facial make-up

Cream make-up or cream rouge

30–60%	color pigment mixture	see § 23.12
40–60%	cream base composed of water, polyol, lipid, surfactant-emulsifier, preservative and perfume	see § 23.2

Fluid make-up or fluid rouge

ca 30%	color pigment mixture	see § 23.12
ca 70%	water	
ca 5%	suspending agent for the pigments	*magnesium aluminum silicate quaternium-18 hectorite*
ca 0.3%	preservative	*quaternium-15*

23.14   Incidence of side effects: Facial make-up cosmetics (see § 20.17)

	% of total	
US manufacturers' file:	6.2	(519/8399)
US hospitals' file:	2.2	(15/698)
FDA pilot study:	2.7	(16/589)*
Spanish study:	10.8	(21/210)
Dutch file:	3.5	(7/202)
British consumers' report:	no date available	
Strassburg study:	10.4	(10/96)**

*0   severe   ** including eye make-up
 4   moderate
 12 mild

23.15   Risk index: Facial make-up cosmetics (see § 20.18)

Facial make-up products are graded as *medium risk* cosmetics according to the following reports:
US manufacturers' file (at 1 experience per 232,000 estimated units distributed)
FDA pilot study (at 1 experience per 2,200 person-brand used cosmetics).

Tabulation of side effects

Side effects of ingredients of facial make-up cosmetics are tabulated in § 23.47.

FACE MASKS

23.16   Masks have been designed to provide intensive care (cleaning and moisturizing) for the face, within a relatively short period of time. Masks are muddy pastes or viscous liquids that will easily adhere to the skin of the face after being applied. There are several types, which may be characterized by the following typical formulas.

23.17   **Face mask formulations**

Mask (paste ready for use)

Ingredients:		Example:
10–40%	water	water
30–80%	powder base	kaolin, magnesium aluminum silicate
ca 3%	binder	hydroxyethyl cellulose
0–5%	abrasive	almond meal
0–30%	active ingredients	methyl nicotinate, allantoin, honey
ca 0.5%	preservative	methylparaben, DMDM-hydantoin

Mask powder (to be mixed with an aqueous fluid, e.g. water, milk, cucumber juice, yoghurt, just before use; preservatives are unnecessary)

Ingredients		Example:
30–80%	powder base	bentonite, yeast
ca 3%	binder	magnesium aluminum silicate
0– 5%	abrasive	bran
0–50%	active ingredients	arnica flowers, wheat flour, oat flour, zinc peroxide

Peeling masks (this is a viscous liquid that will dry to a colorless film, which can be peeled off after use)

Ingredients:		Example:
50–60%	water	water
10–20%	alcohol	ethanol
10–15%	polyvinyl alcohol (PVA)	polyvinyl alcohol
ca 1%	lipid	lanolin oil
ca 1%	surfactant	buteth-45
ca 1%	perfume	perfume

23.18   **Incidence of side effects: Face masks** (see § 20.17)

	% of total	
US manufacturers' file:	0.5	(40/8399)
US hospitals' file:	no data abailable	
FDA pilot study:	no data available	
Spanish study:	0	(0/210)
Dutch file:	2	(4/202)
British consumers' report:	no data available	
Strassburg study:	0	(0/96)

23.19   **Risk index: Face masks** (see § 20.18)

Face masks are graded as *medium risk* cosmetics according to:
US manufacturers' file (at 1 experience per 105,000 estimated units distributed.)
Side effects of ingredients of face masks are tabulated in § 23.47.

AFTERSHAVE

23.20   An aftershave is primarily intended to be a perfume for men. Sometimes ingredients are added for the purpose of adstringency and counterirritancy.

23.21   A typical formula for **aftershave** is:

Ingredients:		*Example:*
25–60%	water	*water*
40–60%	alcohol	*ethanol*
2– 5%	polyol	*glycerol*
ca 0.5%	perfume compound mixture	*perfume*
0.01%	color	*CI 19140*
0– 1%	special additives	*panthenol, allantoin, benzethonium chloride*

23.22   Side effects from aftershave cosmetics are mainly caused by the perfume compound mixture. A typical fragrance ingredient is *musk*. The following synthetic musks may be ingredients of aftershaves:
– acetylhexamethylindane (Phantolide®)
– acetyl-tert-butyldimethylindane (Celestolide®)
– acetylethyltetramethyltetralin (AETT, Versalide®)
   (neurotoxic, use abandoned in 1977)
– ambrettolide
– ethylene brassylate
– hexahydrohexamethylcyclopentabenzopyran (Galaxolide®)
– musk ambrette
– musk ketone
– musk tibetene
– musk xylol

23.23   **Incidence of side effects: aftershaves** (see § 20.17)

	% of total	
US manufacturers' file:	0.8	(70/8399)
US hospitals' file:	1.0	(7/698)***
FDA pilot study:	0.7	(4/589)*
Spanish study:	5.6	(11/210)**
Dutch file:	4.5	(9/202)
British consumers' report:	5.8	(36/626)
Strassburg study:	1.0	(1/96)

*0 severe   **including pre-shaves
 0 moderate   ***including shaving aids
 4 mild

23.24 **Risk index: Aftershaves** (see § 20.18)

Aftershaves are graded as *low risk* cosmetics according to the following reports:
US manufacturers' file (at 1 experience per 1,416,000 estimated units distributed)
FDA pilot study (at 1 experience per 4,200 person-brand used cosmetics)

Tabulation of side effects

Side effects of ingredients of aftershaves are tabulated in § 23.47. See also the chapter on contact allergy to fragrance materials (§ 5.8–§ 5.17).

OTHER SHAVING AIDS

Shaving aids include shaving foams (aerosol) and beard softeners (paste, cream).

23.25 A typical formula for an **aerosol shaving foam** is:

Ingredients:		*Example:*
ca 10%	propellant	*butane, isobutane, propane*
ca 90%	concentrate:	
	ca 90% water	*water*
	ca 5% foam surfactant	*triethanolamine cocoate, lauric diethanolamine*
	ca 3% polyol	*propylene glycol*
	ca 0.2% perfume	*perfume*

23.26 A typical formula for a **cream beard softener is:**

Ingredients:		*Example:*
ca 80%	water	*water*
ca 15%	lipid	*stearic acid*
ca 1%	polyol	*polypropylene glycol*
ca 1%	surfactant: emulsifier	*potassium stearate*
ca 0.2%	preservative	*methylparaben, propylparaben, DMDM-hydantoin*
ca 0.1%	perfume	*perfume*

23.27 Some beard softeners are designed to exert a depilatory effect. The following typical formula for this type of cosmetic is a powder, that is mixed with water to a paste, just before use:

Powder beard softener (depilating)

Ingredients:		*Example:*
ca 80%	powder base	*kaolin, calcium carbonate*
ca 5%	binder	*dextrin*
3– 5%	depilating agent	*strontium thioglycolate, barium sulfide*
ca 1%	surfactant	*nonoxynol-10*
ca 0.5%	perfume	*perfume*

23.28   Shaving aids

23.28   Incidence of side effects: Shaving foams (see § 20.17)

	% of total	
US manufacturers' file:	0.6	(52/8399)
US hospitals' file:	1.0	(7/698)
FDA pilot study:	0.7	(7/589)*
Spanish study:	0	(0/210)
Dutch file:	1.0	(2/202)
British consumers' report:	no data available	
Strassburg study:	0	(0/96)

*0 severe
 0 moderate
 4 mild

23.29   Risk index: Shaving foams (see § 20.18)

Shaving foams are graded as *low risk* cosmetics according to the following reports:
US manufacturers' file (at 1 experience per 1,045,000 estimated units distributed)
FDA pilot study (at 1 experience per more than 5000 person-brand used cosmetics).

Tabulation of side effects

Side effects of ingredients of shaving aids are tabulated in § 23.47.

EYE MAKE-UP

Eye make-up products include eye shadow, eye liner, mascara and eyebrow pencil.
Typical formulas are:

23.30   Eye shadow: compact powder
(This cosmetic has the same basic structure as compact face powder.)

40–60% *talc* as powder base
ca   7% *zinc stearate* for skin adherence
ca   1% *magnesium carbonate* as perfume carrier
ca   5% lipid binder: e.g. *decyl oleate, isopropyl lanolate*
ca   5% *titanium dioxide* to improve covering power
10–30% colored pigments (see § 27.10)
              – green: *chrome oxides* (CI 77288-77289)
              – blue: *ultramarine* or *ferric ferro-cyanide* (CI 77007-77510)
              – red: *carmine, litholrubin B (barium lake)* (CI 75470-15850)
              – brown-black: *iron oxide, carbon black* (CI 77491-77499-77267)
              – yellow: *sunset yellow aluminum lake* (CI 15985)
              – orange: *tartrazine, aluminum lake* (CI 19140)
              – pearl pigments: *titanated* or *bismuthoxychloride-coated micas.*

23.31   Eye shadow: stick
This has the same formula as eye shadow compact powder, but with a considerably higher content of the lipid binder: 60–80%. Examples for the lipid binder are:
mineral oil, petrolatum, paraffin wax, beeswax.

To prevent rancidity of these lipids approximately 0.05% antioxidants are added, for example: butylated hydroxyanisole (see § 27.5 for an extensive list).

23.32   Eye liner fluid:

ca 25%   polymer as an emulsion: (e.g. *styrenebutadiene emulsion*)
ca 10%   pigments (see § 23.30)
ca 3%   suspending agent (e.g.: *magnesium aluminum silicate*)
ca 1%   surfactant
ca 0.5%   preservative

23.33   Mascara: paste or a block
(mascara blocks mix easily with water to form a paste.)

Ingredients:		*Example:*
ca 70%	water (absent in solid block)	*water*
5–10%	pigments (see § 23.29)	*iron oxide, chrome oxide*
ca 5%	surfactants	*TEA-oleate*
ca 3%	suspending agents	*magnesium aluminum silicate*
ca 20%	lipids	*lanolin, carnauba wax, oleic acid*
0–5%	rayon fibers	*polyamide rayon fiber*
0.05–0.3%	preservative	*thimerosal*

23.34   Mascara ('waterproof'): These cosmetics should be removed at night, as otherwise the eyelashes may be pulled out.

Ingredients:		*Example:*
ca 65%	hydrocarbon solvent	*petroleum distillate*
ca 2%	solvent thickener	*aluminum stearate*
ca 20%	lipids	*beeswax, hydroabietyl alcohol, lanolin*
ca 10%	pigments	*carbon black*
ca 0.05%	antioxidants	*BHA*

23.35   Incidence of side effects: Eye make-up cosmetics (see § 20.17)

According to the following reports, with the exception of the Spanish study, eye make-up cosmetics belong to the 'Top-6' products in relation to side effects (!):

	% of total	
US manufacturers' file:	10.0	(842/8399)
US hospitals' file:	12.9	(90/698)
FDA pilot study:	6.8	(40/589)*
Spanish study:	4.3	(9/210)
Dutch file:	15.4	(31/202)
British consumers' report:	14.1	(88/626)
Strassburg study:	10.0	(10/96)**

*0 severe   **including facial make-up
 6 moderate
34 mild

23.36   Risk index: Eye make-up cosmetics (see § 20.18)

Eye make-up products are graded as *medium risk* cosmetics according to the following reports:
US manufacturers' file (at 1 experience per 237,000 estimated units distributed)
FDA pilot study (at 1 experience per 1,900 person-brand used cosmetics)

23.37   Although many patients ascribe their eye complaints to the use of mascara or other eye make-up products, true contact allergic reactions seem to be infrequent. Most cases of complaints are of an irritant character.

Patch test with mascara 'as is' may frequently cause false positive irritant reactions and should therefore be interpreted with care. Testing of the ingredients in the suitable concentrations and vehicles is advisable.

On the other hand in cases of relevant eye cosmetic dermatitis, patch testing with eye cosmetics often gives false negative reactions. It has been suggested to mix the mascara rubbed on to the patch-tester with a drop of dimethyl sulfoxide 50% before patch-testing [41].

Control tests with eye cosmetics are necessary, usage and open tests may be helpful.

Tabulation of side effects

Side effects of ingredients of eye make-up are tabulated in § 23.47.

ANTI-ACNE PRODUCTS

23.38   Though it would clearly be advisable to regard and regulate anti-acne products as drugs, many of them are sold in Europe as over-the-counter cosmetic preparations. They are available as creams, clear lotions, and as gels.

Anti-acne products may contain the following active ingredients:
– allantoin
– benzalkonium chloride
– benzoyl peroxide
– resorcinol
– resorcinol acetate
– salicylic acid
– sulfur (colloidal)
– thioxolone (hydroxy-oxo-benzoxathiole)
– tocopherol acetate
– tretinoin (vitamin A acid)
– triclosan
– Vibenoid® (an aromatic retinoid-amide)

23.39   Typical formulas for the various types of products are:

I. Cream

Ingredients:		*Example:*
40–70%	water	*water*
ca 2%	polyol	*propylene glycol*
30–50%	lipid	*cetearyl alcohol, caprilic/capric triglyceride*
2– 5%	surfactant	*polysorbate 40, sorbitan stearate*
0– 5%	anti-acne agent	*benzoyl peroxide*
0.3%	preservative	*methylparaben*
0.1%	perfume	*perfume*

II. Clear lotion

Ingredients:		*Example:*
50–80%	water	*water*
20–50%	alcohol	*ethanol, isopropanol*
ca 2%	polyol	*glycerol*
1– 2%	surfactant	*cocamidopropylbetaine*
ca 0.5%	organic acid	*citric acid*
ca 1%	anti-acne agent	*salicylic acid, triclosan*

III. Clear gel

Ingredients:		*Example:*
ca 70%	water	*water*
ca 10%	alcohol	*ethanol*
ca 20%	block polymer	*poloxamer 407*
ca 1%	anti-acne agent	*resorcinol, triclosan*

23.40   **Incidence of side effects: Anti-acne and adstringent products** (see § 20.17)

	% of total	
US manufacturers' file:	0.6	(49/8399)
US hospitals' file:	no data available	
FDA pilot study:	0.7	(4/589)*
Spanish study:	0	(0/210)
Dutch file:	0.5	(1/202)
British consumers' report:	no data available	
Strassburg study:	0	(0/96)

*0 severe
 2 moderate
 2 mild

23.41 **Risk index: Anti-acne and adstringent products** (see § 20.18)

Anti-acne and adstringent products are graded as *medium risk* cosmetics according to the following reports:
US manufacturers' file (at 1 experience per 150,000 estimated units distributed)
FDA-pilot study (at 1 experience per 2,000 person-brand used cosmetics),

23.42 Adverse reactions to the various active ingredients (*from other sources*) are mentioned elsewhere in this book.

CAMOUFLAGE AND GREASEPAINT ('SCHMINK')

23.43 These cosmetics are make-up products with a high content of colored pigments in order to obtain a high covering power. Basically they have similar formulations, typical formulas being:

23.44 **Camouflage cream**

Ingredients:		*Example:*
ca 20%	water	*water*
ca 25%	lipid	*stearic acid, acetylated lanolin*
ca 2%	surfactant	*TEA lauryl sulfate*
40–50%	color pigments	*titanium dioxide, iron oxides*
ca 0.2%	preservative	*methylparaben, propylparaben*
		imidazolidinyl urea
0–0.1%	perfume	*perfume*

Greasepaint stick (black)

ca 40%	lipid	*ozokerite, mineral oil, petrolatum*
ca 1%	surfactant	*sorbitan stearate*
ca 60%	color pigments	*carbon black*
ca 0.1%	antioxidant	*BHT*

Theater compact powder
See facial make-up: compact face powder (§ 23.13).

23.45 **Incidence of side effects and risk index**

For this class of cosmetics, there are no data available regarding the incidence of side effects and calculation of the risk index. Only the Dutch file mentioned one case of an adverse reaction to a camouflage product. However, it may probably be assumed that these products are *medium-risk cosmetics,* just as facial and eye make-up products (§ 23.14–15 and § 23.35–36).

TOOTHPASTES AND MOUTHWASHES

23.46 These products and their side effects are discussed in Chapter 13.

23.47   Contact allergy to ingredients of facial cosmetics

Ingredient	Use	Patch test conc. & vehicle (§ 5.2)	Cross-reactions (§ 5.5)	Comment	Ref.
abietol in eye liner	lipid	10% pet.		Sensitization due to prophetic patch testing	
atranorin in aftershave lotion	fragrance	1% pet./ 0.1% acet.	fumarproto-cetraric acid	Present in oak moss perfumes *See also* § 5.16 *and* § 25.53	22
beeswax in cold cream	vehicle constituent	30% pet. and pure		*See also* § 5.39	20
benzoin in 'party' make-up	fragrance	2–10% pet. 10% alc.		*See also* § 5.39, § 22.65, § 25.9 *and* § 26.3 *under* Styrax benzoin	29
benzyl alcohol in aftershave lotion	fragrance	5–10% pet. 10% alc.		*See also* § 5.7, § 5.16 *Cave:* irritant patch test reactions	27
castor oil in make-up remover	cleanser	pure		Has also caused contact allergy in lipstick (§ 23.53) *See also* § 5.22	64
chloracetamide in eye cream	preservative	0.2% pet., 0.1–1% aqua		*See also* § 5.7, § 25.9 *and* § 25.69	4
chloroallyl-hexami-nium chloride in blush-on	preservative	1% pet. 2% aqua		Is a formaldehyde releaser *See also* § 5.7	20
cinnamic alcohol in aftershave lotion	fragrance	2% pet.		*See also* § 5.16	41
colophony in blush-on	binder	20% pet.		*See also* § 5.39 *and* § 22.65	28
colophony in eye shadow	binder	20% pet.		*See also* § 5.39 *and* § 22.65	5 18
DC Red 17 (CI 26100) in blush-on	color	1% pet.		*See also* § 23.53	3
DC Red 17 (CI 26100) in eye cream	color	1% pet.		*See also* § 23.53	
DC Red 31 (Brilliant Lake Red R, CI 15800)	color	1% pet.	related dyes (*see* § 4.3)	Has caused pigmented cosmetic dermatitis (*see* § 4.3) *See also* § 23.53	31 32
DC Red 36 (CI 12085) in face powder	color	1% pet.		Has also caused contact allergy in lipstick (§ 23.53)	3
DC Yellow 11 (CI 47000) in blush-on	color	0.1% pet.	DC Yellow 10 (0.1% pet.) [55]	Patch testing with the dye 1% may sensitize [51] DC Yellow 11 proved to be a sensitizer in human [53, 54] and animal [52] experiments *See also* § 23.53 *and* § 25.25	34 7 51 55

(continued)

23.47 Ingredients of facial cosmetics

(continuation)

Ingredient	Use	Patch test conc. & vehicle (§ 5.2)	Cross-reactions (§ 5.5)	Comment	Ref.
DC Yellow 11 (CI 47000) in eye cream	color	0.1% pet.	DC Yellow 10 (0.1% pet.) [55]	*See also* § 23.53 *and* § 25.25	11 51 55
DC Yellow 11 (CI 47000) in color stick	color	0.1% pet.		Concomitant sensitization to DC Red 17	62
dichlorophene in liquid make-up base	preservative	0.5–1% pet.		*See also* § 5.7	25
dihydroabietyl alcohol (abitol) in mascara	binder	1% pet.	cross-reaction to colophony and abietic acid possible	*See also* § 5.16	23
diisopropanolamine in blush-on	emulsifier	1% aqua			20
diisopropanolamine in eye shadow	emulsifier	1% aqua		25% of the controls reacted to the undiluted ingredient	19
2,5-di-tert.-butyl hydroquinone in eye shadow	antioxidant	1% pet.			6
Eusolex 8021® in moisturizing cream	sunscreen	2% m.o.		Eusolex 8021 is a mixture of 3-(4-methylbenzylidene) camphor and 4-isopropyl dibenzoylmethane The actual allergen was not determined	43
fumarprotocetraric acid in aftershave lotion	fragrance	0.1% acet.	atranorin	Present in oak moss perfumes *See also* § 5.16 *and* § 25.53	22
hydroxycitronellal in aftershave lotion	fragrance	2% pet.	linalool (?) [44]	*See also* § 5.16	41 44
hydroxycitronellal in cream make-up	fragrance	2% pet.		*See also* § 5.16	9
2-(2′-hydroxy-5′-methylphenyl)benzo-triazole (Tinuvin P®) in face cream	sunscreen	1% pet. 5% pet. [49]		*See also* § 24.12 *and* § 25.66 *under* drometrizole	20
imidazolidinyl-urea (Germall 115®) in moisturizing lotion and liquid eye liner	preservative	1% pet. 2% aqua		*See also* § 5.7	35 26
isoeugenol in 'eye-cosmetics'	fragrance	2% pet.		The patient was also allergic to wool wax alcohols *See also* § 5.16	63
lanolin in eye shadow	binder	pure		*See also* § 5.22 *and* § 23.53	38
lanolin in facial cream	binder	pure		*See also* § 5.22 *and* § 23.53	16

(continued)

(continuation)

Ingredient	Use	Patch test conc. & vehicle (§ 5.2)	Cross-reactions (§ 5.5)	Comment	Ref.
linalool in aftershave lotion	fragrance	30% pet.	hydroxycitronellal (?)	Caused facial psoriasis in the reported case *See also § 5.16*	44
methylheptine carbonate in aftershave lotion	fragrance	0.5% pet.		*See also § 5.16 and § 23.53*	41
methylheptine carbonate in facial cream	fragrance	0.5% pet.		*See also § 5.16 and § 23.53*	30
musk ambrette in aftershave lotions	fragrance			*See § 6.5*	
nickel	(contaminant)	5% pet.			42
oak moss in foundation lotion	fragrance	2% pet.		*See § 5.16*	9
parabens in facial cream	preservatives	each 5% pet.		*See also § 5.7, § 25.53 and § 13.40*	39
perfumes				*See § 5.8*	
perfume in eye cream		0.1%?		Contact allergy to e.g. angelica root oil (as is) and alcohol C-8 (as is)	33
perfume in facial tissue				The patient reacted to cinnamic alcohol and cinnamic aldehyde	60
perfume in mascara		1% pet.			8
o-phenylphenol in foundation cream	preservative	1% pet.		*See § 5.7 and § 25.9*	20
potassium sorbate in face powder	preservative	5% pet.	sorbic acid		59
propolis in face cream	moisturizer	natural extract		Composition: 50% resin and vegetable balsam, 30% wax, 10% essential and aromatic oils, 5% pollen, and 5% various other substances [47]. Has also caused contact allergy in toothpaste [48] *See also §5.43*	48
triethanolamine in shaving cream	surfactant	2% aqua/pet.		*See also § 5.22 and § 25.9*	50
triethanolamine cocohydrolyzed protein in facial skin cleanser	mild surfactant	5 and 50% aqua			24
wool alcohols in 'eye-cosmetics'	vehicle ingredient	30% pet.		The patient also reacted to isoeugenol in the cosmetics	63

Irritant dermatitis due to face painting with tempera pigments in a commercial dishwashing liquid was described by Mathias [36]. *Staphylococcus epidermidis* contamination of mascaras may either cause or prolong bacterial blepharitis [56]: some cases of corneal ulceration due to contamination with *Pseudomonas aeruginosa* have been documented [57]. Rouge has caused contact urticaria [58].

331

LIPSTICK AND LIP BALM

23.48   These products intended for the care and the make-up of the lips, are mainly lipid mixtures of suitable composition; they are sufficiently rigid, and can therefore be easily applied to lips.

Indelible lipsticks contain xanthene dyes (acid form; CI numbers start with 45...) which are dissolved in special solvents (castor oil, oleyl alcohol, hexylene glycol, diisopropyladipate). Such solutions are pale-red colored, but streak bright red on the skin or lip, leaving an indelible color.

23.49   Typical formulas are:

Lipstick

Ingredients:		Example:
ca 60%	lipid-wax mixture	carnauba wax, beeswax
ca 30%	lipid solvent for xanthene oleyl alcohol	ricinus oil
5–8%	color and pigments	titanium dioxide, CI 45380-acid, CI 12085, CI-15630-barium
ca 0.05%	antioxidant	p-hydroxyanisole
ca 0.1%	perfume	perfume

Lip balm

Ingredients:		Example:
ca 95%	lipid-wax mixture	lanolin oil, beeswax, jojoba oil
1–2%	UV absorber	benzophenone-2
0.5%	perfume	perfume
0.05%	antioxidant	octyl gallate, BHA

23.50   **Incidence of side effects: Lipstick and lip balms** (see § 20.17)

	% of total	
US manufacturers' file:	1.6	(136/8399)
US hospitals' file:	no data available	
FDA pilot study:	1.2	(7/589)*
Spanish study:	0.5	(1/210)
Dutch file:	1.5	(3/202)
British consumers' report:	3.0	(19/626)
Strassburg study:	3.1	(3/96)

*0 severe
 0 moderate
 7 mild

23.51   Risk index: Lipsticks and lip balms (see § 20.18)

Lipstick and lip balms are graded as *medium risk* cosmetics according to the following reports:
US manufacturers' file (at 1 experience per 651,000 estimated units distributed)
FDA pilot study (at 1 experience per 3,200 person-brand used cosmetics)

23.52   Cheilitis caused by an allergic reaction to one of the ingredients of lipstick has nowadays become rare, mainly because of the use of better purified xanthene dyes, e.g. eosin. Lipstick may be patch-tested 'as is'.

23.53   Contact allergy to lipstick ingredients

Ingredient	Patch test conc. & vehicle (§ 5.2)	Cross-reactions (§ 5.5)	Comment	Ref.
amyl dimethyl p-amino-benzoic acid	1% pet.		Sunscreen	10
azulene	1% pet.			17
bromofluorescein derivatives	?			2
t-butylhydroquinone (TBHQ)	1% pet.			12
carmine in lip salve	pure			37
castor oil in lipstick/cream	pure		The offending chemical probably was ricinoleic acid (30% pet. and pure) Has also caused contact allergy in make-up remover (§ 23.47)	46 65
DC Orange 17 (permanent orange; CI 12075)	1% pet.	possibly other azo-dyes		3
DC Red 17 (Toney Red; Sudan III; CI 26100)	1% pet.	possibly other azo-dyes	*See also* § 23.47	8
DC Red 19 (Rhodamine B; Basic Violet 10; CI 45170)	1% pet.			17
DC Red 21 (CI 45380)			*See under* eosin	
DC Red 31 (Brilliant Lake Red R; CI 15800)	1%	other azo-dyes (*see* § 4.3)	Has caused pigmented cosmetic dermatitis (§ 4.3) *See also* § 23.47	17
DC Red 36 (Permaton Red; Fire Red 2513; CI 12085)	1% pet.		Has also caused contact allergy in a face powder (§ 23.47)	3

(continued)

23.53   Lipstick ingredients

(continuation)

Ingredient	Patch test conc. & vehicle (§ 5.2)	Cross-reactions (§ 5.5)	Comment	Ref.
DC Yellow 11 (quinazoline yellow SS; CI 47000)	0.1% pet.	DC Yellow 10	Patch testing with the dye may sensitize Has also caused contact allergy in rouge and eye cream (§ 23.47) and in soap (§ 25.25)	7 51
eosin (2,4,5,7-tetra-bromofluorescein; DC Red 21; CI 45380)	50% pet.	possibly other bromofluorescein derivatives	Contact allergy very rare nowadays; actual allergen unknown Has caused photo-sensitivity (§ 6.5)	14 2
geraniol	2% pet.		Fragrance compound *See also* § 5.16	13
lanolin	pure		*See also* § 5.22 and § 23.47	38
methylheptine carbonate	0.5% pet.		*See* also § 5.16 and § 23.47	1
p-nitrobenzene-azo-β-naphthol (para-Red Dark)	?	possibly other azo-dyes		40
oleyl alcohol	30% pet.		*See also* § 5.22	15
perfume	*See* § 5.8			17
phenyl salicylate (salol)	2% pet.	other aryl salicylates [45]	Also incorporated in cosmetic creams and sunscreen preparations (§ 25.66) *See also* § 13.3	13 45
propyl gallate	2% pet.		Antioxidant *See also* § 5.7 *under* gallate esters	21
sodium salt of m-xylene-azo-β-naphthol-3,6-disulfonic acid		possibly other azo-dyes		40
1-sulfo-β-naphthalene-azo-β-naphthol		possibly other azo-dyes		40
wool wax alcohols	30% pet.		The two patients reported also had contact allergy to eye cosmetics	63

23.54   REFERENCES

1. Baer, H. L. (1935): Lipstick dermatitis. *Arch. Derm., 32,* 726.
2. Calnan, C. D. (1959): Allergic sensitivity to eosin. *Acta allerg., 13,* 493.
3. Calnan, C. D. (1967): Reactions to artificial colouring materials. *J. Soc. cosmet. Chem., 18,* 215.
4. Calnan, C. D. (1971): Chloroacetamide dermatitis from a cosmetic. *Contact Dermatitis Newsl. 9,* 215.
5. Calnan, C. D. (1971): Colophony in eye-shadow. *Contact Dermatitis Newsl. 10,* 235.

6. Calnan, C. D. (1973): Ditertiary butylhydroquinone in eye-shadow. *Contact Dermatitis Newsl. 14*, 402.
7. Calnan, C. D. (1976): Quinazoline yellow SS in cosmetics. *Contact Dermatitis, 2,* 160.
8. Calnan, C. D. (1976): Dermatocosmetic relations *J. Soc. cosmet. Chem., 27,* 491.
9. Calnan, C. D. (1979): Perfume dermatitis from the cosmetic ingredients oakmoss and hydroxycitronellal. *Contact Dermatitis, 5,* 194.
10. Calnan, C. D. (1980): Amyldimethylamino benzoic acid causing lipstick dermatitis. *Contact Dermatitis, 6,* 233.
11. Calnan, C. D. (1981): Quinazoline yellow dermatitis (D and C Yellow 11) in an eye cream. *Contact Dermatitis, 7,* 271.
12. Calnan, C. D. (1981): Monotertiary butyl hydroquinone in lipstick. *Contact Dermatitis, 7,* 280.
13. Calnan, C. D., Cronin, E. and Rycroft, R. J. G. (1981): Allergy to phenyl salicylate. *Contact Dermatitis, 7,* 208.
14. Calnan, C. D. and Sarkany, I. (1957): Studies in contact dermatitis: II. Lipstick cheilitis. *Trans. St. John's Hosp. derm. Soc. (Lond.), 39,* 28.
15. Calnan, C. D. and Sarkany, I. (1960): Studies in contact dermatitis: XII. Sensitivity to oleyl alcohol. *Trans. St. John's Hosp. derm. Soc. (Lond.), 44,* 47.
16. Cronin, E. (1966): Lanolin dermatitis. *Brit. J. Derm., 78,* 167.
17. Cronin, E. (1967): Contact dermatitis from cosmetics. *J. Soc. cosmet. Chem., 18,* 681.
18. Cronin, E. (1972): Clinical prediction of patch test results. *Trans. St. John's Hosp. derm. Soc. (Lond.), 58,* 153.
19. Cronin, E. (1973): Di-isopropanolamine in an eye-shadow. *Contact Dermatitis Newsl. 13,* 364.
20. Cronin, E. (1980): Cosmetics. In: *Contact Dermatitis,* pp. 93-170. Churchill Livingstone, Edinburgh.
21. Cronin, E. (1980): Lipstick dermatitis due to propylgallate. *Contact Dermatitis, 6,* 213.
22. Dahlquist, I. and Fregert, S. (1980): Contact allergy to atranorin in lichens and perfumes. *Contact Dermatitis, 6,* 111.
23. Dooms-Goossens, A., Degreef, H. and Luytens, E. (1979): Dihydroabietylalcohol (Abitol), a sensitizer in mascara. *Contact Dermatitis, 5,* 350.
24. Emmett, E. A. and Wright, R. C. (1976): Allergic contact dermatitis from tea-coco hydrolyzed protein. *Arch Derm., 112,* 1008.
25. Epstein, E. (1966): Dichlorophene allergy. *Ann. Allergy, 24,* 437.
26. Fisher, A. A. (1975): Allergic contact dermatitis from Germall 115, a new cosmetic preservative. *Contact Dermatitis, 1,* 126.
27. Fisher, A. A. (1975): Allergic paraben and benzyl alcohol hypersensitivity - relationship of the 'delayed' and immediate varieties. *Contact Dermatitis, 1,* 281.
28. Foussereau, J. (1975): A case of allergy to colophony in a facial cosmetic. *Contact Dermatitis, 1,* 259.
29. Hoffmann, T. E. and Adams, R. M. (1978): Contact dermatitis to benzoin in greasepaint makeup. *Contact Dermatitis, 4,* 379.
30. Hoffman, M. J. and Peters, J. (1935): Dermatitis due to facial cream, caused by methyl heptine carbonate *J. Amer. med. Ass., 104,* 1072.
31. Kozuka, T., Tashiro, M., Sano, S., Fujimoto, K., Nakamura, Y., Hashimoto, S. and Nakaminami, G. (1979): Brilliant Lake Red as a cause of pigmented contact dermatitis. *Contact Dermatitis, 5,* 297.
32. Kozuka, T., Tashiro, M., Sano, S., Fujimoto, K., Nakamura, Y., Hashimoto, S. and Nakaminami, G. (1980): Pigmented contact dermatitis from azo dyes. I. Cross-sensitivity in humans. *Contact Dermatitis, 6,* 330.
33. Larsen W. G. (1975): Cosmetic dermatitis due to a perfume. *Contact Dermatitis, 1,* 142.
34. Larsen, W. G. (1975): Cosmetic dermatitis due to a dye (D and C yellow no. 11). *Contact Dermatitis, 1,* 61.
35. Mandy, S. H. (1974): Contact dermatitis to substituted imidazolidinyl-urea - a common preservative in cosmetics. *Arch Derm., 110,* 463.
36. Mathias, C. G. T. (1980): Contact dermatitis in children due to face paints. *Cutis, 26,* 584.
37. Sarkany, I., Meara, R. H. and Everall, J. (1961): Cheilitis due to carmine in lip salve. *Trans St. John's Hosp. derm. Soc. (Lond.), 46,* 39.
38. Schorr, W. F. (1973): Lip gloss and gloss-type cosmetics. *Contact Dermatitis Newsl. 14,* 408.
39. Simpson, J. R. (1978): Dermatitis due to parabens in cosmetic creams. *Contact Dermatitis, 4,* 311.
40. Sulzberger, M. B., Goodman, J., Byrne, L. A. and Mallozzi, E. D. (1938): Acquired specific hypersensitivity to simple chemicals. II. Cheilitis, with special reference to sensitivity to lipsticks. *Arch. Derm. Syph., 37,* 597.
41. Van Ketel, W. G. (1979): Patch testing with eye cosmetics. *Contact Dermatitis, 5,* 402.

42. Van Ketel, W. G. and Liem, D. H. (1981): Eyelid dermatitis from nickel contaminated cosmetics. *Contact Dermatitis, 7*, 217.
43. Woods, B. (1981): Dermatitis from Eusolex 8021 sunscreen agent in a cosmetic. *Contact Dermatitis, 7*, 108.

UPDATE – 2nd Edition

44. De Groot, A. C. and Liem, D. H. (1983): Facial psoriasis caused by contact allergy to linalool and hydroxycitronellal in an after-shave. *Contact Dermatitis, 9*, 230.
45. Marchand, B., Barbier, P., Ducombs, G. et al. (1982): Allergic contact dermatitis to various salols (phenyl salicylates). *Arch. derm. Res., 272*, 61.
46. Sai, S. (1983): Lipstick dermatitis caused by castor oil. *Contact Dermatitis, 9*, 75.
47. Metzner, J. (1978): Studies on the question of potentiating effects of propolis constituents. *Pharmazie, 33*, 465.
48. Monti, M., Berti, E., Carminati, G. and Cusini, M. (1983): Occupational and cosmetic dermatitis from propolis. *Contact Dermatitis, 9*, 163.
49. De Groot, A. C. and Liem, D. H. (1983): Contact allergy to Tinuvin® P. *Contact Dermatitis, 9*, 324.
50. Curtis, G. and Netherton, E. W. (1940): Cutaneous hypersensitivity to triethanolamine. *Arch. Derm. Syph., 41*, 729.
51. Björkner, B. and Magnusson, B. (1981): Patch test sensitization to D & C Yellow no. 11 and simultaneous reaction to Quinoline Yellow. *Contact Dermatitis, 7*, 1.
52. Lamson, S. A., Kong, B. M. and De Salva, S. J. (1982): D & C Yellow Nos. 10 and 11: delayed contact hypersensitivity in the guinea pig. *Contact Dermatitis, 8*, 200.
53. Rapaport, M. J. (1980): Allergy to D & C Yellow No. 11. *Contact Dermatitis, 6*, 364.
54. Weaver, J. E. (1983): Dose response relationships in delayed hypersensitivity to quinoline dyes. *Contact Dermatitis, 9*, 309.
55. Björkner, B. and Niklasson, B. (1983): Contact allergic reaction to D & C Yellow No. 11 and Quinoline Yellow. *Contact Dermatitis, 9*, 263.
56. Ahearn, D. G. and Wilson, L. A. (1976): Microflora of the outer eye and eye area cosmetics. *Devel. Indus. Microbiol., 17*, 23.
57. Wilson, L. A. and Ahearn, D. G. (1977): Pseudomonas-induced corneal ulcers associated with contaminated eye mascaras. *Amer. J. Ophthal., 84*, 112.
58. De Groot, A. C. and Liem, D. H. (1983): Contact urticaria to rouge. *Contact Dermatitis, 9*, 322.
59. Fisher, A. A. (1980): Cutaneous reactions to sorbic acid and potassium sorbate. *Cutis, 25*, 350, 352, 423.
60. Guin, J. D. (1981): Contact dermatitis to perfume in paper products. *J. Amer. Acad. Derm., 4*, 733.
61. Rapaport, M. J. (1980): Sensitization to Abitol. *Contact Dermatitis, 6*, 137.
62. Calnan, C. D. (1973): Allergy to D and C Red 17 and D and C Yellow 11. *Contact Dermatitis Newsl., 14*, 405.
63. Schorr, W. F. (1973): Lip gloss and gloss type cosmetics. *Contact Dermatitis Newsl., 14*, 408.
64. Brandle, I., Boujnah-Khouadja, A. and Foussereau, J. (1983): Allergy to castor oil. *Contact Dermatitis, 9*, 424.
65. Sai, S. (1983): Lipstick dermatitis caused by ricinoleic acid. *Contact Dermatitis, 9*, 524.

24. Nail cosmetics

24.1 The nail-line of cosmetics consists of: lacquer, lacquer remover, hardener, elongator, cuticle softener and cream. Lacquers are the most popular nail cosmetics. Typical formulas are:

24.2 **Nail lacquer**

Ingredients:		*Example:*
ca 15%	film polymer	*nitrocellulose*
ca 7%	polymer resin	*toluene-sulfonamide-formaldehyde resin** *(Santolite MHP or MS®)*
ca 7%	lipid plasticizer	*dibutyl phthalate, camphor, castor oil*
ca 70%	solvent mixture	*toluene, butyl acetate, butanol, ethyl acetate*
0–1%	color pigments mixture	*titanium dioxide, CI 15850 calcium lake, CI 15880 calcium lake*
ca 1%	suspending agent	*quaternium-18 hectorite*

* Toluene-sulfonamide-formaldehyde resins are indispensable in nail lacquer technology; they have outstanding properties. Sensitization, however, has occurred incidentally. There is always a small amount of free formaldehyde present, at least in the preparations available in Holland. The Enschede laboratory found levels of 0.15% free formaldehyde in 22 commercial nail lacquers of different brands, and only in 2 samples was the concentration lower than 0.01%. The presence of toluene-sulfonamide-formaldehyde resins was confirmed by infrared spectroscopy.

24.3 **Nail lacquer remover**

Ingredients:		*Example:*
ca 98%	solvent mixture	*butyl acetate, ethyl acetate, ethoxyethanol (Cellosolve®), acetone*
ca 2%	lipid	*castor oil, lanolin oil*

24.4   **Nail hardener (formaldehyde type)**

Ingredients:		*Example:*
ca 80%	water	*water*
ca 5%	hardening agent	*formaldehyde**
ca 1%	organic acid	*lactic acid*

* Limited to 5% in the *EEG Cosmetic Directive* (1976).

24.5   **Nail elongator** (other names: **nail extender, liquid nails, artificial nail set**)

There are two types: one using plastic nails to be glued with a special glue (e.g. ethylcyanoacryl-type glue), the other type is a dual product of the following typical formulas:

Elongator I (powder)

Ingredients:		*Example:*
ca 97%	acryl-type polymer (powder)	*polymethyl methacrylate*
ca 3%	polymerization initiator	*benzoyl peroxide*

Elongator II (liquid)

Ingredients:		*Example:*
ca 99%	acryl-type monomer	*methyl methacrylate (monomer)*
ca 1%	stabilizer	*hydroquinone*
		p-dimethylaminochlorbenzene

Powder I and liquid II are mixed before use and applied as an extension of the nail. It hardens after ca 15 minutes.

24.6   **Cuticle removers or softeners** are dilute solutions of alkali.

A typical formula is:

Ingredients:		*Example:*
ca 90%	water	*water*
1–5%	softening agent	*potassium hydroxide*
5–1%	thickener	*sorbitol, magnesium aluminum silicate*
0.1%	perfume	*perfume*

24.7   **Nail cream** is an ordinary water-in-oil moisturizing cream, with low water (ca 30%) and a high lipid content (typical lipids: lanolin, propolis, jojoba oil, carrot oil). It is applied to combat brittleness and splitting of the nails.

A typical formula is:

Ingredients:		*Example:*
ca 30%	water	*water*
ca 65%	lipids	*beeswax, lanolin wax, jojoba oil, turtle oil*
ca 2%	surfactant: emulsifier	*sodium lauryl sulfate*
ca 0.2%	preservative	*bromonitropropanediol*

24.8 Dermatitis from nail cosmetics may be localized on:
  – the eyelids
  – the lower part of the face (in the majority of patients)
  – the neck and upper chest
  – the skin around the nails (rare)
  – the external auditory meatus (rare)
  – the skin behind the ears (rare)
  – the pinnae (rare)
  – the lips and the corners of the eyes (rare)
  – perineum and groins (rare);
  It can be also generalized (rare).

24.9 Nail varnish may be tested 'as is,' but should be allowed to dry before patch testing. The majority of contact allergic reactions to nail cosmetics are due to the resins.

24.10 **Incidence of side effects: Nail cosmetics** (see § 20.17)

	% of total	
US manufacturers' file:	2.1	(177/8399)
US hospitals' file:	10.3	(72/698)***
FDA pilot study:	3.4	(20/589)*/+
Spanish study:	23.3	(49/210)
Dutch file:	1.0	(2/202)
British consumers' report:	no data available	
Strassburg study:	20.8	(20/96)

*0 severe   **2 allergic   *** of which 8 were due to nail har-
 4 moderate   0 non-   deners
 16 mild   allergic
+ Of the 20 reported occurrences of side effects, 13 were due to polishes, 4 to hardeners, 2 to removers, 1 to softener and none to base coats.

24.11 **Risk index: Nail cosmetics** (see § 20.18)

Risk grading according to:
US manufacturers' file: *low risk* (at 1 experience per 856,000 estimated units distributed).
FDA pilot study: *medium risk* (at 1 experience per 1700 person-brand used cosmetics).

24.12   Nail cosmetics

Tabulation of side effects

Side effects of ingredients of nail cosmetics are tabulated in § 24.12 (contact allergy) and § 24.13 (other side effects). For a survey of adverse reactions, see also [20, 23].

24.12   Contact allergy to ingredients of nail cosmetics

Ingredient	Use	Patch test conc. & vehicle (§ 5.2)	Cross-reaction (§ 5.5)	Ref.
aryl-sulfonamide resin (p-toluene sulfonamide formaldehyde resin)	polymer resin	10% pet.	sulfanilamide formaldehyde *See also* § 24.2 *and* § 24.13	8 3
drometrizole	UV-absorber in nail varnish	5% pet.	*see also* § 25.66 *and* § 23.47 *under* 2-(2′-hydroxy-5′-methylphenyl)-benzotriazole	18
formaldehyde	nail hardener	2% aqua	*see also* § 5.7, § 22.7, § 24.13 *and* § 25.53	5
glyceryl phthalate resin	polymer resin	10% pet.		3
guanine	pearlescent pigment	pure		15
methacrylic acid esters	monomers		cross-reactions	10
– methyl methacrylate	monomer	1% pet.	between methyl	7
– ethyl methacrylate	monomer	1% pet.	methacrylate	9
– butyl methacrylate	monomer	1% pet.	monomers and acrylic	
– isobutyl methacrylate	monomer	1% pet.	monomers	
– tetrahydrofurfuryl methacrylate	monomer	1% pet.	are possible	
– methacrylic acid	monomer	1% pet.	See for irritant and	
– diethylene glycol dimethacrylate	monomer	1% pet.	allergic reactions to acrylates and	
– trimethylol propane trimethacrylate	monomer	1% pet.	methacrylates also [4] Permanent loss of fingernails and persistent paraesthesia due to contact allergy to methyl methacrylate in an artificial nail has been reported [19]	
nitrocellulose	film polymer	10% aqua		21
p-tertiary butylphenol resin	resin in plastic nail adhesive	1% pet.		16 17
tricresyl ethyl phthalate	plasticizer in artificial nail	5% pet.		17

24.13   **Other side effects of ingredients of nail cosmetics**

Ingredient	Use	Side effects	Comment	Ref.
acrylates	artificial nails	onycholysis	Contact allergy not excluded	22
formaldehyde	nail hardener	paronychia, subungual hyperkeratosis, subungual hemorrhages, leukonychia, onycholysis, lip hemorrhages in nail biters	These effects may be allergic or non-allergic in nature *See also* § 5.7, § 22.7, § 24.12 *and* § 25.53	14 6 11
nail varnish	contact urticaria	causative ingredient not specified	*See* § 7.6	
phenol formaldehyde resin	polymer resin	subungual hemorrhage, red-brown discoloration of the nail plate, onycholysis, subungual hyperkeratosis	These effects may both be allergic or non-allergic in nature	13 16
toluene sulfonamide formaldehyde resin	polymer resin	onycholysis	The validity of this report was questioned by Brauer[1] *See also* § 24.2 *and* § 24.12	12
Transparent Yellow Lake (CI 16901)		orange discoloration of the nail		2

24.14   **REFERENCES**

1. Brauer, E. W. (1980): Letter to the Editor. *Cutis, 26,* 588.
2. Calnan, C. D. (1967): Reactions to àrtificial colouring materials. *J. Soc. cosmet. Chem., 18,* 215.
3. Calnan, C. D. and Sarkany, I. (1958): Studies in contact dermatitis, III. Nail varnish. *Trans. St. John's Hosp. Derm. Soc. (Lond.), 40,* 1.
4. Cavelier, C., Jelen, G., Hervé-Bazin, B. and Foussereau, J. (1981): Irritation et allergie aux acrylates et méthacrylates. *Ann. Derm. Vénéréol. (Paris), 108,* 549.
5. Epstein, E. and Maibach, H. I. (1966): Formaldehyde allergy. *Arch. Derm., 94,* 186.
6. Fisher, A. A. (1979): Current contact news. *Cutis, 23,* 743, 746, 753, 847, 852, 855, 863, 871.
7. Fisher, A. A. (1980): Cross reactions between methyl methacrylate monomer and acrylic monomers presently used in acrylic nail preparations. *Contact Dermatitis, 6,* 345.
8. Keil, H. and van Dijck, L. S. (1944): Dermatitis due to nail polish. *Arch. Derm., 50,* 39.
9. Maibach, H. I. et al. (1978): Butyl methacrylate monomer and ethyl methacrylate monomer – frequency of reaction. *Contact Dermatitis, 4,* 60.
10. Marks Jr., J. F., Bishop, M. E. and Willis, W. P. (1979): Allergic contact dermatitis to sculptured nails. *Arch. Derm., 115,* 100.
11. Mitchell, J. C. (1981): Non-inflammatory onycholysis from formaldehyde-containing nail hardener. *Contact Dermatitis, 7,* 173.
12. Paltzick, R. L. and Enscoe, I. (1980): Onycholysis secondary to toluene sulfonamide formaldehyde resin used in nail hardener mimicking onychomycosis. *Cutis, 25,* 647.

13. Rein, C. R. and Rogin, J. R. (1950): Allergic eczematous reaction of the nail bed due to 'undercoats'. *Arch. Derm., 61,* 971.
14. Rice, E. G. (1968): Allergic reactions to nail hardeners. *Cutis, 4,* 971.
15. Stritzler, C. (1958): Dermatitis of the face caused by guanine in pearly nail lacquer. *Arch. Derm., 78,* 252.

UPDATE–2nd Edition

16. Rycroft, R. J. G., Wilkinson, J. D., Holmes, R. and Hay, R. J. (1980): Contact sensitization to p-tertiary butylphenol (PTBP) resin in plastic nail adhesive. *Clin. exp. Derm., 5,* 441.
17. Burrows, D. and Rycroft, R. J. G. (1981): Contact dermatitis from PTBP resin and tricresyl ethyl phthalate in a plastic nail adhesive. *Contact Dermatitis, 7,* 336.
18. De Groot, A. C. and Liem, D. H. (1983): Contact allergy to Tinuvin® P. *Contact Dermatitis, 9,* 324.
19. Fisher, A. A. (1980): Permanent loss of fingernails from sensitization and reaction to acrylic in a preparation designed to make artificial nails. *J. Derm. surg. Oncol., 6,* 70.
20. Scher, R. K. (1982): Cosmetics and ancillary preparations for the care of nails. *J. Amer. Acad. Derm., 6,* 523.
21. Dobes, W. L. and Nippert, P. H. (1944): Contact eczema due to nail polish. *Arch. Derm. Syph., 49,* 183.
22. Goodwin, P. (1976): Onycholysis due to acrylic nail applications. *Clin. exp. Derm., 1,* 191.
23. Baran, R. (1982): Pathology induced by the application of cosmetics to the nail. In: *Principles of Cosmetics for the Dermatologist,* Chapter 24, pp. 181-184. Eds.: Ph. Frost and S. N. Horwitz. C. V. Mosby company, St. Louis, U.S.A.

25. Cosmetics for the body and parts of the body

BATH AND SHOWER COSMETICS

25.1 These cosmetics, which consist mainly of foam and fragrance, have the following typical formulas:

25.2 **Foam bath (bubble bath), foam shower:** basically a shampoo formulation (see § 22.2) but with the emphasis on the foam building surfactants.

Ingredients:		*Example:*
70–80%	water	*water*
10–20%	surfactant: foam builder	*sodium laureth sulfate, lauric DEA*
0–1%	thickener	*sodium chloride*
ca 1%	perfume	*perfume*
ca 0.2%	preservative	*bromonitropropanediol, methyl-paraben*
ca 0.02%	color	*CI 61570*

25.3 **Bath oil (floating type):** when this bath oil is poured into the bath, oil floats on the water surface and will partly stay on the body after bathing.

Ingredients:		*Example:*
ca 95%	lipid	*oleyl alcohol, mineral oil*
ca 0.5%	surfactant	*polyethylene glycol glyceryl cocoate*
ca 0.5%	perfume	*perfume*
ca 0.05%	antioxidant	*butylated hydroxyanisole*

Bath oil (dispersible type): when poured into the bath, a milky dispersion instantly appears.

Ingredients:		*Example:*
ca 80%	lipid	*decyl oleate, mineral oil*
5–10%	surfactant	*sulfated castor oil, polyethylene glycol-400 dioleate*
1–5%	perfume	*perfume*
ca 0.05%	antioxidant	*butylated hydroxyanisole*

25.4 Bath and shower cosmetics

25.4   **Bath cream:** bath cream has the same properties as dispersible bath oil, but it gives more foam.

Ingredients:		*Example:*
60–70%	water	*water*
ca 5%	lipid	*isopropyl myristate*
ca 5%	surfactant: pearlescent additive	*PEG 8 distearate*
20–30%	surfactant	*TEA lauryl sulfate*
ca 0.3%	preservative	*imidazolidinyl urea, methyl-paraben*
ca 1%	perfume	*perfume*
ca 0.05%	antioxidant	*butylated hydroxyanisole, butylated hydroxytoluene*

25.5   **Bath salt:** bath salts are added to baths to imitate natural mineral water, but most formulas contain only one or more of the following salts: disodium phosphate, magnesium sulfate, sea salt, sodium bicarbonate, sodium carbonate, sodium chloride, sodium iodide, sodium sesquicarbonate, sodium thiosulfate.

Ingredients:		*Example:*
ca 99%	salts (see list above)	*sodium chloride, potassium iodide, sodium bicarbonate*
ca 0.5%	perfume	*perfume*
ca 0.01%	color	*CI 45370*

25.6   **Effervescent bath tablet:** these are added to baths for a steady release of carbon dioxide or oxygen gas.

Ingredients:		*Example:*
10–25%	salts for CO_2 gas release or salts for O_2 gas release	*citric acid, sodium sesquicarbonate* *sodium perborate, manganese sulfate*
ca 20%	filler additives	*sodium chloride, kaolin, talc*
ca 0.5%	perfume	*perfume*
ca 0.01%	color	*CI 45170*

25.7   **Incidence of side effects: Bath and shower cosmetics** (see § 20.17)

	% of total	
US manufacturers' file:	2.8	(237/8399)
US hospitals' file:	1.2	(8/698)
FDA pilot study:	4.2	(25/589)*

*1   severe
 3   moderate
21 mild

Spanish study:	0	(0/210)
Dutch file:	2.5	(5/202)
British consumers' report:	no data available	
Strassburg study:	0	(0/96)

25.8   Risk index: Bath and shower cosmetics (see § 20.18)

Risk grading according to:
US manufacturers' file: *medium risk* (at 1 experience per 432,000 estimated units distributed).
FDA pilot study: *high risk* (at 1 experience per 800 person-brand used cosmetics).

Fragrance materials and their side effects are discussed in Chapter 5. The side effects of bath, shower and body cosmetics are tabulated in § 25.9.

25.9   Contact allergy to ingredients of bath, shower and body cosmetics

Ingredient	Cosmetic	Patch test conc. & vehicle (§ 5.2)	Cross-reactions (§ 5.5)	Comment	Ref.
ammonyx LO® (lauryl-dimethyl-amine oxide) (foam builder)	dish washing detergents, shampoos, foam bath, surgical scrubs	3.7% aqua			35
benzoin (resin)	hand cream	2–10% pet. 10% alc.		*See also* § 5.39, § 22.65, § 23.47 *and* § 26.3 *under* Styrax benzoin	72
chloracetamide (preservative)	hand lotion	0.2% pet. 0.1–1% aqua		*See also* § 5.7, § 23.47 *and* § 25,69	64
p-chloro-m-xylenol (preservative)	body lotion	1–5% pet.		*See also* § 5.7	8
coconut diethanolamide (foam builder)	hand gels	0.5% pet.		Also in handwashing liquids and shampoos	37
monosulfiram (antioxidant)	soap	1% pet.	related thiuram compounds	*See also* § 4.11, § 12.1 *and* § 25.25	16
octyl dodecanol (emollient)	moisturizing lotion	30% pet. 13.5% aqua		*See also* § 5.22	69
o-phenylphenol (preservative)	'medicated cream'	1% pet.		*See also* § 5.7 *and* § 23.47	68
triethanolamine (emulsifier)	hand lotion	2% pet./aqua		*See also* § 5.22 *and* § 23.47	54

Allergic contact urticaria due to a wheat bran bath has been reported in an atopic child, whose eczema improved on a gluten-free diet [86]. Excessive use of bubble baths may lead to urinary tract irritation, especially in children. Vitamin E in baths can produce a follicular eruption [89].

HAND AND BODY LOTION

25.10   These products are popular as 'all-purpose' lotions, but they are especially and very widely used for treating mild 'housewives eczema'. The composition is basically similar to ordinary moisturizing and cleansing milks:

25.11   **Hand and body lotion**

Ingredients:		*Example:*
60–80%	water	*water*
ca 5%	polyol	*sorbitol*
20–30%	lipid	*mineral oil, glyceryl stearate, cetyl alcohol*
2–5%	surfactant: emulsifier	*TEA lauryl sulfate, trioleth-8-phosphate*
ca 0.3%	preservative	*kathon CG®*
ca 0.02%	color	*CI 16185*
ca 0.2%	perfume	*perfume*

25.12   **Incidence of side effects: Hand and body lotion** (see § 20.17)

	% of total	
US manufacturers' file:	2.9	(246/8399)
US hospitals' file:	1.3	(9/698)
FDA pilot study:	1.4	(8/589)*
Spanish study:	no data available	
Dutch file:	11.3	(23/202)**
British consumers' report:	no data available	
Strassburg study:	no data available	

*0 severe   ** one of the 'Top-6'
 1 moderate
 7 mild

25.13   **Risk index: Hand and body lotion** (see § 20.18)

Risk grading according to:
US manufacturers' file: *medium risk* (at 1 experience per 715,000 estimated units distributed)
FDA pilot study: *low risk* (at 1 experience per 5000 person-brand used cosmetics)
For side effects of ingredients of hand and body lotions see § 25.9.

BODY TALC

25.14   Body talc is widely used in the Americas. It is mainly a fragrance product. The formula is very simple, as can be seen from the following example:

Body talc

Ingredients:		*Example:*
90–98%	talc	*talc*
0.5%	silica (fused) to improve free flow	*silica (fused)*
ca 2%	carrier for perfume	*magnesium carbonate*
ca 0.5%	perfume	*perfume*

25.15   Another type of body talcs has additional properties: relief of itching, deodorizing, antiseptic, absorption of perspiration. A typical example is:

Dusting powder

Ingredients:		*Example:*
80–90%	talc	*talc*
0.5%	silica (fused) to improve free flow	*silica (fused)*
ca 10%	active ingredients	*salicylic acid, boric acid, zinc oxide, lanolin*
ca 2%	perfume carrier	*magnesium carbonate*
ca 0.5%	perfume	*perfume*

25.16   **Incidence of side effects: Body talc** (see § 20.17)

	% of total	
US manufacturers' file:	0.4	(32/8399)
US hospitals' file:	1.0	(7/698)
FDA pilot study:	2.9	(17/589)*
Spanish study:	0	(0/210)
Dutch file:	0	(0/202)
British consumers' report:	no data available	
Strassburg study:	0	(0/96)

*1   severe
1   moderate
15 mild

25.17   **Risk index: Body talc** (see § 20.18)

Risk grading according to:
US manufacturers' file: *low risk* (at 1 experience per 1,352,000 estimated units distributed).
FDA pilot study: *medium risk* (at 1 experience per 2100 person-brand used cosmetics).

SOAP

25.18   The classic toilet soap bar, which is still very popular, is almost entirely the sodium salt of fatty acids (either a single salt or a natural mixture).

25.19   A typical formula for **toilet soap bar** is:

Ingredients:		*Example:*
85-95%	sodium salt of fatty acids	*sodium cocoate, sodium tallowate*
ca 0.5%	perfume	*perfume*
ca 0.1%	antioxidant and chelating agent	*o-tolylbiguanide, EDTA*
ca 0.01%	color	*titanium dioxide*

25.20   Various ingredients may be added to obtain special soap types:

Lipids:	lanolin paraffin	Soap type:	superfatty soap
Polyols:	sucrose glycerin		transparent soap
Antimicrobials:	triclocarban hexachlorophene dichlorophene triclosan sulfur (colloidal)		deodorant soap

25.21   **Syndet soap bars** consist entirely or partially of synthetic detergents ('syndets'). The development of these products was largely due to some undesirable properties of soaps such as the alkalinicity, leading to skin irritation, and incompatibility with hard water, leading to precipitation of calcium fatty acid salts.

The use of syndet soap bars has increased considerably, especially for medical use, where frequent hand washing is inevitable. In many countries the term *'soap'* is protected and may be used only for the classic type of soap.

25.22   A typical formula of **syndet soap bars** is:

Ingredients:		*Example:*
50–95%	synthetic surfactant	*dioctyl sodium sulfosuccinate,* *sodium lauryl sulfate,* *cocamidopropylbetaine*
0–50%	soap: sodium salt of fatty acids	*sodium cocoate*
5–20%	additives to aid technologic performance	*kaolin, sorbitol, paraffin, sodium* *silicate, cellulose gum*
1–5%	pH adjusting agent (to a pH of ca 5.5)	*lactic acid, citric acid*
ca 0.1%	antioxidant and chelating agent	*Sopant®, edetic acid*
ca 0.5%	perfume	*perfume*

25.23   **Side effects of soaps** on the skin include:
1. irritant contact dermatitis
2. allergic contact dermatitis (to *ingredients* of soaps)
3. a combination of irritant and allergic reactions.

Irritant side effects

25.24   Soaps exert a weak toxic effect on the skin, thus slightly damaging it; prolonged or repeated contact will lead to irritant dermatitis. This reaction may be provoked by prolonged contact with a soap solution on practically every skin, although there is a great variety in individual susceptibility; atopic individuals are particularly susceptible.

The eruption often starts under a ring, and is associated with wet work (kitchen personnel, hairdressers, housewives, bartenders): it is diagnosed as 'housewives eczema' or 'soap dermatitis'.

Assessment of irritant effects: There is no reliable laboratory method to assess the irritant effects of soaps and consequently results of investigations in this field are often contradictory.

The conventional patch testing technique with soap solutions is inadequate, as it produces a monomorphic erythematous reaction, with only small variations in intensity. Presently the following test methods are in use:
1. Measurements of skin vapor loss before and after exposure to a 1% solution of soap [25].
2. A modified patch test procedure. This test method employs the Duhring chamber, an aluminum cup, 12 mm in diameter. The test entails daily exposures to an 8% solution of soaps [23, 48].

Allergic side effects

25.25   Soaps themselves are not sensitizing, but sometimes chemicals are added that may cause allergic reactions; these include perfumes [75], lanolin, colophony [74] and germicides, e.g. mercury [70]. *Apricot soap* has been reported to cause pruritus ani et vulvae due to contact allergy [61]. *Monosulfiram soap* has caused allergic contact dermatitis in a patient sensitive to tetramethylthiuram disulfide [16]. Patients sensitized to DC Yellow 11 in maximization tests exhibited an allergic contact dermatitis from the use of soap containing this dye [76, 77]. Halogenated salicylanilides have caused epidemics of photoallergic reactions (§ 6.5). Photodermatitis from chlorophenylphenol in soap has been reported in two patients [97]. Contact allergy to chromium in a toilet soap caused 'pigmented cosmetic dermatitis' [99].

25.26   **Incidence of side effects: Soaps** (see § 20.17)

	% of total	
US manufacturers' file:	3.7	(313/8399)
US hospitals' file:	9.5	(66/698)***
FDA pilot study:	12.6	(74/589)*/***
Spanish study:	4.1	(8/210)**
Dutch file:	0.5	(1/202)
British consumers' report:	12.0	(75/626)***
Strassburg study:	0	(0/96)

*1	severe	** shampoos included
4	moderate	*** one of the 'Top-6'
69	mild	

25.27   **Risk index: Soaps** (see § 20.18)

Risk grading according to:
US manufacturers' file: *low risk* (at 1 experience per 3,300,000 estimated units distributed)
FDA pilot study: *medium risk* (at 1 experience per 1600 person-brand used cosmetics)

FLUID SOAP AND HAND CLEANER

25.28   Fluid soaps (particularly in use to clean the hands) have gained in popularity, because they are, when supplied with special dispensing bottles, more hygienic in use than soap bars. Liquid soaps found their way into the medical profession because they can be formulated to a pH in accordance with the skin (ca 5.5); wrongly it has been assumed that this would cause less irritation of the skin, even when used frequently. Because of the hygienic advantages fluid soaps are also gaining in popularity for use in public buildings.

One should be aware that the term *'liquid soap'* is protected in many countries and restricted to pure 'salts of fatty acids'. Therefore, product names like *hand cleaner, hand washing lotion,* etc. are in use. The typical formulas for these products are basically similar to those for shampoos, but special attention is given to the pH of the product (5.5) and surfactants of low skin-irritancy are selected. Examples of such mild acting surfactants are:

25.29   Protein-fatty acid condensates (Lamepon®, Maypon®, different types)
- potassium coco hydrolyzed animal protein (Lamepon POTR®)
- sodium soya hydrolyzed animal protein (Maypon K®)
- triethanolamine coco hydrolyzed animal protein (Lamepon STR®)
- triethanolamine oleoyl hydrolyzed animal protein (Lamepon POTR®)

Amino acid-fatty acid condensates
- sodium cocoyl glutamate (Amisoft CS11®)
- sodium cocoyl sarcosinate (Sarkosine KA®)
- sodium hydrogenated tallow glutamate (Amisoft HS11®)
- sodium lauroyl glutamate (Amisoft LS11®)
- sodium lauroyl sarcosinate (Sarkosyl NL30®, Medialan LD®, Maprosil 30®)
- sodium myristoyl sarcosinate (Hamposyl M30®)
- triethanolamine cocoyl glutamate (Amisoft CT12®)

Phosphate esters
- lecithin
- trilaneth-4 phosphate (Hostaphat KW34ON®)
- trioleth-8 phosphate (Hostaphat KO380®)
- trioleyl phosphate (Hostaphat KO300®)

Amphoteric surfactants (see § 27.15)
- amphoteric-1 (Miranol CMconc®)
- amphoteric-2 (Miranol C2Mconc®)
- amphoteric-6 (Miranol 2MCA®)
- amphoteric-12 (Miranol ISM®)
- cocamidopropyl betaine (Tegobetain L7®)
- cocobetaine (Emcol CC37-18®, Dehyton AB30®, Standapol AB45®)

25.30   A typical formula for a **handwashing lotion (handcleaner)** is:

Ingredients:		Example:
60–80%	water	*water*
ca 15%	surfactant (principal)	*amphoteric-2, disodiummonoundecylen-amido-monoethanolamine sulfo-succinate*
ca 1%	surfactant: foam builder	*lauramide monoethanolamine*

(continued)

350

(continuation)

Ingredients:		*Example:*
ca 1%	thickener	*carbomer-934*
ca 2%	lipid: superfatty agent	*lanolin oil*
ca 1%	organic acid: pH-adjusting agent	*citric acid*
ca 0.3%	preservative	*kathon CG®*
ca 0.01%	color	*CI 19140*
ca 0.3%	perfume	*perfume*

25.31   **Incidence of side effects**

There are no data available on the incidence of side effects and on the risk index of *fluid soaps and hand cleaners.*

DEPILATORY PREPARATIONS

25.32   Hair can be removed by mechanical pulling with the aid of an *epilating wax*. The wax has a melting point near 45°C and is poured on the skin in melted condition. When the wax has solidified, the hair may be pulled off with the wax. Removing hair by mechanical epilation has no permanent effect.

A typical formula for **epilating wax** is:

Ingredients:		*Example:*
ca 70%	colophony	*colophony*
ca 30%	lipids: waxes and oils	*beeswax, linseed oil*
ca 0.2%	perfume	*perfume*

25.33   The most popular method of removing hair is depilating with a paste. The active ingredients are alkali (pH 12.5) and one or more of the following depilating agents: calcium or strontium thioglycolate, barium or calcium sulfide, or sodium stannite. These products are applied as a paste to the skin for 5–10 minutes. Thus the hair is weakened and can be removed, together with the paste, with a spatula. Residual alkali should be rinsed off immediately with water in order to prevent irritation. 'After-depilating' creams, containing lactic acid or citric acid as active ingredients are used to assure the neutralization of alkali. Hair removal by this method is not permanent.

25.34   A typical formula for a **depilating cream/paste** is:

Ingredients:		*Example:*
60–70%	water	*water*
ca 5%	thickener: inorganic	*magnesium aluminum silicate*
20–30%	lipid	*cetyl alcohol, mineral oil*
2–5%	surfactant: emulsifier	*sodium lauryl sulfate*

(continued)

25.34 Depilatory preparations

(continuation)

Ingredients:		*Example:*
ca 2%	alkaline agent to adjust pH to 12.5	*calcium hydroxide*
3–5%	depilating agent	*sodium stannite, calcium thioglycolate*
ca 0.5%	perfume	*perfume*

Other mercapto-type depilating agents are: *thiolactic acid* and *thioglycerol.*

25.35   Permanent removal of hair is claimed by means of enzymatic (protease: papain or keratinase) inactivation of the hair follicle. Pre-removal by epilating the hair is necessary in order to allow contact of the enzyme with the hair papilla. To prevent inactivation of the proteinase enzyme, the product is sold as a powder (containing the enzyme) and a liquid, which are mixed before use. The mixture is applied with a brush and should contact the hair follicle. If the preremoval of the hair is not complete the procedure will fail.

25.36   A typical formula for an **enzymatic depilator** is:

I. Powder

Ingredients:		*Example:*
ca 90%	inert powder	*kaolin*
ca 2%	surfactant: nonionic	*polysorbate 80*
ca 1%	thickener	*pectin*
ca 3%	proteinase	*eratinase*

II. Liquid

Ingredients:		*Example:*
ca 99%	water	*water*
ca 1%	buffering salt for optimum pH	*dipotassium phosphate*

25.37   **Incidence of side effects: Depilatories** (see § 20.17)

	% of total	
US manufacturers' file:	0.9	(73/8399)
US hospitals' file:	1.0	(7/698)
FDA pilot study:	2.2	(13/589)*
Spanish study:	1.0	(2/210)
Dutch file:	2.4	(1/41)**
British consumers' report:	no data available	
Strassburg study:	5.2	(5/96)

*0	severe	**0 allergic
3	moderate	1 non-allergic
10	mild	

25.38   **Risk index: Depilatories** (see § 20.18)

Depilatories are graded as *high-risk* cosmetics according to the following reports:
US manufacturers' file (at 1 experience per 26,000 (as Top-1!) estimated units distributed)
FDA pilot study (at 1 experience per 250 (as Top-1!) person-brand used cosmetics)

SKIN BLEACHING AGENTS

25.39   Skin bleaching agents are applied to the skin of the face and other parts of the body for depigmentation of hyperpigmented lesions, usually for a relatively long period of time. Some of these products are also known as 'summer freckles cream'; the active ingredients in both preparations are the same. Most skin bleaching creams also contain a sunscreen (UV-B absorber) in order to prevent repigmentation of the treated skin. The compounds used in skin bleaching creams are listed in Table 25.41.

25.40   A typical formula of a **skin bleaching cream** is:

Ingredients:		*Example:*
40–70%	water	*water*
ca 5%	polyol	*sorbitol*
30–50%	lipid	*olive oil, lanolin, decyl oleate*
2–5%	surfactant	*TEA-coco hydrolyzed animal protein, TEA oleate*
1–5%	skin bleaching agent	*hydroquinone*
ca 2%	UV-B absorber	*amyldimethyl-PABA*
0.3%	preservative	*methylparaben, dehydroacetic acid*
0.2%	perfume	*perfume*

25.41   **Skin bleaching agents**

ammoniated mercury (prohibited in most countries)	nicotinic acid
ascorbic acid	sodium bisulfite
ascorbyl palmitate	sodium hydrosulfite
ascorbyl-3-phosphate	sodium hypochlorite (may be tested in 0.5% aqua [38])
hydrogen peroxide	sodium metabisulfite
hydroquinone	
monobenzyl ether of hydroquinone	zinc formaldehyde sulfoxylate (Rongalite®)
niacinamide	zinc peroxide

25.42   **Incidence of side effects: Facial skin bleach products** (see § 20.17)

	% of total	
US manufacturers' file:	1.9	(157/8399)
US hospitals' file:	no data available	
FDA pilot study:	no data available	
Spanish file:	0	(0/210)
Dutch file:	0	(0/202)
British consumers' report:	no data available	
Strassburg study:	0	(0/96)

25.43   **Risk index: Facial skin bleach products** (see § 20.18)

Facial skin bleach products are graded as *high-risk* cosmetics according to the following report:
US manufacturers' file (at 1 experience per 55,000 (!) estimated units distributed).

NB: Skin bleaching cosmetics belong to the 'Top-2' most risky cosmetics. This is particularly due to the skin bleaching ingredient hydroquinone.

Side effects of ingredients of skin bleaching agents are tabulated in § 25.44 (contact allergy) and § 25.45 (other side effects).

25.44   **Contact allergy to ingredients of skin bleaching agents**

Ingredient	Patch test conc. & vehicle (§ 5.2)	Cross-reactions (§ 5.5)	Comment	Ref.
ammoniated mercury	1–2% pet.	*see also* § 5.7 *and* § 25.45	Formerly used for the treatment of psoriasis	36
hydroquinone	1% pet.		*See also* § 25.45 *and* § 5.44	3 52 62
monobenzyl ether of hydroquinone (monobenzone)	1% pet.	p-hydroxybenzoic acid ester, bisphenol-A, diethylstilbestrol (?)	Patch test sites have become depigmented *See also* § 5.42 *and* § 25.45	51 6 17

25.45   **Other adverse reactions to ingredients of skin bleaching agents**

Ingredient	Adverse reactions	Comment	Ref.
ammoniated mercury	nephrotic syndrome	Systemic absorption has been studied by Barr et al. [5]	4
	chronic mercury poisoning (for symptoms and signs of mercury poisoning, *see* § 16.56)	Topical use of ammoniated mercury containing drugs has caused pigmentation of the skin (§ 10.1) *See also* § 25.44	60
hydroquinone	irritant dermatitis	Especially with higher concentrations (4–5%)	52 3
	ochronosis	*See also* § 25.44	19 82 83

(continued)

(continuation)

Ingredient	Adverse reactions	Comment	Ref.
	brown discoloration of the nails		84
	pigmented colloid milium		19
			83
	leukoderma		78
monobenzylether of hydroquinone (monobenzone)	irritant dermatitis	*See also* § 5.42 *and* § 25.44	51
	leukoderma		79
monomethyl ether of hydroquinone	leukoderma		80

DEODORANT–ANTIPERSPIRANT

25.46   The use of deodorant-antiperspirants has considerably increased during the last twenty years. In particular the underarm-deo is very popular. Feminine hygiene deodorants ('intimate sprays') were popular some years ago, but they have lost their popularity nowadays, because serious side effects have occurred from their use.

25.47   Deodorant-antiperspirant products are available as *aerosols* (or *pumpsprays*), as viscous liquids *(lotion, roller)* and as *solid sticks*. They often contain one or more of the following active ingredients:

A: **Antiperspirant agents**
 – alcloxa (aluminum chlorohydroxy allantoinate)
 – aldioxa (aluminum dihydroxy allantoinate)
 – aluminum chloride
 – aluminum chlorohydrate
 – aluminum chlorohydrex
 – aluminum zirconium chlorohydrates
 – buffered aluminum sulfate
 – hexamine
 – sodium aluminum chlorohydroxylactates

B: **Anticholinergic agents**
 – propantheline bromide
 – scopolamine bromide
N.B. Anticholinergic agents are very rarely used in market products.

C: **Antimicrobials**
 – chlorhexidine digluconate
 – dichlorophene
 – hexachlorophene
 – triclocarban
 – triclosan

D: **Odor eliminators**
 – citronellyl senecionate (Sinodor®)
 – zinc ricinoleate

E: **perfume;** to mask minor residues of malodor

25.48 Deodorant-antiperspirant

25.48   The following typical formulas will illustrate most types of market products:

Aerosol antiperspirant

Ingredients:		*Example:*
ca 90%	propellant	*chlorofluorocarbon 11 and 12*
ca 10%	concentrate:	
	– ca 30% antiperspirant	*aluminum chlorohydrate*
	– ca 60% carrier liquid	*isopropyl myristate*
	– ca 3% anticaking agent	*quaternium-18 hectorite*
	– ca 1% perfume	*perfume*

Aerosol deodorant

Ingredients:		*Example:*
ca 80%	propellant	*butane, isobutane, chlorofluorocarbon 11*
ca 20%	concentrate:	
	– organic solvent	*ethanol*
	– carrier fluid	*propylene glycol*
	– antimicrobial	*triclosan*
	– perfume	*perfume*

Intimate spray

Ingredients:		*Example:*
ca 95%	propellants	*chlorofluorocarbon 11 and 12*
ca 5%	concentrate:	
	– ca 95% lipid carrier	*isopropyl myristate, wheat germ triglycerides*
	– 1–3% antimicrobial	*triclosan*
	– 1–2% perfume	*perfume*

Deo pumpspray

Ingredients:		*Example:*
5–30%	water	*water*
10–30%	alcohol	*ethanol*
5–15%	lipid	*decyl oleate*
ca 5%	surfactant	*sodium lauryl sulfate*
1– 3%	antimicrobial	*triclosan*
1– 2%	perfume	*perfume*

Deo roller or lotion/cream

Ingredients:		*Example:*
60–80%	water	*water*
ca 5%	polyol	*propylene glycol*
5–15%	lipid	*stearic acid, mineral oil, beeswax*
2– 5%	surfactant (non-ionic)	*polysorbate-40, sorbitan oleate*
ca 10%	antiperspirant	*alcloxa*
1– 3%	antimicrobial	*triclosan*
ca 0.5%	perfume	*perfume*

Deo stick

Ingredients:		*Example:*
ca 10%	ethanol	*ethanol*
ca 60%	polyol	*propylene glycol*
ca 5%	lipid	*stearic acid*
ca 8%	soap surfactant	*sodium stearate*
ca 0.5%	antimicrobial	*triclosan*
ca 10%	antiperspirant	*aldioxa*
ca 1.5%	perfume	*perfume*

25.49   **Incidence of side-effects: Deodorant-antiperspirant** (see § 20.17)

	% of total	
US manufacturers' file:	7.9	(663/8399)**
US hospitals' file:	4.3	(30/698)
FDA pilot study:	30.9	(182/589)*/**
Spanish study:	5.1	(10/210)
Dutch file:	7.9	(16/202)**
British consumers' report:	24.9	(156/626**
Strassburg study:	8.3	(8/96)**

*5   severe   ** one of the 'Top-6'
 11   moderate
164 mild
  2   not reported

25.50   **Risk index: Deodorant-antiperspirant** (see § 20.18)

Risk grading according to:
US manufacturers' file: *medium risk* (at 1 experience per 275,000 estimated units distributed).
FDA pilot study: *high risk* (at 1 experience per 250 (!) person-brand used cosmetics).

25.51   Feminine hygiene cosmetics

25.51   Incidence of side effects: Feminine hygiene cosmetics (see § 20.17)

	% of total	
US manufacturers' file:	0.9	(79/8399)
US hospitals' file:	4.3	(30/698)
FDA pilot study:	1.5	(9/589)*
Spanish study:	no data available	
Dutch file:	0	(0/202)
British consumers' report:	no data available	
Strassburg study:	no data available	

*0 severe
0 moderate
9 mild

25.52   Risk index: Feminine hygiene cosmetics (see § 20.18)

Feminine hygiene cosmetics are graded as *medium risk* cosmetics according to the following reports:
US manufacturers' file (at 1 experience per 215,000 estimated units distributed).
FDA pilot study (at 1 experience per 1200 person-brand used cosmetics).

25.53   Contact allergy to ingredients of deodorants, antiperspirants and feminine hygiene cosmetics

Ingredient	Use	Patch test conc. & vehicle (§ 5.2)	Cross-reactions (§ 5.5)	Comment	Ref.
atranorin	fragrance	1% pet., 0.1% acet.	fumarprotocetraric acid	Present in oak moss perfumes *See also* § 5.16 *and* § 23.47	15
benzethonium chloride*	antimicrobial	0.1% aqua	benzalkonium chloride	*See also* § 5.7	20
cetalkonium chloride	antimicrobial	0.1% aqua		*See also* § 5.7	49
chlorhexidine*	antimicrobial	1% aqua		*See also* § 5.7	20
chlorofluoro-carbon 11	propellant	pure	ethyl chloride (?)	*See also* § 5.22 under chlorofluoromethane *and* § 22.66 under aerosol propellants	55
chlorofluoro-carbon 12	propellant	pure	ethyl chloride (?)	*See also* § 5.22 under chlorofluoromethane *and* § 22.66 under aerosol propellants	55
dibutyl phthalate	vehicle	5–10% pet.	*not* to dimethyl and diethyl phthalate	*See also* § 5.22	50 95
evernic acid	fragrance	0.1% acet.		Present in oak moss perfumes *See also* § 5.16	15
fenticlor	antimicrobial	1–10% pet.		*See also* § 5.7, § 6.5 *and* § 22.65	9
formaldehyde	antiperspirant	2% aqua		*See also* § 5.7, § 22.7, § 24.12 *and* § 24.13	13

(continued)

(continuation)

Ingredient	Use	Patch test conc. & vehicle (§5.2)	Cross-reactions (§5.5)	Comment	Ref.
fumarproto-cetraric acid	fragrance	0.1% acet.	atranorin	Present in oak moss perfumes *See also* § 5.16 *and* § 23.47	15
glutaraldehyde	antimicrobial	1% aqua (not stable)	*not* to formaldehyde	*See also* § 5.7	31
glyceryl stearate	vehicle constituent	30% pet.		*See also* § 5.22	46
isopropyl myristate*	vehicle constituent	5% pet.		*See also* § 5.22	20
isostearyl alcohol	antimicrobial	5% alc.		The patients were sensitized by a Draize test with a pump-spray deodorant	93
lilial	fragrance	1% pet.		*See also* § 5.16	63
paraben	preservative	5% pet.		The patient has previously been sensitized to parabens in a corticosteroid cream *See also* § 5.7, § 13.40 *and* § 23.47	87
perfumes		*see* § 5.8			58
propantheline bromide	anticholinergic agent	1–5% aqua			24 71
propylene glycol	vehicle constituent	1% and 10% aqua		*See also* § 5.22	2
DL-α-tocopherol	antioxidant	0.1% o.o.		*See also* § 5.7 For patch testing, *see also* § 27.5.1	34 1
triclocarban	antimicrobial	1–2% pet.		*See also* § 5.7	2
triclosan	antimicrobial	1–2% pet.		*See also* § 5.7	57 94
zirconium compounds	antiperspirants	patch testing on normal skin is negative; 2–4% veh. (?) on skin, denuded of epidermis; also intra-dermal testing with sodium zirconium lactate 1/1000 and 1/10,000 aqueous		Has caused granulomatous skin reactions (*see also* § 4.8)	18 47

* in feminine hygiene cosmetics

BODY MAKE-UP

25.54 Body make-up is chiefly used at parties and during carnival time. It is applied over large surfaces of the skin (arms, legs, trunk) and therefore preferably formulated as fluids, such as fluid make-up.

A typical formula for **body paint** is:

Ingredients:		*Example:*
ca 75%	water	*water*
ca 15%	color pigment mixture (*see* facial make-up)	*titanium dioxide, iron oxides*
ca 2%	suspending agent	*magnesium aluminum silicate*
ca 1%	surfactant	*dioctyl sodium sulfosuccinate*
ca 0.3%	preservative	*quaternium-15*
ca 0.1%	perfume	*perfume*

25.55 **Incidence of side effects and risk index**

There are no data available for the incidence of side effects and the risk index for body make-up products. It can be assumed, however, that the risk index for body make-up products is the same as for facial make-up and eye make-up (these are classified as *medium-risk* cosmetics).

For side effects of ingredients of body make-up, see § 23.44.

SUN AND SOLARIA COSMETICS

25.56 Sun cosmetics are designated primarily to protect the human skin (white skin in particular) against harmful effects of sunlight, notably premature ageing of the skin, and the induction of premalignant and malignant skin lesions.

Until recently, attention had mainly been focused on protection against short-wave ultraviolet rays (UVB region: 290–320 nm), but in view of recent knowledge of skin photobiology, an increasing tendency is noticeable to extend the protection to the UVA region (320–400 nm) also.

25.57 The active protecting ingredients of sun cosmetics are the so-called 'sunscreens'. Sunscreens fall into two major classes:

1. *Chemical absorbers:* UV-absorbing compounds of organic synthetic nature. Such sunscreens are invisible, and therefore cosmetically elegant. A list of currently used sunscreens is provided in § 27.13. Usually these chemical absorbers are efficient only in the UVB region. The benzophenones, however, may provide protection against UV waves up to 360 nm. Special UVA absorbers are dianisoyl methane and 4-isopropyl dibenzoyl methane (in Eusolex 8021). Anthranilates absorb UVA up to 350 nm.

2. *Reflectors:* These include the white pigments titanium dioxide and zinc oxide, which are effective reflectors and scatterers of both ultraviolet (UVB/UVA) and visible radiation.

Though sunscreens containing reflectors are opaque, they may still have a reasonable cosmetic acceptability, provided care is taken to incorporate in the formulation coloring agents, which can be varied to suit the individual user. Other, less frequently used reflectors are red veterinary petrolatum, talc and iron oxide.

Sunscreens are also used to protect patients suffering from photosensitive dermatoses (§ 25.58). The use of appropriate absorbers or reflectors is an intrinsic part of the management of these affections. The absorption spectra of some sunscreens are listed in § 25.58.

25.58   **Absorption spectra of some sunscreens** [90]

Chemical (class)	Absorption spectrum (nm)	Maximum absorption (nm)
PABA (derivatives)	250–320	288
Salicylates		
homomenthyl salicylate	295–315	306
2-ethylhexyl salicylate	280–320	300
menthyl salicylate	270–330	
Anthranilates	322–350	340
Cinnamates		
2-ethylhexyl-p-methoxy-cinnamate	290–320	307–310
2-ethoxyethyl-p-methoxy-cinnamate	280–320	310
diethanolamine p-methoxy-cinnamate	280–310	285–290
Benzophenones		
oxybenzone	270–350	287–290
Camphor derivatives	280–320	
3-(4-methylbenzylidene)-2′-oxobornylidene camphor	280–315	300
3-(4-methylbenzylidene)-DL-camphor	280–315	300
3-(4-methylbenzylidene)camphor + 4-isopropyldibenzoylmethane	up to 370 nm	
Miscellaneous		
2-phenyl-benzimidazole-5-sulfonic acid	290–320	302
dibenzalazine	up to 330 nm	
digalloyl trioleate	270–320	300

Sun protective factor (SPF) values of various sunscreen classes are given in § 25.59 [98]. It should be appreciated that these values were obtained by indoor testing; the percentage of chemical, bases used, and other factors can influence these values.

25.59   SPF values of sunscreening agents:

PABA	4–8
PABA esters	6–10
Benzophenones	4–6
Cinnamates	4–6
Salicylates	2–6
Anthranilates	2–6
PABA esters-benzophenones	10–15

25.60 **Action spectra of various normal and abnormal responses of human skin to solar radiation** [22, 88]

Condition	Range of effectiveness wavelength (nm)	Maximum reaction (nm)
I. *Normal individuals*		
Sunburn reaction (solar)	290–320	305–307
Sunburn reaction (artificial light source)	250–320	250–
Immediate pigment darkening (IPD) or tanning reaction	320–700	340–380
Delayed tanning (melanogenesis)	290–480	290–320
II. *Photosensitivity*		
A. Phototoxic reaction		
Oral or internal (drugs)	300–400	320–380
Topical or external (drugs)	300–400	320–380
Phytophotodermatitis (plants)	320–400	320–360
Phototoxicity in chemically induced porphyria or hematoporphyrins	380–600	380–420
B. Photoallergic reaction		
Drug photoallergy (delayed hypersensitivity, topical, or systemic)	290–450	320–380
Certain solar urticarias (immediate hypersensitivity)	290–380	290–320 320–400
C. Persistent photosensitivity (persistent light reactions or actinic reticuloid	290–400	290–320
III. *Degenerative and neoplastic*		
Chronic actinic elastosis	290–400	290–320
Actinic keratosis	290–320	290–315
Basal cell epithelioma	290–320	290–315
Squamous cell carcinoma	290–320	290–315
Malignant melanoma (?)	290–320	290–315
IV. *Genetic and metabolic*		
Xeroderma pigmentosum	290–320	290–320
Albinism	290–400	290–320
Ephelides (freckles)	290–400	290–320
Erythropoietic porphyria	390–600	390–420
Erythropoietic protoporphyria	390–600	390–420
Porphyria cutanea tarda	390–600	390–420
Variegate porphyria	390–600	390–420
Vitiligo (macules)	290–320	290–315
Hartnup syndrome	290–320	
Cockayne's syndrome	290–320	
Darier-White disease	290–320	
Bloom's syndrome	290–320	
Rothmund-Thomson syndrome	290–320	
Hailey-Hailey disease	290–320	
V. *Nutritional*		
Kwashiorkor	290–400	
Pellagra	290–400	
VI. *Infections (viral)*		
Lymphogranuloma venereum	290–320	
Herpes simplex	290–320	

(continued)

(continuation)

Condition		Range of effectiveness wavelength (nm)	Maximum reaction (nm)
VII.	*Miscellaneous* (light and abnormal skin or diseases)		
	Hydroa aestivale	290–400 infrared	290–320
	Hydroa vacciniforme	290–400 infrared	290–320
	Polymorphous photodermatoses, including variants such as papular, plaques, papulovesicular and eczematous eruptions	290–400	290–320
	Disseminated superficial actinic porokeratosis	290–320	290–320
	Discoid lupus erythematosus	290–320	290–320
	Systemic lupus erythematosus	290–230	
	Dermatomyositis	290–320	
	Photosensitive eczema	290–320	

25.61   Sometimes ingredients are added to sun cosmetics for secondary (cosmetic) effects: artificial tanning, sun tan promotion, skin healing, skin moisturizing, insect repelling, local anesthesia. These effects may be obtained by the following compounds:

– dihydroxyacetone	artificial tanner
– walnut extract (Juglans regia)	artificial tanner
– juglon (5-hydroxy-1,4-naphthoquinone)	artificial tanner
– 5-methoxypsoralen	sun tan promoter
– allantoin	skin healing agent
– N,N-diethyl-m-toluamide	insect repellent
– benzocaine	local anesthetic
– lidocaine	local anesthetic
– moisturizing materials: *see* § 23.4	

In some sunscreens oil of bergamot or 5-methoxypsoralen (bergapten) is incorporated. The manufacturers claim that the formulations can stimulate a quick tanning response and subsequently the acquired tan can provide the possible advantages against the harmful effects of sunlight in the form of enhanced photoprotection resulting from the increased melanin pigment. However, the photoreactive 5-MOP is not only cytotoxic and phototoxic to melanocytes, but can also be highly mutagenic and carcinogenic to the epidermal melanocytes and keratinocytes. Therefore it is felt that the widespread use of these sunscreens may provoke unwanted effects similar to those seen in oral photochemotherapy (Ch. 18), notably the risk of cutaneous carcinoma to the normal human population. Their application should therefore be discouraged [88, 91, 92].

25.62   Sun cosmetics are available in various forms: milks/creams (most popular), oils, gels, lotions and aerosol foams. Typical formulas are:

Sun milk-cream

Ingredients:		*Example:*
40–75%	water	*water*
ca 5%	polyol	*propylene glycol*

(continued)

(continuation)

Ingredients:		*Example:*
15–30%	lipid	*lanolin, decyl oleate*
ca 2%	surfactant/emulsifier	*TEA lauryl sulfate*
1–8%	UV absorber	*4-isopropyl dibenzoylmethane*
		methyl benzylidene camphor
0–2%	reflectors	*titanium dioxide*
0–5%	secondary active agents	*allantoin*
ca 0.2%	preservative	*parabens, phenoxetol*
ca 0.1%	perfume	*perfume*

Sun oil

Ingredients:		*Example:*
ca 90%	lipid	*peanut oil, isopropyl myristate*
1–8%	UV absorber	*homomenthyl salicylate,*
		benzophenone 1
ca 0.05%	antioxidant	*Trolox C®*
ca 1%	perfume	*perfume*

Sun gel

Ingredients:		*Example:*
50–60%	water	*water*
ca 5%	polyol	*sorbitol*
ca 2%	thickener: gelling agent	*carbomer 914, TEA*
10–30%	organic solvent	*ethanol*
1–8%	UV absorber	*allantoin-PABA,*
		benzophenone 9
ca 0.05%	perfume	*perfume*
ca 0.2%	preservative	*DMDM hydantoin,*
		methyl-paraben

Sun lotion

Ingredients:		*Example:*
60–95%	water	*water*
10–40%	alcohol	*ethanol*
10–20%	polyol	*glycerol*
5–10%	lipid	*glyceryl stearate, oleic acid*
ca 2%	surfactant: emulsifier	*sodium lauryl sulfate*
1–8%	UV absorber	*amyldimethyl-PABA*
ca 0.2%	preservative	*bromonitropropanediol*
ca 0.1%	perfume	*perfume*

Sun aerosol foam

Ingredients:		*Example:*
ca 10%	propellant	*chlorofluorocarbon 12 & 14*
ca 90%	concentrate:	
	– ca 70% water	*water*
	– ca 5% polyol	*propylene glycol*
	– ca 20% lipid	*acetylated lanolin, stearic acid*
	– ca 2% surfactant:	*TEA lauryl sulfate*
	emulsifier	*polysorbate 40*
1–5%	UV absorber	*2-phenyl-5-methylbenzoxazole, guanine*
ca 1%	other active agents	*polyamino sugar condensate, sodium lactate, dihydroxyacetone*
ca 0.2%	preservative	*quaternium-15, o-phenylphenol*
ca 0.1%	perfume	*perfume*

After sun milk/cream

Ingredients:		*Example:*
40–70%	water	*water*
ca 5%	polyol	*sorbitol*
10–30%	lipid	*lanolin oil, wheat germ glycerides*
2–5%	surfactant: emulsifier	*sodium lauryl sulfate*
ca 2%	moisturizer	*collagen*
ca 2%	skin healing agent	*allantoin*
0–0.5%	local anaesthetics	*benzocaine*
0.2%	preservative	*methylparaben, propylparaben*
0.1%	perfume	*perfume*

Solaria oils are used to prevent drying of the skin from solaria treatments: they contain a UV absorber, and rarely a tanning promoter.

Solaria oil

Ingredients:		*Example:*
ca 98%	lipid	*isopropyl palmitate, caprylic/capric triglyceride*
ca 2%	UV absorber	*methylbenzylidene camphor*
0–75 ppm	UVA tanning promoter	*5-methoxypsoralen*
ca 0.05%	antioxidant	*butylated hydroxyanisole*

25.63   **Side effects of topical sunscreens** include:

1. irritant dermatitis [40]
2. phototoxic dermatitis (though this seems rather paradoxic); see Chapter 6
3. photoallergic dermatitis; see Chapter 6

4. allergic contact dermatitis.
Sunscreens that have caused contact allergy are listed in § 25.66.

25.64   Incidence of side effects: Topical sunscreens (see § 20.17)

	% of total	
US manufacturers' file:	2.1	(174/8399)
US hospitals' file:	0.7	(5/698)
FDA pilot study:	0.9	(5/589)*
Spanish study:	0	(0/210)
Dutch file:	3.0	(6/202)
British consumers' report:	no data available	
Strassburg study:	2.1	(2/96)

*0 severe
 0 moderate
 5 mild

25.65   Risk index: Topical sunscreens (see § 20.18)

Risk grading according to:
US manufacturers' file: *medium risk* (at 1 experience per 216,000 estimated units distributed).
FDA pilot study: *low risk* (at 1 experience per more than 5000 person-brand used cosmetics).

25.66   Contact allergy to topical sunscreens

Drug	Patch test conc. & vehicle (§ 5.2)	EFS (§ 5.4)	Cross-reactions (§ 5.5)	Comment	Ref.
p-aminobenzoic acid (PABA)	5% pet. 1% alc.	3	paraphenylene diamine, procaine, sulfonamides, azo-dyes and other para-compounds	Stains light-colored fabrics Has caused photosensitivity (§ 6.5); systemic eczematous contact-type dermatitis (§ 17.2)	14 29
amyl(isoamyl)-N-dimethyl p-amino-benzoic acid	1–5% pet.	4		Has caused phototoxic reactions (§ 6.5) Has caused burning after sun exposure	33 10 7
benzotriazole derivatives	5% pet.	4		*See also under* drometrizole	30
benzyl salicylate	2% pet.	3		*See also* § 5.16	32
digalloyl trioleate	3.5% pet.	4		Has caused photosensitivity (§ 6.5)	43
dioxybenzone	2% pet.	3	oxybenzone		39
drometrizole	5% pet.	4		UV-absorber in nail varnish in the reported case *See also* § 24.12 *and* § 23.47 *under* 2-(2'-hydroxy-5'-methylphenyl)-benzotriazole *See also under* benzotriazole derivatives	73

(continued)

(continuation)

Drug	Patch test conc. & vehicle (§ 5.2)	EFS (§ 5.4)	Cross-reactions (§ 5.5)	Comment	Ref.
2-ethoxyethyl-p-methoxycinnamate	1% pet.	4	balsam Peru, benzyl cinnamate, methyl cinnamate, cinnamyl alcohol	Has caused photosensitivity (§ 6.5)	12
Eusolex 8021®	2% m.o.	4		Eusolex 8021® is a mixture of 3-(4-methylbenzylidene) camphor and 4-isopropyl-dibenzoylmethane Eusolex 8021® was the sunscreen in a moisturizing cream in the reported case	59
glyceryl-p-amino-benzoate	1.5%–5% pet.	3	benzocaine, other para-compounds (?)	Has caused photosensitivity (§ 6.5)	28 11 44
glyceryl-3-(glyceroxy)-anthranilate	5–10% pet.	4		UVA filter in Contralume Cream®	56
homomenthyl salicylate	2% o.o. 5% pet.	4		Has caused a follicular eruption	42
2,2′-dihydroxy-4-methoxy-benzophenone (benzophenone-8)	2% pet.	4			81
3-(4′-methylbenzylidene) camphor (Eusolex 6300®)	2% pet.	4		*See also under* Eusolex 8021®	85
methyl salicylate	2% o.o.	4?		Patch test sensitization may occur *See also* Chapter 17 *under* salicylic acid	21
oxybenzone (benzophenone-3)	2% pet.	4	dioxybenzone	Has caused photoallergy (§ 6.5, *under* 2-hydroxy-4-methoxy-benzophenone)	39 53
phenyl salicylate	2% pet.	3		Also in cosmetics, mouth washes, toothpaste (§ 13.3) and lip salve (§ 23.53)	27
sulisobenzone (benzophenone-4)	5% aqua 5–10% pet.	3		Also immediate-type urticarial reaction (§ 7.5)	41 80

Contact allergic reactions to commercial sunscreens are not always caused by the UV-absorber; vehicle ingredients which have caused contact allergy include triethanolamine stearate [65] and tertiary butyl alcohol [66].

SPORT AND MASSAGE OILS

25.67   Sport and massage oils and liniments (emulsions) are mainly smooth lipid mixtures, to which rubefacients and counterirritants are added. Typical formulas are:

Sport massage oil

Ingredients:		*Example:*
ca 80–90%	lipid	*mineral oil, isopropyl myristate*
0.5–5%	rubefacient-counterirritant	*glycol salicylate, methyl nicotinate*
0.05%	perfume	*perfume*

Massage liniment

Ingredients:		*Example:*
ca 40–50%	water	*water*
ca 30%	lipid	*caprylic/capric triglyceride, decyl oleate*
ca 2%	surfactant	*sodium lauryl sulfate*
0.5–5%	rubefacient-counterirritant	*ammonia, capsicum oleoresin, camphor*
0.05%	perfume	*pine oil*

Sport massage aerosol

Ingredients:		*Example:*
ca 60%	propellants	*chlorofluorocarbon 11 & 12*
ca 40%	concentrate:	
	– ca 60% solvent	*isopropyl alcohol*
	– ca 35% lipid carrier	*isopropyl myristate*
	– ca 5% rubefacient-counterirritant	*methyl nicotinate, methyl salicylate, arnica extract*
	– ca 0.05% perfume	*camphor oil, pine needle oil*

25.68   The following counterirritants and rubefacients are frequently used in sport massage products:

ammonia	methyl nicotinate
arnica extract	methyl salicylate
camphor oil	pine oil
capsicum oleoresin	rosemary extract
cajuput oil	turpentine
glycol salicylate	

25.69   Side effects

There are no data available for the *incidence of side effects* and the *risk index* for sport and massage cosmetics. Contact allergy to chloracetamide in a body massage cream has been reported [67].

FOOT COSMETICS

25.70 Foot care products have one or more of the following properties: refreshing, antipruritic, callus-softening, deodorizing and antiperspirant, cleansing, moisture absorbing, antiseptic or antifungal.

Various types of products are available: powders, tablets, creams, lotions, aerosols.

25.71 Typical foot cosmetics formulas are:

Foot powder

Ingredients:		*Example:*
80–90%	powder base	*talc, kaolin, starch, boric acid*
0–10%	functional ingredients	*thymol, camphor, menthol, captan*
ca 0.1%	perfume	*pine needle oil*

Foot cream

Ingredients:		*Example:*
40–60%	water	*water*
ca 5%	polyol	*glycerol*
20–40%	lipid	*glyceryl stearate, cetyl alcohol*
ca 2%	surfactant	*TEA lauryl sulfate, polysorbate 20*
0–10%	functional ingredients	*zinc oxide, zinc undecylenate, menthol, alcloxa*
ca 0.2%	preservative	*methylparaben, propylparaben*
ca 0.1%	perfume	*camphor oil*

Foot aerosol

Ingredients:		*Example:*
ca 40%	propellant	*chlorofluorocarbon 11 & 12*
ca 60%	concentrate:	
	– ca 1% functional ingredient	*dichlorophene, triclosan, aluminum chlorohydrate*
	– ca 5% lipid carrier	*isopropyl myristate*
	– 0–10% polyol	*propylene glycol*
	– ca 80% solvent	*ethanol*
	– ca 2% surfactant	*laureth 4*
	– ca 0.1% perfume	*perfume*

25.71　Foot cosmetics

Foot tablet (for foot bath)

Ingredients:		*Example:*
ca 20%	CO_2-generating ingredients	*sodium bicarbonate, citric acid anhydrous*
ca 10%	oxygen-generating salts	*sodium perborate*
10–50%	salts	*magnesium sulfate, sodium chloride*
ca 0.5%	color	*CI 45350 (DC Yellow 8)*
ca 1%	perfume	*pine needle oil*
ca 2%	surfactant	*laureth 4*

25.72　Examples of other typical functional ingredients for foot cosmetics are:

alcloxa	(antiperspirant)	methyl salicylate	(herbal fragrance)
aldioxa	(antiperspirant)	paraben: methyl-ethyl-propyl-butyl	(antimicrobial)
allantoin	(skin-healing agent)	phenol	(antipruritic, antimicrobial)
aluminum chloride	(antiperspirant)		
aluminum chlorohydrate	(antiperspirant)	pine oil	(herbal fragrance)
aluminium hydroxide	(antiperspirant)	salicylic acid	(callus-softening agent)
balsam Peru	(balsamic fragrance, antimicrobial)	sodium borate (borax)	(callus-softening agent)
benzalkonium chloride	(antimicrobial)	sodium perborate	(oxygen-releasing agent)
benzocaine	(antipruritic)		
boric acid	(antimicrobial)	sodium persulfate	oxygen-releasing agent)
camphor	(antipruritic, soothing)	sodium phosphate	(callus-softening agent)
captan	(antifungal)		
chlorhexidine digluconate	(antimicrobial)	sorbic acid	(antifungal)
chlorphenesin	(antifungal)	starch	(moisture absorber)
climbazol	(antifungal)	sulfur (colloidal)	(antifungal)
dehydroacetic acid (DHA)	(antifungal)	thymol	(antipruritic, herbal fragrance)
dichlorophene	(antimicrobial)	triclosan	(antimicrobial)
disodiummonoundecylen-amidomonoethanolamine sulfosuccinate	(antifungal)	undecylenamide diethanolamine	(antifungal)
hexachlorophene	(antimicrobial)	undecylenamide monoetlhanolamine	(antifungal)
kaolin	(moisture absorbent)		
lidocaine	(antipruritic)	undecylic acid	(antifungal)
menthol	(refreshing agent, antipruritic)	zinc oxide	(skin healing, antiphlogistic agent)
methenamine (hexamine)	(antimicrobial)	zinc undecylenate	(antifungal)

25.73   **Incidence of side effects: Foot cosmetics** (see § 20.17)

	% of total	
US manufacturers' file:	0.1	(11/8399)
US hospitals' file:	no data available	
FDA pilot study:	0	(0/589)
Spanish study:	0	(0/210)
Dutch file:	1.5	(3/202)
British consumers' report:	no data available	
Strassburg study:	0	(0/96)

25.74   **Risk index: Foot cosmetics** (see § 20.18)

Foot cosmetics are graded as *low risk* cosmetics according to the following reports:
US manufacturers' file (at 1 experience per 1,170,000 estimated units distributed)
FDA pilot study (at 1 experience per 1700 person-brand used cosmetics)

Contact allergy to Irgasan DP 300® in foot powder has been reported [94].

BARRIER CREAM

25.75   Barrier creams are used to protect the skin against corrosive agents during working conditions. Though mechanical protection of the hands by gloves is more effective, application of barrier creams is more convenient. Such creams should be easy to apply, and easily washed off at the end of the work. As the cream stays in contact with the skin for a long time, the ingredients should be carefully selected on minimal irritation in producing and developing effective barrier creams. Extensive testing is necessary to achieve optimal protection and performance.

25.76   Four main types of barrier creams with typical formulas are:

Cream barrier against dust

Ingredients:		*Example:*
ca 65%	water	*water*
ca 10%	polyol	*glycerol*
ca 20%	active barrier ingredient:	*stearic acid*
	solid lipid and zinc stearate	*zinc stearate*
ca 2%	surfactant: emulsifier	*sodium stearate*
ca 0.3%	preservative	*methylparaben, propylparaben, quaternium-15*
ca 0.05%	perfume	*perfume*

Cream barrier against organic solvents

Ingredients:		*Example:*
ca 50%	water	*water*
ca 2%	polyol	*glycerol*
ca 30%	active barrier ingredient:	*potassium stearate, sodium lauryl*
	soap surfactant, starch	*glutamate, starch*
ca 0.3%	preservative	*methylparaben, propylparaben,*
		phenoxetol
ca 0.05%	perfume	*perfume*

Cream barrier against aqueous solvents

Ingredients:		*Example:*
ca 65%	water	*water*
ca 2%	polyol	*glycerol*
ca 25%	active barrier ingredient:	*petrolatum, beeswax*
	semisolid lipid, silicones	*cyclomethicone*
ca 2%	surfactant	*sodium lauryl sulfate,*
		cocamidopropylbetaine
ca 0.3%	preservative	*bromonitropropanediol*
ca 0.05%	perfume	*perfume*

Ointment (anhydrous type) barrier against aqueous solvents

Ingredients:		*Example:*
ca 99%	active barrier ingredient:	*petrolatum, squalane, beeswax*
	semisolid lipid, zinc stearate	*zinc stearate*
ca 0.05%	antioxidant	*ascorbyl palmitate*
ca 0.05%	perfume	*perfume*

25.77   Barrier creams are advocated as a practical means to prevent the occurrence of (irritant as well as allergic) industrial dermatoses. The invisible protecting glove effect, produced when the cream is applied properly, should prevent the penetration of noxious substances, and facilitate the washing process. The requirements of barrier creams were discussed in detail by Schneider et al. [45]. The usefulness of these creams is still in doubt. The layer formed on the skin by the cream is very thin, and the quantity of protective material is generally insufficient, as compared with the amount of deleterious substance against which it should protect the skin. Besides, part of the applied protective substance gets lost by friction and perspiration. Furthermore, the oily layer might even facilitate the penetration of substances into the epidermis! Thus, the protection offered by barrier creams seems to be small. On the other hand, organic solvents may damage the natural skin barrier by the extraction of epidermal lipids, thus promoting penetration of toxic and allergenic substances. In such circumstances lipid-containing barrier creams might provide a substitute for the lost natural lipids, reestablishing the skin barrier function.

The interest in barrier creams increased with the introduction of silicone oils after the Second World War. However, from the results of a comparative study Herrmann [26] concluded that barrier creams containing silicone oil did not have advantages over those without these oils.

Patch tests with barrier creams under occlusion may cause false positive irritant reactions. This is due to the surfactant fraction. Patch tests with separate ingredients are to be preferred.

25.78   Side effects

There are no data available on the *incidence of side effects* and *risk index* for barrier creams.

Contact allergy to parabens in a barrier cream has been reported [96].

25.79   REFERENCES

1. Aeling, J. L., Panagotacos, P. J. and Andreozzi, R. J. (1973): Allergic contact dermatitis to vitamin E in aerosol deodorant. *Arch. Derm., 108*, 579.
2. Ägren-Jonsson, S. and Magnusson, B. (1976): Sensitization to propantheline bromide, trichlorocarbanilide and propylene glycol in an antiperspirant. *Contact Dermatitis, 2*, 79.
3. Arndt, K. A. and Fitzpatrick, T. B. (1965): Topical use of hydroquinone as a depigmenting agent. *J. Amer. med. Ass., 194*, 965.
4. Barr, R. D., Rees, P. H., Cordy, P. E., Kungu, A., Woodger, B. A. and Cameron, H. M. (1972): Nephrotic syndrome in adult Africans in Nairobi. *Brit. med. J., 2*, 131.
5. Barr, R. D., Woodger, B. A. and Rees, P. H. (1973): Levels of mercury in urine correlated with the use of skin lightening creams. *Amer. J. clin. Path., 59*, 36.
6. Bentley-Phillips, B. and Bayler, M. A. H. (1975): Cutaneous reactions to topical application of hydroquinone. *S. Afr. med. J., 49*, 1391.
7. Blank, H. (1971): Immediate cutaneous reactions to sunscreens. *Arch. Derm., 103*, 461.
8. Calnan, C. D. (1962): Contact dermatitis from drugs. *Proc. roy. Soc. Med., 55*, 39.
9. Calnan, C. D. (1975): Dihydroxydichlorodiphenylmonosulphide in a deodorant. *Contact Dermatitis, 1*, 127.
10. Calnan, C. D. (1980): Amyldimethylaminobenzoic acid causing lipstick dermatitis. *Contact Dermatitis, 6*, 233.
11. Caro, I. (1978): Contact allergy/photoallergy to glycerol PABA and benzocaine. *Contact Dermatitis, 4*, 381.
12. Cronin, E. (1980): Photosensitisers. In: *Contact Dermatitis*, pp. 102 and 454. Churchill Livingstone, Edinburgh.
13. Cronin, E. (1980): Cosmetics. In: *Contact Dermatitis*, p. 109. Churchill Livingstone, Edinburgh.
14. Curtis, G. H. and Crawford, P. F. (1951): Cutaneous sensitivity to monoglycerol para-aminobenzoate: cross-sensitization and bilateral eczematization. *Cleveland Clin. Quart., 18*, 35.
15. Dahlquist, I. and Fregert, S. (1980): Contact allergy to atranorin in lichens and perfumes. *Contact Dermatitis, 6*, 111.
16. Dick, D. C. and Adams, R. H. (1979): Allergic contact dermatitis from monosulfiram (Tetmosol) soap. *Contact Dermatitis, 5*, 199.
17. Dorsey, C. S. (1960): Dermatitic and pigmentary reactions to monobenzyl ether of hydroquinone. *Arch. Derm., 81*, 245.
18. Epstein, W. L. and Allen, J. R. (1964): Granulomatous hypersensitivity after use of zirconium-containing poison oak lotions. *J. Amer. med. Ass., 190*, 940.
19. Findlay, G. H., Morrison, J. G. L. and Simson, I. W. (1975): Exogenous ochronosis and colloid milium from hydroquinone bleaching creams. *Brit. J. Derm., 93*, 613.
20. Fisher, A. A. (1973): Allergic reactions to feminine hygiene sprays. *Arch. Derm., 108*, 801.
21. Fisher, A. A. (1973): The role of patch testing in allergic contact dermatitis. In: *Contact Dermatitis, 2nd Edition*, p. 33. Lea and Febiger, Philadelphia.
22. Fitzpatrick, T. B., Pathak, M. A. and Parrish, J. A. (1974): Protection of human skin against sunburn. In: *Sunlight and Man, Normal and Abnormal Photobiologic Responses*, p. 753. University of Tokyo Press, Tokyo.

373

23. Frosch, P. J. and Kligman, A. M. (1979): The soap chamber test, a new method for assessing the irritancy of soaps. *J. Amer. Acad. Derm., 1*, 35.
24. Hannuksela, M. (1975): Allergy to propantheline in an antiperspirant. *Contact Dermatitis, 1*, 244.
25. Hassing, J. H., Nater, J. P. and Bleumink, E. (1982): The irritancy of low concentrations of soap and synthetic detergents as measured by skin water loss. *Dermatologica (Basel), 164*, 314.
26. Herrmann, W. A. (1957): Barrier creams (1). *Acta derm.-venereol. (Stockh.), 37*, 276.
27. Hindson, C. (1980): Phenylsalicylate (Salol) in a lip salve. *Contact Dermatitis, 6*, 216.
28. Hjorth, N., Wilkinson, D., Magnusson, B., Bandmann, H. J. and Maibach, H. I. (1978): Glyceryl-p-aminobenzoate patch testing in benzocaine-sensitive subjects. *Contact Dermatitis, 4*, 4.
29. Horio, T. and Higuchi, T. (1978): Photocontact dermatitis from p-aminobenzoic acid. *Dermatologica (Basel), 156*, 124.
30. Joó, I. and Simon, N. (1974): Die Benzotriazolderivate als UV-Absorber. *Arch. derm. Forsch., 249*, 13.
31. Jordan, W. P., Dahl, M. V. and Albert, H. L. (1972): Contact dermatitis from glutaraldehyde. *Arch. Derm., 105*, 94.
32. Kahn, G. (1971): Intensified contact sensitization to benzylsalicylate. *Arch. Derm., 103*, 497.
33. Kaidbey, K. H. and Kligman, A. M. (1978): Phototoxicity to a sunscreen ingredient. *Arch. Derm., 114*, 547.
34. Minkin, W., Cohen, H. J. and Frank, S. B. (1973): Contact dermatitis from deodorants. *Arch. Derm., 107*, 775.
35. Muston, H. L., Boss, J. M. and Summerly, R. (1977): Dermatitis from Ammonyx LO, a constituent of a surgical scrub. *Contact Dermatitis, 3*, 347.
36. North American Contact Dermatitis Group (1973): Epidemiology of contact dermatitis in North America: 1972. *Arch. Derm., 108*, 537.
37. Nurse, D. S. (1980): Sensitivity to coconut diethanolamide. *Contact Dermatitis, 6*, 502.
38. Osmundsen, P. E. (1980): Contact dermatitis due to sodium hypochlorite. *Contact Dermatitis, 4*, 177.
39. Pariser, R. J. (1977): Contact dermatitis to dioxybenzone. *Contact Dermatitis, 3*, 172.
40. Parrish, J. A., Pathak, M. A. and Fitzpatrick, T. B. (1975): Facial irritation due to sunscreen products. *Arch. Derm., 111*, 525.
41. Ramsay, D. C., Cohen, H. J. and Baer, R. L. (1972): Allergic reaction to benzophenone. *Arch. Derm., 105*, 906.
42. Rietschel, R. L. and Lewis, C. W. (1978): Contact dermatitis to homomenthylsalicylate. *Arch. Derm., 114*, 442.
43. Sams, W. R. (1956): Contact photodermatitis. *Arch. Derm. Syph., 73*, 142.
44. Satulsky, E. M. (1950): Photosensitization induced by monoglycerol para-aminobenzoate. *Arch. Derm. Syph., 62*, 711.
45. Schneider, W., Tronnier, H. and Wagner, H. (1962): Protektiver Hautschutz. In: *Dermatologie und Venereologie Bd 1/2, 1070.* Editors: H. A. Gottron and W. J. Schönfeld. G. Thieme Verlag, Stuttgart.
46. Schwartzberg, S. (1961): Allergic eczematous contact dermatitis caused by sensitisation by glycerol monostearate. *Ann. Allergy, 19*, 402.
47. Shelley, W. B. and Hurley, H. J. (1958): The allergic origin of zirconium deodorants granulomas in man. *Brit. J. Derm., 70*, 75.
48. Shellow, W. V. R. and Rapaport, M. J. (1981): Comparison testing of soap irritancy using aluminum chamber and standard patch methods. *Contact Dermatitis, 7*, 77.
49. Shmunes, E. and Levy, E. J. (1972): Quaternary ammonium compound contact dermatitis from a deodorant. *Arch. Derm., 105*, 91.
50. Sneddon, I. B. (1972): Dermatitis from dibutylphtalate in an aerosol antiperspirant and deodorant. *Contact Dermatitis Newsl., 12*, 308.
51. Spencer, M. C. (1962): Leukoderma following monobenzyl ether of hydroquinone bleaching. *Arch. Derm., 86*, 615.
52. Spencer, M. C. (1965): Topical use of hydroquinone for depigmentation. *J. Amer. med. Ass., 194*, 962.
53. Thompson, G., Maibach, H. I. and Epstein, J. (1977): Allergic contact dermatitis from sunscreen preparations complicating photodermatitis. *Arch. Derm., 113*, 1252.
54. Thyresson, N., Lodin, A. and Nilzen, A. (1956): Eczema of the hands due to triethanolamine in cosmetic hand lotions for housewives. *Acta derm.-venereol. (Stockh.), 36*, 355.
55. Van Ketel, W. G. (1976): Allergic contact dermatitis from propellants in deodorant sprays in combination with allergy to ethylchloride. *Contact Dermatitis, 2*, 115.
56. Van Ketel, W. G. (1977): Allergic contact dermatitis from an aminobenzoic acid compound used in sunscreens. *Contact Dermatitis, 3*, 283.

57. Wahlberg, J. E. (1976): Routine patch testing with Irgasan DP 300. *Contact Dermatitis, 2*, 292.
58. Wishart, J. M. (1974): Generalized exfoliative dermatitis due to contact with an antiperspirant. *Brit. J. clin. Pract., 28*, 264.
59. Woods, B. (1981): Dermatitis from Eusolex 8021 sunscreen agent in a cosmetic. *Contact Dermatitis, 7*, 168.
60. Wüstner, H., Orfanos, C. E., Steinbach, K., Käferstein, H. and Herpers, H. (1975): Nagelverfärbung und Haarausfall. *Dtsch. med. Wschr., 100*, 1694.
61. Yaffee, H. S. (1978): Apricot allergy. *Schoch Letter, 28*, July, Item 46.

UPDATE – 2nd Edition

62. Romaguera, C. and Grimalt, F. (1983): Dermatitis from PABA and hydroquinone. *Contact Dermatitis, 9*, 226.
63. Larsen, W. G. (1983): Allergic contact dermatitis to the fragrance material lilial. *Contact Dermatitis, 9*, 158.
64. Suhonen, R. (1983): Chloracetamide - a hidden contact allergen. *Contact Dermatitis, 9*, 161.
65. Edwards, E. K. Jr. and Edwards, E. K. (1983): Allergic reaction to triethanolamine stearate in a sunscreen. *Cutis, 31*, 195.
66. Edwards, E. K. Jr. and Edwards, E. K. (1982): Allergic reaction to tertiary butyl alcohol in a sunscreen. *Cutis, 29*, 476.
67. Dooms-Goossens, A., Degreef, H., VanHee, J. et al. (1981): Chlorocresol and chloracetamide: Allergens in medications, glues and cosmetics. *Contact Dermatitis, 7*, 51.
68. Adams, R. M. (1981): Allergic contact dermatitis due to o-phenylphenol. *Contact Dermatitis, 7*, 332.
69. Tucker, W. F. G. (1983): Contact dermatitis to Eutanol G. *Contact Dermatitis, 9*, 88.
70. Alomar, A., Camarasa, J. G. and Barnadas, M. (1983): Addison's disease and contact dermatitis from mercury in a soap. *Contact Dermatitis, 9*, 76.
71. Gall, H. and Kempf, E. (1982): Kontaktallergie auf das lokale Antiperspirant Propanthelinbromid. *Dermatosen Beruf Umw., 30*, 55.
72. Mann, R. J. (1982): Benzoin sensitivity. *Contact Dermatitis, 8*, 263.
73. De Groot, A. C. and Liem, D. H. (1983): Contact allergy to Tinuvin® P. *Contact Dermatitis, 9*, 324.
74. Cooke, M. A. and Kurwa, A. R. (1975): Colophony sensitivity. *Contact Dermatitis, 1*, 192.
75. Rothenborg, H. W. and Hjorth, N. (1968): Allergy to perfumes from toilet soaps and detergents in patients with dermatitis. *Arch. Derm., 97*, 417.
76. Jordan, W. P. Jr. (1981): Contact dermatitis from D & C yellow 11 dye in a toilet bar soap. *J. Amer. Acad. Derm., 4*, 613.
77. Weaver, J. E. (1983): Dose response relationships in delayed hypersensitivity to quinoline dyes. *Contact Dermatitis, 9*, 309.
78. Fisher, A. A. (1982): Can bleaching creams containing 2% hydroquinone produce leukoderma? *J. Amer. Acad. Derm., 7*, 134.
79. Grojean, M. F., Thivolet, J. and Perrot, H. (1982): Leucomélanodermies accidentelles provoquées par les topiques dépigmentants. *Ann. Derm. Vénéréol. (Paris), 109*, 641.
80. Colomb, D. (1982): Dépigmentation en confettis après application de Leucodinine B^R sur un chloasma (Letter). *Ann. Derm. Vénéréol. (Paris), 109*, 899.
81. Eiermann, H. J., Larsen, W., Maibach, H. I. and Taylor, J. S. (1982): Prospective study of cosmetic reactions: 1977-1980. *J. Amer. Acad. Derm., 6*, 909.
82. Cullison, D., Abele, D. C. and O'Quinn, J. L. (1983): Localized exogenous ochronosis. Report of a case and review of the literature. *J. Amer. Acad. Derm., 8*, 882.
83. Findlay, G. H. (1982): Ochronosis following skin bleaching with hydroquinone. *J. Amer. Acad. Derm., 6*, 1092.
84. Mann, R. J. and Harman, R. R. M. (1983): Nail staining due to hydroquinone. *J. Amer. Acad. Derm., 6*, 1092.
85. Hunloh, W. and Goerz, G. (1983): Contact dermatitis from Eusolex^R 6300. *Contact Dermatitis, 9*, 333.
86. Langeland, T. and Nyrud, M. (1982): Contact urticaria to wheat bran bath: A case report. *Acta derm.-venereol. (Stockh.), 62*, 82.
87. Fisher, A. A. (1982): Cortaid cream dermatitis and the 'paraben paradox'. (Letter). *J. Amer. Acad. Derm., 6*, 116.
88. Pathak, M. A. (1982): Sunscreens: Topical and systemic approaches for protection of human skin against harmful effects of solar radiation. *J. Amer. Acad. Derm., 7*, 285.

89.   Fisher, A. A. (1982): Contact dermatitis from topical medicaments. *Semin. Derm., 1,* 49.

90.   Roelandts, R., VanHee, J., Bonamie, A. et al. (1983): A survey of ultraviolet absorbers in commercially available sun products. *Int. J. Derm., 22,* 247.

91.   Cartwright, L. E. and Walter, J. F. (1983): Psoralen-containing sunscreen is tumorigenic in hairless mice. *J. Amer. Acad. Derm., 8,* 830.

92.   Walter, J. F., Gange, R. W. and Mendelson, I. R. (1982): Psoralen-containing sunscreen induces phototoxicity and epidermal ornithine decarboxylase activity. *J. Amer. Acad. Derm., 6,* 1022.

93.   Aust, L. B. and Maibach, H. I. (1980): Incidence of human skin sensitization to isostearyl alcohol in two separate groups of panelists. *Contact Dermatitis, 6,* 269.

94.   Roed-Petersen, J., Auken, G. and Hjorth, N. (1975): Contact sensitivity to Irgasan DP 300. *Contact Dermatitis, 1,* 293.

95.   Calnan, C. D. (1975): Dibutyl phthalate. *Contact Dermatitis, 1,* 388.

96.   Husain, S. L. (1975): Sensitivity to parabens in Codella barrier cream. *Contact Dermatitis, 1,* 395.

97.   Adams, R. M. (1972): Photodermatitis from chlorophenylphenol. *Contact Dermatitis Neswl., 11,* 276.

98.   Rapaport, M. J. (1983): Sunscreening agents and sun protective factors. *Int. J. Derm., 22,* 293.

99.   Mathias, C. G. T. (1982): Pigmented cosmetic dermatitis from contact allergy to a toilet soap containing chromium. *Contact Dermatitis, 8,* 29.

26. Plant products in cosmetics

26.1   Plants and plant-products have been used in cosmetics for many centuries. They are still being used as such, both on rational and irrational grounds; it is sometimes difficult to distinguish between these two in the available literature. It is remarkable that reports on side effects caused by plant components of cosmetics, with the notable exception of fragrances, are rare.

This part of the book contains a review of plants ingredients of which, according to the literature, have been incorporated in cosmetic preparations.

Reports of side effects on the skin (though only in a few cases to plant products as part of cosmetics) have been listed. When plants are patch-tested, control tests are always necessary, as many plants may contain more or less toxic components.

The reader is also referred to Chapter 5 on contact allergy to fragrance materials and topical plant-derived substances, and § 27.7 on fragrance materials.

26.2   **Plants and cosmetics** (see for side effects § 26.3)

Name (common)	Species	Family
Aloë	*Aloe vera*	Liliaceae
Angelica	*Angelica officinalis*	Umbelliferae
Anise	*Pimpinella anisum*	Umbelliferae
Arnica	*Arnica montana*	Compositae
Artichoke	*Cynara scolymus*	Compositae
Balm mint	*Melissa officinalis*	Labiatae
Bergamot orange	*Citrus bergamia*	Rutaceae
Bistort	*Polygonum bistorta*	Polygonaceae
Butterbur	*Petasites hybrides*	Compositae
Caraway	*Carum carvi*	Umbelliferae
Carrot	*Daucus carota*, var. sativa	Umbelliferae
Chamomile	*Matricaria chamomilla*	Compositae
Chamomile	*Anthemis nobilis*	Compositae
Chinese cinnamon (cassia)	*Cinnamomum cassia*	Lauraceae
Clover blossom	*Trifolium pratense*	Papilionaceae
Coconut	*Cocos nucifera*	Palmae

(continued)

26.2 Plants and cosmetics

(continuation)

Name (common)	Species	Family
Coltsfoot	*Tussilago farfare*	Compositae
Comfrey	*Symphytum officinale*	Boraginaceae
Common horsetail	*Equisetum arvense*	Equicetaceae
Common speedwell	*Veronica officinalis*	Scrophulariaceae
Common tormentil	*Potentilla tormentilla*	Rosaceae
Coneflower	*Echinacea pallida*	Compositae
Corn flower	*Centaurea cyanus*	Compositae
Cucumber	*Cucumis sativus*	Cucurbitaceae
Cummin	*Cuminum cyminum*	Umbelliferae
Dandelion	*Taraxatum officinale*	Compositae
Dill	*Anetum graveolens*	Umbelliferae
Elder	*Sambucus nigra*	Caprifoliaceae
Elecampane	*Inula helenium*	Compositae
Fennel	*Foeniculum vulgare*	Umbelliferae
Fenugreek	*Trigonella foenum graecum*	Papilionaceae
Garlic	*Allium sativum*	Liliaceae
Ginger	*Zingiber officinalis*	Zingiberaceae
Ginseng	*Panax ginseng*	Araliaceae
Goat's rue	*Galega officinalis*	Papilionaceae
Goldenrod	*Solidago virgaurea*	Compositae
Great burdock	*Artium lappa*	Compositae
Great plantain	*Plantago major*	Plantaginaceae
Hawthorn	*Crataegus oxycantha*	Rosaceae
Hop	*Humulus lupulus*	Cannabaceae
Horse chestnut	*Aesculus hippocastanum*	Hippocastanaceae
Hyssop	*Hyssopus officinalis*	Labiatae
Indian corn	*Zea mays*	Gramineae
Ivy	*Hedera helix*	Araliaceae
Juniper	*Juniperus communis*	Cupressaceae
Knotgrass	*Polygonum aviculare*	Polygonaceae
Lemon	*Citrus limon*	Rutaceae

(continued)

(continuation)

Name (common)	Species	Family
Levant storax	*Liquidambar orientalis*	Hamamelidaceae
Lily	*Lilium candidum*	Liliaceae
Lovage	*Levisticum officinale*	Umbelliferae
Mallow	*Malva sylvestris*	Malvaceae
Marigold	*Calendula officinalis*	Compositae
Marshmellow	*Althea officinalis*	Malvaceae
Mays	*Zea mays*	Gramineae
Milfoil (= yarrow)	*Achillea millefolium*	Compositae
Mint	*Mentha piperita*	Labiatae
Mistletoe	*Viscum album*	Loranthaceae
Mossy stonecrop	*Sedum acre*	Crassulaceae
Mugwort	*Artemisia vulgaris*	Compositae
Myrtle	*Myrtus communis*	Myrtaceae
Nettle	*Urtica dioica*	Urticaceae
Oak	*Quercus*	Fagaceae
Parsley	*Petroselinum sativum*	Umbelliferae
Pellitory	*Parietaria officinalis*	Urticaceae
Pepper	*Piper nigrum*	Piperaceae
Red Pepper	*Capsicum annuum*	Solanaceae
Rhatany	*Krameria trianda*	Krameriaceae
Rocket	*Eruca sativa*	Cruciferae
Rosemary	*Rosmarinus officinalis*	Labiatae
Rue	*Ruta graveolens*	Rutaceae
Sage	*Salvia officinalis*	Labiatae
Savin	*Juniperus sabina*	Pinaceae
Sea weed	*Fucus vesiculosus*	Phaeophyceae
Shepard's purse	*Capsella bursa-pastoris*	Cruciferae
Silver birch	*Betula alba*	Betulaceae
Snake weed	*Polygonum bistorta*	Polygonaceae
Soapwort	*Saponaria officinalis*	Caryophyllaceae
St. John's wort	*Hypericum perforatum*	Hypericaceae

(continued)

26.2 Plants and cosmetics

(continuation)

Name (common)	Species	Family
Strawflower	*Helichrysum stoechas*	Compositae
Sunflower	*Helianthus annuus*	Compositae
Sweet bay, laurel	*Laurus nobilis*	Lauraceae
Sweet fennel	*Foeniculum*, var. dulce	Umbelliferae
Sweet flag	*Acorus calamus*	Araceae
Sweet meadow	*Spirea ulmaria* = *Filipendula ulmarea*	Rosaceae
Thyme	*Thymus vulgaris*	Labiatae
Traveller's joy	*Clematis vitalba*	Ranunculaceae
Walnut	*Juglans regia*	Juglandaceae
Watercress	*Nasturtium officinale*	Cruciferae
Water fennel	*Oenanthe phellandrium*	Umbelliferae
Wild thyme	*Thymus serpyllum*	Labiatae
Willow	*Salix*	Salicaceae
Witch hazel	*Hamamelis virginiana*	Hamamelidaceae
Wood sage	*Teucrium chamaedrys*	Labiatae
Yarrow (= milfoil)	*Achillea millefolium*	Compositae
Yellow gentian	*Gentiana lutea*	Gentianaceae
Yellow sweet clover	*Melilotus officinalis*	Papilionaceae

26.3 Side effects of some plants and plant products used in cosmetics

Species	Part of the plant	Frequency of use (§ 27.2)	Side effects reported (limited to skin and oral mucosa)	Ref.
Achillea millefolium	herb	88	Irritant dermatitis Allergic dermatitis	54 86
Acorus calamus	root		Contact allergy to calamus oil (?)	48
Aesculus hippocastanum	fruit	5	Dermatitis from ointment and pills containing 'horse chestnut extract compound' *See also* § 5.39 *under* esculin	67
Allium sativum	bulb		Allergic dermatitis Irritant dermatitis Photosensitization (?)	64 11 96 41 21

(continued)

(continuation)

Species	Part of the plant	Frequency of use (§ 27.2)	Side effects reported (limited to skin and oral mucosa)	Ref.
Aloe vera	leaf	95	Allergic dermatitis	87
Althea officinalis	root	11		
Anetheum graveolens	fruit		Plant causes phytophotodermatitis Carvone derived from oil of dill has caused contact allergy (§ 13.3)	73
Angelica officinalis	root		Contact allergy to angelica root and oil of angelica root May cause phototoxic dermatitis	51 32
Anthemis nobilis	herb	5	Allergic dermatitis to chamomile ointment Anaphylactic reaction to chamomile tea *See also* § 5.39	5 9 97 100
Arctium lappa	root		Irritant dermatitis Allergic dermatitis (?)	57
Arnica montana	herb	18	Irritant dermatitis Allergic dermatitis, caused by sesquiterpene lactones	6 79 36 101
Artemisia vulgaris	herb		'Weed dermatitis' Many species cause allergic dermatitis	54 66 50
Betula alba	leaf	54	Contact allergy to oleum betulae phototoxicity (?) Immediate contact allergy to birch leaves and sap (in scratch tests)	78 24 98
Calendula officinalis	flower	11	Irritant dermatitis from the plant and a tincture made from it	7
Capsella bursa-pastoris	herb		Seeds have vesicant and rubefacient properties	7
Capsicum annuum	fruit		Irritant dermatitis	84
Carum carvi	fruit		The plant is a photosensitizer Carvone in caraway oil has caused contact allergy (§ 13.3)	
Centaurea cyanus	flower			86 7
Cinnamonum cassia	leaf and twig		Irritant dermatitis and contact allergy from cinnamon oil (§ 5.16)	15
Cinnamonum zeylanicum	bark		Cinnamon bark oil Ceylon is a sensitizer due to cinnamic aldehyde	15
Citrullus vulgaris, (= citrullus colocynthis)	fruit		Colocynth in alcoholic hair tonics and brillantines has caused eczema	37

(continued)

26.3 Plant products in cosmetics

(continuation)

Species	Part of the plant	Frequency of use (§ 27.2)	Side effects reported (limited to skin and oral mucosa)	Ref.
Citrus bergamia	fruit		Phototoxicity and (photo)allergy from 5-methoxypsoralen	59 34
Citrus limon	fruit		Lemon juice has caused dermatitis Lemon oil is phototoxic	63
Clematis vitalba	leaf		Vesication, redness and ulcers from contact with the plant	74
Cocos nucifera	fruit		Caproic, caprylic and capric acids in coconut oil are skin irritants Soaps containing coconut oil have produced dermatitis Coconut oil is comedogenic (§ 9.2)	32
Crataegus oxycantha	flower, leaf			23
Cucumis sativus	fruit	19		7
Cuminum cyminum	fruit		Undiluted cumin oil is phototoxic	71
Cyanara scolymus	herb		Allergic dermatitis	31 89
Daucus carota, var. sativa	root	10	Irritant and allergic dermatitis from the plant, phototoxicity from carrot seed oil (?) Contact urticaria from carrots	48
Echinacea pallida			Allergic dermatitis	88
Equisetum arvense	stem	33		
Eruca sativa	herb		Allergic dermatitis and photodermatitis from taramira oil expressed from the seeds	7
Foeniculum vulgare	fruit	10	Contact allergy to oil of fennel Phytophotodermatitis from the plant	32 73
Hamamelis virginiana	leaf	147	Allergic contact dermatitis *See also* § 5.17	29
Hedera helix	leaf		Irritant dermatitis Allergic dermatitis	2 76
Helianthus annuus	seed		Allergic contact dermatitis	75
Humulus lupulus	flower	15	Allergic and irritant dermatitis 'Hoprash' in hop-pickers	10 18
Hypericum perforatum	flower ends, leaves, stem head	10	Dermatitis (irritant? allergic?)	25 45
Inula helenium	root		Inula oil (= alantroot oil = elecampane oil) contains alantolactone, which is a sensitizer (§ 5.40)	40

(continued)

(continuation)

Species	Part of the plant	Frequency of use (§ 27.2)	Side effects reported (limited to skin and oral mucosa)	Ref.
Juglans regia	nut		Allergic dermatitis from nutshell and wood	14 4 81
Juniperus communis	herb	13	Oil of juniper berries is irritant to the skin and the respiratory tract	77
Juniperus sabina	herb		Savin oil is toxic, due to sabinol The twigs cause inflammation of the skin	
Krameria triandra	root		Allergic dermatitis, also from topical preparations containing krameria	33
Laurus nobilis	leaf		Contact allergy Laurel oil is a sensitizer (§ 5.16)	103 26
Levisticum officinale	herb		Contact allergy to extracts of lovage	12 32
Liquidamber orientalis	exudate from trunk		Contact allergy to storax (§ 5.39)	
Matricaria chamomilla	flower heads	45	Allergic dermatitis *See also* § 5.39 *under* chamomile oil	68 97
Melilotus officinalis	flower ends		Alopecia due to dicoumarol	45 19
Melissa officinalis	leaf	15		
Mentha piperita	leaf		Contact allergy to oil of peppermint in perfumes and tooth pastes (§ 13.3)	13 35 32
Myrtus communis	leaf		Dermatitis (?)	29
Oenanthe phellandrium	seed		Irritant dermatitis	72
Parietaria officinalis	herb		Allergic contact dermatitis	70
Petasites hybrides	herb	3		
Petroselinum sativum	root		Irritant dermatitis Allergic dermatitis Contact allergy to oil of parsley used in perfumery Phytophotodermatitis (?) Urticaria, angioedema and shock	38 53 42 85 69 99
Pimpinella anisum	seed		Irritant and allergic reactions from oil of aniseed Oil of aniseed contains anethole	39 52 47
Piper nigrum	fruit		Black pepper oil is weakly phototoxic Diluted white pepper oil has caused contact allergy	1

(continued)

383

26.3 Plant products in cosmetics

(continuation)

Species	Part of the plant	Frequency of use (§ 27.2)	Side effects reported (limited to skin and oral mucosa)	Ref.
Plantago major	leaf		Allergic dermatitis from pollen	62 46
Polygonum aviculare	root		Contact dermatitis in 'susceptible' individuals	61
Quercus	bark		Allergic contact dermatitis Irritant dermatitis	93
Rosmarinus officinalis	leaf	40	Irritancy and allergic dermatitis from rosemary oil Photosensitivity from the oil	48 17 60
Ruta graveolens	herb		Irritant dermatitis Photodermatitis	32 27 95 104
			Allergic dermatitis (?)	49
Ruta montana	herb		Rue oil is phototoxic The plant yields 8-methoxypsoralen	73
Salix	bark		Allergic contact dermatitis from willow in propolis	90
Salvia officinalis	leaf	46	Cheilitis and stomatitis from sage tea	94
			Allergic contact dermatitis due to alantolactone	102
Sambucus nigra	flower		Leaves are irritant	55
Saussurea lappa	root		See § 5.16 Costus absolute is an active sensitizer Costus root oil causes contact allergy	65
Solidago virgaurea	herb		Irritant dermatitis Allergic dermatitis	82 88
Spirea ulmaria = *Filipendula ulmarea*	flower ends		Dermatitis not reported	58
Styrax benzoin	balsamic exsudate		Contact allergy to compound tincture of benzoin (§ 5.39, § 22.65, § 23.47 *and* § 25.9)	22
Symphytum officinale	root	5	Leaves have irritant properties	92
Taraxacum officinale	root		Allergic dermatitis	44
Thymus serpyllum	herb		Thyme oil has caused contact allergy in biogaze (§ 5.39)	

(continued)

(continuation)

Species	Part of the plant	Frequency of use (§ 27.2)	Side effects reported (limited to skin and oral mucosa)	Ref.
Thymus vulgaris	herb		Contact allergy to thymol	82
			Cheilitis and glossitis from tooth-paste containing thymol (§ 13.3)	8
			Irritant dermatitis	32
			Contact allergy to thyme oil (§ 5.39)	
			See also § 5.42 *under* biogaze	
Trifolium pratense	flower	24	'Urticaria or skin irritation'	28
Tussilago farfare	herb	37		
Urtica dioica	herb	29	Urtication of the skin	
Viscum album	plant	4	Has irritant properties	91
Zea mays	fruit	50	Irritant dermatitis in corn-pickers	16
			Contact dermatitis from corn flour	56
			Contact sensitivity to maize	80
			Contact urticaria from corn starch	
			Contact allergy to corn starch	
Zingiber officinalis	rhizome		Ginger oil is irritant and allergenic; weakly phototoxic	32

26.4   REFERENCES

1. Agrup, G. (1969): Hand eczema and other hand dermatoses in South Sweden. *Acta derm.-venereol. (Stockh.)*, *49, Suppl. 61*, 1.
2. Allen, P. H. (1943): Poisonous and injurious plants of Panama. *Amer. J. trop. Med., 23, Suppl. 3.*
3. Arctander, S. (1960): *Perfume and Flavor Materials of Natural Origin.* Published by the author, Elizabeth, N. J.
4. Barniske, R. (1957): Dermatitis bullosa, ausgelöst durch den Saft grüner Walnusschalen (Juglans regia L.). *Derm. Wschr., 135,* 189.
5. Beetz, D., Cramer, H. J. and Mehlhorn, H. Ch. (1971): Zur Häufigkeit der epidermalen Allergie gegenüber Kamille in kamillenhaltigen Arzneimitteln und Kosmetica. *Derm. Wschr., 157,* 505.
6. Beetz, D., Würbach, G. and Cramer, A. J. (1971): Allergenanalytische Untersuchungen mit Hilfe der Dünnschichtchromatographie bei Überempfindlichkeit gegenüber Arnika Tinctur. *Allergie u. Immunol. (Leipzig), 17,* 228.
7. Behl, P. N., Captain, R. M., Bedi, B. M. S. and Gupta, S. (1966): *Skin Irritant and Sensitizing Plants Found in India.* P. N. Behl, Irwin Hospital, New Delhi.
8. Beinhauer, L. G. (1940): Cheilitis and dermatitis. *Arch. Derm., 41,* 892.
9. Benner, M. and Lee, H. (1973): Anaphylactic reaction to chamomile tea. *J. Allergy clin. Immunol., 52,* 307.
10. Bettley, F. R. (1953): Hop dermatitis. *Brit. med. J., 2,* 512.
11. Bleumink, E. and Nater, J. P. (1973): Contact dermatitis to garlic: Cross reactivity between garlic, onion and tulip. *Arch. derm. Forsch., 247,* 117.
12. Calnan, C. D. (1969): Lovage sensitivity. *Contact Dermatitis Newsl., 5,* 99.
13. Calnan, C. D. (1970): Oils of Cloves, Laurel, Lavender, Peppermint. *Contact Dermatitis Newsl., 7,* 148.
14. Calnan, C. D. (1970): Avodiré wood sensitivity. *Contact Dermatitis Newsl., 8,* 190.
15. Calnan, C. D. (1970): Oil of cinnamon. *Contact Dermatitis Newsl., 8,* 181.
16. Coca, A. F., Walzer, M. and Thommen, A. A. (1931): *Asthma and Hayfever.* Charles C. Thomas, Springfield, Ill.

17. Collins, M. (1964): *Spices of the World Cookbook*. Mac Cormick, Baltimore.
18. Cookson, J. S. and Lawton, A. (1953): Hop dermatitis in Herefordshire. *Brit. med. J., 2*, 376.
19. Cornbleet, T. and Hoit, L. (1957): Alopecia from coumarin. *Arch. Derm., 75*, 440.
20. *CTFA Cosmetic Ingredients Dictionary* (1977): *2nd Edition*. Editor: N. Estrin. CTFA Inc., Washington DC, USA.
21. Cueva, J. and Duran, C. J. (1955): Dermatitis due to garlic. *Rev. med. Hosp. gen. (Méx.), 18*, 29.
22. Cullen, S. I., Tonkin, A. and May, F. E. (1974): Allergic contact dermatitis to compound tincture of benzoin spray. *J. Trauma, 14*, 348.
23. Duke-Elder, S. and Mac Faul, P. A. (1972): Injuries Part I: Mechanical Injuries. Extra-ocular foreign bodies (pp. 464-467) and Agricultural Injuries (pp. 32-34). In: *System of Ophthalmology, Vol. XIV*. Henry Kimpton, London.
24. Espersen, E. (1952): Berlocque dermatitis. A survey and a case. *Acta derm.-venereol. (Stockh.), 32*, Suppl. 29, 91.
25. Farmer, E. W. (1941): The patch test as means of diagnosis in contact dermatitis. *Med. J. Aust., 1*, 9.
26. Foussereau, J., Benezra, C. and Ourisson, G. (1967): Contact dermatitis from laurel. I and II. *Trans. St. John's Hosp. derm. Soc. (Lond.), 53*, 141 and 147.
27. Garat, B. R. et al (1948): Dermatitis bullosa, Striate dermatitis: 8 cases provoked by Ruta graveolens (Rue). *Rev. argent. Dermatosif., 32*, 15.
28. Gardner, C. A. and Bennetts, H. W. (1956): *The Toxic Plants of Western Australia*. West Australian Newspapers Ltd., Perth.
29. Genner, V. and Bonnevie, P. (1938): Eczematous eruptions produced by leaves of trees and bushes. *Arch. Derm. Syph., 37*, 583.
30. *Gids voor geneeskrachtige planten* (1979): Reader's Digest, Amsterdam.
31. Gougerot, H. and Seringe, J. (1936): Eczéma professionnel: par l'artichaut (?). *Bull. Soc. franç. Derm. Syph., 43*, 1463.
32. Greenberg, L. A. and Lester, D. (1954): *Handbook of Cosmetic Materials*. Interscience Publ. Inc., New York.
33. Grolnick, M. (1938): Dermatitis due to haemorrhoidal ointment containing Krameria and oil of Cade. *J. Amer. med. Ass., 110*, 951.
34. Harber, L. C., Holloway, R. M. and Moragne, M. (1964): Polymorphous light eruption, office diagnosis and management. *N.Y. State J. Med., 64*, 619.
35. Harry, R. G. (1948): *Cosmetic Materials, Vol. II*. Leonard Hill, London.
36. Hausen, B. M., Herrmann, H. D. and Willuhn, G. (1978): The sensitizing capacity of compositive plants, Part 1. *Contact Dermatitis, 4*, 3.
37. Haxthausen, H. (1930): Fall von Koloquinthekzem. *Derm. Wschr., 91*, 1391.
38. Heubschmann, K. and Cupik, J. (1941): Allergic dermatitis with small and large vesicles caused by parsley. *Derm. Wschr., 113*, 725, 744 and 766.
39. Hjorth, N. (1967): Toothpaste sensitivity. *Contact Dermatitis Newsl., 1*, 14.
40. Hjorth, N. (1970): Active sensitization with alantolactone. *Contact Dermatitis Newsl., 8*, 175 and 180.
41. Hjorth, N. and Roed-Petersen, J. (1976): Occupational protein contact dermatitis in food handlers. *Contact Dermatitis, 2*, 28.
42. Hjorth, N. and Weissman, K. (1972): Occupational dermatitis in chefs and sandwich makers. *Contact Dermatitis Newsl., 11*, 301.
43. Hutchinson, J. (1955): *British Wild Flowers*, Vol. I and Vol. II. Penguin Books Ltd. Harmondsworth, Middlesex.
44. Janke, D. (1950): Durch Löwenzahn (Taraxatum officinale) verursachtes Ekzem. *Hautarzt, 1*, 177.
45. Kingsbury, J. M. (1964): *Poisonous Plants of the United States and Canada*. Prentice-Hall Inc., Englewood Cliffs, New Jersey.
46. Kjaer, A. (1960): Naturally derived *iso* Thiocyanates (Mustard Oils) and their parent glucosides. In: *Progress in the Chemistry of Organic Natural Products, Vol. 18*, pp. 122-176. Editor: L. Zechmeister, Springer Verlag, Vienna.
47. Kjaer, A. (1969): The distribution of sulphur compounds. In: *Chemical Plant Taxanomy*, p. 453. Editor: T. Smain. Academic Press, London.
48. Klarmann, E. G. (1958): Perfume dermatitis. *Ann. Allergy, 16*, 425.
49. Klauder, J. V. and Kimmich, J. M. (1956): Sensitisation dermatitis due to carrots. *Arch. Derm., 74*, 149.
50. Kurz, G. and Rapaport, M. J. (1979): External/internal allergy to plants (Artemisia). *Contact Dermatitis, 5*, 407.
51. Larsen, W. G. (1975): Cosmetic dermatitis due to a perfume. *Contact Dermatitis, 1*, 142.

52. Loveman, A. B. (1938): Stomatitis venenata. Report of a case of sensitivity of the skin to oil of anise. *Arch. Derm. Syph., 37*, 50.
53. Luppi, A. and Bucchi, G. (1970): Epidemiological research on the morbosity in a rural district. Note III. A professional dermatosis in horticulture, from celery and parsley. *Igiene mod., 63*, 617.
54. Mackoff, S. and Dahl, A. O. (1951): A botanical consideration of the weed oleoresin problem. *Minn. Med., 34*, 1169.
55. Maiden, J. H. (1909): On some plants which cause inflammation or irritation of the skin. *Agric. Gaz. NSW, 20*, 111 and 1073.
56. Malten, K. E. (1970): Allergic contact dermatitis due to cattle fodder products. *Contact Dermatitis Newsl., 7*, 158.
57. Massey, A. B. (1941): Plant poisoning. *Merck Rep., 50*, 24.
58. McCord, C. P. (1962): The occupational toxicity of cultivated flowers. *Ind. Med. Surg., 31*, 365.
59. Meneghini, C. L., Rantuccio, F. and Lomuto, M. (1971): Additives, vehicles and active drugs as causes of delayed type allergic dermatitis. *Dermatologica (Basel), 143*, 137.
60. *Merck Index* (1976): 9th Edition. Merck and Co. Inc., Rahway, New Jersey.
61. Meunscher, W. C. (1951): *Poisonous Plants of the United States, 2nd Edition.* MacMillan Co., New York.
62. Michelson, H. E. (1936): Dermatitis due to pollen. *Arch. Derm. Syph., 33*, 897.
63. Minami, S. (1968): Dermatitis caused by lemons. *Jap. J. clin. exp. Med., 45*, 11.
64. Mitchell, J. C. (1980): Contact sensitivity to garlick (allium). *Contact Dermatitis, 6*, 356.
65. Mitchell, J. C. and Epstein, W. L. (1974): Contact hypersensitivity to a perfume material, costus absolute. The role of sesquiterpene lactones. *Arch. Derm., 110*, 871.
66. Mitchell, J. C., Geismann, T. A., Dupuis, G. and Towers, G. H. N. (1970): Allergic contact dermatitis caused by Artemisia and Chrysanthemum species. *J. invest. Derm., 56*, 98.
67. Mitchell, J. and Rook, A. (1979): *Botanical Dermatology*, p. 745. Greengrass Ltd., Vancouver.
68. Moslein, P. (1963): Pflanzen als Kontakt-Allergene. *Berufsdermatosen, 11*, 24.
69. Nielsen, B. E. (1970): *Coumarins of Umbelliferous Plants.* The Royal Danish School of Pharmacy, Copenhagen.
70. Noferi, A. (1970): Difficulties and limitations of specific hyposensitization in patients sensitized to Parientaria officinalis. *Folia allerg. (Roma), 17*, 256.
71. Opdijke, D. (1974): Monographs on fragrance raw materials. *Food Cosm. Toxicol., 12*, 807.
72. Pammel, L. H. (1911): *A Manual of Poisonous Plants*, pp. 476-477. Torch Press, Cedar Rapids, Iowa. Reprinted 1965 by Univ. Microfilms Inc., Ann Arbor, Michigan.
73. Pathak, M. A., Daniels, F. and Fitzpatrick, T. B. (1962): Presently known distribution of furocoumarins (Psoralens) in plants. *J. invest. Derm., 39*, 225.
74. Piffard, H. G. (1881): *A Treatise on the Materia Medica and Therapeutics of the Skin.* Wm Wood and Co., New York.
75. Rávnay, T. and Garazsi, M. (1955): Untersuchungen bezüglich Überempfindlichkeit gegenüber Blättern von Helianthus annuus (Sonnenblume). *Z. Haut- u. Geschlkr., 92*, 320.
76. Roed-Petersen, J. (1975): Allergic contact hypersensitivity to ivy (Hedera helix). *Contact Dermatitis, 1*, 57.
77. Rothe, A., Heine, A. and Rebohle, E. (1973): Wacholderbeeröl als Berufsallergen für Haut und Atemtrakt. *Berufsdermatosen, 21*, 11.
78. Rudzki, E. and Baranowska, E. (1974): Contact sensitivity in stasis dermatitis. *Dermatologica (Basel), 148*, 353.
79. Rudzki, E. and Grzywa, Z. (1977): Dermatitis from Arnica montana. *Contact Dermatitis, 3*, 281.
80. Schiefelin et al. (1973): *Almay Hypoallergenic Cosmetics Product Formulary, 8th Edition.* Pharmaceutical Laboratories Division, 5th Avenue, New York.
81. Schleicher, H. (1974): Über phytogene allergische Kontaktekzeme. *Derm. Mschr., 160*, 443.
82. Schwartz, L., Tulipan, L. and Birmingham, D. J. (1957): *Occupational Diseases of the Skin, 3rd Edition.* Lea and Febiger, Philadelphia.
83. Shellard, E. J. (1978): The use of plant products in modern cosmetics. Paper presented at the F.I.P. Congress, Cannes, France.
84. Smith Jr., J. G., Crounse, R. G. and Spence, D. (1970): The effects of capsicain on human skin, liver and epidermal lysosomes. *J. invest. Derm., 54*, 170.
85. Stransky, L. and Tsankov, N. (1980): Contact dermatitis from parsley (Petroselium). *Contact Dermatitis, 6*, 233.
86. Thune, P. O. and Solberg, Y. J. (1980): Photosensitivity and allergy to aromatic lichen acids, compositae oleoresins and other plant substances. *Contact Dermatitis, 6*, 81.

87. Touton, K. (1926): In: *Jadassohn's Handbuch der Haut- und Geschlechtskrankheiten. Vol. 4, Pt. I.,* Springer, Berlin.

88. Underwood, G. B. and Gaul, L. E. (1948): Overtreatment dermatitis in dermatitis venenata due to plants. *J. Amer. med. Ass., 138,* 579.

89. Von Schneider, G. and Thiele, Kl. (1974): Eigenschaften und Bestimmung der Artischoken-Bitter-stoffen, Cynaropicrin. *Planta med. (Stuttg.), 25,* 149.

90. Wanscher, B. (1976): Contact dermatitis from propolis. *Brit. J. Derm., 94,* 451.

91. Watt, J. M. and Breyer-Brandwijk, M. G. (1962): *The Medicinal and Poisonous Plants of Southern Africa, 2nd Edition.* E. and S. Livingstone, Edinburgh.

92. Woods, B. (1962): Irritant Plants. *Trans. St. John's Hosp. derm. Soc. (Lond.), 48,* 75.

93. Woods, B. and Calnan, C. D. (1976): Toxic woods. *Brit. J. Derm., 94, Suppl. 13.*

94. Zakon, S. J., Goldberg, A. L. and Khan, J. B. (1947): Lipstick cheilitis: a common dermatosis: Report of 32 cases. *Arch. Derm. Syph., 56,* 499.

UPDATE – 2nd Edition

95. Heskel, N. S., Amon, R. B., Storrs, F. J. and White, C. R. Jr. (1983): Phytophotodermatitis due to Ruta graveolens. *Contact Dermatitis, 9,* 278.

96. Campolmi, P., Lombardi, P., Lotti, T. and Sertoli, A. (1982): Immediate and delayed sensitization to garlic. *Contact Dermatitis, 8,* 352.

97. Van Ketel, W. G. (1982): Allergy to Matricaria chamomilla. *Contact Dermatitis, 8,* 143.

98. Lahti, A. and Hannuksela, M. (1980): Immediate contact allergy to birch leaves and sap. *Contact Dermatitis, 6,* 464.

99. Kauppinen, K., Kousa, M. and Reunala, T. (1980): Aromatic plants – A cause of severe attacks of angio-edema and urticaria. *Contact Dermatitis, 6,* 251.

100. Benner, M. and Lee, H. (1973): Anaphylactic reaction to chamomile tea. *J. Allergy clin. Immunol., 52,* 307.

101. Hausen, B. M. (1978): Identification of the allergens of *Arnica montana* L. *Contact Dermatitis, 4,* 308.

102. Sertoli, A., Fabbri, P., Campoli, P. and Panconesi, E. (1978): Allergic contact dermatitis to *Salvia Officinalis, Inula Viscosa* and *Conyza Bonariensis. Contact Dermatitis, 4,* 314.

103. Foussereau, J., Muller, J. C. and Benezra, C. (1975): Contact allergy to *Frullania* and *Laurus Nobilis:* cross-sensitization and chemical structure of the allergens. *Contact Dermatitis, 1,* 223.

104. Gawkrodger, D. J. and Savin, J. A. (1983): Phytophotodermatitis due to common rue (*Ruta graveolens*). *Contact Dermatitis, 9,* 224.

27. Tabulation of ingredients of cosmetics

27.1   In this chapter, tabulations are given of the following groups of ingredients of cosmetics:
- Antimicrobials and antioxidants (§ 27.5)
- Fragrance materials (§ 27.7)
- Colors (§ 27.9–11)
- Sunscreens (§ 27.13)
- Lipids and surfactants (§ 27.15)
- Miscellaneous cosmetic ingredients (§ 27.16).

27.2   REFERENCES

The reference numbers given under 'advised patch test concentration, vehicle and reference' and occasionally mentioned elsewhere in this chapter refer to the following sources:

1. Maibach, H. I. et al. (1980): Test concentrations and vehicles for dermatological testing of cosmetic ingredients. *Contact Dermatitis, 6,* 369.
2. Fisher, A. A. (1973): *Contact Dermatitis,* 2nd Edition. Lea and Febiger, Philadelphia.
3. Fregert, S. and Hjorth, N. (1979): In: *Textbook of Dermatology,* 3rd Edition. Editors A. Rook, D. S. Wilkinson and F. J. G. Ebling. Blackwell Scientific Publications, Oxford.
4. NACDG. North American Contact Dermatitis Group. Diagnostic Screening Trays. Cited by Maibach et al. (1980) (Ref. 1).
5. Bandmann, H. and Dohn, W. (1967): *Die Epicutantestung.* Bergmann, München.
6. CIR 1981. Final Reports. *Cosmetic Ingredient Review.* 1110 Vermont Ave. N.W., Suite 8, Washington DC 2008.
7. Fisher, A. A. (1975): Patch testing with perfume ingredients. *Contact Dermatitis, 1,* 166.
8. Rapaport, M. J. (1980): Patch testing of color additives. *Contact Dermatitis, 6,* 231.
9. Kozuka, T., Tashiro, M., Sano, S. et al. (1980): Pigmented cosmetic dermatitis from azo dyes. I. Cross-sensitivity in humans. *Contact Dermatitis, 6,* 330.
10. Fregert, S. (1967): Allergic contact dermatitis from the pesticides captan and phaltan. *Contact Dermatitis Newsl., 2,* 29.
11. Eiermann, H. J. (1980): Regulatory issues concerning AETT and 6–MC. *Contact Dermatitis, 6,* 120.
12. Cronin, E. (1980): *Contact Dermatitis,* p. 97. Churchill Livingstone, Edinburgh.
13. Rudzki, E. (1977): *Contact urticaria from silk. Contact Dermatitis, 3,* 53.
14. Rudzki, E. and Grzywa, Z. (1977): Contact urticaria from egg. *Contact Dermatitis, 3,* 103.
15. Schorr, W. F. (1971): Cosmetic allergy. *Arch. Derm., 104,* 459.
16. Verbov, J. L. (1969): Contact dermatitis from miranols. *Trans. St. John's Hosp. derm. Soc. (Lond.), 55,* 192.

UPDATE–2nd Edition

17. Fregert, S. (1981): *Manual of Contact Dermatitis, 2nd Edition.* Munksgaard, Copenhagen.
18. Cronin, E. (1980): *Contact Dermatitis.* Churchill Livingstone, Edinburgh.
19. Eiermann, H. J., Larsen, W., Maibach, H. I. and Taylor, J. S. (1982): Prospective study of cosmetic reactions: 1977-1980. *J. Amer. Acad. Derm., 6,* 907.

20. Mitchell, J. C., Adams, R. M., Glendenning, W. E. et al. (1982): Results of standard patch tests with substances abandoned. *Contact Dermatitis, 8,* 336.
21. Roed-Petersen, J. (1980): Allergic contact dermatitis from butyl acetate. *Contact Dermatitis, 6,* 55.
22. Larsen, W. G. (1975): Cosmetic dermatitis due to a perfume. *Contact Dermatitits, 1,* 142.
23. Rudzki, E., Grzywa, Z. and Bruo, W. S. (1976): Sensitivity to 35 essential oils. *Contact Dermatitis, 2,* 196.
24. Rudzki, E. and Grzywa, Z. (1976): Sensitizing and irritating properties of star anise oil. *Contact Dermatitis, 2,* 305.

27.3 **Frequency of use** (Freq. use) is defined as frequency of use in 19,000 formulas listed in FDA File – 1976 [1].
Contact allergy: If contact allergy has been reported, this is indicated by a + in the columns headed 'Cont. all.' Reference to the relevant paragraphs is made in the 'Comment' columns.

ANTIMICROBIALS AND ANTIOXIDANTS

27.4 Antimicrobials and antioxidants are tabulated as follows:
– Antioxidants and chelating agents (§ 27.5.1)
– Antimicrobials: acids – esters – alcohols – amides (§ 27.5.2)
– Formaldehyde and donor compounds (§ 27.5.3)
– Mercurials (§ 27.5.4)
– Phenols – halogenated phenols – organohalogen compounds (§ 27.5.5)
– Cationic compounds (§ 27.5.6)
– All other antimicrobials (§ 27.5.7).

Preservatives permitted in the EEC: Agents marked with an * in the 'Comment' columns of the tables are permitted preservatives in the EEC (*Draft List,* 5664/82 April 1982).

27.5.1 Antioxidants and chelating agents

Name	Synonym®	Advised patch test conc. & veh. (§ 5.2) and ref. (§ 27.2)	Freq. use (§ 27.3)	Cont. all. (§ 27.3)	Comment
ascorbic acid		–	45		–
– 5,6-diacetyl		–			–
ascorbyl palmitate		–		–	
butylated hydroxyanisole (BHA)	Tenox BHA	5% pet. [1] 2% pet. [4]	3735	+	*See* § 5.7
butylated hydroxytoluene (BHT)	Ionol, Tenox BHT	5% pet. [1]; 2% pet. [4]	1315	+	*See* § 5.7
t-butylhydroquinone (TBHQ)		1% pet.	116	+	*See* § 23.53
citric acid		1% aqua. [2]	2068		–
diamylhydroquinone	Santovar	–	36		–
dilaurylthiodipropionate		–	60		–

(continued)

(continuation)

Name	Synonym®	Advised patch test conc. & veh. (§ 5.2) and ref. (§ 27.2)	Freq. use (§ 27.3)	Cont. all. (§ 27.3)	Comment
ditert-butyl hydroquinone (DTBHQ)		1% pet.	116	+	*See* § 23.47
2,6-ditert-butyl-4-hydroxymethylphenol	Ionox 100	–		–	
ethylenediamine tetraacetate (EDTA)		1% pet. [1]	1592	+	*See* § 5.7
– EDTA disodium		–			–
– EDTA tetrasodium		–			–
– EDTA trisodium		–			–
erythorbic acid (= isoascorbic acid)		–	180		–
ethoxyquin (= 6-ethoxy-1,2-dihydroxy-2,2,4-trimethyl quinoline)		1% pet. [3] 1% o.o. [17] 0.5% aqua [2]		+	*See* § 5.44
gallates		–			*See* § 5.7 *under* gallate esters
– cetyl gallate		–			–
– dodecyl gallate		1% pet. [3]		+	–
– octyl gallate		1% alc. [3] 0.1% pet. [17]			–
– propyl gallate		2% pet. [1]	1411	+	*See* § 23.53
p-hydroxyanisole (= hydroquinone monomethyl ether)		–	175		*See* § 25.45
hydroxyethylenediamine tetraacetate (HEDTA)		–	53		–
hydroxytetramethylchromane carboxylic acid	Trolox C	6%			–
monosulfiram		1% pet.		+	*See* § 4.11, § 12.1, § 25.9 *and* § 25.25
mono-tert-butylhydroquinone		–			*See* tert-butyl hydroquinone
nordihydroguaiaretic acid (NDGA)		2% pet. [2]; 5% pet. [3]		+	*See* § 5.7
pentasodium pentetate (= pentasodium diethylenetriamine pentaacetate)		–	183		–
stearic hydrazide		–	15		–
tetrasodium etidronate (= tetrasodium hydroxyethane diphosphonate)	Turpinal 4NL	–			–
3,3-thiodipropionic acid (= TDPA)		–			–
tocopherol (mixed isomers)		pure [1,2]; 0.1% o.o. [3]	145	+	*See* § 5.7
tocopheryl acetate		–	66		–
tocopheryl succinate		–			–
o-tolylbiguanide	Sopanox	2% pet. [3]	21		–

(continued)

27.5.1 Antioxidants and chelating agents

(continuation)

Name	Synonym®	Advised patch test conc. & veh. (§ 5.2) and ref. (§ 27.2)	Freq. use (§ 27.3)	Cont. all. (§ 27.3)	Comment
trihydroxybutyrophenone (= THBP)		–			–
trimethyl-tris(di-tert-butylhydroxybenzyl) benzene	Sopant	–			–
trisodium ethylenediamine tetraacetate		–			–
trisodium hydroxyethylenediamine tetraacetate		–	53		–
trisodium nitrilotriacetate		–			–

27.5.2 Antimicrobials: acids, esters, alcohols, amides

Name	Synonym®	Advised patch test conc. & veh. (§ 5.2) and ref. (§ 27.2)	Freq. use (§ 27.3)	Cont. all. (§ 27.3)	Comment (*§ 27.4)
benzoic acid		5% pet. [2]; 10% pet. [1]	248	+	*See § 5.32
benzyl alcohol		10% pet. [1]; 5% pet. [2, 17]; 10% alc. [5]	142	+	*See § 5.7
dehydroacetic acid (DHA)		1% pet. ?	194		*
disodium monoundecylenamide monoethanolamine sulfosuccinate	Steinazid SBU 185	–	17		*
formic acid		1% aqua [2]			*
formic acid sodium salt		–			*
glyceryl laurate		–			
parabens					See § 5.7
– benzylparaben		10% pet. [1]; 3% pet. [3]	41	+	*
– butylparaben		5% pet. [1]	499	+	*
– ethylparaben		5% pet. [1]	39	+	*
– methylparaben		5% pet. [1]	6413	+	*
– propylparaben		5% pet. [1]	6069	+	*
phenoxetol (= phenoxyethanol)		5% pet. [1]	22		*
phenoxypropanol		–			*
potassium sorbate		5% pet.	85	+	*See § 5.7
salicylic acid		2% pet. [1]; 5% aqua [3]	43	+	*See § 5.38
sodium benzoate		5% pet.	149	+	*See § 5.7

(continued)

(continuation)

Name	Synonym®	Advised patch test conc. & veh. (§ 5.2) and ref. (§ 27.2)	Freq. use (§ 27.3)	Cont. all. (§ 27.3)	Comment (*§ 27.4)
sodium dehydroacetate		–	157		*
sorbic acid		5% aqua [3]; 2% pet. [1]	526	+	*See § 5.7
sorbic acid isopropyl ester		–			*
undecylenamide diethanolamine	Steinazid DU 185	–			*
undecylenamide monoethanolamine	Steinazid U 185	–			*
undecylenic acid		2% euc. [5]; pure [2]	14	+	*See § 5.32
usnic acid		1% pet. [2]		+	*See § 5.7
usnic acid copper salt		–			*

27.5.3   Formaldehyde and donor compounds

Name	Synonym®	Advised patch test conc. & veh. (§ 5.2) and ref. (§ 27.2)	Freq. use (§ 27.3)	Cont. all. (§ 27.3)	Comment (*§ 27.4)
benzylformal			–		*
bromonitropropanediol	Bronopol	0.25–0.5% pet./aqua		+	*Some investigators doubt whether this compound releases formaldehyde under usage conditions see § 5.7
chloroallylhexaminium chloride (= quaternium-15)	Dowicil 200	2% aqua [4] 1% pet.	536	+	*See § 5.7
dimethyloldimethylhydantoin (= DMDM hydantoin)	Glydant	1% pet. [20]	15	+	*See § 27.2 [20]
formaldehyde and paraformaldehyde		2% aqua [1]	929	+	*See § 5.7
imidazolidinyl urea	Germall 115 Biopure	2% aqua [4] 1% pet.	1446	+	*See § 5.7
methenamine (= hexamine)		0.15% aqua		+	*See § 5.7
methylolchloracetamide		0.1% aqua		+	*See § 5.7
monomethyloldimethylhydantoin (= MDM hydantoin)		–	9		*
trihydroxyethylhexahydrotriazine	Grotan BK	1% aqua [5]		+	*See § 5.7 *under* hexahydro-1,3,5-tris(2-hydroxyethyl)-triazine

27.5.4 Mercurials

27.5.4 Mercurials

Name	Synonym®	Advised patch test conc. & veh. (§ 5.2) and ref. (§ 27.2)	Freq. use (§ 27.3)	Cont. all. (§ 27.3)	Comment (*§ 27.4)
phenylmercuric acetate		0.05% pet. [2]; 0.01% aqua [3, 17]	61	+	*See § 5.7
phenylmercuric borate		0.1% euc. [5] 0.01% aqua		+	*See § 5.7
phenylmercuric chloride		–			*
phenylmercuric nitrate		0.05% pet. [2]; 0.01% aqua [3]		+	*See § 5.7
thiomersal (= sodium ethyl-mercurithiosalicylate)	Merthiolate	0.1% pet. [1]	6	+	*See § 5.7

27.5.5 Phenols, halogenated phenols, organohalogen compounds

Name	Synonym®	Advised patch test conc. & veh. (§ 5.2) and ref. (§ 27.2)	Freq. use (§ 27.3)	Cont. all. (§ 27.3)	Comment (*§ 27.4)
bithionol		1% pet. [3]		+	See § 5.7
bromochlorophene		2% pet.		+	*See § 5.7
bromonitrodioxane	Bronidox	–			*
bromonitropropanediol	Bronopol				*See § 27.5.3 –
captan	Vancide 89RE	1% aqua [4] 1% pet. [2] 0.1% pet. [17]	41	+	*See [10] and § 22.7 –
chloracetamide		0.1% aqua [3, 17] 1% aqua [2] 0.2% pet. [18]		+	*See § 5.7
chlorhexidine diacetate		–			*
chlorhexidine digluconate	Hibitane	1% aqua (gluconate)	23	+	*See § 5.7
chlorhexidine dihydrochloride		1% alc. [1]			*
chlorobutanol (= trichlorbutanol)		1% pet. [1]	8		*
chlorocresol (= p-chloro-m-cresol, PCMC)		1% pet. [3, 17] 5% pet. [2]		+	*See § 5.7
chlorophene (= 2-benzyl-4-chlorphenol)		–			*
chloroxylenol (p-chloro-m-xylenol, PCMX)		1% pet. [3]; 2% pet. [2]	114	+	*See § 5.7
climbazol (= imidazolyl-chlorphenoxydimethylbutanon)	Baypival	–			*

(continued)

(continuation)

Name	Synonym®	Advised patch test conc. & veh. (§ 5.2) and ref. (§ 27.2)	Freq. use (§ 27.3)	Cont. all. (§ 27.3)	Comment (*§ 27.4)
cloflucarban (= halocarban)	Irgasan CF3	–			*
O-cymene-5-ol	Biosol	–	41		
1,2-dibromo-2,4-dicyanobutane		–			–
dibromohexamidine isethionate		–			*
dibromopropamidine isethionate		–			*See § 5.7
dibromsalan		1% pet. [1]	4		–
2,4-dichlorbenzylalcohol	Myacide SP	–			*
3,4-dichlorbenzylalcohol		–			*
dichlorophene	G-4	0.5% pet. 1% pet. [17]	18	+	*See § 5.7
dichloro-m-xylenol (DCMX)		–			*
fenticlor		1–10% pet. [2]		+	See § 5.7
glyceryl-p-chlorphenyl ether (= chlorofenesin)		0.5–1% pet.		+	*See § 5.32 *under* chlorophenesin
hexachlorophene	G-11	1% pet. [1]	8	+	*See § 5.7
isopropylcresols (mixed isomers)		–	13		–
Kathon CG® (chlormethylisothiazolon + methylisothiazolinon + additives)		0.5% pet.			*
o-phenylphenol – sodium salt		1% pet. [2] 1% pet. [2]	6	+	*See § 5.7 *
tetrabrom-o-cresol		–			*
tribromsalan (TBS)		1% pet. [2]	11		*
trichlorbutanol		–			–
triclocarban (TCC)		2% pet. [3]		+	*See § 5.7
triclosan	Irgasan DP300	1% pet. [1]	90	+	See § 5.7

27.5.6   Cationic compounds

Name	Synonym®	Advised patch test conc. & veh. (§ 5.2) and ref. (§ 27.2)	Freq. use (§ 27.3)	Cont. all. (§ 27.3)	Comment (*§ 27.4)
benzalkonium chloride	Zephiran	0.05% aqua [1] 0.1% aqua [2, 3]	78	+	*See § 5.7 *under* quaternary ammonium compounds
benzethonium chloride	Hyamine 1622	0.1% aqua [3]	85	+	*See § 5.7 *under* quaternary ammonium compounds

(continued)

27.5.6 Cationic compounds

(continuation)

Name	Synonym®	Advised patch test conc. & veh. (§ 5.2) and ref. (§ 27.2)	Freq. use (§ 27.3)	Cont. all. (§ 27.3)	Comment (*§ 27.4)
cetrimonium bromide (= cetrimide)		0.01%–0.1% aqua	17	+	*See § 5.7 *under* quaternary ammonium compounds
cetrimonium chloride		–	16		*
cetylpyridinium chloride		0.05% aqua	25	+	See § 5.7 *under* quaternary ammonium compounds
chlorhexidine		1% aqua (gluconate)	23	+	See § 5.7
dibromohexamidine isethionate		–			See § 27.5.5
dibromopropamidine isethionate		–			See § 27.5.5
dodecylguanidine acetate	Dodine	–			*
hexamidine p-hydroxybenzoate		–			*
hexamidine isethionate	Hexomedine	0.15% aqua		+	*See § 5.7
hexetidine		1% aqua [2] 0.1% pet.		+	*See § 5.32
piroctone olamine	Octopirox	–			*
polyhexamethylenebiguanide chloride	Arlagard C	–			*
(other) quaternary ammonium compounds		0.1% and 0.01% aqua [17]			See § 27.15.3
stearalkonium chloride		1–5% aqua [2]	277		

27.5.7 All other antimicrobials

Name	Synonym®	Advised patch test conc. & veh. (§ 5.2) and ref. (§ 27.2)	Freq. use (§ 27.3)	Cont. all. (§ 27.3)	Comment (*§ 27.4)
chlorquinaldol	Sterosan	5% pet. [3]		+	*See § 5.7
coal tar		5% pet. [1]	5	+	*See § 5.38
diiodohydroxyquin	Diiodoquin	5% pet. [3]		+	See § 5.7
dimethoxane (= acetoxydimethyldioxane)		0.1% aqua [15]	79		*Has caused photosensitivity (§ 6.5)
dimethyloxazolidine	Oxadine A	–			*
ethacridine lactate	Rivanol	2% pet. [3]		+	See § 5.7
glutaraldehyde		1% aqua [2]	30	+	*See § 5.7
2-hydroxypyridine-N-oxide	Oxypyrion	–			–
iodine		0.5% aqua [1], open test	4	+	See § 5.7

(continued)

(continuation)

Name	Synonym®	Advised patch test conc. & veh. (§ 5.2) and ref. (§ 27.2)	Freq. use (§ 27.3)	Cont. all. (§ 27.3)	Comment (*§ 27.4)
iodochlorohydroxyquinoline	Vioform	5% pet. [3]		+	*See* § 5.7 *under* quinoline derivatives
oxyquinoline (= 8-hydroxyquinoline)		5% pet. [3]	5	+	*See* § 5.7 *under* quinoline derivatives
– benzoate (salt)		–			*
– benzoate (ester) (= benzoxyquine)		–	4		*
– sulfate (salt)		–	11		*
povidone-iodine (PVP-iodine)		10% solution		+	*See* § 5.7
proflavine dihydrochloride		1% pet. [2]		+	*See* § 5.7
pyrithiones		–			–
– aluminum pyrithione camsylate		–			*
– pyrithione disulfide	in Omadine MDS	–			*
– sodium pyrithione		–			*
– zinc pyrithione	Zinc Omadine	1% aqua susp., 1–5% pet.	48	+	*See* § 5.7
selenium sulfide		2% aqua		+	*See* § 22.7
sulfur, colloidal		5% pet. [2] 1% pet. [17]	43	+	*See* § 5.38
tyrothricine		0.5% euc. [5]; pure [2]	8	+	*See* § 5.25
undebenzophenone (= ethylene glycophenyl undecyl ether p-hydroxybenzoate)		–			*

FRAGRANCE MATERIALS

27.6   The fragrance materials are tabulated in § 27.7. Sources are:
1. Opdyke, D.L.J.: RIFM Monographs, published in *Food and Cosmetic Toxicology, 1973-April 1981.*
2. Opdyke, D.L.J. and Letizia, C. (1982): RIFM Monographs, published in *Food and Cosmetic Toxicology, 20,* 633–851.
3. *Code of Practice, IFRA.* F. Grundschober, 8 rue Charles-Humbert, CH-1205 Geneva, Switzerland.

The **names of the fragrance ingredients** are given according to the RIFM Monographs nomenclature.

Patch test concentrations and vehicles are non-irritating test concentrations in human maximization tests (see also § 5.2).

Quantitative use: defined as use of fragrances in the USA in thousands of lbs per year, according to the RIFM.

– = no data from RIFM (in the columns on non-irritating patch test conc.)
N = material of natural origin
HMT = human maximization test.

27.7   Fragrance materials

Name	Non-irritating patch test conc. (RIFM) (§ 27.6)	Quant. use (§ 27.6)	Patch test conc. & veh. (§ 5.2) and ref. (§ 27.2)	Cont. all. (§ 27.3)	Comment (N: § 27.6)
Abies alba (cone) oil	20% pet.	1	2% pet.	+	N *See* § 27.2, [23]
Abies alba (needle) oil	20% pet.	1	2% pet.	+	N *see* § 27.2, [23]
acetaldehyde diethyl acetal	10% pet.	1	–		–
acetaldehyde ethyl-trans-3-hexenylacetal	5% pet.	1	–		–
acetate C-7	8% pet.	1	–		–
acetate C-8	8% pet.	5	–		–
acetate C-9	2% pet.	5	–		–
acetate C-10	8% pet.	1	–		–
acetate C-11	8% pet.	1	–		–
acetate C-12	20% pet.	1	–		–
acetoin	10% pet.	1	–		–
acetophenone	2% pet.	10	–		–
acetyl butyrol	4% pet.	1	–		–
acetyl carene	10% pet.	–	–		–
acetyl cedrene	30% pet.	200	–		–
acetylethyltetramethyltetralin (AETT, Versalide®)	4% pet.	100	–		Discontinued in 1977: neurotoxic (*see* § 27.2 [11])
5-acetyl-1,1,2,3,3,6-hexamethylindan (Phantolide®)	4% pet.	6	–		phototoxic
acetyl isovaleryl	5% pet.	< 0.1	–		Sensitizer in HMT
acetyl propionyl	4% pet.	1	–		–
4-acetyl-6-tert-butyl-1,1-dimethylindan (Celestolide®)	4% pet.	5	–		–
alantroot oil (= elecampane oil)	4% pet.	–	do not test		N Sensitizer in HMT (due to alantolactone) *See* § 26.3 *under Inula helenium and* § 5.40
alcohol C-6	1% pet.	1	–		–
alcohol C-7	1% pet.	1	–		–
alcohol C-8	2% pet.	10	pure (?)	+	*See* § 27.2, [22]
alcohol C-9	2% pet.	10	pure (?)	+	*See* § 27.2, [22]

(continued)

(continuation)

Name	Non-irritating patch test conc. (RIFM) (§ 27.6)	Quant. use (§ 27.6)	Patch test conc. & veh. (§ 5.2) and ref. (§ 27.2)	Cont. all. (§ 27.3)	Comment (N: § 27.6)
alcohol C-10	3% pet.	20	–		–
alcohol C-11	1% pet.	10	–		–
alcohol C-11, undecylenic	4% pet.	1	–		–
alcohol C-12	4% pet.	20	–		–
alcohol C-14, myristic	12% pet.	1	–		–
aldehyde C-6	1% pet.	1	–		–
aldehyde C-7	4% pet.	1	pure (?)	+	*See* § 27.2, [22]
aldehyde C-7, dimethyl acetal	8% pet.	1	–		–
aldehyde C-8	0.25% pet.	10	–		–
aldehyde C-9	1% pet.	10	pure (?)	+	*See* § 27.2, [22]
aldehyde C-10	–	25	10% DE [7]		–
aldehyde C-11, undecylenic	1% pet.	20	10% DE [7]		–
aldehyde C-11, undecylic	5% pet.	20	–		–
aldehyde C-12, lauric	1% pet.	20	10% DE [7]		–
aldehyde C-12 MNA (methyl m-nonylacetaldehyde)	4% pet.	35	–		–
aldehyde C-14, myristic	1% pet.	2	–		–
ale oil	20% pet.	1	1% alc./2% pet. [7] 1% pet. [17]		N
allo-ocimenol	8% pet.	–	–		–
allyl-α-ionone*	10% pet.	2	–		–
allyl butyrate*	4% pet.	–	–		Test concentration slightly irritating
allyl caproate*	4% pet.	5	–		–
allyl caprylate*	4% pet.	1	–		–
allyl cinnamate*	0.1% pet.	–	–		Test concentration slightly irritating
allyl cyclohexylacetate*	4% pet.	2	–		–
allyl cyclohexylpropionate*	4% pet.	30	–		–
allyl isovalerate*	1% pet.	–	–		–
allyl phenoxyacetate*	1% pet.	1	–		–

(continued)

*Note on allyl esters: during human testing with allyl esters delayed type of irritation 2 or 3 days after exposure occasionally occurred, which the investigators considered as sensitization. In every case this reaction has been traced to the presence of at least 0.1% of free allyl alcohol.

27.7   Fragrance materials

(continuation)

Name	Non-irritating patch test conc. (RIFM) (§ 27.6)	Quant. use (§ 27.6)	Patch test conc. & veh. (§ 5.2) and ref. (§ 27.2)	Cont. all. (§ 27.3)	Comment (N: § 27.6)
allyl phenylacetate*	1.5% pet.	1	–		Test concentration irritating Sensitizer in HMT
allyl trimethylhexanoate	4% pet.	1	–		–
almond oil bitter	4% pet.	–	almond oil pure [2]; bitter almond oil 10% o.o. [2]	+ (?)	N *See* § 5.40 Crude oil is toxic
almond oil bitter FFPA (= free of prussic acid)	4% pet.	50	–		N
almond oil sweet	4% pet.	1	1% alc./2% pet. [7], 1% pet. [17]		N
ambergris tincture	30% pet.	–	–		N
ambrette seed oil	1% pet.	1	1% alc./2% pet. [7], 1% pet. [17]		N
ambrettolide	1% pet.	1	–		–
amyl benzoate	6% pet.	1	–		–
amyl cinnamate	8% pet.	1	32% pet.	+	*See* § 5.16
amylcinnamic acetate	8% pet.	–	–		–
α-amylcinnamic alcohol	8% pet.	10	2% pet.	+	*See* § 5.16
α-amylcinnamic aldehyde	6% pet.	800	2% pet.	+	*See* § 5.16
amylcinnamic aldehyde diethyl acetal	10% pet.	3	–		–
α-amylcinnamic aldehyde dimethyl acetal	8% pet.	3	–		–
amylcinnamylidene methylanthranilate	8% pet.	1	–		–
4-tert-amylcyclohexamone	8% pet.	10	–		–
amylcyclohexyl acetate (mixed isomers)	12% pet.	–	–		–
amyl formate	3% pet.	1	–		–
amyl isoeugenol	8% pet.	–	–		–
amyl salicylate	10% pet.	600	2% o.o. [2]		–
amyl vinylcarbinol	10% pet.	–	–		–
amyl vinyl carbinyl acetate	10% pet.	5	–		Sensitizer in HMT

(continued)

*Note on allyl esters: during human testing with allyl esters delayed type of irritation 2 or 3 days after exposure occasionally occurred, which the investigators considered as sensitization. In every case this reaction has been traced to the presence of at least 0.1% of free allyl alcohol.

(continuation)

Name	Non-irritating patch test conc. (RIFM) (§ 27.6)	Quant. use (§ 27.6)	Patch test conc. & veh. (§ 5.2) and ref. (§ 27.2)	Cont. all. (§ 27.3)	Comment (N: § 27.6)
amyris oil acetylated	10% pet.	5	1% alc./2% pet. [7], 1% pet. [17]		N
anethole	2% pet.	16	5% pet. [1]; 2% pet. [3, 17], 2% alc. [17]	+	*See* § 13.3
angelica root oil	1% pet.	1	2% pet.	+	*See* § 26.3 *under Angelica officinalis and* § 27.2, [23] N Phototoxic
angelica seed oil	1% pet.	1	–		N Not phototoxic
anise oil	2% pet.	1	anise oil 25% o.o. [7]; 10% o.o. [5]	+	N *See* § 13.3
anise (star anise) oil	4% pet.	1	1% pet.	+	N *See* §13.3 Testing with star anise oil 1% may cause patch test sensitization and irritant patch test reactions. Lower test concentrations give false-negative results (§ 27.2, [24])
anisic aldehyde	10% pet.	50	1% pet. (§ 5.17)		–
anisol	4% pet.	1	0.01% chloroform [5]		–
anisyl alcohol	5% pet.	5	–		–
anisyl n-butyrate	8% pet.	1	–		–
anisyl formate	4% pet.	1	–		–
anisylidene acetone	2% pet.	1	2% pet.	+	*See* § 5.16 Sensitizer in HMT
anisyl phenylacetate	12% pet.	1	–		–
anisyl propionate	4% pet.	1	–		–
armoise oil	12% pet.	5	1% alc./2% pet. [7], 1% pet. [17]		N
artemisia oil (wormwood)	2% pet.	1	1% alc./2% pet. [7], 1% pet. [17]		N
baccartol	4% pet.	–	–		–
balsam Canada	2% pet.	5	25% pet. [1]		N
balsam Copaiba	8% pet.	40	–		N
balsam Peru	8% pet.	–	25% pet.	+	N *See* § 5.16
balsam Tolu	2% pet.	20	1% alc. [2]; 10% alc. [7]	+	N *See* § 5.16
basil oil sweet	4% pet.	2	1% alc./2% pet. [7], 1% pet. [17]		N

(continued)

27.7   Fragrance materials

(continuation)

Name	Non-irritating patch test conc. (RIFM) (§ 27.6)	Quant. use (§ 27.6)	Patch test conc. & veh. (§ 5.2) and ref. (§ 27.2)	Cont. all. (§ 27.3)	Comment (N: § 27.6)
bay oil	10% pet.	10	1% pet. [7]		N
beeswax absolute	4% pet.	–	30% pet. [1]	+	N *See* § 5.39
benzaldehyde	4% pet.	75	10% pet. [1] 5% pet. or 10% alc. [17]	+	*See* § 5.16
benzaldehydedimethyl acetal	4% pet.	1	–		–
benzal glyceryl acetal	4% pet.	1	–		–
benzhydrol	5% pet.	1	–		–
benzoin resinoid	8% pet.	100	2% pet. [1] 10% pet./alc.	+	N *See* § 5.39
benzonitrile	2% pet.	–	–		–
benzophenone	6% pet.	100	–		*See* § 25.66
benzyl acetate	8% pet.	1000	as is [7]		–
benzyl alcohol	10% pet.	250	5–10% pet. 10% alc.	+	*See* § 5.7
benzyl benzoate	30% pet.	500	10% pet. [1]	+	*See* § 5.41 Also used as antiparasitic drug
benzyl butyrate	4% pet.	5	–		–
benzyl cinnamate	8% pet.	20	5–8% pet. [5] 5% pet./10% alc. [17]	+	*See* § 5.16
benzyl formate	10% pet.	2	–		–
benzylidene acetone	2% pet.	–	0.5% pet.	+	*See* § 5.16 Sensitizer in HMT
benzyl isoamyl ether	12% pet.	1	–		–
benzyl isobutyrate	4% pet.	1	–		–
benzyl isoeugenol	5% pet.	1	–		–
benzyl isovalerate	4% pet.	1	–		–
benzyl laurate	30% pet.	1	–		–
benzyl phenylacetate	2% pet.	2	–		–
benzyl propionate	4% pet.	8	–		–
benzyl salicylate	30% pet.	300	2% pet. [7]	+	*See* § 5.16
bergamot oil, expressed	30% pet.	300	bergamot oil 2% pet. [3,17] 10% pet. [7]	+	N Phototoxic; principal phototoxic compound is 5MOP *See* § 5.39 *and* § 27.2, [23]

(continued)

(continuation)

Name	Non-irritating patch test conc. (RIFM) (§ 27.6)	Quant. use (§ 27.6)	Patch test conc. & veh. (§ 5.2) and ref. (§ 27.2)	Cont. all. (§ 27.3)	Comment (N: § 27.6)
bergamot oil, rectified	30% pet.	–			N Free of furocoumarines and non-volatile residues
birch tar oil	2% pet.	1	1% alc./2% pet. [7], 1% pet. [17]		N *See also* § 26.3 *(Betula alba)*
bisabolene	10% pet.	1	–		–
black pepper oil	4% pet.	10	–		N Weakly phototoxic *See* § 26.3 *(Piper nigrum)*
bois de rose, acetylated	12% pet.	30	1% alc./2% pet. [7], 1% pet. [17]		N
bois de rose Brasilian	5% pet.	400	1% alc./2% pet. [7], 1% pet. [17]		N
boldo leaf oil	4% pet.	1	–		N
L-borneol	8% pet.	2	–		–
L-bornyl acetate	2% pet.	3	–		–
bornyl isovalerate	4% pet.	1	–		–
bromstyrol	4% pet.	1	–		Strongly irritant
butyl acetate	4% pet.	8	25% o.o. [2]	+	*See* § 27.2, [19] *and* § 5.44
n-butyl anthranilate	4% pet.	1	–		–
butyl-n-butyrate	4% pet.	2	–		–
butyl butyrolactate	4% pet.	1	–		–
n-butyl cinnamate	4% pet.	1	–		–
butyl cinnamic aldehyde	8% pet.	5	–		–
4-tert-butylcyclohexanol	4% pet.	10	–		–
p-tert-butylcyclohexanone	6% pet.	–	–		–
4-tert-butylcyclohexylacetate	4% pet.	300	–		–
butyl isobutyrate	4% pet.	1	–		–
n-butyl isovalerate	1% pet.	1	–		–
butyl lactate	1% pet.	1	–		–
p-tert-butyl-α-methylhydro-cinnamic aldehyde (Lilial®)	4% pet.	1000	1% pet.	+	*See* § 5.16
butyl oleate	10% pet.	1	–		–
p-tert-butylphenol	1% pet.	2	–		Sensitizer in HMT Causes depigmentation
3-butyl phthalide	2% pet.	–	–		–

(continued)

27.7 Fragrance materials

(continuation)

Name	Non-irritating patch test conc. (RIFM) (§ 27.6)	Quant. use (§ 27.6)	Patch test conc. & veh. (§ 5.2) and ref. (§ 27.2)	Cont. all. (§ 27.3)	Comment (N: § 27.6)
n-butyl propionate	2% pet.	1	–		–
sec-butyl quinoline	2% pet.	4	–		–
n-butyl salicylate	2% pet.	1	–		–
butyl undecylenate	8% pet.	1	–		–
n-butyraldehyde	1% pet.	0.5	–		–
n-butyric acid	1% pet.	–	–		–
cabreuva oil	6% pet.	1	1% alc./2% pet. [7], 1% pet. [17]		N
cade oil rectified (juniper tar)	2% pet.	1	25% c.o. [2]		N *See* § 26.3
cadinene	10% pet.	4	1% pet. [7]		–
cajeput oil	4% pet.	1	1% alc./2% pet. [7], 1% pet. [17]		N
calamus oil	4% pet.	2	1% alc./2% pet. [7], 1% pet. [17]		N
camphene	4% pet.	6	–		–
camphor oil brown	4% pet.	1			N
camphor oil yellow	4% pet.	20	camphor oil 10% pet. [2]		N
camphor oil white	20% pet.	15			N
camphor usp	4% pet.	–	10% pet.	+	N *See* § 5.42
cananga oil	10% pet.	2	2% pet.	+	N *See* § 5.16 *and* § 27.2, [23]
capric acid	1% pet.	1	–		–
caprylic acid	1% pet.	–	–		–
caraway oil	4% pet.	–	caraway seed oil 25% c.o. [2]		N Has caused immediate type hypersensitivity (§ 13.3) Weakly phototoxic *See also* § 7.5
cardamom oil	4% pet.	2	1% alc./2% pet. [7], 1% pet. [17]		N
δ-carene	10% pet.	–	–		Weakly phototoxic
carrot seed oil	4% pet.	1	1% alc./2% pet. [7], 1% pet. [17]		N *See also* § 26.3 (*Daucus carota*)
carvacrol	4% pet.	2	–		–
L-carveol	4% pet.	1	–		–

(continued)

(continuation)

Name	Non-irritating patch test conc. (RIFM) (§ 27.6)	Quant. use (§ 27.6)	Patch test conc. & veh. (§ 5.2) and ref. (§ 27.2)	Cont. all. (§ 27.3)	Comment (N: § 27.6)
D-carvone	2% pet.	3	carvone 5% pet. [1] 2% pet. [3]	+	*See* § 13.3 Sensitizer in HMT
L-carvone	1% pet.	2	–		*See also* § 26.3 *(Anetheum graveolens* and *Carum carvi)*
carvone oxide	–	–	–		Sensitizer in HMT (IFRA, October 1979)
L-carvyl acetate	4% pet.	1	–		–
L-carvyl propionate	4% pet.	1	–		–
caryophyllene	4% pet.	20	5% pet. [7]		–
caryophyllene acetate	4% pet.	4	–		–
caryophyllene alcohol	4% pet.	5	–		–
cascarilla oil	4% pet.	1	1% alc./2% pet. [7], 1% pet. [17]		N
cassia oil	4% pet.	9	2% pet. [3]	+	N Sensitizer due to cinnamic aldehyde *See* § 27.2 [23] Weakly phototoxic Has caused contact urticaria (§ 7.5 under cinnamon oil)
castoreum	4% pet.	20	1% alc./2% pet. [7], 1% pet. [17]		N
cedar leaf oil	4% pet.	10	–		N Has caused phototoxicity (§ 6.5)
cedarwood oil Atlas	8% pet.	25	cedarwood oil 10% o.o. [7]; 10% pet. [3]		N Cedarwood oils have caused phototoxicity (§ 6.5)
cedarwood oil Texas	6% pet.	25			
cedarwood oil Virginia	8% pet.	100			
α-cedrene	5% pet.	–	–		–
cedr-8-ene epoxide	10% pet.	–	–		–
cedrenol	8% pet.	8	–		–
cedrenone	20% pet.	1	–		–
cedrenyl acetate	8% pet.	45	–		–
cedrol	8% pet.	50	–		–
cedrol methyl ether	8% pet.	1	–		–
cedryl acetate	8% pet.	100	–		–
cedryl formate	12% pet.	5	–		–

(continued)

27.7 Fragrance materials

(continuation)

Name	Non-irritating patch test conc. (RIFM) (§ 27.6)	Quant. use (§ 27.6)	Patch test conc. & veh. (§ 5.2) and ref. (§ 27.2)	Cont. all. (§ 27.3)	Comment (N: § 27.6)
celery seed oil	4% pet.	2	1% alc./2% pet. [7], 1% pet. [17]		N *See also* § 26.3 *(Anthemis nobilis)*
cetyl alcohol	12% pet.	1	30% pet.	+	*See* § 5.22
chamomile oil German	4% pet.	1 ⎫	chamomile as is [3] chamomile oil		N *See also* § 26.3 *(Anthemis nobilis) and* § 5.39
chamomile oil Roman	4% pet.	3 ⎭	25% o.o. [2]		N *See also* § 26.3 *(Anthemis nobilis) and* § 5.39
chenopodium oil	4% pet.	1	1% alc./2% pet. [7], 1% pet. [17]		N
cinnamic acid	4% pet.	1	5% pet. [7]; 1% pet. [17] 10% pet. [3]		Has caused contact urticaria (§ 7.5)
cinnamic alcohol	4% pet.	150	1% pet. [17] 2% pet.	+	*See* § 5.16
cinnamic aldehyde		100	2% pet. 1% pet. [17]	+	*See* § 5.16 Sensitizer in HMT
cinnamic aldehyde dimethyl acetal	10% pet.	–	–		–
cinnamic aldehyde methyl anthranilate	12% pet.	1	–		Sensitizer in HMT
cinnamon bark oil Ceylon	8% pet.	4	2% pet.	+	N *See* § 5.16 *under* cinnamon oil Sensitizer due to cinnamic aldehyde. Weakly phototoxic
cinnamon leaf oil Ceylon	10% pet.	4	2% pet.	+	N *See* § 5.16 *under* cinnamon oil
cinnamyl acetate	5% pet.	5	–		–
cinnamyl anthranilate	4% pet.	1	–		Carcinogenic (?)
cinnamyl benzoate	5% pet.	1	10% pet.	+	*See* § 5.16
cinnamyl butyrate	4% pet.	1	–		–
cinnamyl cinnamate	4% pet.	1	8% pet.	+	*See* § 5.16
cinnamyl formate	4% pet.	1	–		–
cinnamyl isobutyrate	4% pet.	1	–		–
cinnamyl isovalerate	2% pet.	1	–		–
cinnamyl nitrile	4% pet.	–	–		–
cinnamyl propionate	4% pet.	1	–		–
cinnamyl tigliate	4% pet.	1	–		–
citral		75	2% pet. [17]	+	*See* § 5.16 Sensitizer in HMT

(continued)

(continuation)

Name	Non-irritating patch test conc. (RIFM) (§ 27.6)	Quant. use (§ 27.6)	Patch test conc. & veh. (§ 5.2) and ref. (§ 27.2)	Cont. all. (§ 27.3)	Comment (N: § 27.6)
citral dimethyl acetal	4% pet.	50	–		–
citral ethylene glycol acetal	5% pet.	–	–		–
citral methyl anthranilate	12% pet.	1	–		–
citronella oil	8% pet.	400	1% pet. [7]; 2% pet. [3, 17]	+	*See* § 5.16
citronellal	4% pet.	4	2–4% pet.	+	*See* § 5.16
citronellic acid	2% pet.	1	–		–
citronellol	6% pet.	150	2% pet. [3] 1% pet. [7]		–
citronellyl acetate	4% pet.	20	–		–
citronellyl n-butyrate	5% pet.	1	–		–
citronellyl crotonate	8% pet.	1	–		–
citronellyl ethyl ether	4% pet.	1	–		–
citronellyl formate	4% pet.	40	–		–
citronellyl isobutyrate	4% pet.	–	–		–
citronellyl nitrile	6% pet.	5	–		–
citronellyl oxyacetaldehyde	8% pet.	4	1% pet. [7]		–
citronellyl phenylacetate	4% pet.	1	–		–
citronellyl propionate	4% pet.	2	–		–
civet absolute	4% pet.	3.5	–		N
civetone	4% pet.	1	–		–
clary sage oil	8% pet.	10	2% pet.	+	N *See* § 27.2, [23] *and* § 12.1
clove bud oil	5% pet.	100	clove oil 2% pet. [1]	+	N
clove leaf oil Madagascar	5% pet.	30			N *See* § 27.2, [19] *and* [23]
clove stem oil	10% pet.	40			N
cognac oil green	4% pet.	1	1% alc./2% pet. [7], 1% pet. [17]		N
coniferyl alcohol		–	2% pet.	+	*See* § 5.16
copaiba oil	8% pet.	33	1% alc./2% pet. [7], 1% pet. [17]		N
coriander oil	6% pet.	10	10% c.o. [2] 2% pet.	+	N *See* § 27.2, [23]

(continued)

27.7 Fragrance materials

(continuation)

Name	Non-irritating patch test conc. (RIFM) (§ 27.6)	Quant. use (§ 27.6)	Patch test conc. & veh. (§ 5.2) and ref. (§ 27.2)	Cont. all. (§ 27.3)	Comment (N: § 27.6)
cornmint oil	8% pet.	1	1% alc./2% pet. [7], 1% pet. [17]		N
costus root essential oil, absolute and concrete	4% pet.	1	1% pet.	+	N *See* § 5.16 Sensitizer in HMT
coumarin	8% pet.	250	5–10% pet. [3] 10% o.o. [17]	+	*See* § 5.16
p-cresol	4% pet.	2	–		–
p-cresyl acetate	4% pet.	1	–		–
p-cresyl caprylate	4% pet.	1	–		–
p-cresyl isobutyrate	4% pet.	1	–		–
p-cresyl methyl ether	2% pet.	10	–		–
p-cresyl phenylacetate	4% pet.	2	–		–
cubeb oil	8% pet.	1	1% alc./2% pet. [7], 1% pet. [17]		N
cuminaldehyde	4% pet.	3	–		–
cumin oil	4% pet.	2	1% alc./2% pet. [7], 1% pet. [17]		N Weakly phototoxic *See* § 26.3 *(Cuminum cyminum)*
cuminyl alcohol	4% pet.	2	–		–
cyclamen alcohol	20% pet.	–	–		Sensitizer in HMT
cyclamen aldehyde	3% pet.	150	–		–
cyclamen aldehyde diethyl acetal	24% pet.	–	–		–
cyclamen aldehyde dimethyl acetal	24% pet.	1	–		–
cyclamen aldehyde ethyleneglycol acetol	24% pet.	1	–		–
cyclamen aldehyde methylanthranilate	6% pet.	–	–		–
cyclamen aldehyde propyleneglycol acetal	24% pet.	–	–		–
cyclohexanol	4% pet.	–	–		–
cyclohexyl acetate	4% pet.	1	–		–
2-cyclohexyl cyclohexanone	20% pet.	35	–		–
cyclohexylethyl acetate	4% pet.	–	–		–
cyclohexylethyl alcohol	4% pet.	–	–		–

(continued)

(continuation)

Name	Non-irritating patch test conc. (RIFM) (§ 27.6)	Quant. use (§ 27.6)	Patch test conc. & veh. (§ 5.2) and ref. (§ 27.2)	Cont. all. (§ 27.3)	Comment (N: § 27.6)
cyclopentadecanolide	10% pet.	3	–		–
cyclopentadecanone	10% pet.	1	–		–
cyclopentanone	10% pet.	1	–		–
p-cymene	4% pet.	9	1% pet. [7]		–
cypress oil	5% pet.	1	1% alc./2% pet. [7], 1% pet. [17]	N	
cyste absolute	4% pet.	1	–	N	
davana oil	4% pet.	1	1% alc./2% pet. [7], 1% pet. [17]	N	
2,4-decadienal	5% pet.	1	–		–
decahydro-β-naphthol	2% pet.	4	–		–
decahydro-β-naphthyl acetate	12% pet.	1	–		–
decahydro-β-naphthyl formate	12% pet.	1	–		–
γ-decalactone	10% pet.	1	–		–
δ-decalactone	1% pet.	1	–		–
decanal dimethylacetal	4% pet.	1	–		–
2-decen-1-al	4% pet.	–	–		–
cis-4-decen-1-al	1% pet.	1	–		–
9-decenyl acetate	12% pet.	1	–		–
decylenic alcohol	2% pet.	20	–		–
decyl methyl ether	4% pet.	1	–		–
deertongue absolute	5% pet.	1	–	N	
deertongue incolore	5% pet.	1	–	N	
deobase (deodorized kerosine)	12% pet.	150	–		–
diacetyl	2% pet.	1	1% aqua [5]		–
dibenzyl	8% pet.	–	–		–
dibenzyl ether	4% pet.	1	2% euc. anh. [5]		
dibutyl sulfide	8% pet.	1	–		–
diethylene glycol monoethyl ether	20% pet.	5	–		–
diethylene glycol monomethyl ether	20% pet.	5	–		–

(continued)

27.7   Fragrance materials

(continuation)

Name	Non-irritating patch test conc. (RIFM) (§ 27.6)	Quant. use (§ 27.6)	Patch test conc. & veh. (§ 5.2) and ref. (§ 27.2)	Cont. all. (§ 27.3)	Comment (N: § 27.6)
diethyl maleate	4% pet.	1	–		Sensitizer in HMT
diethyl malonate	4% pet.	1	–		–
diethyl sebacate	4% pet.	1	20% alc.	+	*See § 5.22 and § 5.16*
diethyl succinate	4% pet.	1	–		–
dihexyl fumarate	4% pet.	1	–		–
dihydroanethole	10% pet.	1	–		–
dihydrocarveol	4% pet.	1	–		–
dihydrocarvone	20% pet.	1	–		–
dihydrocoumarin	20% pet.	10	5% pet.	+	*See § 5.16* Sensitizer in HMT
dihydroeugenol	8% pet.	2	–		–
dihydro-α-ionone	12% pet.	1	–		–
dihydro-isojasmone	4% pet.	1	–		–
dihydrojasmone	4% pet.	1	–		–
dihydromethyl-α-ionone	4% pet.	2	–		–
dihydromyrcenol	4% pet.	1	–		–
dihydrosafrole	12% pet.	2	–		–
dihydro-α-terpineol	10% pet.	1	–		–
2,4-dihydroxy-3-methyl-benzaldehyde	–	–	–		Sensitizer (IFRA, February 1980)
dihydroterpinyl acetate	12% pet.	10	–		–
dill seed oil, Indian	4% pet.	1	1% alc./2% pet. [7], 1% pet. [17]		N
dill weed oil	4% pet.	1	1% alc./2% pet. [7], 1% pet. [17]		N
dimethyl anthranilate	10% pet.	1	–		Phototoxic
dimethylbenzyl carbinol	8% pet.	2	–		–
dimethylbenzyl carbinyl acetate	4% pet.	50	–		–
dimethylbenzyl carbinyl butyrate	10% pet.	1	–		–
dimethylbenzyl carbinyl propionate	10% pet.	1	–		–
4,6-dimethyl-8-tert-butylcoumarin	8% pet.	–	–		Photoallergic

(continued)

(continuation)

Name	Non-irritating patch test conc. (RIFM) (§ 27.6)	Quant. use (§ 27.6)	Patch test conc. & veh. (§ 5.2) and ref. (§ 27.2)	Cont. all. (§ 27.3)	Comment (N: § 27.6)
dimethyl carbonate	4% pet.	1	–		–
dimethyl citraconate	12% pet.	–	–		Sensitizer in HMT
dimethylheptenal	4% pet.	3	–		–
dimethylheptenol	10% pet.	1	–		–
dimethylhydroquinone	4% pet.	2	–		–
dimethylionone	4% pet.	–	–		–
dimethyl malonate	8% pet.	1	–		–
3,6-dimethyl-3-octanol	20% pet.	200	–		–
3,7-dimethyl-1-octanol	8% pet.	10	2% pet. [7]		–
3,6-dimethyloctan-3-yl acetate	20% pet.	30	–		–
3,7-dimethyloctanyl acetate	8% pet.	3	–		–
3,7-dimethyloctanyl butyrate	10% pet.	1	–		–
dimethylphenylcarbinol	4% pet.	1	–		–
dimethylphenylethyl carbinol	4% pet.	7	–		–
dimethylphenylethylcarbinyl acetate	4% pet.	1	–		–
dimethyl succinate	4% pet.	2	–		–
dimethyl sulfide	1% pet.	1	–		–
dimyrcetol	4% pet.	3	–		–
dipentene (D,L-limonene)	20% pet.	1	2% pet. [3]		–
diphenylamine	1% pet.	1	–		–
diphenylmethane	8% pet.	4	–		–
diphenyl oxide	4% pet.	100	–		–
dipropylene glycol	20% pet.	50	–		–
γ-dodecalactone	12% pet.	–	–		–
δ-dodecalactone	12% pet.	1	–		–
eau de brouts absolute	4% pet.	1	1% alc./2% pet. [7], 1% pet. [17]		N
elemi oil	4% pet.	1	1% alc./2% pet. [7], 1% pet. [17]		N
estragon oil	4% pet.	2	1% alc./2% pet. [7], 1% pet. [17]		N

(continued)

27.7   Fragrance materials

(continuation)

Name	Non-irritating patch test conc. (RIFM) (§ 27.6)	Quant. use (§ 27.6)	Patch test conc. & veh. (§ 5.2) and ref. (§ 27.2)	Cont. all. (§ 27.3)	Comment (N: § 27.6)
p-ethoxybenzaldehyde	4% pet.	1	–		–
ethyl acetate	10% pet.	2	10% pet. [1]		–
ethyl acetoacetate	8% pet.	8	–		–
ethyl acrylate	4% pet.	1	–		Sensitizer in HMT
ethyl amyl ketone	2% pet.	2	–		–
ethyl anisate	4% pet.	1	–		–
ethyl anthranilate	4% pet.	1	–		–
ethyl benzene	10% pet.	–	–		–
ethyl benzoate	8% pet.	5	–		–
ethyl butyl ketone	4% pet.	1	–		–
ethyl butyrate	5% pet.	51	–		–
ethyl caprate	2% pet.	1	–		–
ethyl caproate	4% pet.	3	–		–
ethyl caprylate	2% pet.	1	–		–
ethyl cellulose	12% DEP	1	–		–
ethyl cinnamate	4% pet.	1	–		–
ethyl citral	4% pet.	1	–		–
ethyl crotonate	4% pet.	1	–		–
ethylene brassylate	30% pet.	2000	–		–
ethyl formate	4% pet.	3	–		–
ethyl heptoate	4% pet.	1	–		–
2-ethylhexanol	4% pet.	25	–		–
2-ethyl hexyl acetate	4% pet.	10	–		–
ethyl hexyl palmitate	4% pet.	1	–		–
ethyl hexyl salicylate	4% pet.	1	–		–
ethyl isobutyrate	8% pet.	1	–		–
ethyl isovalerate	2% pet.	1	–		–
ethyl lactate	8% pet.	10	–		–
ethyl laevulinate	4% pet.	< 1	–		–
ethyl laurate	12% pet.	1	–		–

(continued)

(continuation)

Name	Non-irritating patch test conc. (RIFM) (§ 27.6)	Quant. use (§ 27.6)	Patch test conc. & veh. (§ 5.2) and ref. (§ 27.2)	Cont. all. (§ 27.3)	Comment (N: § 27.6)
ethyl linalool	30% pet.	2	–		–
ethyl linalyl acetate	4% pet.	< 1	–		–
ethyl maltol	10% pet.	–	–		–
ethyl methylphenylglycidate	1% pet.	5	–		–
ethyl myristate	12% pet.	1	–		–
ethyl octine carbonate	2% pet.	–	–		–
ethyl oleate	8% pet.	< 1	–		–
ethyl pelargonate	12% pet.	1	–		–
ethyl phenylacetate	8% pet.	2	–		–
ethyl phenylglycidate	4% pet.	2	–		–
ethyl propionate	2% pet.	16	–		–
ethyl salicylate	12% pet.	5	–		–
ethyl stearate	12% pet.	1	–		–
ethyl undecylenate	8% pet.	< 1	–		–
ethyl vanillin	2% pet.	28	10% pet. [1]		Has caused contact urticaria (§ 7.5)
eucalyptol	16% pet.	5	5% o.o. [5]		–
eucalyptus oil	10% pet.	32	1% pet. [7]; 2% pet. [3, 17]	+	N *See* § 27.2, [23]
eugenol	8% pet.	100	2% pet. [17]	+	*See* § 5.16
eugenyl acetate	20% pet.	5	–		–
eugenyl formate	12% pet.	< 1	–		–
eugenyl phenylacetate	12% pet.	1	–		–
farnesol	not yet published	–	4% pet.	+	*See* § 5.16 Sensitizer, if not sufficiently pure
fenchone	4% pet.	1	–		–
fenchyl acetate	5% pet.	1	–		–
fenchyl alcohol	4% pet.	1	–		–
fennel oil	4% pet.	4	–	+	N *See* § 26.3 *(Foeniculum vulgare)*
fennel oil bitter	4% pet.	1	1% alc./2% pet. [7], 1% pet. [17]		N
fenugreek absolute	2% pet.	1			N

(continued)

27.7   Fragrance materials

(continuation)

Name	Non-irritating patch test conc. (RIFM) (§ 27.6)	Quant. use (§ 27.6)	Patch test conc. & veh. (§ 5.2) and ref. (§ 27.2)	Cont. all. (§ 27.3)	Comment (N: § 27.6)
fig leaf absolute	5% pet.	< 1			N Sensitizer; extremely phototoxic (IFRA, October 1980)
fir balsam Oregon	8% pet.	1			N
fir needle oil Canadian	10% pet.	35 ⎫	1% alc./2% pet. [7], 1% pet. [17]		N
fir needle oil Siberian	2–5% pet.	35 ⎭			N
flouve oil	4% pet.	1	1% alc./2% pet. [7], 1% pet. [17]		N
foin absolute	4% pet.	1	–		N
furfural	2% pet.	1	–		–
galbanum oil	4% pet.	15	10% alc. [5] 1–2% pet. [7, 17]		N
genet absolute	12% pet.	1	–		N
geranial	1% pet.	–	1–5% pet.	+	Sensitizer in HMT *See* § 5.16
geranic acid	4% pet.	1	–		–
geraniol	6% pet.	800	5% pet. [1], 2% pet.	+	*See* § 5.16 Sensitizer in HMT
geranium oil Algerian	10% pet.	100 ⎫			N
geranium oil Bourbon	10% pet.	100 ⎬	2% pet.	+	N *See* § 5.16 *and* § 27.2, [23]
geranium oil Moroccan	10% pet.	100 ⎭			N
geranyl acetate	4% pet.	100	–		–
geranyl acetoacetate	4% pet.	–	–		–
geranyl acetone	10% pet.	1	–		–
geranyl benzoate	2% pet.	2	–		–
geranyl butyrate	4% pet.	2	–		–
geranyl caproate	6% pet.	–	–		–
geranyl crotonate	10% pet.	1	–		–
geranyl ethyl ether	4% pet.	< 1	–		–
geranyl formate	2% pet.	10	–		–
geranyl isobutyrate	10% pet.	1	–		–
geranyl isovalerate	2% pet.	6	–		–

(continued)

(continuation)

Name	Non-irritating patch test conc. (RIFM) (§ 27.6)	Quant. use (§ 27.6)	Patch test conc. & veh. (§ 5.2) and ref. (§ 27.2)	Cont. all. (§ 27.3)	Comment (N: § 27.6)
geranyl nitrile	12% pet.	–	–		–
geranyl oxyacetaldehyde	4% pet.	1	–		–
geranyl phenylacetate	4% pet.	5	–		–
geranyl propionate	4% pet.	5	–		–
geranyl tiglate	6% pet.	1	–		–
ginger oil	4% pet.	2	1% pet. [7]		N Weakly phototoxic *See* § 26.3 *(Zingiber officinalis)*
grapefruit oil, expressed	10% pet.	18	1% alc./2% pet. [7], 1% pet. [17]		N
grisalva	1% pet.	–	–		N
guaiacol	2% pet.	< 1	–		N
guaiac wood acetate	8% pet.	30 ⎫	guaiacol 5% pet. [5]		–
guaiac wood oil	8% pet.	50 ⎭	2% pet.	+	N *See* § 27.2, [23]
guaiene	2% pet.	–	–		–
gurjun balsam	12% pet.	1	–		N
gurjun oil	8% pet.	1	1% alc./2% pet. [7], 1% pet. [17]		N
helichrysum oil	4% pet.	1	1% alc./2% pet. [7], 1% pet. [17]		N +
heliotropin (piperonal)	6% pet.	150	1% pet. [7]	+	*See* § 27.2, [22]
γ-heptalactone	4% pet.	< 4	–		Weak sensitizer in HMT
2-n-heptyl cyclopentanone	10% pet.	1	–		–
heptyl formate	12% pet.	1	–		–
heptylidene methyl anthranilate	12% pet.	< 1	–		–
hexadecanolide	4% pet.	1	–		–
hexahydrocoumarin	–	–	–		Sensitizer in HMT (IFRA, February 1980)
1,3,4,6,7,8-hexahydro-4,6,6,7,8,8-hexamethylcyclopenta-γ-2-benzopyran (Galaxolide®)	15% pet.	50	–		–
γ-hexalactone	12% pet.	1	–		–
δ-hexalactone	4% pet.	< 1	–		Weak sensitizer in HMT

(continued)

(continuation)

Name	Non-irritating patch test conc. (RIFM) (§ 27.6)	Quant. use (§ 27.6)	Patch test conc. & veh. (§ 5.2) and ref. (§ 27.2)	Cont. all. (§ 27.3)	Comment (N: § 27.6)
cis-3-hexenal	2% pet.	–	–		–
hexen-2-al	4% pet.	1	–		–
cis-3-hexenol	4% pet.	20	–		–
trans-2-hexenol	4% pet.	3	–		–
2-hexenyl acetate	10% pet.	1	–		–
cis-3-hexenyl acetate	10% pet.	2	–		–
cis-3-hexenyl anthranilate	10% pet.	< 1	–		–
cis-3-hexenyl benzoate	10% pet.	1	–		–
hexenyl cyclopentanone	10% pet.	–	–		–
cis-3-hexenyl formate	10% pet.	1	–		–
cis-3-hexenyl isobutyrate	10% pet.	1	–		–
cis-3-hexenyl oxyacetaldehyde	4% pet.	1	–		–
cis-3-hexenyl phenylacetate	10% pet.	1	–		–
cis-3-hexenyl propionate	10% pet.	1	–		–
trans-2-hexenyl propionate	10% pet.	1	–		–
cis-3-hexenyl salicylate	3% pet.	–	3% pet.	+	*See* § 5.16
cis-3-hexenyl tiglate	12% pet.	1	–		–
hexoxyacetaldehyde dimethylacetal	10% pet.	1	–		–
hexyl acetate	4% pet.	1	–		–
hexyl benzoate	3% pet.	5	–		–
hexyl butyrate	12% pet.	1	–		–
hexyl caproate	1% pet.	1	–		–
hexyl caprylate	4% pet.	–	–		–
hexyl cinnamic aldehyde	12% pet.	300	2% pet. [7]		–
hexyl crotonate	10% pet.	< 1	–		–
2-hexyl-2-decenal	10% pet.	< 1	–		–
hexyl ethyl acetoacetate	4% pet.	1	–		–
hexyl isobutyrate	4% pet.	5	–		–
hexyl 2-methylbutyrate	10% pet.	< 1	–		–

(continued)

(continuation)

Name	Non-irritating patch test conc. (RIFM) (§ 27.6)	Quant. use (§ 27.6)	Patch test conc. & veh. (§ 5.2) and ref. (§ 27.2)	Cont. all. (§ 27.3)	Comment (N: § 27.6)
hexyl neopentanoate	4% pet.	< 1	–		–
hexyl salicylate	3% pet.	–	–		–
hexyl tiglate	12% pet.	1	–		–
hibawood oil	12% pet.	1	1% alc./2% pet. [7], 1% pet. [17]		N
ho leaf oil	10% pet.	50	1% alc./2% pet. [7], 1% pet. [17]		N
hyacinth absolute	8% pet.	1	–		N
hydratropic acetate	12% pet.	1	–		–
hydratropic alcohol	6% pet.	1	–		–
hydratropic aldehyde	2% pet.	25	–		–
hydratropic aldehyde dimethyl acetal	4% pet.	1	–		–
hydroabietyl alcohol (Abitol®)	10% pet.	9	1% pet.	+	Sensitizer in HMT *See* § 23.47
hydroxycitronellal	5% pet.	500	4–10% pet; 1% pet. [7]	+	*See* § 5.16
hydroxycitronellal dimethylacetal	10% pet.	4	–		–
hydroxycitronellal methylanthranilate	6% pet.	20	–		–
hydroxycitronellol	10% pet.	1	–		–
4-(4-hydroxy-4-methylpentyl)-3-cyclohexene-1-carboxaldehyde (Lyral®)		–	–		–
4-(p-hydroxyphenyl)-2-butanone	12% pet.	1	–		–
hyssop oil	4% pet.	1	1% alc./2% pet. [7], 1% pet. [17]		N
immortelle absolute	2% pet.	1	–		N
indole	1% pet.	4	–		–
ionone	8% pet.	200	2% pet. [3]	+	*See* § 5.16
α-irone	10% pet.	1	–		–
isoamyl alcohol	8% pet.	1	–		–
isoamyl butyrate	3% pet.	2	–		–
isoamyl caproate	2% pet.	1	–		–

(continued)

27.7   Fragrance materials

(continuation)

Name	Non-irritating patch test conc. (RIFM) (§ 27.6)	Quant. use (§ 27.6)	Patch test conc. & veh. (§ 5.2) and ref. (§ 27.2)	Cont. all. (§ 27.3)	Comment (N: § 27.6)
isoamyl caprylate	2% pet.	1	–		–
isoamyl formate	3% pet.	1	–		–
isoamyl geranate	8% pet.	1	–		–
isoamyl isovalerate	2% pet.	1	–		–
isoamyl phenylacetate	2% pet.	1	–		–
isoamyl propionate	4% pet.	1	–		–
isoborneol	10% pet.	10	–		–
isobornyl acetate	10% pet.	200	–		–
isobornyl formate	2% pet.	1	–		–
isobornyl propionate	10% pet.	2	–		–
isobutyl acetate	2% pet.	5	–		–
isobutyl benzoate	2% pet.	2	–		–
isobutyl butyrate	12% pet.	1	–		–
isobutyl caproate	20% pet.	1	–		–
isobutyl cinnamate	8% pet.	1	–		–
isobutyl furylpropionate	2% pet.	1	–		–
isobutyl heptylate	2% pet.	1	–		–
isobutyl isovalerate	1% pet.	< 1	–		–
isobutyl linalool	20% pet.	1	–		–
isobutyl phenylacetate	4% pet.	1	–		–
isobutyl quinoline	2% pet.	2	–		–
isobutyl salicylate	10% pet.	3	–		–
isocamphyl cyclohexanol (mixed isomers)	20% pet.	25	–		–
isocyclocitral	4% pet.	1	–		–
isoeugenol	8% pet.	40	2% pet.	+	*See* § 5.16
isoeugenyl acetate	10% pet.	1	–		–
isohexenyl cyclohexenyl carboxaldehyde	3% pet.	12	–		–
isojasmone	8% pet.	2	–		–
isomenthone	8% pet.	3	–		–

(continued)

(continuation)

Name	Non-irritating patch test conc. (RIFM) (§ 27.6)	Quant. use (§ 27.6)	Patch test conc. & veh. (§ 5.2) and ref. (§ 27.2)	Cont. all. (§ 27.3)	Comment (N: § 27.6)
p-isopropylcyclohexanol	5% pet.	1	–		–
6-isopropyl-2-decalol	–	–	–		Sensitizer in HMT (IFRA, June 1979)
2-isopropyl-5-methyl-2-hexene-1-al	10% pet.	1	–		–
2-isopropyl-5-methyl-2-hexene-1-ol	10% pet.	5	–		–
2-isopropyl-5-methyl-2-hexene-1-yl acetate	10% pet.	20	–		–
isopropyl myristate (IPM)	20% pet.	100	10% alc./2% pet.		*See* § 5.17
isopropyl palmitate	8% pet.	120	2% pet.	+	*See* § 5.22
p-isopropyl phenylacetaldehyde	4% pet.	1	–		–
isopropyl quinoline	2% pet.	1	pure		*See* § 5.17
isopropyl tiglate	10% pet.	1	–		–
isopulegol	8% pet.	3	–		–
isopulegol acetate	8% pet.	2	–		–
isosafrole	8% pet.	1	–		Carcinogenic?
isovaleric acid	1% pet.	1	–		–
jasmine absolute	3% pet.	1	jasmin oil 2% pet. [7]		N
juniper berry oil	8% pet.	2	2% pet.	+	N *See* § 26.3 *and* § 27.2, [23]
labdanum oil	8% pet.	5	1% alc./2% pet. [7], 1% pet. [17]		N
laevulinic acid	4% pet.	1	–		–
laurel leaf oil	10% pet.	–	laurel oil 2% pet. pure [17]	+	*See* § 5.16 *and* § 26.3 (*Laurus nobilis*)
lavandin oil	5% pet.	500	2% pet.	+	N *See* § 27.2, [23]
lavandulyl acetate	10% pet.	1	–		–
lavender absolute	10% pet.	5	–		N
lavender oil	16% pet.	100	1–2% pet. [17]	+	N *See* § 5.16 *See also* § 27.2, [23]
lavender (spike lavender) oil	8% pet.	100	1% alc./2% pet. [7], 1% pet. [17]		N
lemon grass oil East Indian	4% pet.	50 ⎫	lemon grass oil 1% pet. [7],	+	⎰ N *See* § 5.16
lemon grass oil West Indian	4% pet.	250 ⎭	2% pet. [3]		⎱ N *See* § 5.16
lemon oil distilled	10% pet.	–			N *See* § 5.16 *under* lemon oil

(continued)

(*continuation*)

Name	Non-irritating patch test conc. (RIFM) (§ 27.6)	Quant. use (§ 27.6)	Patch test conc. & veh. (§ 5.2) and ref. (§ 27.2)	Cont. all. (§ 27.3)	Comment (N: § 27.6)
lemon oil expressed	10% pet.	150	1–2% pet.	+	N *See* § 5.16 *under* lemon oil. Phototoxic
lemon petitgrain oil	10% pet.	1	–		N Has caused phototoxicity (§ 6.5)
lilial	1% pet.	–	1% pet.	+	*See* § 5.16
lilial-methylanthranilate (Schiff base)	12% pet.	–	–		–
lime oil distilled	15% pet.·	50	1% alc./2% pet. [7], 1% pet. [17]		N Lime oil has caused phototoxicity (§ 6.5)
lime oil expressed	no test concentration	50	1% alc./2% pet. [7], 1% pet. [17]		N Phototoxic (§ 6.5)
D-limonene	8% pet.	150 ⎫	1–5% o.o. [5]; 2% pet. [2, 17]	+	*See* §5.39 *under* thyme oil
L-limonene	4 pet.	1 ⎭		+	*See* § 5.39 *under* thyme oil
linaloe wood oil	8% pet.	1	1% alc./2% pet. [7], 1% pet. [17]		N
linalool	20% pet.	200	30% pet.	+	*See* § 5.16
linalyl anthranilate	8% pet.	1	–		–
linalyl benzoate	8% pet.	3	–		–
linalyl butyrate	8% pet.	1	–		–
linalyl cinnamate	8% pet.	3	–		–
linalyl formate	10% pet.	1	–		–
linalyl isobutyrate	8% pet.	1	–		–
linalyl isovalerate	20% pet.	1	–		–
linalyl methyl ether	5% pet.	1	–		–
linalyl phenylacetate	4% pet.	1	–		–
linalyl propionate	8% pet.	10	–		–
litsea cubeba oil	8% pet.	<1	2% pet.	+	N *See* § 27.2, [23]
lovage oil	2% pet.	1	–		N
mace oil	8% pet.	2	1% alc./2% pet. [7], 1% pet. [17]		N
maltol	10% pet.	–	–		–
marjoram oil, Spanish	6% pet.	2 ⎫	1% alc./2% pet. [7] 1% pet. [17]		N
marjoram oil sweet	6% pet.	1 ⎭			N
L-(p-menthen-6-yl)-1-propanone	4% pet.	50	–		–

(*continued*)

(continuation)

Name	Non-irritating patch test conc. (RIFM) (§ 27.6)	Quant. use (§ 27.6)	Patch test conc. & veh. (§ 5.2) and ref. (§ 27.2)	Cont. all. (§ 27.3)	Comment (N: § 27.6)
L-menthol	8% pet.	50	menthol 2% pet. [1]		*See* § 5.38
menthol racemic	8% pet.	5			*See* § 5.38
menthone racemic	8% pet.	1	–		–
L-menthyl acetate	8% pet.	3	–		–
menthyl acetate racemic	8% pet.	3	–		–
menthyl acetoacetate	8% pet.	< 1	–		–
menthyl isovalerate	1% pet.	< 1	–		–
p-methoxyacetophenone	6% pet.	2	–		–
o-methoxybenzaldehyde	4% pet.	1	–		–
o-methoxycinnamic aldehyde	4% pet.	1	4% pet.	+	*See* § 5.16
methoxycitronellal	10% pet.	–	1% pet.	+	*See* § 5.16
7-methoxycoumarin	–	–	–		Sensitizer and photosensitizer (IFRA, June 1979) *See also* § 6.5.
p-methoxyphenylacetone	4% pet.	1	–		–
4-(p-methoxyphenyl)butan-2-one	5% pet.	1	–		–
methyl abietate	2% pet.	25	–		–
methyl acetate	10% pet.	–	–		–
methyl acetoacetate	8% pet.	1	–		–
p-methylacetophenone	6% pet.	30	–		–
methyl n-amyl ketone	4% pet.	1	–		–
α-methylanisalacetone	8% pet.	1	–		Sensitizer in HMT. Test conc. may be irritating
methyl anisate	4% pet.	1	4% pet.	+	*See* § 5.16
methyl anthranilate	10% pet.	50	–		–
methyl benzoate	4% pet.	15	1% pet. [3]		–
methylbenzylcarbinyl acetate	6% pet.	< 1	–		–
5-methyl-3-butyltetrahydropyran-4-yl acetate	8% pet.	1	–		–
α-methyl butyraldehyde	1% pet.	< 1	–		–
methyl butyrate	8% pet.	< 1	–		–
methyl caproate	4% pet.	< 1	–		–

(continued)

27.7   Fragrance materials

(continuation)

Name	Non-irritating patch test conc. (RIFM) (§ 27.6)	Quant. use (§ 27.6)	Patch test conc. & veh. (§ 5.2) and ref. (§ 27.2)	Cont. all. (§ 27.3)	Comment (N: § 27.6)
methyl chavicol	3% pet.	4	–		–
methyl cinnamate	10% pet.	25	–		–
methylcinnamic alcohol	2% pet.	5	–		–
α-methylcinnamic aldehyde	8% pet.	5	–		–
6-methylcoumarin	4% pet.	1	1% alc.	+	See § 27.2 [4] and § 5.16 Photoallergic (§ 6.5)
7-methylcoumarin	8% pet.	–	–		Has caused photoallergy (§ 6.5) (IFRA, February 1979)
methyl crotonate	6% pet.	1	–		Sensitizer in HMT
3-methylcyclopentadecanone	30% pet.	1	–		–
methyl cyclopentenolone	3% pet.	1	–		–
γ-methyl decalactone	2% pet.	–	–		–
methyl diphenyl ether	2% pet.	2	–		–
methyl ester of rosin (partially hydrogenated)	10% pet.	200	–		–
4-methyl-7-ethoxycoumarin	–	–	–		Photosensitizer (IFRA, June 1979)
methyl ethyl ketone	20% pet.	50	pure		–
methyl eugenol	8% pet.	50	–		–
5-methylfurfural	2% pet.	< 1	–		–
methyl furoate	10% pet.	1	–		–
methyl heptenol	2% pet.	1	–		–
methyl heptenone	3% pet.	2	–		–
methyl heptine carbonate	2% pet.	3	0.5% pet.	+	See § 5.16 Sensitizer in HMT
methylhexylacetaldehyde	10% pet.	< 1	–		–
methyl hexyl ketone	4% pet.	6	–		–
p-methyl hydratropaldehyde	4% pet.	7	–		–
methylionone	10% pet.	250	1% pet. [7] 10% pet.	+	See § 5.16
methyl isoeugenol	8% pet.	3	–		–
methyl isopropyl ketone	10% pet.	–	–		–

(continued)

(continuation)

Name	Non-irritating patch test conc. (RIFM) (§ 27.6)	Quant. use (§ 27.6)	Patch test conc. & veh. (§ 5.2) and ref. (§ 27.2)	Cont. all. (§ 27.3)	Comment (N: § 27.6)
α-methyl naphthyl ketone	2% pet.	5	–		–
β-methyl naphthyl ketone	2% pet.	50	–		–
3-methyl-2(3)-nonenenitrile	10% pet.	–	–		Sensitizer in HMT (IFRA, February 1980)
methyl nonylenate	20% pet.	1	–		–
methyl nonyl ketone	5% pet.	–	–		–
3-methyloctan-3-ol	10% pet.	–	–		–
3-methyl-1-octen-3-ol	10% pet.	–	–		Weak sensitizer in HMT
methyl octine carbonate	2% pet.	1	–		–
methyl octyl acetaldehyde	10% pet.	–	–		–
2-methylpentanoic acid	2% pet.	–	–		–
methyl phenylacetate	8% pet.	5	–		–
methylphenylcarbinyl acetate	4% pet.	10	–		–
methyl propionate	2% pet.	< 1	–		–
p-methylquinoline	2% pet.	1	–		–
methyl salicylate	8% pet.	90	1% pet. [1], 2% pet. [2, 17]	+	*See* § 5.42
methyl p-toluate	8% pet.	1	–		–
methyl undecylenate	12% pet.	< 1	–		–
mimosa absolute	1% pet.	1	–		N
musk ambrette	20% pet.	100	1–3% alc./pet.	+	*See* § 5.16 Photosensitizer (§ 6.5) (IFRA, June 1981)
musk ketone	5% pet.	50	10% pet. [7]		Has caused photoallergy (§ 6.5)
musk tibetene	2% pet.	1	–		–
musk xylol	5% pet.	150	–		–
β-myrcene	4% pet.	2	1% pet. [7]		
myrcenol	4% pet.	–	–		–
myrcenyl acetate	4% pet.	10	–		–
myrrh oil	8% pet.	5	myrrh 10% alc. [5] 1–2% pet. [7, 17]		N
β-naphthyl ethyl ether	2% pet.	10	–		–
β-naphthyl methyl ether	4% pet.	5	–		–

(continued)

27.7 Fragrance materials

(continuation)

Name	Non-irritating patch test conc. (RIFM) (§ 27.6)	Quant. use (§ 27.6)	Patch test conc. & veh. (§ 5.2) and ref. (§ 27.2)	Cont. all. (§ 27.3)	Comment (N: § 27.6)
narcissus absolute	2% pet.	1	–		N
neral	1% pet.	–	–		Sensitizer in HMT
nerol	4% pet.	20	–		–
neroli oil Tunesian	4% pet.	1	neroli oil 10% o.o. [2], 2% pet. [3, 17]		N Has caused phototoxicity (§ 6.5) *See also* § 5.17
nerolidol	4% pet.	1	–		–
nerolidyl acetate	12% pet.	1	–		–
neryl acetate	10% pet.	2	–		–
neryl formate	6% pet.	1	–		–
neryl isovalerate	6% pet.	1	–		–
neryl propionate	6% pet.	1	–		–
nitrobenzene (mirbane oil)	–	–	10% o.o. (?)		Dermatotoxic (IFRA, June 1979)
2,6-nonadienal	2% pet.	1	–		–
2,6-nonadienol	1% pet.	–	–		–
γ-nonalactone	10% pet.	7	–		–
δ-nonalactone	10% pet.	1	–		–
1,3-nonanediol acetate (mixed esters)	8% pet.	50	–		–
2-nonenal	4% pet.	1	–		–
cis-6-nonenal	1% pet.	<0.1	–		–
2-nonyn-1-al dimethylacetal	4% pet.	–	–		–
nootkatone	–	–	–		Sensitizer (IFRA, October 1980) (not if highly purified)
nopol	8% pet.	10	–		–
nopyl acetate	10% pet.	200	–		–
nutmeg oil East Indian	2% pet.	10	1% alc./2% pet. [7], 1% pet. [17]		N
oakmoss concrete	10% pet.	75	2% pet.	+	N *See* § 5.7
ocimene	5% pet.	3	–		–
ocimenol	4% pet.	–	–		–
ocimenyl acetate	4% pet.	1	–		–

(continued)

(continuation)

Name	Non-irritating patch test conc. (RIFM) (§ 27.6)	Quant. use (§ 27.6)	Patch test conc. & veh. (§ 5.2) and ref. (§ 27.2)	Cont. all. (§ 27.3)	Comment (N: § 27.6)
ocotea cymbarum oil	20% pet.	–	1% alc./2% pet. [7], 1% pet. [17]		N
octahydrocoumarin	8% pet.	< 1	–		–
γ-octalactone	12% pet.	–	–		–
δ-octalactone	12% pet.	< 1	–		–
octanol-3	12% pet.	5	–		–
octyl isobutyrate	2% pet.	1	–		N
octyl formate	2% pet.	1	–		–
octyl salicylate	5% pet.	–	2% o.o. [2]		–
oil lavandin acetylated	10% pet.	20	1% alc./2% pet. [7], 1% pet. [17]		N
olibanum absolute	8% pet.	–	–		N
olibanum gum	8% pet.	10	olibanum 2% pet. [3]		N
opoponax	–	–	–		N Sensitizer (not the alcoholic extract) (IFRA, March 1978)
orange flower absolute	20% pet.	4	–		N
orange (bitter orange) oil	10% pet.	20	1% pet. [7], 2% pet. [3, 17]	+	N *See* § 5.16 Phototoxic For sweet orange oil *see* § 27.2, [23]
orange oil expressed	8% pet.	200			
origanum oil	2% pet.	6	origanum 2% pet. [3]		N
orris absolute	3% pet.	1	–		N
11-oxahexadecanolide	10% pet.	< 3	–		–
12-oxahexadecanolide	10% pet.	3	–		–
palmarosa oil	8% pet.	30	1% alc./2% pet. [7], 1% pet. [17]		N
parsley seed oil	2% pet.	1	1% alc./2% pet. [7], 1% pet. [17]		N *See* § 26.3 under *Petroselinum sativum*
patchouly oil	10% pet.	300	1–2% pet.	+	N *See* § 5.16
pelargonic acid	12% pet.	–	–		–
pennyroyal oil Eurafrican	6% pet.	11	1% alc./2% pet. [7], 1% pet. [17]		N
1,1,3,3,5-pentamethyl-4,6-dinitroindane	10% pet.	50	–		–
pentylcyclopentanonepropanone	20% pet.	–	–		–

(continued)

27.7 Fragrance materials

(continuation)

Name	Non-irritating patch test conc. (RIFM) (§ 27.6)	Quant. use (§ 27.6)	Patch test conc. & veh. (§ 5.2) and ref. (§ 27.2)	Cont. all. (§ 27.3)	Comment (N: § 27.6)
pentylidene cyclohexanone	10% pet.	1	–		Strong sensitizer in HMT (IFRA, February 1979)
perilla aldehyde	4% pet.	–	–		Sensitizer in HMT (IFRA, October 1979)
Peru balsam oil	8% pet.	14	1% alc./2% pet. [7], 1% pet. [17]		N
petitgrain Paraguay oil	7% pet.	300	10% o.o.		N Sensitizer in HMT *See* § 5.17 Has caused phototoxicity (*see* § 6.5)
α-phellandrene	4% pet.	12	–		–
phenoxyacetaldehyde	4% pet.	1	–		–
phenoxyacetic acid	2% pet.	–	–		–
phenoxyethyl isobutyrate	4% pet.	4	–		–
phenoxyethyl propionate	10% pet.	4	–		–
phenylacetaldehyde	2% pet.	18	2% pet.	+	*See* § 5.16 Sensitizer in HMT
phenylacetaldehyde dimethyl acetal	2% pet.	6	–		–
phenylacetaldehyde ethyleneglycol acetal	6% pet.	–	–		–
phenylacetaldehyde glyceryl acetal	3% pet.	6	–		–
phenylacetic acid	2% pet.	7	–		–
phenyl acetyl nitrile	2% pet.	1	–		–
phenylethyl acetate	10% pet.	50	1% pet. [7]		–
phenylethyl alcohol	8% pet.	1000	1% pet. [7]		–
phenylethyl anthranilate	10% pet.	1	–		–
phenylethyl benzoate	8% pet.	1	–		–
phenylethyl butyrate	8% pet.	2	–		–
phenylethyl cinnamate	2% pet.	3	–		–
phenylethyl formate	6% pet.	1	–		–
phenylethyl isobutyrate	2% pet.	20	–		–
phenylethyl isovalerate	2% pet.	1	–		–
phenylethyl methyl ether	8% pet.	< 1	–		–

(continued)

(continuation)

Name	Non-irritating patch test conc. (RIFM) (§ 27.6)	Quant. use (§ 27.6)	Patch test conc. & veh. (§ 5.2) and ref. (§ 27.2)	Cont. all. (§ 27.3)	Comment (N: § 27.6)
phenylethyl methyl ethyl carbinol	10% pet.	1	–		–
phenylethyl methylethylcarbinyl acetate	10% pet.	–			–
phenylethyl phenylacetate	2% pet.	10	–		–
phenylethyl propionate	8% pet.	5	–		–
phenylethyl salicylate	8% pet.	10	–		–
phenylethyl tiglate	6% pet.	1	–		–
phenylpropyl acetate	8% pet.	10	–		–
phenylpropyl alcohol	8% pet.	5	–		–
phenylpropyl aldehyde	8% pet.	10	–		–
phenylpropyl cinnamate	4% pet.	3	–		–
phenylpropyl formate	8% pet.	1	–		–
3-phenylpropyl isobutyrate	8% pet.	1	–		–
phenylpropyl propionate	8% pet.	< 1	–		Weak sensitizer in HMT
phenyl salicylate	6% pet.	1	as is [2], 3% alc. [7], 1% pet. [3]	+	*See* § 23.53
phytol	10% pet.	1	–		Weak sensitizer in HMT
pimenta berry oil	8% pet.	1	1% alc./2% pet. [7], 1% pet. [17]		N
pimenta leaf oil	12% pet.	5	1% alc./2% pet. [7], 1% pet. [17]		N
pinacol	8% pet.	1	–		–
α-pinene	10% pet.	6	1% pet. [7], 15% o.o. [3]	+	*See* § 5.39 *under* turpentine *and* § 5.40
β-pinene	12% pet.	15	–		Toxic
pinus pumilio oil	12% pet.	1 ⎱	pine oil 5% pet. [1], pure [7]		N For contact allergy to pine needle oil, *see* § 27.2, [23]
pinus sylvestris oil	12% pet.	1 ⎰			
piperitone	10% pet.	1	–		*See under* heliotropine
piperonal			–		
piperonyl acetate	8% pet.	1	–		–
piperonyl acetone	4% pet.	1	–		–

(continued)

(continuation)

Name	Non-irritating patch test conc. (RIFM) (§ 27.6)	Quant. use (§ 27.6)	Patch test conc. & veh. (§ 5.2) and ref. (§ 27.2)	Cont. all. (§ 27.3)	Comment (N: § 27.6)
prenol	10% pet.	–	–		–
prenyl acetate	20% pet.	< 1	–		–
prenyl benzoate	20% pet.	< 1	–		–
prenyl salicylate	20% pet.	< 10	–		–
n-propyl acetal	10% pet.	1	–		–
propylidene phthalide	4% pet.	1	–		–
propyl propionate	20% pet.	1	–		–
d-pulegone	10% pet.	1	–		–
rhodinyl acetate	12% pet.	2	–		–
rhodinyl butyrate	12% pet.	1	–		–
rhodinyl formate	4% pet.	2	–		–
rhodinyl isobutyrate	4% pet.	1	–		–
rhodinyl propionate	4% pet.	1	–		–
rose absolute French	2% pet.	4	–		N
rosemary oil	10% pet.	50	1% alc./2% pet. [7], 1% pet. [17]		N § 26.3 (*Rosmarinus officinalis*)
rose oil Bulgarian	2% pet.	2	} rose oil 2% pet. 1% alc. [7]	+	N *See* § 5.16
rose oil Moroccan	2% pet.	2			
rose (oil rose) Turkish	2% pet.	2			
rose oxide levo	2% pet.	5	–		–
rue oil	1% pet.	1	1% alc./2% pet. [7], 1% pet. [17]		N Phototoxic
safrole	8% pet.	50	–		Carcinogenic (?)
sage clary oil, Russian	8% pet.	< 3	1% alc./2% pet. [7], 1% pet. [17]		N *See* § 26.3 (*Salvia officinalis*)
sage oil, Dalmatian	8% pet.	20	1% alc./2% pet. [7], 1% pet. [17]		N *See* § 26.3 (*Salvia officinalis*)
sage oil, Spanish	8% pet.	4	1% alc./2% pet. [7], 1% pet. [17]		N *See* § 26.3 (*Salvia officinalis*)
salicylaldehyde	2% pet.	1	–		–
sandalwood oil, East Indian	10% pet.	48	1–2% pet.	+	N *See* § 5.16 *See also* § 27.2, [23]

(continued)

(continuation)

Name	Non-irritating patch test conc. (RIFM) (§ 27.6)	Quant. use (§ 27.6)	Patch test conc. & veh. (§ 5.2) and ref. (§ 27.2)	Cont. all. (§ 27.3)	Comment (N: § 27.6)
α-santalol	20% pet.	4	–		–
santalyl acetate	20% pet.	1	–		–
sassafras oil	4% pet.	–	1% alc./2% pet. [7], 1% pet. [17]		N *See* § 5.17
savin oil	–	–	1% alc./2% pet. [7], 1% pet. [17]		N Plant origin determines sensitizing capacity (IFRA, May 1980)
savory oil (summer variety)	6% pet.	1	1% alc./2% pet. [7], 1% pet. [17]		N
schinus molle oil	4% pet.	1	1% alc./2% pet. [7], 1% pet. [17]		N
skatole	2% pet.	1	–		–
snakeroot oil Canadian	4% pet.	1	1% alc./2% pet. [7], 1% pet. [17]		N
spearmint oil	4% pet.	25	1% alc. [2], 2% pet. [3, 17]	+	N *See* § 13.3
stearic acid	7% pet.	–	1% aqua [2]	+	Has comedogenic properties (*See* § 9.2) *See also* § 27.2, [19]
styrallyl alcohol	8% pet.	10	–		–
styrax (= storax)	–	–	2% pet.	+	N *See* § 5.39 *and* § 26.3 *(Liquid-amber orientalis)* Sensitizer (not if purified with alkali) (IFRA, May 1980)
sucrose octaacetate	4% pet.	–	–		–
sweet birch oil	4% pet.	1	1% alc./2% pet. [7], 1% pet. [17]		N
tagetes oil	2% pet.	< 1	1% alc./2% pet. [7], 1% pet. [17]		N
tangelo oil	8% pet.	–	1% alc./2% pet. [7], 1% pet. [17]		N
tangerine oil	5% pet.	16	1% alc./2% pet. [7], 1% pet. [17]		N
tansy oil	4% pet.	1	1% alc./2% pet. [7], 1% pet. [17]		N
α-terpinene	5% pet.	1	–		–
γ-terpinene	5% pet.	1	–		–
4-terpinenol	5% pet.	10	–		–

(continued)

27.7 Fragrance materials

(continuation)

Name	Non-irritating patch test conc. (RIFM) (§ 27.6)	Quant. use (§ 27.6)	Patch test conc. & veh. (§ 5.2) and ref. (§ 27.2)	Cont. all. (§ 27.3)	Comment (N: § 27.6)
terpineol	12% pet.	1000	α-terpineol 5% o.o. [7]; cis-β-terpineol 25% BL [7]	+	*See* § 5.39
terpinolene	20% pet.	50	1% pet. [7]		–
terpinyl acetate	5% pet.	1000	–		Has caused contact urticaria (§ 7.5)
terpinyl formate	2% pet.	1	–		–
terpinyl propionate	4% pet.	10	–		–
tetrahydrolinalool	4% pet.	1	–		–
tetrahydromuguol	4% pet.	35	–		–
tetrahydromugyl acetate	4% pet.	1	–		–
3,3,5,5-tetramethyl-4-ethoxyvinyl-cyclohexanone	10% pet.	1	–		–
thyme oil red	8% pet.	7	oil of thyme 25% c.o. [2], 1% alc., 10% pet.	+	N *See* § 5.39 *and* § 26.3 *(Thymus vulgaris) See also* § 27.2, [23]
tiglic acid	1% pet.	< 1	–		–
tobacco leaf absolute	1% pet.	–	–		N
tolualdehyde	4% pet.	3	–		–
tolualdehyde glyceryl acetal	10% pet.	–	–		–
p-tolyl acetaldehyde	2% pet.	1	–		–
p-tolyl alcohol	4% pet.	< 1	–		–
tonka absolute	8% pet.	1	–		N
tree moss concrete	10% pet.	35	–		N
triacetin	20% pet.	20	–		–
trichlormethylphenylcarbinyl acetate	1% pet.	40	–		–
tricyclodecen-4-yl 8-acetate	8% pet.	50	–		–
tricyclodecenyl propionate	20% pet.	–	–		–
triethyl citrate	20% pet.	–	–		–
triethylene glycol	20% pet.	10	–		–
triethyl orthoformate	4% pet.	–	–		–
3,5,5-trimethylcyclohexanol	4% pet.	2	–		–

(continued)

(continuation)

Name	Non-irritating patch test conc. (RIFM) (§ 27.6)	Quant. use (§ 27.6)	Patch test conc. & veh. (§ 5.2) and ref. (§ 27.2)	Cont. all. (§ 27.3)	Comment (N: § 27.6)
3,5,5-trimethylhexanal	4% pet.	1	–		–
3,5,5-trimethylhexyl acetate	4% pet.	15	–		–
γ-undecalactone	2% pet.	15	–		–
δ-undecalactone	2% pet.	–	–		–
undecylenic acid	4% pet.	1	5% pet.	+	*See* § 5.32 Also used as antimycotic drug
undecylenic aldehyde digeranyl acetal	10% pet.	< 1	–		–
undecylenic aldehyde (mixed isomers)	5% pet.	< 10	–		–
n-valeraldehyde	2% pet.	1	–		–
γ-valerolactone	10% pet.	< 1	–		–
vanilla tincture	10% pet.	160	–		N
vanillin	2% pet.	250	10% pet. [1]		–
veratraldehyde	15% pet.	–	–		–
vetiver acetate	20% pet.	75	–		Sensitizer in HMT to impurities of technical product
vetiver oil	8% pet.	75	2% pet.	+	N *See* § 27.2, [23]
vetiverol	8% pet.	3	–		–
violet leaf absolute	2% pet.	1	–		N
ylang-ylang oil	10% pet.	76	2–5% pet.	+	N *See* § 5.16
zingerone	8% pet.	< 1	–		–

COLORS

27.8   This section contains the following information on colors:
– Conversion of CTFA/FDA names to Color Index numbers (§ 27.9)
– Tabulation of colors (§ 27.10)
– Tabulation of color ingredients of hair dye preparations (§ 27.11)
Color Index numbers refer to the *Color Index, 3rd Edition*, 1971.

Colors permitted in the EEC: Colors marked with an * in the 'Comment' column of § 27.10 are permitted colors for cosmetics in the EEC, as defined in the *EEC Cosmetic Directive* of 27 July 1976 (76/768/EEC).

27.9 **Conversion of CTFA/FDA names to Color Index numbers (CI)**

CTFA/FDA name	CI	CTFA/FDA name	CI
Acid Black 2	50420	DC Red 33	17200
Acid Orange 3	10385	DC Red 34	15880
Acid Violet 43	60730	DC Red 36	12085
Acid Yellow 3	47005	DC Red 37	45170
Alumina	77002	DC Violet 2	60725
Aluminum powder	77000	DC Yellow 5	19140
Anatto	75120	DC Yellow 6	15985
Apocarotenal	40820	DC Yellow 7	45350
		DC Yellow 8	45350
Barium sulfate	77120	DC Yellow 10	47005
Basic Blue 9	52015	DC Yellow 11	47000
Basic Violet 1	42535	Direct Black 38	30235
Basic Violet 3	42555	Direct Black 131	30270
Bismuth oxychloride	77163	Direct Brown 2	22311
Bronze powder	77400	Direct Brown 31	35660
		Direct Red 81	28160
Calcium carbonate	77220	Disperse Blue 1	64500
Canthaxanthin	40850		
Carbon black	77266	Ext. DC Yellow 1	13065
Carmine	75470	Ext. DC Yellow 7	10316
Carotene	75130		
Chlorophyl	75810	FDC Blue 1	42090
Chlorophyllins	75810	FDC Blue 2	73015
Chlorophyllin-copper	75810	FDC Green 3	42053
Chromium hydroxide	77289	FDC Red 2	16185
Chromiumoxide green	77288	FDC Red 3	45430
Copper powder	77400	FDC Red 4	14700
		FDC Red 40	16035
DC Blue 1	42090	FDC Yellow 5	19140
DC Blue 4	42090	FDC Yellow 6	15985
DC Blue 6	73000	Ferric ferrocyanide	77510
DC Brown 1	20170		
DC Green 5	61570	Graphite	77265
DC Green 6	61565	Guanine	75170
DC Green 8	59040		
DC Orange 4	15510	Iron oxides	77489
DC Orange 5	45370		77491
DC Orange 10	45425		77492
DC Orange 17	12075		77499
DC Red 2	16185		
DC Red 3	45430	Kaolin	77004
DC Red 6	15850		
DC Red 7	15850	Magnesium carbonate	77713
DC Red 8	15585	Manganese Violet	77742
DC Red 9	15585	Mica	77019
DC Red 10	15630		
DC Red 11	15630	Solvent Black 5	50415
DC Red 12	15630		
DC Red 13	15630	Talc	77718
DC Red 17	26100	Titanium dioxide	77891
DC Red 19	45170		
DC Red 21	45380	Ultramarine blue	77007
DC Red 22	45380	Ultramarine pink	77007
DC Red 27	45410	Ultramarine violet	77007
DC Red 28	45410	Ultramarine green	77007
DC Red 30	73360		
DC Red 31	15800	Zinc oxide	77947

27.10   Colors

Color Index no. (§ 27.8)	Common name/ Color Index name	Lakes or salts	USA-FDA name for certified batches	EEC color no.	Freq. use (§ 27.3)	Patch test conc. & veh. (§ 5.2) and ref. (§ 27.2)	Cont. all. (§ 27.3)	Comment (* § 27.8)
Nitroso and nitro dyes								
10006	Pigment Green 8		–	–		–		*
10020	Acid Green 1		Ext. DC-green 1	–	50	–		*
10025	Acid Green 4		–	–		–		*
10316	Acid Yellow 1		Ext. DC-yellow 7	–	70	–		*
		-aluminum lake	–	–	12	–		*
10385	Acid Orange 3		–	–	33	–		–
Azo-dyes								
11000	Solvent Yellow 1		–	–		–		–
11005	Disperse Orange 3		–	–		–		–
11110	Disperse Red 1		–	–		–		–
11210	Disperse Red 17		–	–		–		*
11390	Yellow OB		Solvent Yellow 6	–		1% pet. [9]	+	See § 4.3
11680	Pigment Yellow 1		–	–		–		*
11710	Pigment Yellow 3		–	–		–		*
11720	Pigment Yellow 9		–	–		–		*
11725	Pigment Orange 1		–	–		–		*
11730	Pigment Yellow 2		–	–		–		*
11765	Pigment Yellow 49		–	–		–		*
11850	Solvent Yellow 11		–	–		–		*
11855	Disperse Yellow 3		–	–		–		*
11860	Solvent Yellow 12		–	–		–		*
11870	Solvent Yellow 9		–	–		–		*
11920	Solvent Orange 1		–	–		–		*
12010	Solvent Red 3		–	–		–		*
12055	Solvent Yellow 14, Sudan I		–	–		0.1% pet. [9]	+	* See § 4.3
12075	Pigment Orange 5		DC Orange 17	–	57	1% pet.	+	* See § 23.53
		-lake	–	–	492	–		*

(continued)

27.10 Colors

(continuation)

Color Index no. (§ 27.8)	Common name/ Color Index name	Lakes or salts	USA-FDA name for certified batches	EEC color no.	Freq. use (§ 27.3)	Patch test conc. & veh. (§ 5.2) and ref. (§ 27.2)	Cont. all. (§ 27.3)	Comment (* § 27.8)
12085	Pigment Red 4, Flaming Red		DC Red 36	–	104	1% pet.	+	* See § 23.53 and § 23.47
		-lake	–	–	51	20% aqua [8]		*
12090	Pigment Red 6		–	–		–		*
12100	Solvent Orange 2		Ext. DC Orange 4	–		1% pet. [9]	+	See § 4.3
12120	Pigment Red 3, Toluidine Red		–	–		1% pet. [9]		*
12140	Solvent Orange 7, Sudan II		–	–		1% pet. [9]	+	* See § 4.3
12145	–		–	–		–		*
12150	Solvent Red 1		–	–		–		*
12155	Solvent Red 17		–	–		–		*
12156	Solvent Red 80		Citrus Red 2	–		–		–
12170	Solvent Red 4		–	–		–		*
12175	Solvent Orange 8, Vacanceine Red		–	–		1% pet. [9]	+	See § 4.3
12196	Solvent Violet 1		–	–		–		*
12310	Pigment Red 2		–	–		–		*
12315	Pigment Red 22		–	–		–		*
12335	Pigment Red 8		–	–		–		*
12350	Pigment Red 18		–	–		–		*
12370	Pigment Red 112		–	–		–		*
12385	Pigment Red 12		–	–		–		*
12420	Pigment Red 7		–	–		–		*
12430	Pigment Red 11		–	–		–		*
12440	Pigment Red 10		–	–		–		*
12459	–		–	–		–		*
12460	Pigment Red 9		–	–		–		*
12480	Pigment Brown 1		–	–		–		*
12490	Pigment Red 5		–	–		–		*
12700	Disperse Yellow 16		–	–		–		*
12740	Solvent Yellow 18		–	–		–		*

(continued)

(continuation)

Color Index no. (§ 27.8)	Common name/ Color Index name	Lakes or salts	USA-FDA name for certified batches	EEC color no.	Freq. use (§ 27.3)	Patch test conc. & veh. (§ 5.2) and ref. (§ 27.2)	Cont. all. (§ 27.3)	Comment (* § 27.8)
12770	Disperse Yellow 4		–	–		–		*
12790	Disperse Yellow 5		–	–		–		*
13015	Acid Yellow 9		–	–		–		*
13020	Acid Red 2		–	–		–		*
13065	Acid Yellow 36		Ext. DC Yellow 1	–	178	–		*
13900	Acid Yellow 99		–	–		–		*
14270	Acid Orange 6		–	–		–		*
14600	Acid Orange 20		–	–		–		*
14700	Food Red 1, Ponceau SX		FDC Red 4	–	604	–		*
14720	Acid Red 14, Azorubin		–	E-122		–		*
14805	Acid Brown 4		–	–		–		*
14815	Scarlet GN		–	E-125		–		*
14895	Acid Red 7		–	–		–		*
14905	Acid Red 5		–	–		–		*
15500	Pigment Red 50		–	–		–		*
		-barium salt (15500:1)	–	–		–		*
15510	Acid Orange 7		DC Orange 4	–	333	–		*
		-aluminum lake	DC Orange 4	–	44	–		*
15525	Pigment Red 68		–	–		–		*
15575	Acid Orange 8		–	–		–		*
15580	Pigment Red 51		–	–		–		*
15585	Pigment Red 53		DC Red 8	–	66	–		*
		-sodium salt	DC Red 8	–	39	20% aqua [8]		*
		-barium salt (15585:1)	DC Red 9	–	62	–		*
		-barium lake	DC Red 9	–	1007	30% o.o. [1]		*
		-barium/stron- tium lake	DC Red 9	–	4	–		*
		-zirconium lake	DC Red 9	–	16	–		*

(continued)

27.10 Colors

(continuation)

Color Index no. (§ 27.8)	Common name/ Color Index name	Lakes or salts	USA-FDA name for certified batches	EEC color no.	Freq. use (§ 27.3)	Patch test conc. & veh. (§ 5.2) and ref. (§ 27.2)	Cont. all. (§ 27.3)	Comment (* § 27.8)
15620	Acid Red 88		–	–		–		*
15630	Pigment Red 49, Lithol red		DC Red 10	–	25	1% pet. [9]		*
		-aluminum lake	DC Red 10	–	26	20% aqua [8]		*
		-sodium salt	DC Red 10	–	77	–		*
		-calcium salt (15630:2)	DC Red 11	–	15	–		*
		-calcium lake	DC Red 11	–	104	20% aqua [8]		*
		-barium salt (15630:1)	DC Red 12	–	29	–		*
		-barium lake	DC Red 12	–	150	20% aqua [8]		*
		-strontium salt (15630:3)	DC Red 13	–	23	–		*
		-strontium lake	DC Red 13	–	109	20% aqua [8]		*
15685	Acid Red 184		–	–		–		*
15800	Pigment Red 64, Brilliant Lake Red R		DC Red 31	–	5	1% pet.	+	* *See* § 4.2, § 23.53 *and* § 23.47
		-calcium lake (15800:1)	DC Red 31	–	5	–		*
15850	Pigment Red 57, Lithol Rubin B		DC Red 6	–	16	20% aqua [8]		*
		-barium lake	DC Red 6	–	517	–		*
		-calcium salt (15850:1)	DC Red 7	–	45	–		*
		-barium lake	DC Red 7	– 10	–			*
		-calcium lake	DC Red 7	–	702	–		*
		-zirconium lake	DC Red 7	–	11	–		*
15865	Pigment Red 48		–		–			*
15880	Pigment Red 63, calcium lake		DC Red 34	–	27	–		*
15970	Acid Orange 12		–	–		–		*
15975	Mordant Red 60		–	–		–		*
15980	Food Orange 2		–	E-111		–		*

(continued)

(continuation)

Color Index no. (§ 27.8)	Common name/ Color Index name	Lakes or salts	USA-FDA name for certified batches	EEC color no.	Freq. use (§ 27.3)	Patch test conc. & veh. (§ 5.2) and ref. (§ 27.2)	Cont. all. (§ 27.3)	Comment (* § 27.8)
15985	Food Yellow 3, Sunset Yellow		FDC Yellow 6	E-110	462	2% pet. [2]		*
		-aluminum lake	FDC Yellow 6	–	56	–		*
		-aluminum lake	DC Yellow 6	–	196	–		*
16035	Allura Red		FDC Red 40	–	34	–		*
16045	Food Red 4		–	–		–		*
16140	Acid Red 24		–	–		–		*
16155	Food Red 6, HC Red 6		–	–	4	–		*
16180	Acid Red 17		–	–		–		*
16185	Food Red 9, Amaranth		FDC Red 2	E-123	359	20% aqua [8]		*
		-aluminum lake (16185:1)	FDC Red 2	–	17	–		*
		-aluminum lake	DC Red 2	–	60	–		*
16230	Food Orange 4		–	–		–		*
16250	Acid Red 44		–	–		–		*
16255	Food Red 7, Cochenille Red A		–	E-124		–		*
16290	Food Red 8		–	–		–		*
16580	Acid Violet 3		–	–		–		*
17200	Food Red 12		DC Red 33	–	374	–		*
17580	Acid Black 31		–	–		–		*
18000	Acid Red 108		–	–		–		*
18050	Food Red 10		–	–		–		*
18055	Food Red 11		–	–		–		*
18065	Acid Red 35		–	–		–		*
18125	Acid Violet 5		–	–		–		*
18130	Acid Red 155		–	–		–		*
18690	Acid Yellow 121		–	–		–		*
18736	Acid Red 180		–	–		–		*
18745	Acid Orange 74		–	–		–		*

(continued)

27.10 Colors

(continuation)

Color Index no. (§ 27.8)	Common name/ Color Index name	Lakes or salts	USA-FDA name for certified batches	EEC color no.	Freq. use (§ 27.3)	Patch test conc. & veh. (§ 5.2) and ref. (§ 27.2)	Cont. all. (§ 27.3)	Comment (* § 27.8)
18820	Acid Yellow 11		–	–	–		*
18900	Acid Yellow 29		–	–	–		*
18965	Acid Yellow 17		–	–	–		*
19120	Acid Yellow 13		–	–	–		*
19130	Acid Yellow 27		–	–	–		*
19140	Food Yellow 4, Tartrazine		FDC Yellow 5	E-102	1920	2% pet. [2]		*
		-aluminum lake	FDC Yellow 5	–	246	20% aqua [8]		*
		-aluminum lake	DC Yellow 5	–	282	–		*
		-zirconium lake	DC Yellow 5	–	176	–		*
19235	Acid Orange 137, Orange B		–	–		–		–
19555	Direct Yellow 28		–	–		–		*
20170	Acid Orange 24		DC Brown 1	–	15	–		*
20285	Food Brown 3		–	–		–		*
20470	Acid Black 1		–	–		–		*
21010	Basic Brown 4		–	–		–		*
21090	Pigment Yellow 12		–	–		–		*
21096	Pigment Yellow 55		–	–		–		*
21100	Pigment Yellow 13		–	–		–		*
21108	–		–	–		–		–
21110	Pigment Orange 13		–	–		–		*
21115	Pigment Orange 34		–	–		–		*
21230	Solvent Yellow 29		–	–		–		*
22311	Direct Brown 2		Direct Brown 2	–	6	–		–
22910	Acid Yellow 42		–	–		–		*
24790	Acid Red 163		–	–		–		*
25135	Acid Yellow 38		–	–		–		*
25220	Direct Yellow 15		–	–		–		*
25410	Direct Violet 47		–	–		–		*
26090	Disperse Yellow 7		–	–		–		*

(continued)

(continuation)

Color Index no. (§ 27.8)	Common name/ Color Index name	Lakes or salts	USA-FDA name for certified batches	EEC color no.	Freq. use (§ 27.3)	Patch test conc. & veh. (§ 5.2) and ref. (§ 27.2)	Cont. all. (§ 27.3)	Comment (* § 27.8)
26100	Solvent Red 23, Sudan III, Toney Red		DC Red 17	–	231	1% pet. [9]	+	* See § 23.53 and § 23.47
26105	Solvent Red 24		–	–		–		*
26360	Acid Blue 113		–	–		–		*
27290	Acid Red 73		–	–		–		*
27300	Acid Red 47		–	–		–		*
27306	Solvent Red 31		–	–		–		*
27755	Food Black 2		–	E-152		–		*
27905	Direct Violet 51		–	–		–		*
28160	Direct Red 81		Direct Red 81	–	6	–		*
28440	Food Black 1, Brilliant Black BN		–	E-151		–		*
29020	Direct Yellow 33		–	–		–		*
30045	Direct Brown 1		–	–		–		*
30235	Direct Black 38		Direct Black 38	–	7	–		–
30270	Direct Black 131		Direct Black 131	–	4	–		–
35660	Direct Brown 31		Direct Brown 31	–	4	–		–
Stilbene dyes								
40215	Direct Orange 34		–	–		–		*
40625	–		–	–		–		*
40640	Fluorescent brightener 48		–	–		–		*
Carotenoid dyes								
40820	Apocarotenal (red)		–	E-160e	9	–		*
40825	Ethyl ester of apocarotenal		–	E-160f		–		*
40850	Canthaxanthin (red)		–	E-160g		–		–
Diphenylmethane dyes								
41000	Basic Yellow 2		–	–		–		*

(continued)

27.10 Colors

(continuation)

Color Index no. (§ 27.8)	Common name/ Color Index name	Lakes or salts	USA-FDA name for certified batches	EEC color no.	Freq. use (§ 27.3)	Patch test conc. & veh. (§ 5.2) and ref. (§ 27.2)	Cont. all. (§ 27.3)	Comment (* § 27.8)
Triarylmethane dyes								
42040	Basic Green 1		–	–		–		*
42045	Acid Blue 1		–	–		–		*
42050	Acid Green 8		–	–		–		*
42051	Acid Blue 3, Food Blue 5, Patent Blue V		–	E-131		–		*
42052	Acid Blue 5		–	–		–		*
42053	Food Green 3		FDC Green 3	–	266	–		*
42080	Acid Blue 7		–	–		–		*
42085	Acid Green 3		–	–		–		*
42090	Acid Blue 9, Brilliant Blue FCF		FDC Blue 1	–	1547	–		*
		-aluminum lake	FDC Blue 1	–	285	–		*
		-aluminum lake	DC Blue 1	–	37	–		*
		-NH$_4$-salt	DC Blue 4	–	6	–		*
42095	Food Green 2		–	–		–		*
42100	Acid Green 9		–	–		–		*
42140	Basic Blue 5		–	–		–		*
42170	Acid Green 22		–	–		–		*
42510	Basic Violet 14		–	–		–		*
42520	Basic Violet 2		–	–		–		*
42525	Acid dye (violet)		–	–		–		*
42535	Basic Violet 1, Gentian Violet		Basic Violet 1	–	13	1–2% aqua	+	* See § 5.7
42555	Basic Violet 3, Crystal Violet		Basic Violet 3	–	4	1–2% aqua	+	* See § 5.7
42571	Acid Blue 13		–	–		–		*
42580	Acid Violet 21		–	–		–		*
42640	Acid Violet 49		(formerly) FDC-Violet 1	–		–		*
42650	Acid Violet 17		–	–		–		*
42735	Acid Blue 104		–	–		–		*

(continued)

(continuation)

Color Index no. (§ 27.8)	Common name/ Color Index name	Lakes or salts	USA-FDA name for certified batches	EEC color no.	Freq. use (§ 27.3)	Patch test conc. & veh. (§ 5.2) and ref. (§ 27.2)	Cont. all. (§ 27.3)	Comment (* § 27.8)
42755	Acid Blue 22		–	–		–		*
43625	–		–	–		–		*
44025	Acid green 16		–	–		–		*
44040	Basic Blue 11		–	–		–		*
44045	Basic Blue 26		–	–		–		*
44090	Food Green 4, Wool Green BS		–	E-142		–		*
Xanthene dyes								
45100	Acid Red 52		–	–		–		*
45160	Basic Red 1		–	–		–		*
45170	Basic Violet 10, Rhodamine B		DC Red 19	–	1066	1% pet.; 30% o.o. [1]	+	* See § 23.53
		-aluminum lake	DC Red 19	–	493	–		*
		-barium lake	DC Red 19	–	5	–		*
		-zirconium lake	DC Red 19	–	31	–		*
		-stearate	DC Red 37	–	16	–		*
45220	Acid Red 50		–	–		–		*
45340	–		–	–		–		*
45350	Acid Yellow 73, Uranin (acid)		DC Yellow 7	–	20	–		*
		-natrium salt	DC Yellow 8	–	53	–		*
45370	Acid Orange 11 (acid)		DC Orange 5	–	441	–		*
		-aluminum lake	DC Orange 5	–	109	–		*
		-zirconium lake	DC Orange 5	–	66	–		*
45376	Acid dye		–	–		–		*
45380	Acid Red 87, Eosin yellowish (acid)		DC Red 21	–	404	50% aqua [5]; pure [2]	+	* See § 23.53
		-aluminum lake	DC Red 21	–	138	–		*
		-zirconium lake	DC Red 21	–	95	–		*
		-natrium salt	DC Red 22	–	7	50% aqua [5]		*
45395	Solvent dye (yellowish orange)		–	–		–		*

(continued)

27.10 Colors

(continuation)

Color Index no. (§ 27.8)	Common name/ Color Index name	Lakes or salts	USA-FDA name for certified batches	EEC color no.	Freq. use (§ 27.3)	Patch test conc. & veh. (§ 5.2) and ref. (§ 27.2)	Cont. all. (§ 27.3)	Comment (* § 27.8)
45405	Acid Red 98, Phloxine	–	–	–	–		*
45410	Acid Red 92, Phloxine B (acid)		DC Red 27	–	59	–		*
		-aluminum lake	DC Red 27	–	152	20% aqua [8]		*
		-zirconium lake	DC Red 27	–	146			*
		-natrium salt	DC Red 28	–	12	–		*
45425	Acid Red 95 (acid)		DC Orange 10	–	16	–		*
45430	Food Red 14, Erythrosine		DC Red 3	–		–		* Has caused photosensitivity See § 5.5
		-aluminum lake	DC Red 3	–	244	–		*
		-erythrosine	FDC Red 3	E-127	81	2% pet. [2]		*
		-aluminum lake	FDC Red 3	–	172	–		*
45440	Acid Red 94, Rose Bengal		–	–	–	–		–
Acridine dyes								
46500	Pigment Violet 19		–	–	–	–		*
Quinoline dyes								
47000	Solvent Yellow 33		DC Yellow 11	–	230	0.1% pet.	+	* See § 23.47, § 23.53 and § 25.25
47005	Acid Yellow 3, Quinoline Yellow		–	E-104	21	–		*
			DC Yellow 10	–	363	0.1% pet.	+	* See § 23.47 under DC Yellow 11
		-aluminum lake	DC Yellow 10	–	4	–		*
47035	Acid Yellow 5		–	–	–	–		*
Methine dyes								
48013	Basic Violet 16		–	–	–	–		*
48040	Basic Orange 22		–	–	–	–		*
48055	Basic Yellow 11		–	–	–	–		*

(continued)

(continuation)

Color Index no. (§ 27.8)	Common name/ Color Index name	Lakes or salts	USA-FDA name for certified batches	EEC color no.	Freq. use (§ 27.3)	Patch test conc. & veh. (§ 5.2) and ref. (§ 27.2)	Cont. all. (§ 27.3)	Comment (* § 27.8)
Azine dyes								
50240	Basic Red 2		–	–		–		*
50315	Acid Blue 59		–	–		–		*
50320	Acid Blue 102		–	–		–		*
50400	Solvent Blue 7		–	–		–		*
50405	Acid Blue 20		–	–		–		*
50415	Solvent Black 5		Solvent Black 5	–	4	–		–
50420	Acid Black 2		Acid Black 2	–	6	–		–
Oxazine dyes								
51175	Basic Blue 6		–	–		–		*
51319	Pigment Violet 23		–	–		–		*
Thiazine dyes								
52015	Basic Blue 9, Methylene blue		Basic Blue 9	–	13	–		*
52020	Basic Green 5		–	–		–		*
52030	Basic Blue 24		–	–		–		*
Aminoketone dyes, hydroxyketone dyes								
56205	Acid Yellow 7		–	–		–		*
57020	Mordant dye		–	–		–		*
Anthraquinone dyes								
58000	Mordant Red 11		–	–		–		*
59040	Solvent Green 7, Pyranine		DC Green 8	–	50	–		*
60505	Disperse Red 9		–	–		–		*
60710	Disperse Red 15		–	–		–		*
60725	Solvent Violet 13		DC Violet 2	–	113	–		*
60730	Acid Violet 43		Acid Violet 43	–	6	–		*
			Ext. DC Violet 2	–	13	–		*
61100	Disperse Violet 1		–	–		–		*
61105	Disperse Violet 4		–	–		–		*

(continued)

27.10 Colors

(continuation)

Color Index no. (§ 27.8)	Common name/ Color Index name	Lakes or salts	USA-FDA name for certified batches	EEC color no.	Freq. use (§ 27.3)	Patch test conc. & veh. (§ 5.2) and ref. (§ 27.2)	Cont. all. (§ 27.3)	Comment (* § 27.8)
61505	Disperse Blue 3		–	–		–		*
61554	–		–	–		–		*
61565	Solvent Green 3		DC Green 6	–	160	–		*
61570	Acid Green 25		DC Green 5	–	247	–		*
61585	Acid Blue 80		–	–		–		*
61705	Solvent Violet 14		–	–		–		*
61710	Acid Violet 31		–	–		–		*
61800	Acid Violet 34		–	–		–		*
62015	Disperse Red 11		–	–		–		*
62030	Disperse Violet 8		–	–		–		*
62045	Acid Blue 62		–	–		–		*
62085	Acid Blue 47		–	–		–		*
62095	Acid Blue 49		–	–		–		*
62100	Solvent Blue 12		–	–		–		*
62105	Acid Blue 78		–	–		–		*
62125	Acid Blue 40		–	–		–		*
62130	Acid Blue 41		–	–		–		*
62500	Disperse Blue 7		–	–		–		*
62550	Acid Green 38		–	–		–		*
62560	Acid Green 41		–	–		–		*
63000	Acid Blue 43		–	–		–		*
63010	Acid Blue 45		–	–		–		*
63165	–		–	–		–		*
63615	Mordant Black 13		–	–		–		*
64500	Disperse Blue 1		–	–		–		*
69800	Vat Blue 4, Indanthrone		–	E-130		–		*
69825	Vat Blue 6		DC Blue 9	–		–		*
71105	Pigment Orange 43		–	–		–		*
71255	–		–	–		–		*

(continued)

(continuation)

Color Index no. (§ 27.8)	Common name/ Color Index name	Lakes or salts	USA-FDA name for certified batches	EEC color no.	Freq. use (§ 27.3)	Patch test conc. & veh. (§ 5.2) and ref. (§ 27.2)	Cont. all. (§ 27.3)	Comment (* § 27.8)
Indigoid dyes								
73000	Vat Blue 1		DC Blue 6	–	16	–		*
73015	Food Blue 1, Indigotine		FDC Blue 2	E-132	7	–		*
73300	Vat Red 41, Thio Indigo Red B		–	–	–	–		*
73360	Vat Red 1, Helindone Pink		DC Red 30	–	33	–		–
		-lake	DC Red 30	–	184	–		–
73385	Vat Violet 2		–	–	–	–		*
Phthalocyanine dyes								
74100	Pigment Blue 16		–	–	–	–		*
74160	Pigment Blue 15		Phthalocyaninato copper	–	–	–		*
74180	Direct Blue 86		–	–	–	–		*
74220	Acid Blue 249		–	–	–	–		*
74260	Pigment Green 7		–	–	–	–		*
74350	Solvent Blue 25		–	–	–	–		*
Natural dyes								
75100	Natural Yellow 6, Crocetin		–	–	–	–		*
75120	Natural Orange 4, Bixine, Norbixine, Anatto		–	E-160b	14	5% pet. [1]		*
75125	Natural Yellow 27, Lycopene		–	E-160d	–			*
75130	Natural Yellow 26, β-Carotene, Carotene		–	E-160a	20	50% pet.	+	* Has caused photoallergy (§ 6.5)
75135	Natural Yellow 27, Rubixanthin		–	E-160d	–	–		*
75170	Natural White 1, Guanine		–	–	121	pure	+	* See § 24.12
75300	Natural Yellow 3, Curcumine		–	E-100	–	–		

(continued)

27.10   Colors

(continuation)

Color Index no. (§ 27.8)	Common name/ Color Index name	Lakes or salts	USA-FDA name for certified batches	EEC color no.	Freq. use (§ 27.3)	Patch test conc. & veh. (§ 5.2) and ref. (§ 27.2)	Cont. all. (§ 27.3)	Comment (* § 27.8)
75470	Natural Red 4, Carminic acid		–	E-120		–		*
		-aluminum lake	Carmine	–	198	pure [2]		*
75480	Natural Orange 6, Lawsone (from Henna leaves)		–	–		1% aqua, prick test	+	* Has caused immediate-type allergy (§ 22.28)
75580	Natural Yellow 1, Apigenin		–	–		–		–
75810	Natural Green 3		Chlorophyl		5	–		*
			Chlorophyllin	E-140	7	–		*
			Chlorophyllin copper	E-141	9	–		*

Inorganic pigments

77000	Aluminum powder		Aluminum powder	E-173	101	–		*
77002	Alumina (aluminum oxide)		Alumina	–	6	–		*
77004	Kaolin, China clay		Kaolin	–	1110	–		*
77005	–		–	–		–		*
77007	Ultramarine		Ultramarine blue	–	1386	–		*
			Ultramarine green	–	5	–		–
			Ultramarine violet	–	260	–		–
			Ultramarine pink	–	262	–		–
77019	Mica		Mica	–	3005	–		*
77120	Barium sulfate, blanc fixe		Barium sulfate	–	15	–		*
77163	Bismuth oxychloride		Bismuth oxy-chloride	–	1774	?	+	* See § 27.2, [19]
77220	Calcium carbonate		Calcium carbonate	E-170	451	–		*
77231	Calcium sulfate		–	–		–		*
77266	Graphite		Graphite	–	13	–		*
77267	Carbon black		Carbon black	–	510	–		*
77288	Chrome oxide green		Chromium oxide green	–	433	–		*
77289	Chrome hydroxide		Chromium hydroxide	–	575	Bichromate	+	§ 4.4

(continued)

446

(continuation)

Color Index no. (§ 27.8)	Common name/ Color Index name	Lakes or salts	USA-FDA name for certified batches	EEC color no.	Freq. use (§ 27.3)	Patch test conc. & veh. (§ 5.2) and ref. (§ 27.2)	Cont. all. (§ 27.3)	Comment (* § 27.8)
77343	Chrome-cobalt-aluminum oxide (bluish green)	–	–	–	–	–		–
77346	Cobalt aluminate (blue)	–	–	–	–			*
77400	Bronze powder		Bronze powder	–	20	–		*
	Copper powder		Copper powder	–	5	–		–
77480	Gold powder		–	E-175		–		*
77489	Iron (II) oxide (black)		Iron oxide	E-172		–		*
77491	Iron (III) oxide (red-brown)		Iron oxide	E-172		20% aqua [8]		*
77492	Hydrated iron (III) oxide, (yellow)		Iron oxide	E-172		–		*
77499	Iron (II-III) oxide (black)		Iron oxide	E-172		–		*
	All iron oxides				5987	–		
77510	Ferric ferrocyanide, Prussian blue		Ferric ferrocyanide	–	346	–		*
77520	Ammonium ferric ferrocyanide		–	–		–		*
77713	Magnesium carbonate		Magnesium carbonate	–	556	–		*
77718	Talc		Talc	–	4129	–		* Has caused granulomas (§ 4.9)
77742	Manganese ammonium pyrophosphate		Manganese Violet	218		–		*
77745	Manganese phosphate (pink)		–	–		–		*
77820	Silver powder		–	E-174		–		*
77891	Titanium dioxide		Titanium dioxide	E-171	6399	–		*
77947	Zinc oxide		Zinc oxide	–	556	pure	+	* *See* § 5.22

Colors without color index numbers

–	Lactoflavin (yellow), Vitamin B2		–	E-101		–		*
–	Caramel (brown)		–	E-150	69	–		*

(continued)

27.10 Colors

(continuation)

Color Index no. (§ 27.8)	Common name/ Color Index name	Lakes or salts	USA-FDA name for certified batches	EEC color no.	Freq. use (§ 27.3)	Patch test conc. & veh. (§ 5.2) and ref. (§ 27.2)	Cont. all. (§ 27.3)	Comment (* § 27.8)
–	Capsanthine (orange-red)		–	E-160c		–		*
–	Vegetable black		–	E-153		–		*
–	Acid Black 107		–	–	41	–		Syn: Irgalan Black BGL®
–	Acid Blue 168		–	–	12	–		Syn: Irgalan Blue BL®
–	Acid Blue 170		–	–	20	–		Syn: Irgalan Blue BRL®
–	Acid Brown 19		–	–	30	–		Syn: Irgalan Brown BL®
–	Acid Brown 46		–	–	4	–		Syn: Irgalan Brown 3BL®
–	Acid Brown 48		–	–	7	–		Syn: Irgalan Dark Brown 5R®
–	Acid Brown 224		–	–	8	–		Syn: Lanamid Brown 2GL®
–	Acid Orange 88		–	–	11	–		Syn: Irgalan Orange RL®
–	Acid Red 211		–	–	7	–		Syn: Irgalan Red 2GL®
–	Acid Red 252		–	–	18	–		Syn: Irgalan Brilliant Red BL®
–	Acid Red 259		–	–	18	–		Syn: Irgalan Red 4GL®
–	Acid Violet 73		–	–	5	–		Syn: Irgalan Violet 5RL®
–	Acid Yellow 114		–	–	4	–		Syn: Irgalan Yellow GL®
–	Acid Yellow 127		–	–	13	–		Syn: Irganol Brilliant Yellow 3GLS®
–	Azulene (blue)		–	–	71	1% pet.	+	See §23,53
–	Calamine		–	–	4	–		–
–	Disodium EDTA-copper (green)		–	–	6	–		–

(continued)

(continuation)

Color Index no. (§ 27.8)	Common name/ Color Index name	Lakes or salts	USA-FDA name for certified batches	EEC color no.	Freq. use (§ 27.3)	Patch test conc. & veh. (§ 5.2) and ref. (§ 27.2)	Cont. all. (§ 27.3)	Comment (* § 27.8)
–	Solvent Brown 43		–	–	5	–		Syn: Irgacet Brown 2RL®
–	Disperse Black 9		–	–	54	–		Syn: Amacel Black 3G®
–	Disperse Violet 11		–	–	71	–		Syn: Eastman Violet 5RLF®

27.11   Color ingredients of hair dye preparations

Ingredient	Synonym	Patch test conc. & veh. (§ 5.2) and ref. (§ 27.2)	Freq. use (§ 27.3)	Cont. all. (§ 27.3)	Comment
2-amino-6-chloro-4-nitrophenol		–			–
p-aminodiphenylamine,					*See* N-phenyl-p-phenylenediamine
2-amino-4-nitrophenol		2% pet. [1]	13		–
2-amino-5-nitrophenol		2% pet. [1]	17		–
4-amino-2-nitrophenol		2% pet. [1]	74		*See* § 22.29
m-aminophenol	MAP	2% pet. [1]	195	+	*See* § 22.28
o-aminophenol	OAP	2% pet. [1]	176		–
p-aminophenol	PAP	2% pet. [1]	256	+	*See* § 22.28
N,N-bis(hydroxyethyl)-p-phenylenediamine		–			–
bismuth citrate		–			–
chamomile oil		25% o.o. [2]	5		–
2-chloro-p-phenylenediamine		2% pet. [1]	31		–
4-chlororesorcinol		–	25		–
2,4-diaminoanisole		–			*See* methoxyphenylenediamine
2,4-diaminodiphenylamine		–			–
4,4'-diaminodiphenylamine		–			–
2,4-diaminophenol		2% pet. [1]	9		–
2,6-diaminopyridine		–			–
Disperse Blue 1	CI 64500	–	37		–

(continued)

27.11 Hair dye preparations

(continuation)

Ingredient	Synonym	Patch test conc. & veh. (§ 5.2) and ref. (§ 27.2)	Freq. use (§ 27.3)	Cont. all. (§ 27.3)	Comment
Disperse Violet 4	CI 61105	–			–
Disperse Violet 8	CI 62030	–			–
HC Blue 1	N',N'-bis(2-hydroxyethyl)-N'-methyl-2-nitro-p-phenylenediamine	–	55		For percutaneous penetration under usage conditions, *see* § 22.29
HC Blue 2	N,N,N-tris(2-hydroxyethyl)-2-nitro-p-phenylene-diamine	–	16		–
HC Blue 3		–	4		–
HC Blue 4		–			–
HC Blue 5		–			–
HC Orange 1	2-nitro-4'-hydroxy-diphenylamine	–	4		–
HC Red 1	4-amino-2-nitrodi-phenylamine	–	6		–
HC Red 3	N'-(2-hydroxy-ethyl)-2-nitro-p-phenylenediamine	–	47		–
HC Red 6	CI 16155 (formerly FDC Red 1)	–	4		–
HC Yellow 2	N-(2-hydroxyethyl)-2-nitroaniline		40		–
HC Yellow 3	N'-tris(hydroxy methyl)methyl-4-nitro-o-phenyl-ene diamine	–	21		–
HC Yellow 4	N,N-bis(2-hydroxy-ethyl)-2-amino-5-nitrophenol	–	43		–
HC Yellow 5	N-(2-hydroxy-ethyl)- 4-nitro-o-phenylenediamine	–	7		–
henna (dried leaves of *Lawsonia alba*)		10 mg in 100 ml aqua-ether-ethanol		+	*See* § 22.28
hydroquinone		1% pet.		+	*See* § 25.44 *and* § 25.45
hydroxynaphthoquinone					*See* lawson
lawson	2-hydroxy-1,4-naphthoquinone	–			–
lead acetate		1% aqua	9	+	*See* § 22.28

(continued)

(continuation)

Ingredient	Synonym	Patch test conc. & veh. (§ 5.2) and ref. (§ 27.2)	Freq. use (§ 27.3)	Cont. all. (§ 27.3)	Comment
4-methoxy-m-phenylenediamine	4-MMPD; 2,4-diaminoanisole; 24-DAA	2% pet. [1]	70		*See* § 22.29
4-methoxy-m-phenylenediamine sulfate	4-MMPD-sulfate	2% pet. [1]	229		–
5-methoxy-p-phenylenediamine	5-MPPD; 2,5-diaminoanisole; 25-DAA	–			–
4-methoxytoluene-2,5-diamine		–			–
p-methylaminophenol sulfate	metol	1% aqua [5]; 2% aqua [3]	13		–
1,5-naphthalenediol		–	12		–
1,3-naphthalenediol		–			–
2,7-naphthalenediol		–			–
1-naphthol	α-naphthol	5% o.o. [5]; 0.1% pet. [3]; 1% alc. [3]	64		–
2-nitro-p-phenylenediamine	2-NPPD	2% pet. [1]	281	+	*See* § 22.28
4-nitro-m-phenylenediamine		2% pet. [1]	12		–
4-nitro-o-phenylenediamine	4-NOPD	2% pet. [1]	212		*See* § 22.29
m-phenylenediamine	MPD	2% pet. [1]	30		*See* § 22.29
o-phenylenediamine	OPD		–		–
p-phenylenediamine	PPD	2% pet. [1]; 1% pet. [4]	329	+	*See* § 22.28 *and* § 22.29 Has also caused photoallergy [§ 6.5]
N-phenyl-p-phenylenediamine	p-aminodiphenyl-amine	0.25% pet. [3]; 2% pet. [1]		+	*See* § 22.28
phloroglucinol	1,3,5-trihydroxy-benzene	–	42		–
picramic acid (sodium salt)	2-amino-4,6-dinitro-phenol	–	8		–
pyrocatechol	catechol, pyrocatechin	2% pet. [3]; 2% aqua [3]	40		–
pyrogallol	1,2,3-trihydroxy-benzene	3% aqua [2]; 1% pet. [3]	141		–
resorcinol		2% pet. [1]	372	+	*See* § 22.28, § 5.38 *and* § 22.65
sodium picramate,					*See* picramic acid

(continued)

451

27.11 Hair dye preparations

(continuation)

Ingredient	Synonym	Patch test conc. & veh. (§ 5.2) and ref. (§ 27.2)	Freq. use (§ 27.3)	Cont. all. (§ 27.3)	Comment
2,4,5-toluenetriol		–			–
toluene-2,4-diamine	m-toluenediamine, 24TDA	1% pet. [1]	5	+	*See § 22.28 and § 22.29*
toluene-2,5-diamine and sulfate	p-toluenediamine, 25TDA	2% pet. [1]	143	+	*See § 22.28 and § 22.29*

SUNSCREENS

27.12   Sunscreens (UV-absorbers) are tabulated in § 27.13.
Sunscreens permitted in the USA and the EEC are indicated in the 'Comment' column:

a = permitted in the USA (*Cat. I. OTC Sunscreen Drugs, Federal Register*, 25 August 1978)
b = permitted in the EEC (*Draft List of Permitted Sunscreens in the EEC,* February 1982, 32/6).

27.13   Sunscreens (UV-absorbers)

Sunscreen	Synonym®	Patch test conc. & veh. (§ 5.2) and ref. (§ 27.2)	Freq. use (§ 27.3)	Cont. all. (§ 27.3)	Comment (a/b: § 27.12)
PABA series (p-aminobenzoic acid)					
allantoin-PABA	Alpaba	5% pet. [3]			–
p-aminobenzoic acid	PABA	1% alc. 5% pet. [3]		+	a, b *See* § 25.66
amyl (isoamyl) N-dimethyl PABA	Escalol 506 Padimate A	5% pet. [1] 1% pet. [3]	181	+	a, b *See* § 25.66 –
ethyl N-dihydroxypropyl PABA	Amerscreen P N-propoxylated ethyl PABA	5% pet. [3]			a, b
ethyl N-dimethyl PABA		5% pet. [3]			b
ethyl N-ethoxylated PABA	Lusanthan 25 PEG-25 benzocaine	5% pet. [3]			b
glyceryl mono-PABA	Escalol 106	5% pet. [3]		+	a, b *See* § 25.66
octyl N-dimethyl PABA	Escalol 507, Padimate 0	5% pet. [1]	24		a, b

(continued)

(continuation)

Ingredient	Synonym	Patch test conc. & veh. (§ 5.2) and ref. (§ 27.2)	Freq. use (§ 27.3)	Cont. all. (§ 27.3)	Comment
Anthranilates series (o-aminobenzoic acid)					
glyceryl-3-(glyceroxy)anthranilate (= α-glycerol ester of orthoamino-meta(2,3-dihydroxypropoxy)benzoic acid	UV-A filter in Contralum cream	5–10% pet.		+	*See* § 25.66
homomenthyl N-acetyl anthranilate	in Parsol Ultra	2% pet.			b
menthyl anthranilate		–			a
Salicylates series					
benzyl-4-isopropyl salicylate		–			b
benzyl salicylate		2% pet. [2]		+	b *See* § 25.66
homomenthyl salicylate (= homosalate)	Filtrosol A	5% pet. [1]	49	+	a, b *See* § 25.66
menthyl salicylate	Filtrol	–			b
octyl salicylate	Sunarome WMO	2% o.o. [3]	185		a, b
phenyl salicylate		2% pet.		+	b *See* § 25.66, § 23.53 *and* § 13.3
polypropylene glycol 2 salicylate		–	5		a
triethanolamine salicylate	Sunarome	–	5		a, b
Cinnamates series					Have caused photosensitivity (§ 6.5)
cyclohexyl-p-methoxycinnamate	in Parsol Ultra	–			b
diethanolamine-p-methoxycinnamate		–			a, b
2-ethoxyethyl-p-methoxycinnamate	Cinoxate, GivTan F	1% pet.		+	b *See* § 25.66
ethyldiisopropyl-p-methoxycinnamate	in Neo Heliopan	–			b
isopropyl-p-methoxycinnamate	in Neo Heliopan	–			b
2-octyl-a-cyano-b-phenylcinnamate (= 2-ethylhexyl-2-cyano-3,3-diphenylacrylate)	Uvinul N-539	–			a, b
octyl p-methoxycinnamate	Neo Heliopan AV, Parsol MCX	7.5% pet.			a, b
potassium cinnamate		–			b
potassium p-methoxycinnamate	Solprotex II	–			b
n-propyl p-methoxycinnamate	Solprotex I, II, III	–			b

(continued)

(continuation)

Sunscreen	Synonym®	Patch test conc. & veh. (§ 5.2) and ref. (§ 27.2)	Freq. use (§ 27.3)	Cont. all. (§ 27.3)	Comment (a/b § 27.12)
Benzophenone series					
benzophenone 1 (= 2,4-dihydroxy-)	Uvinul 400	–	138	–	
benzophenone 2 (= 2,2′,4,4′-tetrahydoxy-)	Uvinul D-50	–	254	b	
benzophenone 3 (= 2-hydroxy-4-methoxy-)	Uvinul M-40, Eusolex 4360, oxybenzone	2% pet.	60	+	a, b *See* § 25.66
benzophenone 4 (= 2-hydroxy-4-methoxy-5-sulfonic acid)	sulisobenzone, Uvinul MS-40, Uvistat 1121	5–10% pet. [3]	244	+	a, b *See* § 25.66
benzophenone 5 (= natrium salt of benzophenone 4)		–	11		a, b
benzophenone 6 (2,2′-dihydroxy-4,4′-dimethoxy-)	Uvinul D-49	–	122		b
benzophenone 7 (5-chloro-2-hydroxy-)	Dow HCB	–			–
benzophenone 8 (2,2′-dihydroxy-4-methoxy-)	Dioxybenzone, Uvistat 24	2% pet.	5	+	a *See* § 25.66 *under* dioxybenzone
benzophenone 9 (2,2′-dihydroxy-4,4′-dimethoxy-5-sulfonate sodium)	Uvinul DS-49	–	89		b
benzophenone 10 (= 2-hydroxy-4-methoxy-4′-methyl-)	Mexenone, Uvistat 2211	–			b Has caused photosensitivity *See* § 6.5 *under* mexenone
benzophenone 11 (= mixture of benzophenone 6 and 2)	Uvinul 490	–	139		–
benzophenone 12 (= 2-hydroxy-4-n-octoxy-)	Cyasorb UV 531	–			b
benzophenone, 4-phenyl-	Eusolex 3490	–			–
benzophenone, 4′-phenyl-2-octyl-carboxylate	Eusolex 3573	–			b
Camphor series					
3-benzylidene camphor	Ultracyd, Ultren BK	–			b
3-(4′-methylbenzylidene) camphor	Eusolex 6300	2% pet.		+	b *See* § 25.66
3-(4′-sulfobenzylidene) camphor		–			b
3-(3′-sulfo-4′-methylbenzylidene) camphor		–			b
3-(4-trimethylammoniumbenzylidene) camphor methosulfate		–			b

(continued)

(continuation)

Sunscreen	Synonym®	Patch test conc. & veh. (§ 5.2) and ref. (§ 27.2)	Freq. use (§ 27.3)	Cont. all. (§ 27.3)	Comment (a/b: § 27.12)
Other UV-absorbers					
t-butyl-4-methoxy-4-dibenzoyl methane		–			b
dianisoyl methane	Parsol DAM	10% pet.			b
dibenzalazine	Eusolex 6653	–			b
digalloyl trioleate	in Solprotex I	3.5% pet. [5]		+	a, b *See* § 25.66
5-(3,3-dimethyl-2-norbornylidene)-3-pentene-2-on	Prosolal S9 bornelone	–			b
drometrizole	Tinuvin P	5% pet.		+	*See* § 24.12, § 25.66 *and* § 23.47 (*under* 2-(2′-hydroxy-5′-methyl-phenyl)benzotriazole)
guanine		pure [2]	121	+	b *See* § 24.12
4-isopropyl dibenzoyl methane	in Eusolex 8021 with methylbenzyl-idene camphor	2% m.o.		+	b *See* § 23.47 *and* § 25.66
lawsone + dihydroxyacetone		dihydroxyacetone 10% alc. [1]	8 (DHA)	a	
methoxy benzylidene cyanic acid n-hexyl ester		–			b
2-phenyl-benzimidazole-5-sulfonic acid	Eusolex 232, Novantisol	–			a, b
2-phenyl-5-methyl benzoxazole	Witisol	–			b
1-phenyl-3-(3-pyridyl)-1,3-propanedione		–			b
red petrolatum		pure			a
sodium 3,4-dimethoxyphenyl glyoxilate	Eusolex 161	–			b
p-tolyl benzoxazole		–			b
urocanic acid ethyl ester		–			b

LIPIDS AND SURFACTANTS

27.14   In the following paragraphs, tabulations are given of:
  – Lipids (§ 27.15.1)
  – Anionic surfactants (§ 27.15.2)
  – Cationic surfactants (§ 27.15.3)
  – Non-ionic surfactants (§ 27.15.4)
  – Amphoteric surfactants (§ 27.15.5)
  – Amines – aminoalkanols (§ 27.15.6)
  – Polyols (§ 27.15.7)

27.15.1 Lipids

27.15.1 **Lipids (hydrocarbons, fatty acids, fatty alcohols, esters and silicones)**

Name	Synonym®	Patch test conc. & veh. (§ 5.2) and ref. (§ 27.2)	Freq. use (§ 27.3)	Cont. all. (§ 27.3)	Comment
acetylated lanolin		30% pet. [1]	289		–
acetylated lanolin alcohol		30% pet. [1]	285		Comedogenic (§ 9.2)
almond oil, sweet		pure [2]	248		–
apricot kernel oil		–	11		–
avocado oil		pure [6]	257		–
beeswax		30% pet. [1], pure	2429	+	*See § 5.39 and § 23.47*
butyl myristate		–	122		–
butyl stearate		–	141		Comedogenic (§ 9.2)
C 12–13 alcohol		–	31		–
C 12–15 alcohols lactate		–	6		–
C 15–18 glycol		–	8		–
C 10–13 isoparaffin		–	24		–
C 13–16 isoparaffin		–	5		–
candelilla wax		41% m.o. [1]	1350		–
caprylic/capric triglyceride		–	578		–
carnauba wax		48% m.o. [1]	1967		–
castor oil		pure	2621	+	*See § 5.22*
ceresin		pure [2]	373		–
cetearyl alcohol		–	133		–
cetearyl alcohol + sodium cetearyl sulfate (90 + 10)	Lanette N	20% pet.		+	*See § 5.22*
cetearyl octanoate		–	157		–
cetyl alcohol		30% pet. [1]	1426	+	*See § 5.22*
cetyl lactate		5% aqua [6]	185		–
cetyl palmitate		2.5% cream [6]	377		–
cetyl stearate		–	31		–
cholesterol		–	218		–
cocoa butter		–	361		Comedogenic (§ 9.2)
coconut acid		–	76		–

(continued)

(continuation)

Sunscreen	Synonym®	Patch test conc. & veh. (§ 5.2) and ref. (§ 27.2)	Freq. use (§ 27.3)	Cont. all. (§ 27.3)	Comment (a/b: § 27.12)
coconut oil		pure [2]	132		*See also* § 26.3 *(Cocos nucifera)* Comedogenic (§ 9.2)
cod liver oil		–	7		–
corn oil		–	1091		Comedogenic (§ 9.2)
cottonseed oil		pure [2]	19		–
cyclomethicone		–	32		–
decyl oleate		5.5% pet. [6], 10% o.o.	201	+	*See* § 27.2 [20]
dibutyl phthalate		10% pet. [1], 5% pet. [17]	553	+	*See* § 5.22
dicetyl adipate		–	8		–
diethyl phthalate		10% pet. [1], 2% pet. [7]	104		–
dihydroabietyl alcohol	Abitol	1% pet.	8	+	*See* § 5.16
dimethicone		–	778		–
dimethicone copolyol		–	160		–
dimethyl phthalate		2% pet. [1]	30		–
emulsifying wax		30% pet. [1]	85		Contact allergy to ingredients has been reported (*See* § 5.22)
ethyl linoleate		–	7		–
glyceryl erucate		–	5		–
glyceryl isostearate		–	14		–
glyceryl linoleate		–	7		–
glyceryl oleate		30% pet. [2]	495	+	*See* § 5.22
glyceryl ricinoleate		–	15		–
glyceryl stearate		30% pet. [2, 3]	1455	+	*See* § 5.22
glyceryl stearate SE		–	243		–
glyceryl triacetyl ricinoleate		–	14		–
glycol distearate		50% m.o. [6]	30		–
glycol stearate		–	425		–
grape seed oil		–	6		–
hexyl laurate		–	17		–

(continued)

27.15.1 Lipids

(continuation)

Sunscreen	Synonym®	Patch test conc. & veh. (§ 5.2) and ref. (§ 27.2)	Freq. use (§ 27.3)	Cont. all. (§ 27.3)	Comment (a/b: § 27.12)
hybrid safflower oil		–	14		–
hydroabietyl alcohol	Abitol	1% pet.	8	+	*See* § 5.16 *under* dihydroabietyl alcohol
hydrogenated castor oil		–	18		–
hydrogenated coconut oil		–	102		–
hydrogenated cottonseed oil		–	59		–
hydrogenated lanolin		30% pet. [1]	76		–
hydrogenated lard glycerin		–	92		–
hydrogenated menhaden acid		–	19		–
hydrogenated soybean oil		–	8		–
hydrogenated tallow glycerides		–	26		–
hydrogenated vegetable oil		–	181		–
hydroxylated lanolin		30% pet. [1]	22		–
isocetyl alcohol		–	50		–
isocetyl palmitate		–	9		–
isocetyl stearate		–	93		–
isodecyl isononanoate		–	4		–
isodecyl oleate		pure [6]	27		–
isopropyl isostearate		–	22		Comedogenic (§ 9.2)
isopropyl lanolate		20% pet. [6]	1315		–
isopropyl linoleate		–	23		–
isopropyl myristate		5% pet. [1]	2246	+	*See* § 5.22
isopropyl palmitate		45% pet. [6], 2% pet.	747	+	*See* § 5.22
isopropyl stearate		–	42		–
isostearic acid		–	100		–
isostearyl alcohol		pure, 5% alc.	38	+	*See* § 25.53
isostearyl isostearate		–	11		–
isostearyl neopentanoate		–	97		–
Japan wax		–	150		–

(continued)

458

(continuation)

Sunscreen	Synonym®	Patch test conc. & veh. (§ 5.2) and ref. (§ 27.2)	Freq. use (§ 27.3)	Cont. all. (§ 27.3)	Comment (a/b: § 27.12)
lanolin		pure [1]	2951	+	*See* § 5.22
lanolin acid		–	54		–
lanolin alcohol (wool alcohols)		30% pet. [1]	1454	+	*See* § 5.22
lanolin oil		30% pet. [1]	1648	+	*See* § 27.2, [19]
lanolin wax		–	106		–
lard glyceride		–	4		–
lauric acid		–	19		–
lauryl alcohol		5% pet. [2]	26	+	Comedogenic (§ 9.2)
lauryl lactate		–	11		–
linseed oil		pure [2]	6		Comedogenic (§ 9.2)
methyl oleate		–			Comedogenic (§ 9.2)
methyl rosinate		–	15		–
microcrystalline wax		?	932	+	*See* § 27.2, [19]
mineral oil		–	5932		–
mink oil		–	71		–
montan wax		–	377		–
myristic acid		–	33		–
myristyl alcohol		5% pet. [2]	28		–
myristyl lactate		13.8% pet. [6]	193		–
myristyl myristate		–	170		Comedogenic (§ 9.2)
octyl dodecanol	Eutanol G®	30% pet. [2]	128	+	*See* § 5.22
octyl palmitate		50% pet. [6]	396		–
octyl stearate		–	61		–
oleic acid		–	578		Comedogenic (§ 9.2)
oleyl alcohol		30% pet. [2]	1063	+	*See* § 5.22
olive oil		pure [1]	74	+	*See* § 5.22 Comedogenic (§ 9.2)
ozokerite		pure [2]	1301		–
palmitic acid		–	14		–
paraffin		pure [2]	1290		–

(continued)

(continuation)

Sunscreen	Synonym®	Patch test conc. & veh. (§ 5.2) and ref. (§ 27.2)	Freq. use (§ 27.3)	Cont. all. (§ 27.3)	Comment (a/b: § 27.12)
peach kernel oil		–	24		–
peanut oil		–	14		Comedogenic (§ 9.2)
penta-erythritol rosinate		–	33		–
penta-erythritol tetraoctanoate		–	7		–
persic oil		–	11		–
petrolatum		pure [2]	1746	+	*See* § 5.22
petrol wax		–	295		*See under* paraffin *or* microcrystalline wax
phenyldimethicone		–	118		–
polybutene		30% pet. [6]	109		–
propylene glycol		1 and 10% aqua [17]	5729	+	*See* § 5.22
propylene glycol dicaprylate/dicaprate		–	91		–
propylene glycol dicocoate		–	70		–
propyleneglycol diperlargonate		–	36		–
propyleneglycol laurate		–	81		–
propyleneglycol myristate		–	4		–
propyleneglycol ricinoleate		–	13		–
propyleneglycol stearate		–	365		–
propyleneglycol stearate SE		–	146		–
ricinoleic acid		30% pet. and pure	19	+	*See* § 5.22
safflower glyceride		–	8		–
safflower oil		–	62		Comedogenic (§ 9.2)
sesame oil		50% o.o. [2], pure	172	+	*See* § 5.22
simethicone		–	114		–
soybean oil		–	11		–
spermaceti		pure [2]	215		–
squalane		20% pet. [6]	280		–
squalene		pure [6]	16		–
stearic acid		1% aqua [2] 30% pet. (RIFM)	2635		Comedogenic (§ 9.2)
stearoxy dimethicone		–	56		–

(continued)

(continuation)

Ingredient	Synonym	Patch test conc. & veh. (§ 5.2) and ref. (§ 27.2)	Freq. use (§ 27.3)	Cont. all. (§ 27.3)	Comment
stearyl alcohol		30% pet. [1]	524	+	*See* § 5.22
stearyl heptanoate		–	17		–
stearyl stearate		–	22		–
synthetic beeswax		–	180		–
synthetic spermaceti		–	150		–
synthetic wax		–	455		–
tall oil		–	60		–
tall oil acid		–	32		–
tallow		–	17		–
tallow acid		–	4		–
triethyl citrate		–	4		–
trihydroxy stearin		–	29		–
trilaurin		–	19		–
trilinolein		–	7		–
triolein		–	7		–
turtle oil		–	23		–
undecylenic acid		2% euc. [5], 2–5% pet.	14	+	*See* § 5.32
vegetable oil		–	11		–
wheat germ glycerides		2% lipstick base [6]	449		–
wheat germ oil		50% m.o. [6]	125		–

27.15.2   Anionic surfactants

Name	Synonym®	Patch test conc. & veh. (§ 5.2) and ref. (§ 27.2)	Freq. use (§ 27.3)	Cont. all. (§ 27.3)	Comment
ammonium laureth sulfate		–	80		–
ammonium lauryl sulfate		–	110		–
ammonium myreth sulfate		–	4		–
ammonium nonoxynol-4 sulfate		–	85		–
ammonium oleate		–	16		–

(continued)

27.15.2 Anionic surfactants

(continuation)

Ingredient	Synonym	Patch test conc. & veh. (§ 5.2) and ref. (§ 27.2)	Freq. use (§ 27.3)	Cont. all. (§ 27.3)	Comment
diethanolamine laureth sulfate	–	–	4		–
diethanolamine lauryl sulfate	–	–	19		–
diethanolamine oleth-3 phosphate	–	–	4		–
dioctyl sodium sulfosuccinate	Aerosol OT	5% aqua [2]	52		Test concentration irritant
disodium monocetearyl sulfosuccinate	–	–	6		–
disodium monococamidosulfosuccinate	–	–	123		–
disodium monolauramidosulfosuccinate	–	–	4		–
disodium monooleamidosulfosuccinate	–	–	132		–
disodium monoricinoleoamido monoethanolamine sulfosuccinate	–	–	9		–
disodium monoundecylenamido monoethanolamine sulfosuccinate	–	–	17		–
dodecyl benzene sulfonic acid	–	–	9		–
nonyl nonoxynol-10 phosphate	–	–	4		–
potassium cocoate	–	–	9		–
potassium lauryl sulfate	–	–	7		–
potassium octoxynol-12 phosphate	–	–	11		–
potassium oleate	–	–	5		–
sodium C14-16 olefin sulfonate	–	–	60		–
sodium C16-18 olefin sulfonate	–	–	5		–
sodium cetearyl sulfate	–	–	80		–
sodium cetyl sulfate	–	–	24		–
sodium cocoate	–	–	35		–
sodium cocoyl isethionate	–	–	6		–
sodium diethylaminopropyl cocoaspartamide	–	–	35		–
sodium dihydroxy ethylglycinate	–	–	20		–
sodium dodecyl benzene sulfonate	–	–	63		–
sodium lauramino dipropionate	–	–	19		–
sodium laureth sulfate		1% aqua	280	+	*See* § 22.7
sodium lauroyl sarcosinate		2% aqua [2]	13		–

(continued)

(continuation)

Name	Synonym®	Patch test conc. & veh. (§ 5.2) and ref. (§ 27.2)	Freq. use (§ 27.3)	Cont. all. (§ 27.3)	Comment
sodium lauryl ether sulfate		2% aqua	–	+	*See* § 22.7
sodium lauryl sulfate		0.1% aqua [1]	937	+	*See* § 5.22
sodium lauryl sulfoacetate		–	140		–
sodium methyl cocoyl laurate		–	10		–
sodium methyl naphthalene sulfonate		–	7		–
sodium methyl oleoyl laurate		–	37		–
sodium myreth sulfate		–	65		–
sodium m-nitrobenzene sulfonate		–	23		–
sodium nonoxynol-1 sulfate		–	4		–
sodium octoxynol-3 sulfonate		–	10		–
sodium oleate		–	54		–
sodium palmitate		–	4		–
sodium polynaphthalene sulfonate		–	35		–
sodium stearate		–	103		–
sodium tallowate		–	42		–
sodium xylene sulfonate		–	21		–
sulfated castor oil		5% aqua	278		–
trideceth-7 carboxylic acid		–	16		–
triethanolamine dodecylbenzene sulfonate		–	75		–
triethanolamine lauryl sulfate		–	451		–
triethanolamine monooleamido sulfosuccinate		–	5		–
triethanolamine stearate		5% pet.	31	+	*See* § 5.22

27.15.3   Cationic surfactants

Name	Synonym®	Patch test conc. & veh. (§ 5.2) and ref. (§ 27.2)	Freq. use (§ 27.3)	Cont. all. (§ 27.3)	Comment
behentrimonium chloride (behenyltrimethylammonium chloride)		–			Quaternary ammonium compounds may be tested 0.1% and 0.01% aqua [17]

(continued)

27.15.3 Cationic surfactants

(continuation)

Name	Synonym®	Patch test conc. & veh. (§ 5.2) and ref. (§ 27.2)	Freq. use (§ 27.3)	Cont. all. (§ 27.3)	Comment
benzalkonium chloride	Zephiran	0.1% aqua [2], 0.05% aqua [1]	78	+	*See* § 5.7 *under* quaternary ammonium compounds
benzethonium chloride	Hyamine 1622	0.1% aqua [3]	85	+	*See* § 5.7 *under* quaternary ammonium compounds
benzyltrimethylammonium hydrous-anhydrous protein		–			Quaternary ammonium compounds may be tested 0.1% and 0.01% aqua [17]
cetalkonium chloride (cetyldimethylbenzylammonium chloride)		0.1% aqua	4	+	*See* § 5.7 *under* quaternary ammonium compounds
cetrimonium bromide (cetyltrimethylammonium bromide)	Cetavlon, Cetrimide	0.01–0.1% aqua	17	+	*See* § 5.7 *under* quaternary ammonium compounds
cetrimonium chloride		–	16		Quaternary ammonium compounds may be tested 0.1% and 0.01% aqua [17]
cetylpyridinium chloride		0.05% aqua	25	+	*See* § 5.7 *under* quaternary ammonium compounds
coco-trimonium chloride (coco-trimethylammonium chloride)		–			Quaternary ammonium compounds may be tested 0.1% and 0.01% aqua [17]
denatonium benzoate	Bitrex	–			Has caused contact urticaria (§ 7.5)
domiphen bromide (dodecyldimethyl-2-phenoxy-ethylammonium bromide)		0.1% aqua		+	*See* § 5.7
lauralkonium chloride (lauryldimethylbenzyl ammonium chloride)		–			Quaternary ammonium compounds may be tested 0.1% and 0.01% aqua [17]
laurtrimonium chloride		–			Quaternary ammonium compounds may be tested 0.1% and 0.01% aqua [17]
laurylisoquinolinium bromide	Dodecin	–	17		Quaternary ammonium compounds may be tested 0.1% and 0.01% aqua [17]
laurylpyridinium chloride		–	7		Quaternary ammonium compounds may be tested 0.1% and 0.01% aqua [17]
methylbenzethonium chloride	Hyamine 10X	–	44		Quaternary ammonium compounds may be tested 0.1% and 0.01% aqua [17]
myristalkonium chloride		–	18		Quaternary ammonium compounds may be tested 0.1% and 0.01% aqua [17]

(continued)

(continuation)

Name	Synonym®	Patch test conc. & veh. (§ 5.2) and ref. (§ 27.2)	Freq. use (§ 27.3)	Cont. all. (§ 27.3)	Comment
myrtrimonium bromide		–	16		Quaternary ammonium compounds may be tested 0.1% and 0.01% aqua [17]
olealkonium chloride		–			Quaternary ammonium compounds may be tested 0.1% and 0.01% aqua [17]
polyethylene glycol 2 cocoyl quaternium-4		–			Quaternary ammonium compounds may be tested 0.1% and 0.01% aqua [17]
polyethylene glycol 15 cocoyl quaternium-4		–			Quaternary ammonium compounds may be tested 0.1% and 0.01% aqua [17]
polyethylene glycol 2 oleyl quaternium-4		–			Quaternary ammonium compounds may be tested 0.1% and 0.01% aqua [17]
polyethylene glycol 15 oleyl quaternium-4		–			Quaternary ammonium compounds may be tested 0.1% and 0.01% aqua [17]
polyethylene glycol 2 stearyl quaternium-4		–			Quaternary ammonium compounds may be tested 0.1% and 0.01% aqua [17]
polyethylene glycol 15 stearyl quaternium-4		–			Quaternary ammonium compounds may be tested 0.1% and 0.01% aqua [17]
quaternium-2 (N-soya-N-ethyl-morpholinium ethosulfate)		–	10		Quaternary ammonium compounds may be tested 0.1% and 0.01% aqua [17]
quaternium-3 (alkyldimethylbenzyl-saccharinate)		–	9		Quaternary ammonium compounds may be tested 0.1% and 0.01% aqua [17]
quaternium-4 (ethoxylated quats mixture)		–			Quaternary ammonium compounds may be tested 0.1% and 0.01% aqua [17]
quaternium-5 (dimethyldistearylammonium chloride)		–	19		Quaternary ammonium compounds may be tested 0.1% and 0.01% aqua [17]
quaternium-6 (polypropylene glycol 9 methyldiethylammonium chloride)		–	26		Quaternary ammonium compounds may be tested 0.1% and 0.01% aqua [17]
quaternium-7 (N-stearoyl cocaminoformyl-methylpyridinium chloride)		–	39		Quaternary ammonium compounds may be tested 0.1% and 0.01% aqua [17]
quaternium-8 (alkyldimethylethylbenzyl-ammonium chloride)		–			Quaternary ammonium compounds may be tested 0.1% and 0.01% aqua [17]

(continued)

27.15.3 Cationic surfactants

(continuation)

Name	Synonym®	Patch test conc. & veh. (§ 5.2) and ref. (§ 27.2)	Freq. use (§ 27.3)	Cont. all. (§ 27.3)	Comment
quaternium-9 (soya alkyltrimethyl-ammonium chloride)		–	10		Quaternary ammonium compounds may be tested 0.1% and 0.01% aqua [17]
quaternium-12 (dodecyldimethylammonium chloride)		–			Quaternary ammonium compounds may be tested 0.1% and 0.01% aqua [17]
quaternium-14 (dodecyldimethylethyl-benzylammoniumchloride)		–	12		Quaternary ammonium compounds may be tested 0.1% and 0.01% aqua [17]
quaternium-15 (chloroallylhexaminium chloride)	Dowicil 200	2% aqua [4], 1% pet.	536	+	*See § 5.7 and § 23.47*
quaternium-16 (trihydroxyethylstearyl-ammonium chloride)		–			Quaternary ammonium compounds may be tested 0.1% and 0.01% aqua [17]
quaternium-17 (cetyldimethylammonium bromide)		–			Quaternary ammonium compounds may be tested 0.1% and 0.01% aqua [17]
quaternium-18 (dimethyl dihydrogenated tallow ammonium chloride)		–	26		Quaternary ammonium compounds may be tested 0.1% and 0.01% aqua [17]
quaternium-18 bentonite		pure	9		Quaternary ammonium compounds may be tested 0.1% and 0.01% aqua [17]
quaternium-18 hectorite		pure	309		Quaternary ammonium compounds may be tested 0.1% and 0.01% aqua [17]
quaternium-18 magnesium silicate		–	43		Quaternary ammonium compounds may be tested 0.1% and 0.01% aqua [17]
quaternium-19	Polymer JR	–	56		Quaternary ammonium compounds may be tested 0.1% and 0.01% aqua [17]
quaternium-20 (propylene glycol 25 methyldiethylammonium chloride)		–			Quaternary ammonium compounds may be tested 0.1% and 0.01% aqua [17]
quaternium-21 (propylene glycol 40 methyl-diethylammonium chloride)		–			Quaternary ammonium compounds may be tested 0.1% and 0.01% aqua [17]
quaternium-22 (gluconamidopropyl-dimethyl-2-hydroxyethylammonium chloride)		–	24		Quaternary ammonium compounds may be tested 0.1% and 0.01% aqua [17]
quaternium-23	Gafquat 734	–	94		Quaternary ammonium compounds may be tested 0.1% and 0.01% aqua [17]

(continued)

(continuation)

Name	Synonym®	Patch test conc. & veh. (§ 5.2) and ref. (§ 27.2)	Freq. use (§ 27.3)	Cont. all. (§ 27.3)	Comment
quaternium-24 (decyloctyldimethylammonium chloride)		–			Quaternary ammonium compounds may be tested 0.1% and 0.01% aqua [17]
quaternium-25 (cetylethylmorpholinium ethosulfate)		–			Quaternary ammonium compounds may be tested 0.1% and 0.01% aqua [17]
quaternium-26 (minkamidopropyldimethyl-dihydroxyethylammonium chloride)		–	8		Quaternary ammonium compounds may be tested 0.1% and 0.01% aqua [17]
quaternium-27	Varisoft 475	–			Quaternary ammonium compounds may be tested 0.1% and 0.01% aqua [17]
quaternium-28 (dodecylbenzyltrimethyl-ammonium chloride)		–			Quaternary ammonium compounds may be tested 0.1% and 0.01% aqua [17]
quaternium-29 (dodecylxylyl-bis[trimethyl-ammonium chloride])		–			Quaternary ammonium compounds may be tested 0.1% and 0.01% aqua [17]
quaternium-30 (dodecylbenzyltrihydroxy-ethylammonium chloride)		–			Quaternary ammonium compounds may be tested 0.1% and 0.01% aqua [17]
quaternium-31 (dicetyldimethylammonium chloride)		–	49		Quaternary ammonium compounds may be tested 0.1% and 0.01% aqua [17]
quaternium-32	Monaquat ISIES	–			Quaternary ammonium compounds may be tested 0.1% and 0.01% aqua [17]
quaternium-34 (dicoco-dimethylammonium chloride)		–	5		Quaternary ammonium compounds may be tested 0.1% and 0.01% aqua [17]
quaternium-35 (mink amidopropyldiethyl-hydroxyethylammonium chloride)		–			Quaternary ammonium compounds may be tested 0.1% and 0.01% aqua [17]
quaternium-36 (stearyldihydroxyethoxy-ethylhydroxyethylammonium chloride)		–			Quaternary ammonium compounds may be tested 0.1% and 0.01% aqua [17]
quaternium-37 (ethylmethacrylate/abietyl-methacrylate/diethylaminoethylmetha-crylate/quaternized with dimethylsulfate)		–			Quaternary ammonium compounds may be tested 0.1% and 0.01% aqua [17]
quaternium-38 (ethylmethacrylate/oleyl-methacrylate/diethylaminoethylmetha-crylate/quaternized with dimethylsulfate)		–			Quaternary ammonium compounds may be tested 0.1% and 0.01% aqua [17]

(continued)

27.15.3 Cationic surfactants

(continuation)

Name	Synonym®	Patch test conc. & veh. (§ 5.2) and ref. (§ 27.2)	Freq. use (§ 27.3)	Cont. all. (§ 27.3)	Comment
quaternium-39 (copolymer of acrylamide and β-methacrylyloxyethyltrimethyl-ammonium methosulfate)		–	8		Quaternary ammonium compounds may be tested 0.1% and 0.01% aqua [17]
quaternium-40 (polymeric quaternary ammonium salt)	Merquat 100	–	6		Quaternary ammonium compounds may be tested 0.1% and 0.01% aqua [17]
quaternium-41 (polymeric quaternary ammonium salt)	Merquat 550	–			Quaternary ammonium compounds may be tested 0.1% and 0.01% aqua [17]
quaternium-42 (methylstearyldiethylamino-ethyl methacrylate quaternized with dimethyl sulfate)		–			Quaternary ammonium compounds may be tested 0.1% and 0.01% aqua [17]
quaternium-43 (coco-amidopropyldimethyl-acetamidoammonium chloride)		–			Quaternary ammonium compounds may be tested 0.1% and 0.01% aqua [17]
quaternium-44 (cetyldimethylhydroxyethyl-ammonium chloride)		–			Quaternary ammonium compounds may be tested 0.1% and 0.01% aqua [17]
quaternium-45	Luminex	–			Quaternary ammonium compounds may be tested 0.1% and 0.01% aqua [17]
quaternium-46	Miramin SH	–			Quaternary ammonium compounds may be tested 0.1% and 0.01% aqua [17]
quaternium-47 (dilauryldimethylammonium chloride)		–	4		Quaternary ammonium compounds may be tested 0.1% and 0.01% aqua [17]
quaternium-48 (di-tallow dimethyl-ammonium chloride)		–			Quaternary ammonium compounds may be tested 0.1% and 0.01% aqua [17]
quaternium-49 (polydimethylaminoethyl-methacrylate quaternized with methyl bromide)		–			Quaternary ammonium compounds may be tested 0.1% and 0.01% aqua [17]
quaternium-51	Takanal	–			Quaternary ammonium compounds may be tested 0.1% and 0.01% aqua [17]
quaternium-52	Dehyquart SP	–			Quaternary ammonium compounds may be tested 0.1% and 0.01% aqua [17]
quaternium-54 (ethyl cocammonium ethoxylate (15) sulfate)		–			Quaternary ammonium compounds may be tested 0.1% and 0.01% aqua [17]
soya trimonium chloride		–	5		Quaternary ammonium compounds may be tested 0.1% and 0.01% aqua [17]

(continued)

(continuation)

Name	Synonym®	Patch test conc. & veh. (§ 5.2) and ref. (§ 27.2)	Freq. use (§ 27.3)	Cont. all. (§ 27.3)	Comment
stearalkonium chloride		1–5% aqua [2]	277		Quaternary ammonium compounds may be tested 0.1% and 0.01% aqua [17]
stearalkonium hectorite		–	122		Quaternary ammonium compounds may be tested 0.1% and 0.01% aqua [17]
steartrimonium chloride		–			Quaternary ammonium compounds may be tested 0.1% and 0.01% aqua [17]
tallow trimonium chloride		–			Quaternary ammonium compounds may be tested 0.1% and 0.01% aqua [17]

27.15.4   Non-ionic surfactants

Name	Synonym®	Patch test conc. & veh. (§ 5.2) and ref. (§ 27.2)	Freq. use (§ 27.3)	Cont. all. (§ 27.3)	Comment
capramide diethanolamine		5% aqua [2]	6		–
ceteareth 5		–	52		–
ceteareth 15		–	13		–
ceteareth 17		–	4		–
ceteareth 20		–	65		–
ceteth 2		–	23		–
ceteth 10		–	10		–
ceteth 20		–	30		–
chlorodeceth 14		–	4		–
choleth 24		–	152		–
cocamide		–	15		–
cocamide diethanolamine (cocamide DEA)		5% aqua [2], 0.5% pet.	621	+	*See* § 27.2, [20] *and* § 25.9 *under* coconut diethanolamine
cocamide monoethanolamine (cocamide MEA)		–	15		–
cocamide oxide		–	6		–
coceth 8		–	9		–
dihydrocholeth 30		–	5		–

(continued)

469

27.15.4 Non-ionic surfactants

(continuation)

Name	Synonym®	Patch test conc. & veh. (§ 5.2) and ref. (§ 27.2)	Freq. use (§ 27.3)	Cont. all. (§ 27.3)	Comment
glycereth 26		–	8		–
isostearamide diethanolamine		–	9		–
isosteareth 10		–	12		–
laneth 5		–	48		–
laneth 10 acetate		–	232		–
laneth 15		–	11		–
laneth 16		–	58		–
laneth 25		–	9		–
laneth 27		–	6		–
laneth 40		–	13		–
lauramide		–	19		–
lauramide diethanolamine		1% aqua [5]	656		–
lauramide monoethanolamine		–	10		–
lauramide monoisopropanolamine		–	14		–
lauramine oxide	Ammonyx LO	3.7% aqua	33	+	*See § 25.9 under Ammonyx LO*
laureth 3		–	13		–
laureth 4		–	146		–
laureth 12		–	6		–
laureth 23		–	210		–
linolamide diethanolamine		–	67		–
myreth-3 myristate		–	11		–
myristamide diethanolamine		–	27		–
myristamine oxide		–	23		–
nonoxynol 2		5% aqua [2]	33		–
nonoxynol 4		5% aqua [2]	239		–
nonoxynol 6		5% aqua [2]	4		–
nonoxynol 7		5% aqua [2]	21		–
nonoxynol 8		5% aqua [2]	4		–
nonoxynol 9		5% aqua [2]	124		–
nonoxynol 10		5% aqua [2]	53		–

(continued)

(continuation)

Name	Synonym®	Patch test conc. & veh. (§ 5.2) and ref. (§ 27.2)	Freq. use (§ 27.3)	Cont. all. (§ 27.3)	Comment
nonoxynol 12		5% aqua [2]	10	–	
nonoxynol 14		5% aqua [2]	15	–	
octoxynol 1		–	188	–	
octoxynol 9		5% aqua [2]	136	–	
octoxynol 13		–	29	–	
oleamide diethanolamine		–	59	–	
oleamide monoisopropanolamine		–	15	–	
oleth 2		–	47	–	
oleth 3		–	37	–	
oleth 3 phosphate		–	23	–	
oleth 5		–	15	–	
oleth 10		–	100	–	
oleth 10 phosphate		–	41	–	
oleth 15		–	14	–	
oleth 20		–	103	–	
oleth 25		–	6	–	
pareth 15-3		–	31	–	
pareth 15-9		–	36	–	
pareth 25-12		–	23	–	
polyethylene glycol 7 betanaphthol		–	4	*	
polyethylene glycol 40 castor oil		–	74	*	
polyethylene glycol 15 cocoate		–	11	*	
polyethylene glycol 4 dilaurate		–	5	*	
polyethylene glycol 8 dilaurate		–	6	*	
polyethylene glycol 8 dioleate		–	16	*	
polyethylene glycol 8 distearate		–	65	*	
polyethylene glycol 150 distearate		–	34	*	
polyethylene glycol 7 glyceryl cocoate		–	8	*	
polyethylene glycol 25 hydrogenated castor oil		–	5	*	

* polyethylene glycol is abbreviated PEG in CTFA nomenclature

(continued)

27.15.4   Non-ionic surfactants

(continuation)

Name	Class	Patch test conc. & veh. (§ 5.2) and ref. (§ 27.2)	Freq. use (§ 27.3)	Cont. all. (§ 27.3)	Comment
polyethylene glycol 40 hydrogenated castor oil		–	9	*	
polyethylene glycol 60 hydrogenated castor oil		–	13	*	
polyethylene glycol 24 hydrogenated lanolin		–	4	*	
polyethylene glycol 70 hydrogenated lanolin		–	4	*	
polyethylene glycol lanolate		–	16	*	
polyethylene glycol 20 lanolin		–	29	*	
polyethylene glycol 27 lanolin		–	13	*	
polyethylene glycol 30 lanolin		–	5	*	
polyethylene glycol 40 lanolin		–	26	*	
polyethylene glycol 50 lanolin		–	21	*	
polyethylene glycol 60 lanolin		–	4	*	
polyethylene glycol 75 lanolin	Solulan 75	–	174	*	
polyethylene glycol 85 lanolin		–	30	*	
polyethylene glycol 75 lanolin oil		–	26	*	
polyethylene glycol 75 lanolin wax		–	22	*	
polyethylene glycol 4 laurate		–	9	*	
polyethylene glycol 8 laurate		–	41	*	
polyethylene glycol 4 octanoate		–	15	*	
polyethylene glycol 2 oleate		–	16	*	
polyethylene glycol 4 oleate		–	19	*	
polyethylene glycol 32 oleate		–	6	*	
polyethylene glycol 6 palmitate		–	4	*	
polyethylene glycol 8 propylene glycol cocoate		–	5	*	
polyethylene glycol 25 propylene glycol stearate		–	6	*	
polyethylene glycol 20 sorbitan beeswax		–	23	*	
polyethylene glycol 20 sorbitan isostearate		–	9	*	

* polyethylene glycol is abbreviated PEG in CTFA nomenclature

(continued)

(continuation)

Name	Class	Patch test conc. & veh. (§ 5.2) and ref. (§ 27.2)	Freq. use (§ 27.3)	Cont. all. (§ 27.3)	Comment
polyethylene glycol 75 sorbitan lanolate		–	5		*
polyethylene glycol 10 sorbitan laurate		–	15		*
polyethylene glycol 40 sorbitan peroleate		–	52		*
polyethylene glycol 2 stearate		–	119		*
polyethylene glycol 2 stearate SE		–	11		*
polyethylene glycol 6-32 stearate		–	5		*
polyethylene glycol 8 stearate		–	33		*
polyethylene glycol 20 stearate		–	29		*
polyethylene glycol 30 stearate		–	21		*
polyethylene glycol 32 stearate		–	9		*
polyethylene glycol 40 stearate	Myrj 52	–	157		*
polyethylene glycol 50 stearate		–	18		*
polyethylene glycol 100 stearate	Myrj 59	–	113		*
polyethylene glycol 50 tallow amide		–	34		*
polyglyceryl 3 diisostearate		–	7		–
polyglyceryl 4 oleate		–	5		–
polyglyceryl 2 oleylether		–	31		–
polyglyceryl 4 oleylether		–	29		–
polyglyceryl 10 tetraoleate		–	25		–
polyglyceryl-2-tetrastearate		–	7		–
polysorbate 20	Tween 20	5% aqua [2]	805		–
polysorbate 21		–	6		–
polysorbate 40	Tween 40	5% pet.	57	+	*See* § 5.22
polysorbate 60	Tween 60	–	614		–
polysorbate 61		–	17		–
polysorbate 80	Tween 80	5% aqua and pure [2], 5% pet.	187	+	*See* § 5.22
polysorbate 81		–	17		–
polysorbate 85		–	31		–

* polyethylene glycol is abbreviated PEG in CTFA nomenclature

(continued)

27.15.4 Non-ionic surfactants

(continuation)

Name	Class	Patch test conc. & veh. (§ 5.2) and ref. (§ 27.2)	Freq. use (§ 27.3)	Cont. all. (§ 27.3)	Comment
polypropylene glycol 2-buteth-3		–	5		**
polypropylene glycol 12-buteth-16		–	46		**
polypropylene glycol 33-buteth-45		–	9		**
polypropylene glycol 12-buteth-16		–	46		**
polypropylene glycol 5 butyl ether		–	7		**
polypropylene glycol 18 butyl ether		–	6		**
polypropylene glycol 33 butyl ether		–	21		**
polypropylene glycol 40 butyl ether		–	48		**
polypropylene glycol 5-ceteth-20		–	23		**
polypropylene glycol 28 cetyl ether		–	8		**
polypropylene glycol 30 cetyl ether		–	10		**
polypropylene glycol 10 cetyl ether phosphate		–	6		**
polypropylene glycol 24 glycereth-24		–	13		**
polypropylene glycol 27 glyceryl ether		–	8		**
polypropylene glycol 2 lanolin ether		–	11		**
polypropylene glycol 26 oleate		–	35		**
polypropylene glycol 36 oleate		–	19		**
polypropylene glycol 23 oleyl ether		–	7		**
polypropylene glycol 12 polyethylene glycol 50 lanolin		–	6		**
polypropylene glycol 2 salicylate		–	5		**
polypropylene glycol 11 stearyl ether		–	13		**
polypropylene glycol 15 stearyl ether		–	72		**
sorbitan laurate	Span 20	5% aqua [2]	223	+	*See* § 5.22
sorbitan oleate	Span 80	5% aqua [2]	91	+	*See* § 5.22
sorbitan palmitate		–	26		–
sorbitan sesquioleate	Arlacel 83	5% aqua [2], 20% pet.	592	+	*See* § 5.22
sorbitan stearate	Span 60	5% aqua	269	+	*See* § 5.22
sorbitan trioleate		–	49		–

** polypropylene glycol is abbreviated PPG in CTFA nomenclature

(continued)

(continuation)

Name	Class	Patch test conc. & veh. (§ 5.2) and ref. (§ 27.2)	Freq. use (§ 27.3)	Cont. all. (§ 27.3)	Comment
sorbitan tristearate		–	30	–	
stearamide		–	5	–	
stearamide diethanolamine		–	44	–	
stearamide dihydroxyisobutylamine stearate		–	58	–	
stearamide monoethanolamine		–	50	–	
stearamide monoethanolamine stearate		–	18	–	
stearamine oxide		–	20	–	
steareth 2		–	78	–	
steareth 10		–	7	–	
steareth 20		–	57	–	
sucrose distearate		–	7	–	
tallowamidopolypropylamine oxide		–	7	–	
talloweth 6		–	5	–	
trideceth 9		–	6	–	
trideceth 10		–	5	–	
trideceth 12		–	7	–	
trideceth 15		–	8	–	
trilaneth 4 phosphate		–	5	–	
trimethylolpolypropane triisostearate		–	4	–	

27.15.5   Amphoteric surfactants

Name	Synonym®	Patch test conc. & veh. (§ 5.2) and ref. (§ 27.2)	Freq. use (§ 27.3)	Cont. all. (§ 27.3)	Comment
amphoteric 1 (coco-amphoglycinate or propionate)	Miranol CM conc.	1% aqua [12]	59		*
amphoteric 2 (coco-amphocarboxy-glycinate)	Miranol C2M conc.	1% aqua [12]	82		*
amphoteric 3		–			–
amphoteric 4		–			–
amphoteric 5 (coco-amphocarboxyglycinate + trideceth sulfate + hexylene glycol)	Miranol 2MCT	1% aqua [12]	8		*

*Miranols may be patch-tested in 1% aqua; patch-testing in 3% conc. may cause sensitization (§ 27.2. [16]).

(continued)

27.15.5 Amphoteric surfactants

(continuation)

Name	Class	Patch test conc. & veh. (§ 5.2) and ref. (§ 27.2)	Freq. use (§ 27.3)	Cont. all. (§ 27.3)	Comment
amphoteric 6	Miranol 2MCA	1% aqua [12]	35		*
amphoteric 7	Sandopan TFL	–	6		–
amphoteric 8	Miranol SHD	1% aqua [12]	12		*
amphoteric 9 (coco-amfocarboxyglycinate + sodium lauryl sulfate + sodium laureth sulfate + propyleneglycol)	Miranol 2MCAS	1% aqua [12]	5		*
amphoteric 10 (lauramphocarboxy-glycinate)	Miranol BM conc.	1% aqua [12]	6		*
amphoteric 11	Monateric CA 35	–			–
amphoteric 12 (isostearoamphopropionate)	Miranol ISM	1% aqua [12]	16		*
amphoteric 13	Amphoterge KS	–	7		–
amphoteric 14 (lauramphocarboxyglycinate + sodium trideceth sulfate + hexylene glycol)	Miranol 2MHT	1% aqua [12]	7		*
amphoteric 15		–			–
amphoteric 16 (stearoamphoglycinate)	Miranol DM	1% aqua [12]			*
amphoteric 17 (lauramphoglycinate + sodium trideceth sulfate)	Miranol MHT	1% aqua [12]			*
amphoteric 18	Monateric 805	–			–
amphoteric 19 (lauramphocarboxyglycinate + sodium trideceth sulfate)	Miranol BT	1% aqua [12]			*
amphoteric 20 (lauramphoglycinate)	Miranol HM	5% aqua [12]			–
cocamidopropyl betaine	Tegobetaine L7	–	47		–
cocoamidopropyl sultaine	Lonzaine CS	–			–
cocobetaine	Standapol AB45	2% aqua	21	+	*See* § 22.7
oleyl betaine	Standapol OLB50	–	4		–
pecithin		–	558		–

27.15.6 Amines – aminoalkanols

Name	Patch test conc. & veh. (§ 5.2) and ref. (§ 27.2)	Freq. use (§ 27.3)	Cont. all. (§ 27.3)	Comment
aminomethyl propanediol (AMPO)	–	91	–	
aminomethyl propanol (AMP)	–	143	–	

(continued)

(continuation)

Name	Patch test conc. & veh. (§ 5.2) and ref. (§ 27.2)	Freq. use (§ 27.3)	Cont. all. (§ 27.3)	Comment
bis(3-aminopropyl)amine	–	17		–
diethanolamine (DEA)	0.1% aqua [2]	39		–
diisopropanolamine	1% aqua	92	+	*See* § 23.47
dimethylaminopropylamine	0.5% acet. [5]	–		–
dimethylstearamine	–	24		–
ethanolamine (mono-) (MEA)	–	76		*See* § 22.66 *and* § 17.04
ethylene diamine	1% pet.		+	*See* § 5.22 *and* § 22.66
hydroxybenzomorpholine	–	6		–
hydroxymethylaminoethanol	–	5		–
isopropanolamine	–	20		–
morpholine	–	50		–
oleamidopropyl dimethylamine	–	5		–
palmitamidopropyl dimethylamine	–	9		–
polyethylene glycol 2 cocamine	–	34		–
polyethylene glycol 15 cocamine	–	34		–
polyethylene glycol 5 soyamine	–	7		–
polyethylene glycol 2 tallowamine	–	32		–
polyethylene glycol 8 tallowamine	–	47		–
stearamidoethyl diethylamine	–	24		–
stearamidopropyl dimethylamine	–	9		–
triethanolamine (TEA)	2% pet./aqua	3021	+	*See* § 5.22
triisopropanolamine (TIPA)	–	34		–

27.15.7 Polyols (polyalcohols)

Name	Patch test conc. & veh. (§ 5.2) and ref. (§ 27.2)	Freq. use (§ 27.3)	Cont. all. (§ 27.3)	Comment
butylene glycol	–	284		–
diethylene glycol	–	7		–
dipropylene glycol	–	80		–

(continued)

27.15.7 Polyols

(continuation)

Name	Patch test conc. & veh. (§ 5.2) and ref. (§ 27.2)	Freq. use (§ 27.3)	Cont. all. (§ 27.3)	Comment
ethoxydiglycol	10% aqua [2]	387		–
ethylhexanediol	pure [2]	6		–
glycerin	pure [2]; 1% aqua	1924	+	*See* § 5.22
glycol	10% aqua [2], 5% alc. [3]	19		–
hexylene glycol	–	110		Comedogenic (§ 9.2)
inositol	–	154		–
mannitol	–	7		–
polyethylene glycol 4	10% aqua [2] and pure [2, 3]	18		*
polyethylene glycol 6	10% aqua [2] and pure [2, 3]	15		*
polyethylene glycol 6-32	10% aqua [2] and pure [2, 3]	138		*
polyethylene glycol 8	10% aqua [2] and pure [2, 3]	267		*
polyethylene glycol 20	pure [2, 3]	15		*
polyethylene glycol 32	pure [2, 3]	41		*
polyethylene glycol 75	pure [2, 3]	44		*
polyethylene glycol 150	pure [2, 3]	76		*
polyethylene glycol 2M	–	5		*
polyethylene glycol 6M	–	6		*
polyethylene glycol 7M	–	10		*
polyethylene glycol 14M	–	59		*
polyethylene glycol 90M	–	4		*
polyvinyl alcohol	–	65		–
polypropylene glycol 9	–	4		**
polypropylene glycol	5–10% aqua [2], 5% alc. [3]	5279	+	*See* § 5.22 **
sorbitol	10% aqua [2]	379		
triethylene glycol	–	5		–

* polyethylene glycol is abbreviated PEG in CTFA nomenclature
** polypropylene glycol is abbreviated PPG in CTFA nomenclature

27.16   Miscellaneous cosmetic ingredients

Name	Class	Patch test conc. & veh. (§ 5.2) and ref. (§ 27.2)	Freq. use (§ 27.3)	Cont. all. (§ 27.3)	Comment
acacia (gum arabic)	thickener	as is [2]	15		–
acetamide monoethanolamine	solvent	–	8		–
acetic acid	acidic agent	3% aqua [2]	19		–
acetone	solvent	10% o.o. [2]	39		–
acrylate acrylamide copolymer	polymer (film)	–	22		–
acrylic acrylate copolymer	polymer (film)	–	66		–
adipic acid/epoxypropyl diethylenetriamine copolymer	polymer	–	8		–
alanine	aminoacid	2% pet. [1]	11		–
alcloxa (= aluminum chlorhydroxy allantoinate)	antiperspirant	–	36		–
alcohol (= ethanol)	solvent	alcohol: 10% aqua [1] alcohol denatured: pure [1]	4184	+	*See* § 5.7
aldioxa (= aluminum dihydroxy allantoinate)	antiperspirant	–	44		–
algin (= sodium alginate)	thickener	pure [2]	12		–
allantoin	skin healing agent	0.5% aqua [2]	741	+	*See* § 27.2, [19]
allantoin acetylmethionine	skin healing agent	–	23		–
allantoin calcium pantothenate	skin healing agent	–	8		–
allantoin galacturonic acid	skin healing agent	–	6		–
allantoin polygalacturonic acid	skin healing agent	–	29		–
almond meal	skin abrasive	–	17		–
aloe	skin healing agent	–	44		*See* § 26.3 (*Aloë vera*)
aloe extract	skin healing agent	–	17		*See* § 26.3 (*Aloë vera*)
aloe juice	skin healing agent	–	34		*See* § 26.3 (*Aloë vera*)
althea extract	thickener	–	11		–
aluminum chloride	antiperspirant	2% aqua [2]	36		–
aluminum chlorhydrex	antiperspirant	–	7		–
aluminum chlorohydrate	antiperspirant	10% aqua [2]	243		–
aluminum distearate	thickener	pure [2]	51		–

(continued)

27.16   Miscellaneous cosmetic ingredients

(continuation)

Name	Class	Patch test conc. & veh. (§ 5.2) and ref. (§ 27.2)	Freq. use (§ 27.3)	Cont. all. (§ 27.3)	Comment
aluminum hydroxide	antiperspirant	–	89		–
aluminum silicate	powder filler	–	29		–
aluminum starch octenylsuccinate	powder flow aid	–	8		–
aluminum stearate	thickener (for hydrocarbons)	pure [2]	136		–
aluminum tristearate	thickener (for hydrocarbons)	pure [2]	69		–
aluminum zirconium tetrachlorhydrex gly	antiperspirant	*See* § 25.53	–	+	*See* § 25.53
ammoniated glycyrrhizate	sweetener	–	55		–
ammonium acetate	buffering salt	–	32		–
ammonium alum	adstringent	–	11		–
ammonium bicarbonate	buffering salt	–	18		–
ammonium carbonate	buffering salt	5% aqua [5]	12		–
ammonium chloride	buffering salt	–	19		–
ammonium hydroxide	alkaline agent	–	684		–
ammonium persulfate	peroxide	1% aqua [3]	19	+	*See* § 22.65, § 22.66, *and* § 7.5
ammonium styrene/acrylate copolymer	polymer	–	8		–
ammonium sulfate	buffering salt	–	17		–
ammonium thioglycolate	hair waving agent	2% aqua [5]	187	+	*See* § 22.65 *and* § 22.66
ammonium vinyl acetate/acrylate copolymer	polymer (film)	–	21		–
arnica extract	counterirritant	20% alc. [2, 17], pure [3]	18	+	*See* § 5.39; *also* § 26.3 *(Arnica montana)*
ascorbic acid	vitamin	–	45		–
aspartic acid	acidic agent	–	11		–
attapulgite	adsorbent	–	7		–
azulene	anti-inflammatory agent	1% pet.	71	+	*See* § 23.53
balm mint extract	counterirritant	–	15		–
barium sulfide	depilating agent	2% aqua [2]	5		–
beer	hair conditioner	–	5		*See* § 22.8 *under* ethyl alcohol
bentonite	suspending agent	–	128		–

(continued)

(continuation)

Name	Class	Patch test conc. & veh. (§ 5.2) and ref. (§ 27.2)	Freq. use (§ 27.3)	Cont. all. (§ 27.3)	Comment
benzocaine	counterirritant	5% pet. [2, 3]	14	+	*See* § 5.20
betaine	amphoteric agent	–	15		–
biotin	vitamin	–	28		–
birch leaf extract	adstringent	–	27		*See* § 26.3 *(Betula alba)*
birch sap	adstringent	–	–		*See* § 26.3 *(Betula alba)*
brucine (incl. sulfate)	alcohol denaturant	1% pet. [2]	47		–
butane	aerosol propellant	–	35		–
butoxyethanol (= butyl Cellosolve®)	solvent	–	71		–
butyl acetate	solvent	5–25% o.o. [2]	715	+	*See* § 27.2, [21]
n-butyl alcohol	solvent	–	80		Has caused contact urticaria (§ 7.5)
t-butyl alcohol	solvent	70% aqua	47	+	*See* § 25.66 Has caused contact urticaria (§ 7.5)
butylester of PVM/MA copolymer (Gantrez ES425®)	polymer (film)	–	63		–
butylphthalyl butylglycolate	plasticizer	–	17		–
calamine color pigment	–	4		–	
calcium hydroxide	alkaline agent	pure [2]	26		–
calcium oxide	alkaline agent	do not test	5		–
calcium pantothenate	vitamin	–	57		–
calcium saccharin	sweetener	–	4		–
calcium silicate	suspending agent	–	192		–
calcium stearate	adhesive aid	pure [2]	22		–
calcium thioglycolate	depilating agent	5% aqua [2]	14		–
calendula extract	natural ingredient	–	11	+	*See* § 26.3 *(Calendula officinalis)*
capsicum oleoresin	rubefacient	1% alc. [2]	6		*See* § 26.3 *(Capsicum annuum)*
carbomer 934	thickener	} pure and 10% aqua (CIR 1981)	412		–
carbomer 940	thickener		373		–
carbomer 941	thickener		229		–
carboxyvinylpolymer	thickener	–	170		–

(continued)

27.16 Miscellaneous cosmetic ingredients

(continuation)

Name	Class	Patch test conc. & veh. (§ 5.2) and ref. (§ 27.2)	Freq. use (§ 27.3)	Cont. all. (§ 27.3)	Comment
carrageenan	thickener	pure [2]	18		–
carrot oil	color (natural)	–	10	+ (?)	*See* § 26.3 (*Daucus carota*)
cellulose	powder filler	pure	4		–
chlorofluorocarbon 11S	aerosol propellant	–	4		*See* § 5.22
chlorofluorocarbon 11	aerosol propellant	pure	491	+	*See* § 5.22
chlorofluorocarbon 12	aerosol propellant	pure	1246	+	*See* § 5.22
chlorofluorocarbon 114	aerosol propellant	–	907		–
chloroform	flavor (toothpaste)	40% o.o. [2]	5		–
cholecalciferol	vitamin	–	4		–
citric acid	acidic agent	1% aqua [2]	2068		–
clover blossom extract	natural ingredient	–	24		*See* § 26.3 (*Trifolium pratense*)
coconut milk	natural ingredient	–	8		*See* § 26.3 (*Cocos nucifera*)
cod liver oil	skin healing agent	–	7		–
colloidal silica	powder flow aid	–	39		–
colocynth	natural ingredient	–	9		*See* § 26.3 (*Citrullus vulgaris*)
coltsfoot extract	natural ingredient	1% alc. [5]	37		*See* § 26.3 (*Tussilago farfare*)
comfrey	natural ingredient	–	5		*See* § 26.3 (*Symphytum officinale*)
corn cob meal (milled cobs of Zea mays)	skin abrasive	–	6		*See* § 26.3 (*Zea mays*)
corn flour (Zea mays)	adsorbent	–	9		*See* § 26.3 (*Zea mays*)
corn starch (Zea mays)	adsorbent	–	35		Corn starch is considered to be a known allergen *See* § 26.3 (*Zea mays*)
cucumber juice	natural ingredient	–	19		*See* § 26.3 (*Cucumis sativus*)
cysteine	aminoacid	–	4		–
diethanolamine-styrene/acrylates/divinyl-benzene copolymer	polymer	–	23		–
deodorized kerosine	solvent	–	5		–
dextrin	adhesive aid	–	12		–
diacetone alcohol	solvent	–	5		–
diammonium phosphate	buffering salt	–	20		–

(continued)

(continuation)

Name	Class	Patch test conc. & veh. (§ 5.2) and ref. (§ 27.2)	Freq. use (§ 27.3)	Cont. all. (§ 27.3)	Comment
diatomaceous earth	adsorbent	–	14		–
dicalcium phosphate dihydrate	abrasive (dental)	–	37		–
diethyl aspartate	solvent	–	4		–
diethyl glutamate	solvent	–	4		–
N,N-diethyl-m-toluamide	insect repellent	5% alc. [2]	4		Has caused contact urticatia *(See* § 7.5) and systemic side effects (§ 16.23)
dihydroxyacetone	skin tanning agent	10% alc. [1]	8		–
dimethyl hydantoin formaldehyde resin (DMHF)	polymer (resin)	–	19		
dimethyl octynediol	solvent	–	7		–
disodium phosphate	buffering salt	–	12		–
disodium pyrophosphate		–	6		–
egg (whole egg)	natural ingredient	–	18		Has caused contact urticaria (§ 27.2 [14])
egg oil	natural ingredient	–	6		–
egg powder (dried whole chicken egg)	natural ingredient	–	20		–
ergocalciferol	vitamin	–	70		–
ethane	aerosol propellant	–	6		–
ethanolamine dithiodiglycolate	depilating agent	–	5		–
ethanolamine thioglycolate	hair waving agent	–	14		–
ethoxydiglycol (Carbitol®)	solvent	–	387		–
ethoxyethanol (Cellosolve®)	solvent	–	9		–
ethyl acetate	solvent	10% pet. [1], 5% MEK [2]	561		–
ethyl aspartate	solvent	–	6		–
ethyl cellulose (Ethocel®)	thickener	–	4		–
ethylene dichloride	solvent	50% o.o. [2]	11		–
ethylester of PVM/MA	polymer	–	41		–
ethyl glutamate	solvent	–	6		–
ethyl hexanediol	solvent	pure [2]	6		–
ethyl hydroxymethyl oleyl oxazoline	solvent	–	6		–

(continued)

27.16 Miscellaneous cosmetic ingredients

(continuation)

Name	Class	Patch test conc. & veh. (§ 5.2) and ref. (§ 27.2)	Freq. use (§ 27.3)	Cont. all. (§ 27.3)	Comment
fennel extract	natural ingredient	–	10		*See* § 26.3 *(Foeniculum vulgare)*
ferric citrate	color	–	7		–
fluorescent brightener 47	whitening agent	–	5		–
fluorocarbon 152A	aerosol propellant	–	12		–
folic acid	vitamin	–	24		–
fructose	humectant	–	9		–
gelatin	thickener	pure	33	+	*See* § 5.42
gentian extract	natural ingredient	–	6		*See* § 26.3 *(Gentiana lutea)*
glucose	humectant	–	10		–
glucose glutamate	humectant	–	13		–
glutamic acid	aminoacid	–	11		–
glyceryl phthalate resin	polymer resin	10% pet.	–	+	*See* § 24.12
glycine	aminoacid	–	23		–
glycolic acid	acidic agent	–	24		–
guar gum	thickener	–	6		–
hayflower extract	natural ingredient	–	6		–
hectorite	suspending agent	–	15		–
hinokitiol (β-thujaplicin)	antiseborrheic agent	0.1% alc.	–	+	*See* § 22.65
honey	humectant	–	55		–
hops extract	natural ingredient	–	14		*See* § 26.3 *(Humulus lupulus)*
horse chestnut extract	natural ingredient	–	5	+	*See* § 5.39 *and* § 26.3 *(Aesculus hippocastanum)*
horsetail extract	natural ingredient	–	33		*See* § 26.3 *(Equisetum arvense)*
hydrated silica	abrasive (dental); thickener	–	99		–
hydrochloric acid	acidic agent	do not test	82		–
hydrochlorofluorocarbon 142B	aerosol propellant	–	7		–
hydrogen peroxide	oxidizing agent	3% aqua [2]	59		–
hydroxyethylcellulose (HEC)	thickener	–	367		–

(continued)

(continuation)

Name	Class	Patch test conc. & veh. (§ 5.2) and ref. (§ 27.2)	Freq. use (§ 27.3)	Cont. all. (§ 27.3)	Comment
hydroxyphenyl glycinamide	solvent	–	9		–
hydroxypropyl cellulose (HPC)	thickener	–	106		–
hydroxypropylmethyl cellulose	thickener	–	188		–
hypericum extract	natural ingredient	–	10		*See* § 26.3 *(Hypericum perforatum)*
Ineral® (dimethylol ethylene thiourea)	hair strengthener	10% aqua, 10% pet.		+	*See* § 22.65
inositol	humectant	–	154		–
isobutane	aerosol propellant	–	192		–
isopropyl alcohol	solvent	pure [2], 10% aqua [18]	1437	+	*See* § 5.22 *and* § 5.7 *under* alcohol, isopropyl
juniper extract	natural ingredient	–	7		*See* § 26.3 *(Juniperus communis)*
juniper tar (cade oil)	thickener	25% c.o. [2]	6		*See* § 5.38 *and* § 26.3 *(Juniperus communis)*
karaya gum	natural ingredient	pure [2]	4	+	*See* § 5.39
lauryl aminopropylglycine		–	13		–
lauryl diethylenediaminoglycine		–	13		–
lemon extract *(Citrus limon)*	natural ingredient	–	9		*See* § 26.3 *(Citrus limon)*
lemon juice *(Citrus limon)*	natural ingredient	–	26		*See* § 26.3 *(Citrus limon)*
lithium stearate	adhesive aid		128		–
magnesium aluminum silicate (Veegum)	thickener; suspending agent	–	1305		–
magnesium carbonate	perfume carrier	pure [2]	556		–
magnesium carbonate hydroxide	perfume carrier	–	4		–
magnesium oxide	adhesive aid		5		–
magnesium silicate	adsorbent	–	391		–
magnesium sulfate	salt	–	51		–
magnesium trisilicate	adsorbent	–	17		–
malic acid	acidic agent	–	27		–
malt extract	natural ingredient	–	5		–
mannitol	humectant	–	7		–

(continued)

485

27.16   Miscellaneous cosmetic ingredients

(continuation)

Name	Class	Patch test conc. & veh. (§ 5.2) and ref. (§ 27.2)	Freq. use (§ 27.3)	Cont. all. (§ 27.3)	Comment
matricaria extract	hair dye	–	40	+	*See* § 5.39 (chamomile oil); *also* § 26.3 (*Matricaria chamomila*)
methanol	solvent	pure [2]	34		–
methionine	aminoacid	–	22		–
methoxyethanol (Methylcellosolve®)	solvent	–	5		–
methylcellulose (Methocel®)	thickener	pure [2]	95		–
methylene chloride (dichloromethane)	solvent	–	49		–
methylethylketone (MEK)	solvent	pure [1]	15		–
milk protein	natural ingredient	–	16		–
mineral spirits (Ligroin)	solvent	pure [1]	128		–
mistletoe extract	natural ingredient	–	4		*See* § 26.3 (*Viscum album*)
monobenzone	depigmenting agent	1% pet.	–	+	*See* § 5.42 *and* § 25.44 *under* monobenzylether of hydroquinone *See also* § 10.1
montmorrilonite	suspending agent	–	12		–
nettle extract	natural ingredient	–	29		*See* § 26.3 (*Urtica dioica*)
niacinamide	vitamin; rubefacient	–	25		–
nitrocellulose	polymer (nail film)	10% aqua	873	+	*See* § 27.2, [19] *and* § 24.12
nitrogen	inert gas	–	7		–
nitrous oxide	aerosol propellant	–	11		–
non-fat dry milk	natural ingredient	–	82		–
nylon	polymer (rayon)	–	27		–
oat flour	adsorbent; abrasive (skin)	–	28		–
octylacrylamide/acrylates/butylaminoethyl methacrylate copolymer (Amphomer®)	polymer	–	8		–
pectin	thickener	–	21		–
pentasodium triphosphate	chelating agent	–	81		–
petroleum distillate	–	solvent pure [1], 25% o.o. [2]	48		–
phenacetine	hydrogen peroxide stabilizer	1% pet. [3]	21		–

(continued)

(continuation)

Name	Class	Patch test conc. & veh. (§ 5.2) and ref. (§ 27.2)	Freq. use (§ 27.3)	Cont. all. (§ 27.3)	Comment
phenyl methyl pyrazolone	hydrogen peroxide stabilizer	–	13		–
phosphoric acid	acidic agent	do not test	466		–
pine needle extract	natural ingredient	–	6		–
pine tar oil (rectified pine tar)	natural ingredient	pine oil 5% pet. [1], pure [7]	6		–
poloxamer 182	polymer; thickener	–	6		–
poloxamer 184	polymer; thickener	–	15		–
poloxamer 188	polymer; thickener	–	8		–
poloxamer 212	polymer; thickener	–	10		–
poloxamer 238	polymer; thickener	–	6		–
poloxamer 401	polymer; thickener	–	18		–
poloxamer 407	polymer; thickener	–	5		–
polyacrylamide (Gelamide®)	polymer (film)	–	6		–
polybutene	polymer	–	109		–
polyethylacrylate	polymer	–	5		–
polyethylene	polymer	–	120		–
polymethylmethacrylate	polymer	pure [2]	7		–
polystyrene	polymer	–	10		–
polyvinyl acetate	polymer	–	6		–
polyvinyl alcohol	polymer (film)	–	65		–
polyvinyl butyral	polymer	–	6		–
potassium alum	adstringent	10% aqua [2]	9		–
potassium bicarbonate	buffering salt	–	4		–
potassium carbonate	alkaline agent	1% aqua [2]	12		–
potassium chloride	salt	–	38		–
potassium hydroxide	alkaline agent	do not test	208		–
potassium persulfate	oxidizing agent	2.5% aqua [2], 5% aqua [3]	20		–
propane	aerosol propellant	–	46		–
propantheline bromide	antiperspirant	1–5% aqua	–	+	*See* § 25.53

(continued)

487

(continuation)

Name	Class	Patch test conc. & veh. (§ 5.2) and ref. (§ 27.2)	Freq. use (§ 27.3)	Cont. all. (§ 27.3)	Comment
propenyl methyl guaethol		–	5		–
propylene carbonate	solvent	–	96		–
pumice	abrasive (skin)	–	18		–
polyvinylmethylether/maleic anhydride copolymer	polymer (film)	–	56		–
PVP (polyvinylpyrrolidone)	polymer (film)	pure [2]	512		*See* § 22.66
PVP/VA (polyvinylpyrrolidone/vinylacetate) copolymer	polymer (film)	–	80		–
pyridoxine	vitamin	10% pet. [3]	4		–
pyridoxine dioctanoate	antiseborrheic agent	1% pet.	–	+	*See* § 22.65
pyridoxine hydrochloride	vitamin	10% aqua [2], 1% pet.	26		has cross-reacted to pyridoxine 3,4-dioctanoate (§ 22.65)
pyroxylin	polymer (film, nail)	–	62		–
quince seed	thickener	pure [5]	8		–
rayon	polymer (rayon)	–	26		–
resorcinol acetate	keratolytic agent	5% aqua [2]	4	+	*See* § 5.38
retinol (vitamin A acid)	vitamin	0.1% pet. [2]	122	+	*See* § 5.38
retinyl palmitate	vitamin	–	39		–
rice starch	adsorbent	–	5		–
rosemary	natural ingredient	–	4		*See* § 26.3 (*Rosmarinus officinalis*)
rosemary extract	natural ingredient	–	36		*See* § 26.3 (*Rosmarinus officinalis*)
rose water	natural ingredient	–	6		–
rosin (colophony)	natural ingredient	20% pet. [1]	17	+	*See* § 5.39, § 22.65 *and* § 23.47
rye flour	adsorbent	–	5		–
saccharin	sweetener	–	53		–
sage extract	natural ingredient	–	42		*See* § 26.3 (*Salvia officinalis*)
selenium sulfide	antidandruff agent	2% aqua	–	+ (?)	*See* § 22.7 *and* § 22.8
serine	aminoacid	–	17		–

(continued)

(continuation)

Name	Class	Patch test conc. & veh. (§ 5.2) and ref. (§ 27.2)	Freq. use (§ 27.3)	Cont. all. (§ 27.3)	Comment
shellac	natural ingredient	pure [2], 20% alc. [3]	110		–
silica	powder flow aid	–	435		–
silk powder	natural ingredient, color pigment	–	18		Silk has caused contact urticaria (§ 27.2 [13])
sodium acetate	buffering salt	–	10		–
sodium aluminum chlorohydroxy lactate	antiperspirant	–	4		–
sodium bicarbonate	buffering salt	–	30		–
sodium bisulfate	acidic agent	–	14		–
sodium bisulfite	reducing agent	10% aqua [2]	84		–
sodium borate	alkaline agent	satur. aq. sol. [2]	524		–
sodium bromate	oxidizing agent	–	62		–
sodium carbonate	alkaline agent	10% aqua [2]	23		–
sodium carrageenan	thickener	–	19		–
sodium chloride	salt; thickener (for surfactants)	–	627		–
sodium citrate	buffering salt	–	59		–
sodium hexametaphosphate	chelating agent	–	38		–
sodium hydrosulfite	reducing agent	–	139		–
sodium hydroxide	alkaline agent	do not test	339		–
sodium isethionate	acidic agent	–	5		–
sodium magnesium silicate (Laponite®)	suspending agent, adsorbent	–	13		–
sodium metabisulfite	reducing agent	–	4		–
sodium metasilicate	powder filler	–	17		–
sodium perborate	oxidizing agent	pure [2]	6		–
sodium persulfate	oxidizing agent	–	5		–
sodium phosphate	buffering salt	–	50		–
sodium saccharin	sweetener	–	132		–
sodium sesquicarbonate	CO_2-releasing agent	–	136		–
sodium silicate	thickener	–	41		–
sodium sorbitol borate		–	4		–

(continued)

27.16   Miscellaneous cosmetic ingredients

(continuation)

Name	Class	Patch test conc. & veh. (§ 5.2) and ref. (§ 27.2)	Freq. use (§ 27.3)	Cont. all. (§ 27.3)	Comment
sodium stannate	depilating agent	–	10		–
sodium styrene/acrylates/divinylbenzene copolymer	polymer	–	13		–
sodium styrene/polyethyleneglycol 10 maleate/nonoxynol-10 maleate/acrylate copolymer	polymer	–	7		–
sodium sulfate	salt filler	–	117		–
sodium sulfite	depilating agent	–	310		–
sodium thiosulfate	reducing agent	5% aqua [2]	12		–
starch	adsorbent	–	79		–
starch diethylaminoethyl ether	thickener	–	7		–
strontium hydroxide	alkaline agent	do not test	5		–
styrene/acrylamide copolymer	polymer	–	37		–
styrene/acrylate/ammonium methacrylate copolymer	polymer	–	13		–
styrene/maleic anhydride copolymer	polymer	–	4		–
styrene/PVP (polyvinylpyrrolidone) copolymer	polymer	–	16		–
sucrose	humectant	–	28		–
sucrose acetate isobutyrate	alcohol denaturant	–	65		–
sulfuric acid	acidic agent	do not test	33		–
tartaric acid	acidic agent	–	7		–
p-tert-butylphenol resin	resin	1% pet.	–	+	See § 24.12
tetrasodium pyrophosphate	chelating agent	–	38		–
thiamine hydrochloride	vitamine	10% aqua [3], 50% aqua [2]	28	+	See § 5.44
thiodiglycol	depilating agent	–	4		–
thioglycolic acid	hairwaving agent	10% aqua [2]	26		–
toluene	solvent	50% o.o. [2]	698		–
toluenesulfonamide/formaldehyde resin (Santolite®)	polymer (nail, resin)	10% pet.	485	+	See § 24.12, § 24.13 and § 24.2
tragacanth gum	thickener	1% aqua [2]	41		–
tricalcium phosphate	abrasive (dental)	–	34		–

(continued)

(continuation)

Name	Class	Patch test conc. & veh. (§ 5.2) and ref. (§ 27.2)	Freq. use (§ 27.3)	Cont. all. (§ 27.3)	Comment
trichlorethane	solvent	–	4		–
trichloroethylene	solvent	5% o.o. [2]	4		–
tricresyl ethyl phthalate	plasticizer	5% pet.	–	+	*See* § 24.12
tris(hydroxymethyl)nitromethane	antimicrobial	–	6		–
trisodium phosphate	buffering salt	2% aqua [2]	20		–
uric acid		–	5		–
vinegar	natural ingredient	–	6		–
vinyl acetate/crotonic acid copolymer	polymer (film, hair)	–	87		–
vinyl acetate/crotonic acid/methacryloxy-benzophenone 1 polymer	polymer	–	7		–
vinyl acetate/crotonic acid/vinyl neo-decanoate polymer	polymer	–	20		–
vinylpyrrolidone/styrene copolymer	polymer	–	48		–
wheat germ extract	natural ingredient	–	26		–
wheat starch	adsorbent	–	4		–
wild thyme extract	natural ingredient	–	6		*See* § 26.3 (*Thymus serpyllum*)
witch hazel	natural ingredient	pure [2]	18		*See* § 26.3 (*Hamamelis virginiana*)
witch hazel distillate	natural ingredient	–	116		*See* § 26.3 (*Hamamelis virginiana*)
witch hazel extract	natural ingredient	–	13		*See* § 26.3 (*Hamamelis virginiana*)
xanthan gum thickener	thickener	–	133		–
xylene	solvent	50% o.o. [2]	9		–
yarrow extract	natural ingredient	–	88		*See* § 26.3 (*Achillea millefolium*)
yeast extract	natural ingredient	–	4		–
zinc formaldehyde sulfoxylate	reducing agent	–	14		–
zinc phenolsulfonate	adstringent	–	72		–
zinc stearate	adhesive aid	pure [2]	1359		–
zinc sulfate	adstringent	5% aqua [2]	13		*See* § 5.22

Index

The figures refer to paragraph numbers

Index

Index

496

Index

Index

Index

Index

506

Index

Index

511

Index

Index

519

Index

Index